Stem Cell Therapy for Vascular Diseases

Tulio Pinho Navarro
Lara Lellis Navarro Minchillo Lopes
Alan Dardik

Editors

Stem Cell Therapy for Vascular Diseases

State of the Evidence and Clinical Applications

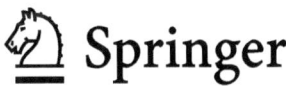 Springer

Editors
Tulio Pinho Navarro
Department of Surgery
Vascular Surgery Section
Federal University of Minas Gerais
Belo Horizonte
Minas Gerais
Brazil

Lara Lellis Navarro Minchillo Lopes
Postgraduate Program in Sciences Applied
to Surgery
Federal University of Minas Gerais
Belo Horizonte
Minas Gerais
Brazil

Alan Dardik
Vascular Biology and Therapeutics Program
and the Departments of Surgery and
Cellular and Molecular Physiology
Yale University School of Medicine
New Haven, CT
USA

ISBN 978-3-030-56953-2   ISBN 978-3-030-56954-9   (eBook)
https://doi.org/10.1007/978-3-030-56954-9

This Springer imprint is published by the registered company Springer Nature Switzerland AG
The registered company address is: Gewerbestrasse 11, 6330 Cham, Switzerland

Preface

Despite major medical and scientific advances in the last 50 years, vascular disease continues to challenge us. Aneurysms, atherosclerosis, heart failure, stroke, malformations, fistulae, and vasculitis all continue to provide diagnostic and therapeutic challenges that keep vascular disease the leading the cause of death and a major source of morbidity and suffering in modern society. Physicians and surgeons continue to treat vascular disease with the technology at hand. Early advances with cautery and suture have been supplemented by stents, wires, and coils to give modern practitioners a range of therapeutic options. But there is still room to improve. What is next? It is likely to be exciting.

Understanding the biology of stem cells has been a tremendous advance in modern medicine and has captured the imagination of many people. The initial requirement to derive stem cells from embryonic cells prompted ethical concerns that limited utility and clinical translation of therapy. However, advances in understanding the biology of stem cells continue to open new possibilities. In 2012, the Nobel Prize was awarded to Drs. Yamanaka and Gurdon for the discovery that somatic cells could be reprogrammed into induced pluripotent stem cells. This groundbreaking discovery has completely changed our view of development and cellular specialization, opening new frontiers in biology; stem cell therapy is not far behind. Although some roadside clinics claim to offer stem cell therapy, a safe and effective therapy must be based on solid science and understanding of biology and developed into consistent products that are tested rigorously through adequately powered clinical trials with reasonable endpoints that are then published in peer-reviewed literature. You and I want this, and our patients deserve this.

The goal of this book is to describe the current status of stem cell biology and therapy as related to the cardiovascular system and vascular diseases. The editors have been involved with stem cell research for over 30 years and are involved with human clinical trials using stem cells; this endeavor capitalizes on their long-term friendship and collaboration that has stood the test of time and distance. The authors are recognized experts in their fields with relevant and real world experience. We hope you will enjoy this book as much as we have enjoyed putting it together.

Belo Horizonte, Brazil   Tulio Pinho Navarro, MD, PhD
Belo Horizonte, Brazil   Lara Lellis Navarro Minchillo Lopes, MD
New Haven, CT, USA   Alan Dardik, MD, PhD

Contents

Contributors

Brian H. Annex, MD Division of Cardiology and Department of Medicine, Medical College of Georgia at Augusta University, Augusta, GA, USA

Vishal Arora, MD Division of Cardiology and Department of Medicine, Medical College of Georgia at Augusta University, Augusta, GA, USA

Ramesh K. Batra, MBBS Yale School of Medicine, Yale University, Yale New Haven Transplant Center, New Haven, CT, USA

Shlomo Baytner, MD Sanz Medical Center, Laniado Hospital, Netanya, Israel

Michael Belkin, MD Sanz Medical Center, Laniado Hospital, Netanya, Israel
Tel Aviv University, Tel Aviv, Israel

Monique Bethel, MD Division of Cardiology and Department of Medicine, Medical College of Georgia at Augusta University, Augusta, GA, USA

Akshaar N. Brahmbhatt, MD Diagnostic Radiology - Department of Imaging Sciences, University of Rochester, Rochester, NY, USA

Luke Brewster, MD, PhD Emory University, Department of Surgery, Vascular Surgery and Endovascular Therapy, Atlanta, GA, USA
Atlanta VA Medical Center, Surgical and Research Services, Decatur, GA, USA
Georgia Institute of Technology, Institute for Bioengineering and Bioscience, Atlanta, GA, USA

Shlomo Bulvik, MD Sanz Medical Center, Laniado Hospital, Netanya, Israel

Pollyana Ribeiro Castro, MD Physiology and Biophysics, Federal University of Minas Gerais (UFMG), Belo Horizonte, Brazil

Angela Cheng, MD Emory University, Department of Surgery, Division of Plastic and Reconstructive Surgery, Atlanta, GA, USA

Lucíola da Silva Barcelos, PhD Physiology and Biophysics, Federal University of Minas Gerais (UFMG), Belo Horizonte, Brazil

Alan Dardik, MD, PhD Vascular Biology and Therapeutics Program and the Departments of Surgery and Cellular and Molecular Physiology, Yale University School of Medicine, New Haven, CT, USA

Biraja C. Dash, PhD Department of Surgery, Division of Plastic Surgery, Yale School of Medicine, Yale University, New Haven, CT, USA

Arash Fereydooni, MD Yale School of Medicine, New Haven, CT, USA

Michael Frogel, MD Cohen's Children's Medical Center, New Hyde Park, NY, USA

Kathy Gonzalez, MD Division of Vascular Surgery, University of Pittsburgh Medical Center, Pittsburgh, PA, USA

Jolanta Gorecka, MD Vascular Biology and Therapeutics Program and the Department of Surgery, Yale University School of Medicine, New Haven, CT, USA

Martin Grajower, MD Albert Einstein College of Medicine, Bronx, NY, USA

Yongquan Gu, MD Department of Vascular Surgery, Xuan Wu Hospital of Capital Medical University, Beijing, China

Stanton C. Honig, MD Department of Urology, Yale School of Medicine, New Haven, CT, USA

Justin R. King, MD Indiana Center for Vascular Biology and Medicine, Indiana University School of Medicine, Indianapolis, IN, USA

Department of Surgery, Indiana University School of Medicine, Indianapolis, IN, USA

Center for Regenerative Medicine, Richard L. Roudebush Veterans Administration Medical Center, Indianapolis, IN, USA

Nicolle Kränkel, PhD Department of Cardiology, Campus Benjamin Franklin, Charité – Universitätsmedizin Berlin, Berlin, Germany

John Langford, MD Department of Surgery, Yale University School of Medicine, New Haven, CT, USA

Shin-Rong Lee, MD, PhD Yale School of Medicine, New Haven, CT, USA

Lianming Liao, MD, PhD Department of Laboratory Medicine, Fujian Medical University Union Hospital, Fuzhou, China

Roman Liberson, MD, PhD Sanz Medical Center, Laniado Hospital, Netanya, Israel

Zhao-Jun Liu, MD, PhD University of Miami Leonard M. Miller School of Medicine, Miami, FL, USA

C. Matouk, MD Department of Neurosurgery, Yale University School of Medicine, New Haven, CT, USA

Dylan McLaughlin, MD Emory University, Department of Surgery, Vascular Surgery and Endovascular Therapy, Atlanta, GA, USA

Lara Lellis Navarro Minchillo Lopes, MD Federal University of Minas Gerais, Belo Horizonte, Minas Gerais, Brazil

Sanjay Misra, MD Department of Radiology, Mayo Clinic, Rochester, MN, USA

Michael P. Murphy, MD Indiana Center for Vascular Biology and Medicine, Indiana University School of Medicine, Indianapolis, IN, USA

Department of Surgery, Indiana University School of Medicine, Indianapolis, IN, USA

Center for Regenerative Medicine, Richard L. Roudebush Veterans Administration Medical Center, Indianapolis, IN, USA

Tulio Pinho Navarro, MD, PhD Department of Surgery, Vascular Surgery Section, Federal University of Minas Gerais, Belo Horizonte, Minas Gerais, Brazil

Marcio Bittar Nehemy, MD, PhD Department of Ophthalmology, Federal University of Minas Gerais, Belo Horizonte, MG, Brazil

Mark Niven, MD Sanz Medical Center, Laniado Hospital, Netanya, Israel

Yael Porat, PhD BioGenCell, Ltd., Laniado Hospital, Netanya, Israel

Benjamin Press, MD Yale School of Medicine, New Haven, CT, USA

Hallie J. Quiroz, MD University of Miami Leonard M. Miller School of Medicine, Miami, FL, USA

Caio Vinicius Regatieri, MD, PhD Department of Ophthalmology, Federal University of São Paulo, São Paulo, Brazil

Department of ophthalmology, Tufts Medical School, Boston, MA, USA

S. M. Robert, MD, PhD Department of Neurosurgery, Yale University School of Medicine, New Haven, CT, USA

Louis Shenkman, MD Tel Aviv University, Tel Aviv, Israel

Galit Sivak, MD Rabin Medical center, Tel Aviv University, Tel Aviv, Israel

Elisabeth Tamara Straessler, MD Department of Cardiology, Campus Benjamin Franklin, Charité – Universitätsmedizin Berlin, Berlin, Germany

Gregory T. Tietjen, PhD Department of Surgery, Yale University School of Medicine, New Haven, CT, USA

Department of Biomedical Engineering, Yale University, New Haven, CT, USA

Department of Surgery – Transplant Section, Yale School of Medicine, New Haven, CT, USA

Edith Tzeng, MD VA Pittsburgh Healthcare System and University of Pittsburgh, Pittsburgh, PA, USA

Division of Vascular Surgery, University of Pittsburgh Medical Center, Pittsburgh, PA, USA

Frank Veith, MD NYU-Langone Medical Center, New York, NY, USA

The Cleveland Clinic, Cleveland, OH, USA

Omaida C. Velazquez, MD DeWitt Daughtry Department of Surgery, University of Miami Leonard M. Miller School of Medicine, Miami, FL, USA

Augusto Vieira, MD Department of Ophthalmology, Federal University of São Paulo, São Paulo, Brazil

Jie Xie, MD, PhD Indiana Center for Vascular Biology and Medicine, Indiana University School of Medicine, Indianapolis, IN, USA

Department of Surgery, Indiana University School of Medicine, Indianapolis, IN, USA

Chapter 1
Introduction to Stem Cell Therapy and Its Application in Vascular Diseases

Lara Lellis Navarro Minchillo Lopes, Tulio Pinho Navarro, and Alan Dardik

1.1 Introduction

1.1.1 Brief History of Stem Cells

Stem cells are undifferentiated cells capable of both self-renewal and differentiation into various specialized cells [1]. Stem cell therapy is the therapeutic administration of stem cells to repair or replace tissue function [2]. The term "stem cell" was proposed by Alexander Maksimov in 1908 when developing "the unitarian theory of hematopoiesis," which proposed a common stem cell progenitor for all blood elements (Fig. 1.1) [3]. However, it was only in 1961 that the existence of murine cells capable of self-renewal was proven by Till et al. while assessing radiation sensitivity of bone marrow tissue [4].

In 1962, John Gurdon performed a classic experiment in frogs, in which he replaced the immature cell nucleus in an egg cell with the nucleus from a mature intestinal cell, resulting in a normal tadpole; this experiment showed that the DNA of the mature cell had all the information needed to develop all cells in the organism, challenging the dogma that the specialized cell is irreversibly committed to its fate [5].

In 1968, Friedenstein et al. reported the discovery of a human bone marrow cell population with high proliferative potential and osteogenic activity in vivo [6]. In the same year, Thomas et al. performed the first hematopoietic stem cell

L. L. N. M. Lopes
Federal University of Minas Gerais, Belo Horizonte, Minas Gerais, Brazil

T. P. Navarro (✉)
Department of Surgery, Vascular Surgery Section, Federal University of Minas Gerais, Belo Horizonte, Minas Gerais, Brazil

A. Dardik
Vascular Biology and Therapeutics Program and the Departments of Surgery and Cellular and Molecular Physiology, Yale University School of Medicine, New Haven, CT, USA

© Springer Nature Switzerland AG 2021
T. P. Navarro et al. (eds.), *Stem Cell Therapy for Vascular Diseases*,
https://doi.org/10.1007/978-3-030-56954-9_1

1

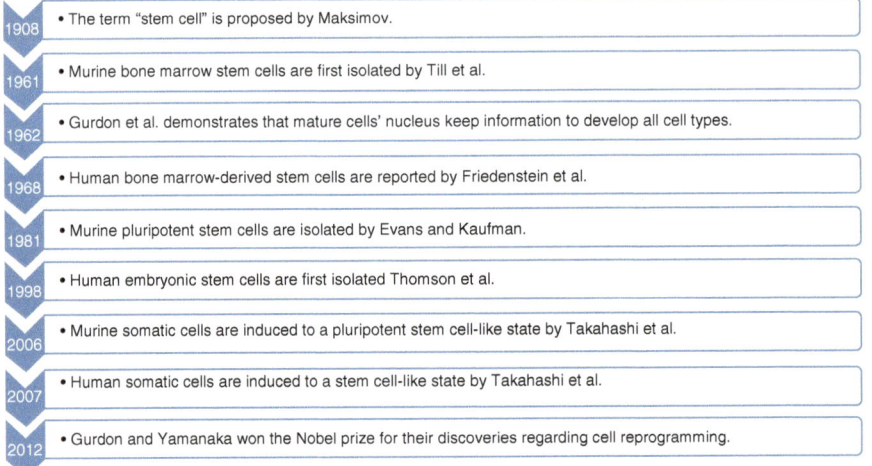

1908 • The term "stem cell" is proposed by Maksimov.

1961 • Murine bone marrow stem cells are first isolated by Till et al.

1962 • Gurdon et al. demonstrates that mature cells' nucleus keep information to develop all cell types.

1968 • Human bone marrow-derived stem cells are reported by Friedenstein et al.

1981 • Murine pluripotent stem cells are isolated by Evans and Kaufman.

1998 • Human embryonic stem cells are first isolated Thomson et al.

2006 • Murine somatic cells are induced to a pluripotent stem cell-like state by Takahashi et al.

2007 • Human somatic cells are induced to a stem cell-like state by Takahashi et al.

2012 • Gurdon and Yamanaka won the Nobel prize for their discoveries regarding cell reprogramming.

Fig. 1.1 Timeline with the main events related to stem cell therapy history

transplantation for the treatment of leukemia [7]. Since then, theoretical implications of human stem cells and their potential clinical applications have been extensively studied.

In 1981, Evans and Kaufman reported the isolation of murine pluripotent embryonic stem cells, and this was followed by the report of Thomson et al., who first isolated human embryonic stem cells in 1998 [8, 9]. Shinya Yamanaka and Kazutoshi Takahashi identified several genes that kept cells immature while performing research on murine embryonal stem cells in 2006. After that, they were able to reprogram fibroblasts into immature stem cells; these resulting induced pluripotent stem cells (iPSC) could develop into mature cell types such as fibroblasts, nerve cells, and gut cells, demonstrating that intact, mature cells could be reprogrammed into pluripotent stem cells [10]. Later, in 2007, they reported induction of human fibroblasts into a pluripotent state [11]. Takahashi's experiments reinforced the concept of using iPSC as a novel technological frontier in stem cell therapy perspectives. In 2012, the Nobel Prize was awarded to John B. Gurdon and Shinya Yamanaka in recognition of their findings showing that mature, specialized cells could be reprogrammed, creating new opportunities to study diseases and to develop new methods for diagnosis and treatment [12].

1.1.2 Mesenchymal Stem Cells vs Mesenchymal Stromal Cells and Cell Markers

In 1991, the term "mesenchymal stem cell" (MSC) was proposed by Caplan et al. to designate adult stem cells capable of differentiating into cells of mesodermal origin [13]. However, as these cells showed limited capacity for self-renewal, thus they failed to meet the criteria to be called stem cells. As such, the term "mesenchymal stromal cell," also abbreviated MSC, was then suggested as a more appropriate designation to these regenerative cells [14].

In 2005, the International Society for Cell and Gene Therapy (ISCT) declared that the terms "stem cell" and "stromal cell" were not equivalent [15]. Furthermore, the term "stem cell" should be limited to a population of cells with demonstrable self-renewal and differentiation capacities, while the term "stromal cell" referred to cells with notable secretory, immunomodulatory, and homing features [16]. In addition, the ISCT provided the following minimal criteria to identify mesenchymal stromal cells: being adherent to plastic; capable of differentiation into adipocyte, chondrocyte, and osteoblast lineages; expression of CD73, CD90, and CD105; and lack of expression of CD11b, CD14, CD19, CD34, CD45, CD79a, and HLA-DR (Fig. 1.2).

Since then, stromal cell surface markers were shown to be plastic and influenced by microenvironmental conditions and stem cell origin among other variables [16–18]. Therefore, there are no specific and unambiguous cell surface markers to distinguish stem cells from stromal cells [16]. Ironically, since the aforementioned ISCT statement, the interchangeable use of the terms "stromal" and "stem" cells by the scientific community has spread. A search in the US National Library of Medicine database (clinicaltrials.gov), performed in November 21, 2019, reported 1009 clinical trials related to the term "mesenchymal stem cell," while only 211 results were related to the term "mesenchymal stromal cell" [19]. Few authors have reported complete mesenchymal stromal cell characterization in both preclinical and clinical publications, and the use of the term "mesenchymal stem cell" remains controversial [16]. Hence, for the purpose of this chapter, the abbreviation "MSC" will be employed to designate populations of regenerative adult mesenchymal cells.

Most of the available data on clinical stem cell therapy relies on adult stem cells and most frequently MSC. Moreover, the use of embryonal stem cells and induced

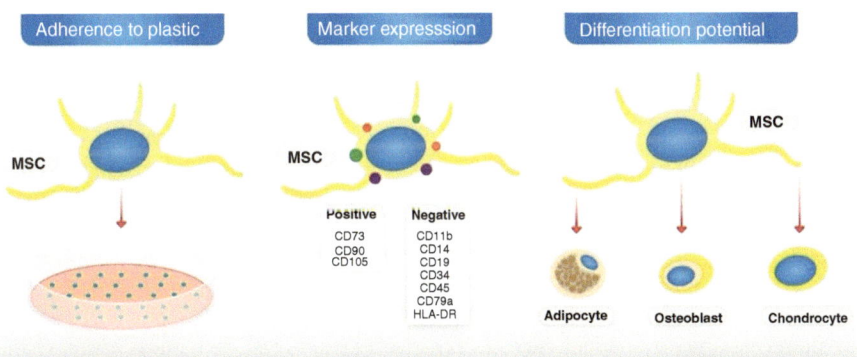

Fig. 1.2 MSC criteria according to the International Society for Cell and Gene Therapy

pluripotent stem cells raises important ethical and safety concerns that impair the use of these two cell types in clinical situations. Therefore, MSC are the main focus of this chapter.

1.2 Differentiation Potential

Stem cells can be classified according to their differentiation potential into totipotent, pluripotent, multipotent, and oligopotent cells. Totipotent stem cells are found in the zygote and can differentiate in both embryonic and extraembryonic cells. Pluripotent cells are also capable of giving rise to any type of embryonic cell, but not to extraembryonic tissue. Multipotent cells give rise to multiple cells of the same lineage whereas oligopotent stem cells have a narrower differentiation spectrum within a same lineage [1].

1.3 Stem Cell Types

Stem cells can be classified into embryonic stem cells (ESC), adult stromal cells, and iPSC according to their origin (Fig. 1.3). The diverse characteristics, advantages, and limitations of these groups (Fig. 1.4) lead to different clinical applications.

1.3.1 Embryonic Stem Cells (ESC)

ESC are stem cells derived from the embryonic inner cell mass and possess unlimited self-renewal capability as well as the ability to differentiate into any type of somatic cell. Even though these cells have potential clinical application, clinical use of these cells is scarce due to ethical conflicts involving the harvest and manipulation of human embryos to obtain these cells. Additionally, embryonic stem cells' unlimited

Fig. 1.3 Stem cell types

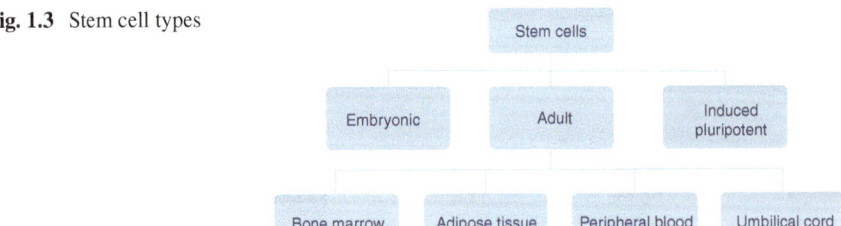

	Stem Cell Type					
	Adult Stem Cells				Embryonic	IPSC
	BM-MSC	PB-MSC	UC-MSC	ADSC		
Advantages	• Donor-specific therapy • Lower malignancy risk • Cell-lineage committed (targeting differentiation) • No ethical conflict	• Donor-specific therapy • Lower malignancy risk • Cell-lineage committed (targeting differentiation) • No ethical conflict • Relatively disposable tissue • Vein puncture has low surgical risk • Simple cell harvesting protocol	• Future donor-specific therapy • Lower malignancy risk • Cell-lineage committed (targeting differentiation) • Disposable tissue • UC tissue harvesting has low surgical risk • Donor UCB banking storage	• Donor-specific therapy • Lower malignancy risk • Cell-lineage committed (targeting differentiation) • No ethical conflict • Disposable tissue • Liposuction has low surgical risk	• High differentiation potential (pluripotent)	• High differentiation potential (pluripotent) • Somatic-cell memory (targeting differentiation) • Donor-specific therapy • No ethical conflict • Disposable tissue • Low cell harvesting procedure risk
Disadvantages	• Cell lineage committed • Biopsy high surgical risk • Non-disposable tissue • Low stem cell concentration • Cell concentration and performance influenced by comorbities	• Cell lineage committed • Cell concentration and performance influenced by comorbities • G-CSF administration needed	• Cell lineage committed • Immuno incompatibility • Ethical conflict • Low stem cell concentration • Need of UCB banking	• Cell lineage committed • Cell concentration and performance influenced by comorbities	• Increased malignancy risk • Immuno incompatibility • Ethical conflicts	• Increased malignancy risk • Complex induction protocol • Somatic-cell memory (biased differentiation)

Fig. 1.4 Stem cell types, advantages and disadvantages [36]

differentiation potential lead to a higher risk of malignancy and requires immuno-modulation as the use of allogeneic cells is mandatory for clinical therapy [20, 21].

1.3.2 Adult Stem Cells (ASC)

ASC are partially undifferentiated cells that can be found within nearly any organ or tissue. Peripheral blood, umbilical cord, bone marrow, and adipose tissue are the most common sources of such cells. Endometrium, amniotic fluid and membrane, placenta, dental tissues, thymus, and spleen are unconventional sources of ASC. ASC may be isolated from the same patient in whom the cell therapy will be applied (donor-specific therapy) with no risk of immune rejection. There is no ethical con-flict regarding the origin of these adult-derived cells or their isolation; however, isolation protocols for ASC can be laborious, and a significant quantity of tissue is frequently needed to obtain high stem cell counts [20].

ASC are lineage-committed multipotent cells, being able to differentiate only into cells of the same germ layer [20]. This feature accounts for the lower malignancy potential of ASC, and therefore these cells may be desirable to be used in therapies that target specific cell differentiation, such as host tissue replacement.

1.3.3 Induced Pluripotent Stem Cells (iPSC)

iPSC are stem cells generated through somatic cell reprogramming into an embry-onic stem cell-like state, first reported in 2006 [10]. In theory, iPSC can be generated from any somatic cell, and thus the use of these cells is emerging as an abundant and accessible source of donor-specific stem cells free of ethical conflicts. These totipo-tent cells demonstrate a broad differentiation potential, being capable of generating any somatic or trophoblastic cell, but they also have a high malignant potential [22].

Because iPSC show advantages of both ASC, e.g., donor-specific therapy and absence of ethical conflicts, and ESC, e.g., differentiation potential, this novel source of stem cells is considered very promising. Nonetheless, strategies to enhance the yield of cell induction into the stem cell-like state and simultaneously control cell differentiation with absence of malignancy are still hurdles to be overcome.

1.4 Stem Cell Origin

Stem cell therapy can be classified according to the cell origin as either autologous, allogeneic, or xenogeneic transplantation (Fig. 1.5).

Stem cell origin

	Autologous	Allogeneic	Xenotransplantation
Advantages	• Immunoincompatibility • No ethical conflict • No infection transmission risk	• Healthy stem cell source • No cell harvesting risk for the host patient • Donor banking creation	• No ethical conflict • Heathy stem cell source • No cell harvesting risk for host patient • Donor baking creation
Disadvantages	• Lower stem cell concentration and limited healing potential • Cell harvestmg procedural risk	• Relative immunoincompatibility • Need of disease screening • Ethical conflict	• High immunoincompatibility • Need of disease screening

Fig. 1.5 Stem cell origins, advantages, and disadvantages [36]

1.4.1 Autologous Transplantation

Autologous transplantation involves the administration of the recipient's own cells, typically using either ASC or iPSC. Autologous cells have the advantages of being immunocompatible, having no risk of infectious disease transmission and involving no ethical or legal issues. On the other hand, donor characteristics such as advanced age, diabetes, obesity, and atherosclerosis exert negative impact on stem cell function, potentially decreasing the effectiveness of cell therapy [23–27]. Therefore, past medical history and advanced patient age may be some of the limitations to the use of autologous ASC for cell therapy.

1.4.2 Allogeneic Transplantation

Allogeneic cell transplantation is the exchange of cells between a donor and a recipient of the same species. The use of cells isolated from a healthier or younger donor could enhance the efficacy of stem cell therapy. However, allogeneic transplantation has the drawbacks of lower immunocompatibility, risk of disease transmission, and potential legal issues regarding exchange of biomaterials.

It has been hypothesized that allogeneic MSC are immunoprivileged. Nonetheless, further research has shown that allogeneic MSC are not privileged, but demonstrate diminished immunogenicity compared with other allogeneic cell types [28]. The therapeutic implications of allogeneic MSC immunogenicity are controversial as cell apoptosis is crucial for immunomodulatory effects but reduces therapeutic cell longevity and engraftment [29].

Strict donor screening is needed to avoid disease transmission by allogeneic cell therapy [2]. The use of cadaveric cells may be an alternative to enhance donor availability and to avoid the risks associated to tissue harvesting therapeutic cells [30].

1.4.3 Xenotransplantation

Xenotransplantation involves the administration of either nonhuman live cells or human biological material that has had ex vivo contact with live nonhuman animal cells [31]. The use of animal stem cells has the potential to increase availability of donors and to reduce the financial burden related to stem cell transplantation. However, this source raises concerns regarding immunologic rejection and disease transmission.

1.5 Stem Cell Isolation and Induction Protocols

The tissue source of stem cells is the main determinant of the required isolation protocol and influences MSC phenotypes and function [14]. Here we discuss basic aspects of stem cell isolation and induction protocols and their clinical implications.

1.5.1 Adult Stem Cells

1.5.1.1 Bone Marrow-Derived MSC (BM-MSC)

BM-MSC are isolated from the bone marrow by density gradient centrifugation, washing, and seeding on culture dishes. BM-MSC can be selected by survival in minimum essential media with fetal bovine serum and by their adherence to plastic [14, 32]. However, these isolation protocols usually result in a heterogeneous cell population, contaminated by other cells [33].

Bone marrow tissue is not a disposable tissue and is necessarily obtained by bone marrow aspiration. The aspiration is an invasive procedure, which leads to higher risks to the donor when compared to other MSC isolation protocols.

1.5.1.2 Adipose-Derived Stem Cells (ADSC)

Adipose tissue is a relatively disposable cell source and can be easily accessed by lipoaspiration, which is considered a minimally invasive procedure. Adipose tissue processing leads to a heterogenic population termed the "stromal vascular fraction" (SVF). The SVF is composed of adipose-derived stem cells (ADSC), pericytes, endothelial cells, pre-adipocytes and immune cells as well as other cell types [34].

Isolation of the SVF may be performed either by enzymatic or mechanical protocols that generally comprise washes, agitation, centrifugation, and collagenase digestion (in enzymatic protocols) [35]. Currently, semi-automated SVF isolation devices are commercially available [34]. ADSC and SVF have been used in clinical trials, but ADSC isolation protocols frequently fail to exclude the other components of the SVF, leading to questions of reproducibility and translatability [14, 34].

1.5.1.3 Peripheral Blood-Derived MSC (PB-MSC)

Peripheral blood is a relatively disposable stem cell source and can be obtained by venipuncture, a minimally invasive procedure. Peripheral blood-derived MSC (PB-MSC) are isolated by centrifugation and dilution protocols. PB-MSC usually circulate in low concentrations; therefore, bone marrow stimulation by granulocyte colony-stimulating factor (G-CSF) is an important adjunct to mobilize PB-MSC into the circulation before collecting blood [36].

G-CSF administration itself is effective in the treatment of diabetic foot ulcers [36]. Thus, the administration of G-CSF may be a confounding variable in study interpretation as well as its associated financial cost.

1.5.1.4 Other Adult Stem Cell Sources

Umbilical cord blood, placenta, Wharton's jelly, amniotic fluid, dental pulp, synovial fluid, and skin are also MSC sources, although less commonly used.

1.5.2 Embryonic Stem Cells (ESC)

The isolation of human embryonic stem cells (hESC) implies the destruction of the embryo. Due to associated ethical and political concerns, research involving the use of these cells has been deferred if not banned. Nevertheless, isolation, culture, and characterization protocols for hESC have been developed [37].

hESC are found in the inner cell mass of both fresh and frozen embryos. Several isolation techniques are described in the literature including mechanical dissection, laser dissection, and immunosurgery [9, 38, 39]. There is no consensus regarding the best method as each of these techniques have specific advantages and disadvantages regarding success rate and financial and time constraints [37].

1.5.3 Induced Pluripotent Stem Cells (iPSC)

iPSC are stem cells induced from somatic cells; as such they are not isolated per se. The use of iPSC has obviated ethical conflicts regarding the use of hESC and has provided insights into early embryo development. The first method to successfully induce human iPSC was the use of four transcription factors Oct3/4, Sox2, Klf4, and c-Myc, under ES cell culture conditions [11]. Currently, several induction methods have been used to generate iPSC including integrating vectors, non-integrating vectors, non-DNA reprogramming, and small molecules [40]. Pluripotency induction and maintenance are based on the interaction of both extrinsic and intrinsic factors [41]. The extrinsic factors involve cytokines, growth factors, and extracellular matrix; extrinsic elements influence intrinsic pathways that reverse epigenetic programming of differentiated somatic cells, such as octamer-binding transcription factor 4 (Oct4) and sex-determining region Y-box 2 (Sox2) [42].

The low cell reprogramming yield (0.01–0.02% when first described), expression of transgenic viral genes, and tumorigenesis by overexpression of oncogenes (c-Myc, kfl4) are major concerns of iPSC induction protocols [11, 43]. Further advances on cell reprogramming techniques are required to enable iPSC use in clinical scenarios.

1.6 Stem Cell Culture and Priming

Culture conditions such as media composition, oxygen tension, and extracellular structure affect stem cell survival, differentiation, and function [14, 43]. Furthermore, several cell priming techniques have been proposed as strategies to enhance stem cell therapeutic effects. Understanding and electing the best cell culture and priming protocol is important not only to enhance their regenerative potential but also for reproducible cell expansion after low yield isolation protocols and target differentiation.

1.6.1 Culture Media

Medium containing either fetal bovine serum (FBS), human AB serum (HABS), human platelet lysate (HPL), or chemically defined media (CMD) is commonly used in MSC culture [14]. FBS is the most common supplement, although it carries the risk of xenogeneic immune reaction and has a variable composition [44]. HABS and HPL are derived from peripheral blood that have been proposed as human-derived immunocompatible alternatives to FBS. However, their composition is also highly variable, and there is a risk of infection transmission [45]. In addition, HPL has pro-inflammatory factors and may alter MSC cell markers, affecting its functionality [14, 46]. Serum-free, xenobiotic-free CMD can improve cell expansion and differentiation and is considered a desirable alternative for MSC culture for clinical use [47].

1.6.2 Hypoxia

Hypoxic culture conditions (1–10% O_2 partial pressure) mimic hypoxic areas within the bone marrow where BM-MSC can be found physiologically (4–7% O_2 tension) [14]. However, hypoxia affects stem cells from other sources by influencing cell metabolism, proliferation, differentiation, and the secretome [48]. Since hypoxia intensity is variable among stem cell studies that use hypoxic conditioning, conclusions regarding the effects of hypoxia need to be cautiously interpreted.

Low oxygen availability lowers metabolism and production of reactive oxygen species (ROS), a mechanism that is thought to be responsible for reduced stem cell injury [48]. In addition, the decrease in ROS added to hypoxia-mediated upregulation of c-jun leads to delayed stem cell senescence and increases immunosuppression [49].

Upregulation of hypoxia-inducible factors 1α and 2α (HIF-1α and HIF-2α), vascular endothelial growth factor (VEGF), and angiopoietin-1 (Ang-1) lead to increase angiogenic potential [50, 51]. This feature is especially desirable when treating ischemic and inflammatory pathologies. Moreover, HIF-2α inhibits p53, increasing the regenerative potential of stem cells [51].

Hypoxic-cultured MSC (2% O_2 tension) were reported to be more proliferative when compared to MSC cultured in normoxic conditions (20%) [52]. The increased cell proliferation compensates for the initial hypoxia-mediated MSC apoptosis in subsequent cell passages. Furthermore, hypoxia favors maintenance of stem cells' undifferentiated state and increases cell motility [50, 53].

1.6.3   Culture Matrices and Devices

Stem cells are often cultured in plastic containers such as T-flasks and well plates. However, these two-dimensional devices are associated with alteration of cell markers as well as reduced capacity for differentiation and proliferation [54, 55]. As a result, a variety of three-dimensional culture systems and matrices composed of collagen, hyaluronic acid, glycosaminoglycan, polyethylene glycol, and alginate have been investigated as alternative matrices for stem cell culture [14, 56].

In an attempt to reproduce the three-dimensional native environment of MSC, spinner flasks, wavy-walled cultures, and bioreactors were proposed and developed as three-dimensional culture systems. Bioreactors demonstrate important advantages besides cost: faster cell expansion, reduced risk of contamination, higher rate of cytokine production, rigorous monitoring, and control of culture parameters [57–59].

Besides three-dimensional structure, the inherent material properties of the cell culture system, such as rigidity and composition, directly influence expression of MSC markers, the cell secretome, and cell viability and are considered as part of the strategy to target stem cell differentiation into specific cell populations [60]. MSC marker expression shifts from neurogenic toward myogenic or osteogenic markers as rigidity increases from low to intermediate and high stiffness, respectively [61]. In addition, the use of extracellular matrix as a surface for cell growth enhances VEGF and glial-derived neurotropic factor production while decreasing synthesis of interleukin-6 when compared to the use of tissue-culture plastic [62].

Besides the aforementioned inherent properties of the culture systems, the mechanism of cell release from the matrix and the route of cell administration need to be considered when choosing an optimal culture matrix, as they affect cell yield and viability. Stem cells cultured in biocompatible microcarriers, such as poly-ε-caprolactone, can be directly administrated without the need of enzymatic release [63]. The administration of cells associated with these types of carriers preserves yield and functionality while providing a microarchitecture design for tissue regeneration [63, 64].

Another trypsin-free alternative is the use of thermoresponsive polymers, such as poly-N-isopropylacrilamide, which are able to reversibly expand and adhere according to the temperature. Hydrogels composed of these polymers are able to transit in aqueous solutions upon temperature increase [65]. Thermoresponsive polymers have been investigated as an alternative to increase stem cell yield, homing, and engraftment.

1.6.4   Stem Cell Priming

Cell priming refers to techniques used to trigger stem cell "memory," inducing cell activity toward a specific therapeutic purpose. Stem cells may be primed for different therapeutic purposes such as to promote immunomodulation, cell homing, target differentiation, and decrease apoptosis [14]. Priming techniques include the use of various stimuli such as pharmaceutical (valproic acid, progesterone), interleukins (IL-1, IFN-γ), genetic (dsRNA), and environmental (three-dimensional structure, hypoxia), among others [14].

Priming is an important strategy to enhance the overall effectiveness of stem cell therapy. Nonetheless, it is especially important when guiding and limiting ESC and iPSC proliferation and differentiation as these pluripotent stem cells demonstrate increased oncogenicity.

1.7   Routes of Stem Cell Administration

Cell delivery is a crucial step in stem cell therapy since administration routes can enhance cell survival and functionality, increasing stem cell therapy effectiveness in hostile microenvironmental conditions [66]. Intravascular administration is considered systemic therapy, whereas injections into a particular site and topical administration are local delivery methods (Fig. 1.6). Both systemic (intravascular) and local delivery methods have demonstrated effectiveness in the treatment of vascular pathologies [67]. Various diseases and clinical scenarios require different cell mechanisms of action, and there are a lack of studies comparing cell delivery methods [68]. Accordingly, no consensus regarding the optimal administration route has been achieved.

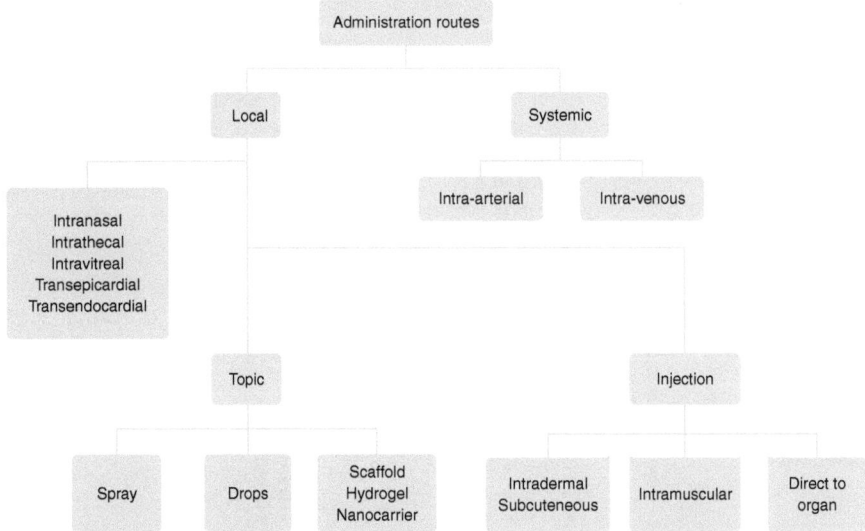

Fig. 1.6 Routes of stem cell administration

Since treating different diseases requires several cell-induced regenerative pathways and proper cell homing, understanding the advantages and disadvantages of different cell delivery methods is critical to better address the disease and tissue of interest (Fig. 1.7).

1.7.1 Local Administration Routes

Injections into the diseased site and topical administration are the main local stem cell delivery techniques. Local delivery methods enhance cell homing, a key feature in the treatment of patients with peripheral vascular diseases, which by definition prevents robust intravascular cell delivery [69].

Topical delivery typically consists of administration of a cell suspension directly to the target lesion using a spray or drops. This is a local, simple, and painless delivery method that has been used as tissue replacement strategy for chronic wound and burn treatment [68]. Topical cell delivery is a lower-risk alternative to local injections and systemic routes and enhances engraftment at the site of interest [68]. However, preliminary procedures to optimize cell homing, such as debridement, may be unavoidable [66]. Moreover, inaccurate cell density and spacing and the lack of extracellular protective environment lead to premature cell differentiation and increased cell mortality [66].

Intramuscular, intradermal, and translesional injections are safe and simple local administration routes [36]. Intramuscular administration is associated with a higher cell dwell time and provides a highly vascular support for the therapeutic

Stem cell administration route

Topic	Systemic		Local		
	Intraarterial	Intravenous	Spray or drops	Hydrogel, scaffold or nanocarrier	Injection
Advantages	• Can be performed during angioplasty angioplasty • Possible immunomodulation and glucose homeostasis optimizing effect	• Can be performed during angioplasty angioplasty • Possible immunomodulation and glucose homeostasis optimizing effect	• Painless • Simple • Low risk • Inexpensive	• Low risk • Cell density and spacing control • Better retention and engraftment • Mechanical anchorage • Stem cell behavior modulation	• Simple • Low risk • Inexpensive • Better vascular support • Crosses anatomical barriers
Disadvantages	• High surgical risk • Low addressing and poor engraftment • Thrombosis/embolia • Expensive	• High surgical risk • Low addressing and poor engraftment • Thrombosis/embolia • Expensive • Lung entrapping	• High cell death • Low addressing and poor engraftment • No cell density and spacing control • Premature differentiation	• High protocol complexity • Expensive	• High cell death • Low addressing and poor engraftment • No cell density and spacing control • Infection risk • Ectopic stem cell transformation

Fig. 1.7 Stem cell administration routes, advantages, and disadvantages [36]

cells, enhancing local and systemic flow of cytokines [70]. Direct injections into the target tissue have the potential to overcome delivery obstacles such as the blood-brain barrier. Nonetheless, ectopic stem cell transformation and increased surgical risk can be associated with direct injections. Additionally, intraparenchymal cell injection leads to decreased systemic response and can result in tissue trauma [68].

Bioscaffolds, fibrin, nanofibers, and other exogenous support systems have been extensively investigated as local stem cell therapy adjuvants [71, 72]. The use of these components is a strategy to modulate stem cell behavior and provide mechanical anchorage, ultimately enhancing the efficiency of local administration [69, 73].

1.7.2 Systemic Administration Routes

Intra-arterial and intravenous infusion are the main routes of systemic stem cell administration. Systemic cell delivery leads to enhanced interaction with the host immune system and regeneration signaling pathways and is appropriate to treat systemic conditions or large areas of pathology not amenable to local treatment [68].

Intra-arterial infusion enables cell delivery to the site of interest with lower cell loss when compared to intravenous delivery [74]. Thrombi and emboli formation raise concerns regarding the intra-arterial route, especially in intra-coronary and intra-carotid infusion [68]. These complications can be avoided by controlling infusion speed, cell dosage, and size [75].

Intravenous infusion may be a more accessible and safer route compared with intra-arterial infusion, as microthrombi can be captured by the lungs with fewer significant clinical consequences [68]. However, intravenous infused cells are retained in lung vasculature, at up to 90% in animal models, and therefore may be removed by the host immune system [76]. After being entrapped in the lung, stem cells are phagocytosed by monocytes, which switch toward immunoregulatory phenotype and are redistributed systemically [77]. As a result, a reduced number of therapeutic cells may reach the organ of interest by this administration route, even though there is the potential to have systemic immunomodulation.

1.7.3 Other Administration Routes

Intranasal and intrathecal stem cell administration have been investigated in the treatment of neurologic pathologies such as subarachnoid hemorrhage and neuropathic pain [78, 79]. Intravitreal stem cell infusion was described as therapeutic alternative to diabetic retinopathy and retinal vein occlusion [80]. Transepicardial and transendocardial routes are important local administration routes used in stem cell therapy for ischemic cardiomyopathy [81, 82].

1.8   Stem Cell-Mediated Mechanisms of Regeneration

The therapeutic potential of stem cells was originally accredited to the cells' broad differentiation capability and potential for host tissue replacement by cell engraftment. However, substantial evidence regarding direct cell interaction and trophic paracrine effects has challenged the importance of stem cell differentiation in tissue regeneration [83, 84]. This evidence was further supported by studies demonstrating low MSC engraftment in both clinical settings and in vivo models [85–87]. As such, the focus of stem cell therapeutic potential has shifted from direct differentiation toward secondary signaling effector cells. Cytokines, growth factors, and chemokines released by stem cells induce angiogenesis, immunomodulation, neuroregeneration, and extracellular matrix production while reducing cell apoptosis and fibrosis [83, 88].

In recent years, investigations demonstrated that inactivated, apoptotic, and fragmented mesenchymal stem cells retain some immunomodulatory capacity and are potentially regenerative [89–91]. Nonetheless, direct stem cell differentiation continues to play an important role in specific therapeutic scenarios such as tissue engineering and tissue replacing therapies [92, 93].

1.8.1   Immunomodulation

Stromal cells are associated with a spectrum of different immunomodulatory mechanisms, attained via both soluble factors and direct cell-cell interaction [77]. Host microenvironmental characteristics, stromal cell source, culture, and administration conditions influence the expression of surface markers and the profile of secreted cytokines [94–96]. Although a clear picture of stem cell-induced immunomodulation is not well understood, some pathways are consistent.

1.8.1.1   Monocytes and Macrophages Interaction

Mesenchymal stem cells inhibit monocyte and macrophage differentiation into the type 1 phenotype and dendritic cells, inducing type 2 anti-inflammatory and immunoregulatory differentiation by secreting interleukin-1 receptor antagonist (IL-1 RA) [97]. These induced anti-inflammatory monocytes play an important role in MSC-mediated beneficial effects in the treatment of sepsis and induction of tolerance against alloimmunity and autoimmunity by secreting high levels of IL-10 and suppressing T-cell activity, respectively [98, 99].

Recent investigations in asthma and peritonitis animal models show that MSC phagocytosis by host monocytes induces anti-inflammatory type 2 differentiation in a cytokine-independent pathway [100, 101]. Furthermore, stromal cells increase monocyte count and phagocytic activity besides inhibiting dendritic cell maturation and migration [100, 102, 103].

1.8.1.2 T-Cell, B-Cell, and Natural Killer Cell Interaction

Mesenchymal stromal cells suppress T-cell proliferation and induce a shift from Th1 pro-inflammatory to Th2 anti-inflammatory subtypes [104]. MSC induce conventional T-cell differentiation into regulatory T-cells (T-reg), important mediators of graft immune tolerance and prevention of autoimmunity [105, 106]. Stromal cells inhibit proliferation of alloreactive CD4+ and CD8+ T-cells [107].

MSC suppress plasmablast production and induce regulatory B-cell (B-reg) formation, which promotes immunological tolerance [108, 109]. These effects are thought to be promoted by direct cell-cell contact, whereas inhibition of B-cell proliferation and differentiation by MSC is ascribed to soluble factors such as IFN-γ and IL-1 RA [94, 110]. Natural killer cell activity and proliferation are also inhibited by MSC via secretion of prostaglandin E2, TGF-β, nitric oxide, and other factors [111–113].

1.8.1.3 Complement and Coagulation Systems

MSC exert procoagulant activity by triggering both host coagulation and the innate immune system, increasing C3 activation, D-dimer, and thrombin-antithrombin complex formation while decreasing platelet counts [68, 114, 115]. Christy et al. demonstrated increased tissue factor expression in MSC that varies according to the cell source [116]. BM-MSC express less tissue factor compared to ADSC, which are highly procoagulant [116]. Thus, theoretically, BM-MSC may be preferable in the treatment of ischemic conditions and in systemic MSC infusion, whereas ADSC may be preferable in the treatment of hemorrhagic conditions.

Procoagulant MSC activity increases with increased cell passages and can be reduced by cell dilution, heparin, or tissue factor blockers [117, 118]. Adverse thrombotic events reported by clinical studies will be discussed below.

1.8.2 Angiogenesis

Angiogenesis is the growth of blood vessels from pre-existing vessels. The angiogenic potential of MSC has been the focus not only in investigations involving diseases caused by limited angiogenesis, such as peripheral arterial disease, myocardial ischemia, and stroke, but also in pathologic angiogenesis associated with tumors [87]. Since MSC engraftment is typically low, the pro-angiogenic effects of MSC are generally attributed to paracrine activity of secreted factors. The MSC secretome is composed of various soluble factors such as vascular endothelial growth factor (VEGF), fibroblast growth factor 2 (FGF-2), angiopoietin-1 (ang-1), interleukin-6 (IL-6), and monocyte chemoattractant protein-1 (MCP-1), among others. Investigations using the chicken chorioallantoic membrane and mouse matrigel plug assay showed that BM-MSC induce angiogenesis in vitro [119, 120].

VEGF and FGF-2 are critical factors for wound healing and are capable of inducing endothelial cell (EC) proliferation, migration, and remodeling of the extracellular matrix [121]. Hypoxic conditions, conditioned medium from tumor necrosis factor α (TNF-α), and lipopolysaccharide (LPS) enhance human MSC production of VEGF, FGF-2, and insulin-like growth factor (IGF-1) and, therefore, are potential strategies to enhance MSC-induced angiogenesis [122].

However, evidence regarding MSC differentiation in endothelial cells as a mechanism of angiogenesis is scarce [87]. However, the use of MSC conditioned by EC-differentiation medium significantly increased differentiation into a more angiogenic cell type, leading to better therapeutic outcomes in wire injury model and in vivo angiogenesis assay [123, 124]. MSC differentiation toward EC phenotype is especially promising for vascular graft tissue engineering and intima replacing therapies. The potential of MSC angiogenesis to form tumors remains controversial and will be discussed below.

1.8.3 Apoptotic, Inactivated, and Fragmented Stem Cells

In 2005, Thum et al. proposed "the dying stem cell hypothesis," suggesting that apoptosis of therapeutic stem cells was responsible for modulation of host immune reactivity [125]. Recent studies showed that immunomodulation of mesenchymal stem cells not only occur by soluble mediators but also rely on cell-cell interaction; since these interactions do not require intact cell metabolism, cell viability is not a prerequisite for the therapeutic effects of stem cells [126].

Sun et al. demonstrated that cytotoxic activity against mesenchymal stem cells was a vital step in inducing immunomodulation [29]. In addition, the need for the host cytotoxic response could be bypassed by using apoptotic MSC. Moreover, apoptotic adipose-derived MSC were more effective in reducing oxidative stress, inflammation, and apoptosis compared with living MSC in a sepsis animal model [127].

Heat inactivated stem cells exhibited similar effects on monocyte function as living MSC in an ischemic kidney model despite lack of proliferative and metabolic activities [91]. MSC membrane particles retained immunomodulatory capacity by inducing selective apoptosis of pro-inflammatory monocytes [90].

1.8.4 Mesenchymal Stem Cell-Derived Extracellular Vesicles (MSC-EV)

MSC-derived microvesicles and exosomes are extracellular vesicles secreted by mesenchymal stromal cells containing proteins, miRNA, and mRNA. These structures are involved in cell-cell communication acting on regenerative pathways such as coagulation, inflammation, angiogenesis, and immune responses [83]. The therapeutic potential of MSC extracellular vesicles has been demonstrated in several disease models such as acute kidney injury, liver fibrosis, myocardial ischemia-reperfusion, and stroke [128–131]. MSC-EV have been proposed as a promising non-cellular therapy since their biological activity is similar to that of MSC [132].

1.8.5 Stem Cells as a Delivery System

Stem cells are considered an innovative drug and gene delivery system due to their affinity to travel to injured tissue and tumors [133]. MSC can take up drugs such as paclitaxel, doxorubicin, and gemcitabine and release these drugs at a specific site of interest [134]. Studies performed using in vitro pancreatic adenocarcinoma showed the ability of MSC to deliver these three drugs [134, 135]. Moreover, MSC loaded with paclitaxel impaired tumor growth and angiogenesis in vivo, using a murine leukemia model [136]. In addition, MSC loaded with organic and inorganic nanoparticles have been proposed as photothermal cancer drugs and as diagnostic agents for laser-induced thermal ablation and magnetic resonance imaging [137–139].

Stem cells have also emerged as a gene therapy alternative. MSC transduced by vectors or three-dimensional/reverse transfection systems express genes for cytokines, drugs, and cell receptors and other proteins [133]. However, transient gene expression and carcinogenesis are important issues in stem cell-mediated gene therapy [133]. All in all, current studies suggest that stem cell therapy may be a promising gene and target drug delivery system, capable of increasing the effectiveness of therapy and reducing side effects.

1.9 Stem Cell Therapy Safety and Adverse Events

Stem cell therapy potential adverse events are various and depend on multiple factors such as disease to be treated, donor medical history, stem cell characteristics, the cell manufacturing process, administration route, and host response to the therapy. Here, we summarize main safety concerns regarding stem cell therapy safety (Fig. 1.8).

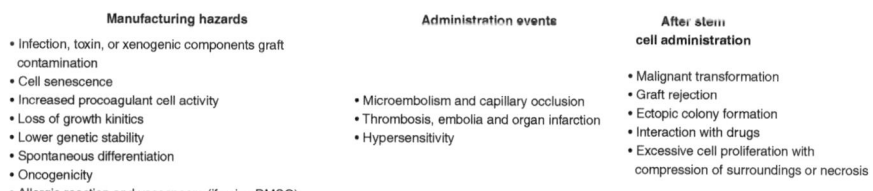

Fig. 1.8 Stem cell therapy risks

1.9.1 Stem Cell Manufacturing Hazards

Stem cell isolation and induction and cell culture and priming can all potentially lead to adverse clinical events. Allogeneic transplantation with inadequate donor screening and suboptimal culture conditions may lead to transplantation of cells contaminated by xenogenic components, toxins, and infectious microorganisms [14, 140]. Dimethylsulfoxide (DMSO), a cell protectant used in cryopreservation protocols, is associated with allergic reactions and vasospasm [141, 142].

Stem cell quality diminishes with age, a process termed cell senescence that is characterized by several genetic, phenotypic, and functional modifications that result in loss of the state of "stemness" [143]. Advanced donor age and in vitro stem cell expansion are associated with cell senescence [144]. Furthermore, prolonged stem cell culture is associated with increased procoagulant activity as well as loss of growth kinetics and immunomodulatory properties [145, 146]. After the fifth passage, MSC show significant drop of differentiation potential [145]. Moreover, late stem cell passages show lower genetic stability, leading to spontaneous cell differentiation and oncogenicity [14].

Rigorous donor screening, control of isolation, induction, and culture conditions and the use of automated systems are effective alternatives to reduce the risk of infections. DMSO use should be avoided in cryopreservation for therapeutic purposes. Limited cell passage, the cytokinesis-block micronucleus assay, and monitoring of miRNA and proteins are recommended in order to avoid adverse effects of stem cell aging in clinical therapeutic scenarios [14, 147].

1.9.2 Stem Cell Administration Adverse Events

Stem cell administration is specially challenging since, unlike therapeutic drugs, these cellular therapies tend to aggregate in specific sites, depending on the route of administration [148]. As previously discussed, MSC exert procoagulant activity, which is especially worrisome in systemic stem cell administration. Large cell size, high infusion speed, and ADSC cell type are variables related to increased procoagulant properties [116].

Intravenous and intra-arterial stem cell infusion may cause microembolism, although generally without clinical sequelae [140]. Nonetheless, several studies have reported thrombotic events such as pulmonary embolism, pulmonary infarction, and venous thrombosis of brachial and portal veins as major complications of intravenous MSC infusion [149–151]. Intra-arterial stem cell delivery can cause not only capillary obstruction but also occlusion at the precapillary level, raising concerns especially when treating high oxygen consumption organs such as heart and brain [152]. Microvascular obstruction after intra-coronary BM-MSC administration has also been reported [153].

Acosta el al. reported peripheral microthrombosis following intra-arterial administration of autologous ADSC in the treatment of critical limb ischemia [154]. Importantly, this report showed that MSC from diabetic patients have decreased fibrinolytic activity, raising concerns regarding intravascular infusion of autologous stromal cells in diabetic patients [154].

The risk of thrombotic complications following intra-arterial infusion can be reduced by controlling infusion speed, cell dosage, and size [75]. Nonetheless, lower MSC concentration may be ineffective in avoiding pulmonary microthrombosis following intravenous stem cell administration [140]. Heparin, bivalirudin, and other anticoagulant drugs can prevent cell priming and limit progression of MSC-mediated thrombogenic events [155].

There are several reports of hypersensitivity reactions following systemic administration of allogeneic placenta-derived MSC and ADSC [115, 156–158]. It remains unclear, however, if the reported events were related to anti-donor immune responses [159].

1.9.3 Adverse Events After Stem Cell Administration

Uncontrolled stem cell differentiation is a key obstacle that needs to be solved in order to ensure the safety of stem cell therapy. Excessive cell proliferation may result in compression of the surrounding structures and cell necrosis among other detrimental effects [140]. Depending on the route of administration, transplanted cells may migrate and form undesired ectopic colonies that can differentiate in ectopic tissue or tumors [160]. Pluripotent cells such as ESC and iPSC are particularly concerning due to their unlimited proliferation capacity that can cause neoplastic formation in animal models [161, 162]. Interestingly, neoplasia may arise from malignant transformation of host cells surrounding the graft after administration of senescent stem cells [163].

Graft rejection and graft versus host disease are potential complications of allogeneic and xenogeneic cell transplantation. Major histocompatibility complex (MHC) matching and the use of less immunogenic stem cells have been proposed as alternatives to avoid these reactions [164]. This recommendation is, however, highly controversial since recent studies suggest the importance of host immune reaction in the effectiveness of MSC therapy.

Stem cell interaction with host drugs is an under-explored theme. Murine in vivo studies have reported that MSC infusion may abolish the effects of G-CSF [165]. Corticosteroid administration was reported to inhibit MSC-mediated immunomodulation in a cirrhosis model and, therefore, should be avoided while performing stem cell therapy [166]. Further investigation regarding medication interactions with transplanted stem cells are needed.

Tumor formation and adverse immune reactions can be avoided by using autologous stem cells and following safety recommendations mentioned above.

1.10   Stem Cell Therapy for Vascular Diseases

Vascular disorders are frequently chronic conditions characterized by impaired blood flow; the general goal of stem cell therapy for these diseases is to restore blood flow, improving the perfusion and function of the ischemic end organ. Stem cell therapy was shown to be safe and effective to treat some vascular disorders such as diabetic foot ulcers [36] and is considered a promising alternative for other diseases such as vasculitis and lymphedema.

1.10.1   The Vascular Patient

The potential for stem cell therapy to induce regeneration relies on the interaction between stem cells and the host. The high prevalence of risk factors that impact stem cell therapy, including age, diabetes, hypertension, smoking, dyslipidemia, obesity, and coagulation and immunity disorders, remains a key challenge in the treatment of vascular patients.

Lower cell yield, hostile administration site microenviroment, and decreased and dysfunctional cell activity are important limitations and barriers of autologous stem cell therapy in vascular patients. Stem cells from diabetic patients show decreased fibrinolytic activity, leading to higher risk of adverse events. It is not clear whether other metabolic disorders are associated with higher risk of complications.

The management of chronic diseases frequent requires the use multiple medications whose interactions with stem cell therapy are yet to be discovered. The inhibition of MSC-mediated immunomodulation by corticosteroids is a special concern for patients diagnosed with immunological disorders. The use of allogeneic cells and strict clinical management of comorbidities is essential to optimize stem cell therapy in vascular patients. Further investigation regarding the interactions of stem cell therapy with medications is needed (Fig. 1.9).

1.10.2   Stem Cell Manufacturing and Administration for Vascular Diseases

Several strategies have been developed to enhance stem cell therapy-induced angiogenesis in the treatment of vascular disease. Regarding cell manufacturing, hypoxic preconditioning and pretreatment with curcumin and angiotensin II increased VEGF secretion and angiogenesis to treat myocardial ischemia [87, 167–169]. Another strategy is the use of EC-conditioned differentiation medium to increase MSC differentiation into a more angiogenic cell type [123, 124].

Blood flow impairment and organ ischemia caused by vascular disorders hinders stem cell delivery, engraftment, and function. Recently, Liu et al. showed the use of

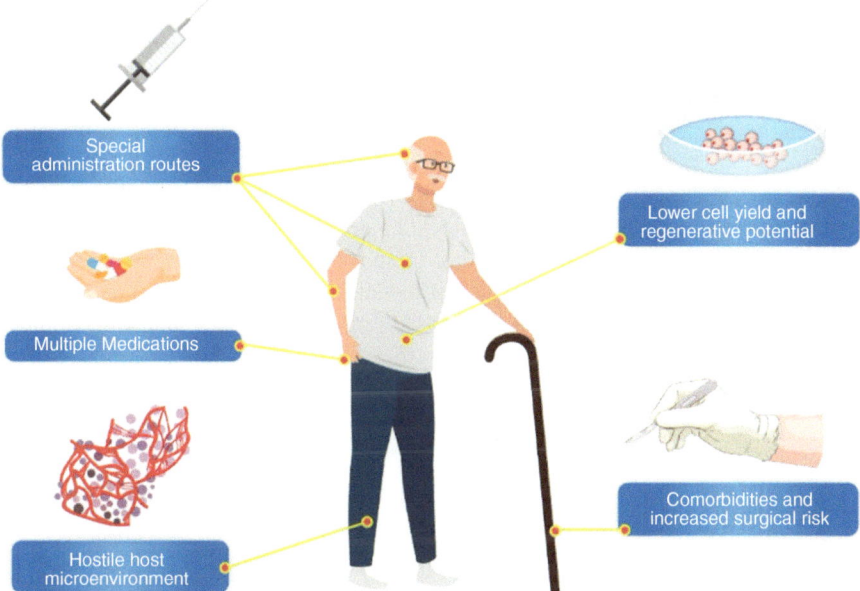

Fig. 1.9 Particularities of stem cell therapy for vascular diseases

BM-MSC coated with dendrimer nanocarriers modified with adhesion molecules to increase stem cell anchoring, transendothelial migration, extravasation, and homing to the targeted tissues [170].

Both local and systemic routes of administration have several advantages and disadvantages. Specific administration routes have been studied in the treatment of stroke (intranasal and intrathecal) [78, 79], ophthalmic (intravitreal), and cardiovascular [81, 82] diseases (transepicardial and transendocardial). Individualized decisions based on the disease and/or organ to be treated are essential to choose the appropriate administration route and adjuvants and to avoid suboptimal therapy.

1.11   Conclusion

Stem cell therapy has emerged as a promising therapeutic option for several clinical conditions. In addition to embryos, stem cells can be isolated from several adult tissues, particularly bone marrow, peripheral blood, adipose tissue, and umbilical cord derivatives. Along with adult cells, induced pluripotent stem cells are ethical alternatives for stem cell therapy and enhance the availability of therapeutic cells. Autologous tissue is a safe therapeutic cell origin, whereas allogeneic and xenogeneic stem cells raise concerns regarding disease transmission and immunogenicity.

The mechanisms of regeneration induced by stem cells are yet to be fully understood. As various protocols for isolation, culture, priming, and administration result in different therapeutic effects, understanding the effect of these processes remains particularly challenging. Stem cell therapy is generally safe, demonstrating limited risks which rely particularly on the stem cell type and administration route. Treatment of vascular diseases is especially challenging due to the presence of patient-associated comorbidities that frequently impair stem cell-induced regeneration.

Stem cell therapy comprises a spectrum of cell-based regenerative strategies characterized by three sets of variables: (1) stem cell intrinsic properties (origin, type, isolation/induction, culture, and priming features); (2) therapy protocol (dose, concentration, administration route, adjuvants); and (3) patient characteristics (medical history, immune reaction, disease of interest). Understanding and controlling the effects and interactions between these variables is the key for progress in clinical stem cell therapy.

References

1. Zakrzewski W, Dobrzyński M, Szymonowicz M, Rybak Z. Stem cells: past, present, and future. Stem Cell Res Ther. 2019;10(1):68.
2. Kirby GTS, Mills SJ, Cowin AJ, Smith LE. Stem cells for cutaneous wound healing. Biomed Res Int. 2015;2015:285869.
3. Konstantinov IE. In search of Alexander a. Maximow: the man behind the unitarian theory of hematopoiesis. Perspect Biol Med. 2000;43(2):269–76.
4. Till JE, McCulloch EA. A direct measurement of the radiation sensitivity of normal mouse bone marrow cells. Radiat Res. 1961;14(2):213–22.
5. Gurdon JB. The developmental capacity of nuclei taken from intestinal epithelium cells of feeding tadpoles. J Embryol Exp Morphol. 1962;10:622–40.
6. Friedenstein AJ, Piatetzky S II, Petrakova KV. Osteogenesis in transplants of bone marrow cells. J Embryol Exp Morphol. 1966;16(3):381–90.
7. de la Morena MT, Gatti RA. A history of bone marrow transplantation. Hematol Oncol Clin North Am. 2011;25(1):1–15.
8. Evans MJ, Kaufman MH. Establishment in culture of pluripotential cells from mouse embryos. Nature. 1981;292(5819):154–6.
9. Thomson JA, Itskovitz-Eldor J, Shapiro SS, Waknitz MA, Swiergiel JJ, Marshall VS, et al. Embryonic stem cell lines derived from human blastocysts. Science. 1998;282(5391):1145–7.
10. Takahashi K, Yamanaka S. Induction of pluripotent stem cells from mouse embryonic and adult fibroblast cultures by defined factors. Cell. 2006;126(4):663–76.
11. Takahashi K, Tanabe K, Ohnuki M, Narita M, Ichisaka T, Tomoda K, et al. Induction of pluripotent stem cells from adult human fibroblasts by defined factors. Cell. 2007;131(5):861–72.
12. NobelPrize.org. The Nobel prize in physiology or medicine 2012. [cited 2020 04 April]; Available from: https://www.nobelprize.org/prizes/medicine/2012/press-release/.
13. Caplan AI. Mesenchymal stem cells. J Orthop Res. 1991;9(5):641–50.
14. Yin JQ, Zhu J, Ankrum JA. Manufacturing of primed mesenchymal stromal cells for therapy. Nat Biomed Eng. 2019;3(2):90–104.
15. Horwitz EM, Le Blanc K, Dominici M, Mueller I, Slaper-Cortenbach I, Marini FC, et al. Clarification of the nomenclature for MSC: the International Society for Cellular Therapy position statement. Cytotherapy. 2005;7(5):393–5.
16. Viswanathan S, Shi Y, Galipeau J, Krampera M, Leblanc K, Martin I, et al. Mesenchymal stem versus stromal cells: International Society for Cell & Gene Therapy (ISCT(R)) mes-

enchymal stromal cell committee position statement on nomenclature. Cytotherapy. 2019;21(10):1019–24.

17. Lin CS, Ning H, Lin G, Lue TF. Is CD34 truly a negative marker for mesenchymal stromal cells? Cytotherapy. 2012;14(10):1159–63.

18. Bellagamba BC, Grudzinski PB, Ely PB, Nader PJH, Nardi NB, da Silva Meirelles L. Induction of expression of CD271 and CD34 in mesenchymal stromal cells cultured as spheroids. Stem Cells Int. 2018;2018:7357213.

19. Available from: https://clinicaltrials.gov/ct2/results?cond=&term=mesenchymal+stem+cell&cntry=&state=&city=&dist=.

20. Leeper NJ, Hunter AL, Cooke JP. Stem cell therapy for vascular regeneration: adult, embryonic, and induced pluripotent stem cells. Circulation. 2010;122(5):517–26.

21. Blum B, Benvenisty N. The tumorigenicity of human embryonic stem cells. Adv Cancer Res. 2008;100:133–58.

22. Mali P, Ye Z, Hommond HH, Yu X, Lin J, Chen G, et al. Improved efficiency and pace of generating induced pluripotent stem cells from human adult and fetal fibroblasts. Stem Cells (Dayton, Ohio). 2008;26(8):1998–2005.

23. Choudhery MS, Badowski M, Muise A, Pierce J, Harris DT. Donor age negatively impacts adipose tissue-derived mesenchymal stem cell expansion and differentiation. J Transl Med. 2014;12:8.

24. Beane OS, Fonseca VC, Cooper LL, Koren G, Darling EM. Impact of aging on the regenerative properties of bone marrow-, muscle-, and adipose-derived mesenchymal stem/stromal cells. PLoS One. 2014;9(12):e115963.

25. Duscher D, Rennert RC, Januszyk M, Anghel E, Maan ZN, Whittam AJ, et al. Aging disrupts cell subpopulation dynamics and diminishes the function of mesenchymal stem cells. Sci Rep. 2014;4:7144.

26. Hequet O. Hematopoietic stem and progenitor cell harvesting: technical advances and clinical utility. J Blood Med. 2015;6:55–67.

27. Serena C, Keiran N, Ceperuelo-Mallafre V, Ejarque M, Fradera R, Roche K, et al. Obesity and type 2 diabetes alters the immune properties of human adipose derived stem cells. Stem Cells. 2016;34(10):2559–73.

28. Berglund AK, Fortier LA, Antczak DF, Schnabel LV. Immunoprivileged no more: measuring the immunogenicity of allogeneic adult mesenchymal stem cells. Stem Cell Res Ther. 2017;8(1):288.

29. Galleu A, Riffo-Vasquez Y, Trento C, Lomas C, Dolcetti L, Cheung TS, et al. Apoptosis in mesenchymal stromal cells induces in vivo recipient-mediated immunomodulation. Sci Transl Med. 2017;9(416):3–4.

30. Hodgetts SI, Stagg K, Sturm M, Edel M, Blancafort P. Long live the stem cell: the use of stem cells isolated from post mortem tissues for translational strategies. Int J Biochem Cell Biol. 2014;56:74–81.

31. Administration FUSFD. Xenotransplantation. 2017 [updated 04/28/2017; cited 2017 12/05/2017]; Available from: https://www.fda.gov/BiologicsBloodVaccines/Xenotransplantation/.

32. Hass R, Kasper C, Bohm S, Jacobs R. Different populations and sources of human mesenchymal stem cells (MSC): a comparison of adult and neonatal tissue-derived MSC. Cell Commun Signal. 2011;9:12.

33. Murray IR, West CC, Hardy WR, James AW, Park TS, Nguyen A, et al. Natural history of mesenchymal stem cells, from vessel walls to culture vessels. Cell Mol Life Sci. 2014;71(8):1353–74.

34. Andia I, Maffulli N, Burgos-Alonso N. Stromal vascular fraction technologies and clinical applications. Expert Opin Biol Ther. 2019;19(12):1289–305.

35. Gentile P, Calabrese C, De Angelis B, Pizzicannella J, Kothari A, Garcovich S. Impact of the different preparation methods to obtain human adipose-derived stromal vascular fraction cells (AD-SVFs) and human adipose-derived mesenchymal stem cells (AD-MSCs): enzymatic digestion versus mechanical centrifugation. Int J Mol Sci. 2019;20(21):4–7.

36. Lopes L, Setia O, Aurshina A, Liu S, Hu H, Isaji T, et al. Stem cell therapy for diabetic foot ulcers: a review of preclinical and clinical research. Stem Cell Res Ther. 2018;9(1):188.
37. Khan FA, Almohazey D, Alomari M, Almofty SA. Isolation, culture, and functional characterization of human embryonic stem cells: current trends and challenges. Stem Cells Int. 2018;2018:1429351.
38. Tanaka N, Takeuchi T, Neri QV, Sills ES, Palermo GD. Laser-assisted blastocyst dissection and subsequent cultivation of embryonic stem cells in a serum/cell free culture system: applications and preliminary results in a murine model. J Transl Med. 2006;4:20.
39. Strom S, Inzunza J, Grinnemo KH, Holmberg K, Matilainen E, Stromberg AM, et al. Mechanical isolation of the inner cell mass is effective in derivation of new human embryonic stem cell lines. Hum Reprod. 2007;22(12):3051–8.
40. Hayes M, Zavazava N. Strategies to generate induced pluripotent stem cells. Methods Mol Biol. 2013;1029:77–92.
41. Yeo JC, Ng HH. The transcriptional regulation of pluripotency. Cell Res. 2013;23(1):20–32.
42. Zhang S, Cui W. Sox2, a key factor in the regulation of pluripotency and neural differentiation. World J Stem Cells. 2014;6(3):305–11.
43. Dakhore S, Nayer B, Hasegawa K. Human pluripotent stem cell culture: current status, challenges, and advancement. Stem Cells Int. 2018;2018:7396905.
44. Gstraunthaler G, Lindl T, van der Valk J. A plea to reduce or replace fetal bovine serum in cell culture media. Cytotechnology. 2013;65(5):791–3.
45. Burnouf T, Strunk D, Koh MB, Schallmoser K. Human platelet lysate: replacing fetal bovine serum as a gold standard for human cell propagation? Biomaterials. 2016;76:371–87.
46. Abdelrazik H, Spaggiari GM, Chiossone L, Moretta L. Mesenchymal stem cells expanded in human platelet lysate display a decreased inhibitory capacity on T- and NK-cell proliferation and function. Eur J Immunol. 2011;41(11):3281–90.
47. Oikonomopoulos A, van Deen WK, Manansala AR, Lacey PN, Tomakili TA, Ziman A, et al. Optimization of human mesenchymal stem cell manufacturing: the effects of animal/xeno-free media. Sci Rep. 2015;5:16570.
48. Ejtehadifar M, Shamsasenjan K, Movassaghpour A, Akbarzadehlaleh P, Dehdilani N, Abbasi P, et al. The effect of hypoxia on mesenchymal stem cell biology. Adv Pharmaceut Bullet. 2015;5(2):141–9.
49. Nold P, Hackstein H, Riedlinger T, Kasper C, Neumann A, Mernberger M, et al. Immunosuppressive capabilities of mesenchymal stromal cells are maintained under hypoxic growth conditions and after gamma irradiation. Cytotherapy. 2015;17(2):152–62.
50. Rosova I, Dao M, Capoccia B, Link D, Nolta JA. Hypoxic preconditioning results in increased motility and improved therapeutic potential of human mesenchymal stem cells. Stem Cells. 2008;26(8):2173–82.
51. Das B, Bayat-Mokhtari R, Tsui M, Lotfi S, Tsuchida R, Felsher DW, et al. HIF-2alpha suppresses p53 to enhance the stemness and regenerative potential of human embryonic stem cells. Stem Cells. 2012;30(8):1685–95.
52. Grayson WL, Zhao F, Izadpanah R, Bunnell B, Ma T. Effects of hypoxia on human mesenchymal stem cell expansion and plasticity in 3D constructs. J Cell Physiol. 2006;207(2):331–9.
53. Basciano L, Nemos C, Foliguet B, de Isla N, de Carvalho M, Tran N, et al. Long term culture of mesenchymal stem cells in hypoxia promotes a genetic program maintaining their undifferentiated and multipotent status. BMC Cell Biol. 2011;12:12.
54. Roobrouck VD, Vanuytsel K, Verfaillie CM. Concise review: culture mediated changes in fate and/or potency of stem cells. Stem Cells. 2011;29(4):583–9.
55. Shekaran A, Sim E, Tan KY, Chan JKY, Choolani M, Reuveny S, et al. Enhanced in vitro osteogenic differentiation of human fetal MSCs attached to 3D microcarriers versus harvested from 2D monolayers. BMC Biotechnol. 2015;15(1):102.
56. Haugh MG, Heilshorn SC. Integrating concepts of material mechanics, ligand chemistry, dimensionality and degradation to control differentiation of mesenchymal stem cells. Curr Opin Solid State Mater Sci. 2016;20(4):171–9.

57. Mo M, Zhou Y, Li S, Wu Y. Three-dimensional culture reduces cell size by increasing vesicle excretion. Stem Cells. 2018;36(2):286–92.
58. Petrenko Y, Sykova E, Kubinova S. The therapeutic potential of three-dimensional multipotent mesenchymal stromal cell spheroids. Stem Cell Res Ther. 2017;8(1):94.
59. Rashedi I, Talele N, Wang XH, Hinz B, Radisic M, Keating A. Collagen scaffold enhances the regenerative properties of mesenchymal stromal cells. PLoS One. 2017;12(10):e0187348.
60. Murphy WL, McDevitt TC, Engler AJ. Materials as stem cell regulators. Nat Mater. 2014;13(6):547–57.
61. Engler AJ, Sen S, Sweeney HL, Discher DE. Matrix elasticity directs stem cell lineage specification. Cell. 2006;126(4):677–89.
62. Shakouri-Motlagh A, O'Connor AJ, Brennecke SP, Kalionis B, Heath DE. Native and solubilized decellularized extracellular matrix: a critical assessment of their potential for improving the expansion of mesenchymal stem cells. Acta Biomater. 2017;55:1–12.
63. Carrier-Ruiz A, Evaristo-Mendonca F, Mendez-Otero R, Ribeiro-Resende VT. Biological behavior of mesenchymal stem cells on poly-epsilon-caprolactone filaments and a strategy for tissue engineering of segments of the peripheral nerves. Stem Cell Res Ther. 2015;6:128.
64. Lam A, Li J, Toh J, Sim E, Chen A, Chan J, et al. Biodegradable poly-ε-caprolactone microcarriers for efficient production of human mesenchymal stromal cells and secreted cytokines in batch and fed-batch bioreactors. Cytotherapy. 2016;19:8–12.
65. Jun I, Lee YB, Choi YS, Engler AJ, Park H, Shin H. Transfer stamping of human mesenchymal stem cell patches using thermally expandable hydrogels with tunable cell-adhesive properties. Biomaterials. 2015;54:44–54.
66. Duscher D, Barrera J, Wong VW, Maan ZN, Whittam AJ, Januszyk M, et al. Stem cells in wound healing: the future of regenerative medicine? A mini-review. Gerontology. 2016;62(2):216–25.
67. Isakson M, de Blacam C, Whelan D, McArdle A, Clover AJP. Mesenchymal stem cells and cutaneous wound healing: current evidence and future potential. Stem Cells Int. 2015;2015:831095.
68. Caplan H, Olson SD, Kumar A, George M, Prabhakara KS, Wenzel P, et al. Mesenchymal stromal cell therapeutic delivery: translational challenges to clinical application. Front Immunol. 2019;10:1645.
69. O'Loughlin A, O'Brien T. Topical stem and progenitor cell therapy for diabetic foot ulcers. In: Gholamrezanezhad DA, editor. Stem cells clinic and research. Published online: InTech; 2011. p. 578–604.
70. Hamidian Jahromi S, Davies JE. Concise review: skeletal muscle as a delivery route for mesenchymal stromal cells. Stem Cells Transl Med. 2019;8(5):456–65.
71. Qazi TH, Mooney DJ, Duda GN, Geissler S. Biomaterials that promote cell-cell interactions enhance the paracrine function of MSCs. Biomaterials. 2017;140:103–14.
72. Jenkins TL, Little D. Synthetic scaffolds for musculoskeletal tissue engineering: cellular responses to fiber parameters. NPJ Regen Med. 2019;4:15.
73. Falanga V, Iwamoto S, Chartier M, Yufit T, Butmarc J, Kouttab N, et al. Autologous bone marrow-derived cultured mesenchymal stem cells delivered in a fibrin spray accelerate healing in murine and human cutaneous wounds. Tissue Eng. 2007;13(6):1299–312.
74. Watanabe M, Yavagal DR. Intra-arterial delivery of mesenchymal stem cells. Brain Circ. 2016;2(3):114–7.
75. Janowski M, Lyczek A, Engels C, Xu J, Lukomska B, Bulte JW, et al. Cell size and velocity of injection are major determinants of the safety of intracarotid stem cell transplantation. J Cereb Blood Flow Metab. 2013;33(6):921–7.
76. Fischer UM, Harting MT, Jimenez F, Monzon-Posadas WO, Xue H, Savitz SI, et al. Pulmonary passage is a major obstacle for intravenous stem cell delivery: the pulmonary first-pass effect. Stem Cells Dev. 2009;18(5):683–92.

77. de Witte SFH, Luk F, Sierra Parraga JM, Gargesha M, Merino A, Korevaar SS, et al. Immunomodulation by therapeutic Mesenchymal Stromal Cells (MSC) is triggered through phagocytosis of MSC by Monocytic cells. Stem Cells. 2018;36(4):602–15.
78. Nijboer CH, Kooijman E, van Velthoven CT, van Tilborg E, Tiebosch IA, Eijkelkamp N, et al. Intranasal stem cell treatment as a novel therapy for subarachnoid hemorrhage. Stem Cells Dev. 2018;27(5):313–25.
79. Vaquero J, Zurita M, Rico MA, Aguayo C, Bonilla C, Marin E, et al. Intrathecal administration of autologous mesenchymal stromal cells for spinal cord injury: safety and efficacy of the 100/3 guideline. Cytotherapy. 2018;20(6):806–19.
80. Park SS. Cell therapy applications for retinal vascular diseases: diabetic retinopathy and retinal vein occlusion. Invest Ophthalmol Vis Sci. 2016;57(5):ORSFj1–ORSFj10.
81. van der Spoel TI, Vrijsen KR, Koudstaal S, Sluijter JP, Nijsen JF, de Jong HW, et al. Transendocardial cell injection is not superior to intracoronary infusion in a porcine model of ischaemic cardiomyopathy: a study on delivery efficiency. J Cell Mol Med. 2012;16(11):2768–76.
82. Kanelidis AJ, Premer C, Lopez J, Balkan W, Hare JM. Route of delivery modulates the efficacy of mesenchymal stem cell therapy for myocardial infarction: a meta-analysis of preclinical studies and clinical trials. Circ Res. 2017;120(7):1139–50.
83. Keshtkar S, Azarpira N, Ghahremani MH. Mesenchymal stem cell-derived extracellular vesicles: novel frontiers in regenerative medicine. Stem Cell Res Ther. 2018;9(1):63.
84. Caplan AI, Dennis JE. Mesenchymal stem cells as trophic mediators. J Cell Biochem. 2006;98(5):1076–84.
85. Caplan AI, Correa D. The MSC: an injury drugstore. Cell Stem Cell. 2011;9(1):11–5.
86. Wu Y, Chen L, Scott PG, Tredget EE. Mesenchymal stem cells enhance wound healing through differentiation and angiogenesis. Stem Cells. 2007;25(10):2648–59.
87. Bronckaers A, Hilkens P, Martens W, Gervois P, Ratajczak J, Struys T, et al. Mesenchymal stem/stromal cells as a pharmacological and therapeutic approach to accelerate angiogenesis. Pharmacol Ther. 2014;143(2):181–96.
88. Kean TJ, Lin P, Caplan AI, Dennis JE. MSCs: delivery routes and engraftment, cell-targeting strategies, and immune modulation. Stem Cells Int. 2013;2013:732742.
89. Chang CL, Leu S, Sung HC, Zhen YY, Cho CL, Chen A, et al. Impact of apoptotic adipose-derived mesenchymal stem cells on attenuating organ damage and reducing mortality in rat sepsis syndrome induced by cecal puncture and ligation. J Transl Med. 2012;10:244.
90. Goncalves FDC, Luk F, Korevaar SS, Bouzid R, Paz AH, Lopez-Iglesias C, et al. Membrane particles generated from mesenchymal stromal cells modulate immune responses by selective targeting of pro-inflammatory monocytes. Sci Rep. 2017;7(1):12100.
91. Luk F, de Witte SF, Korevaar SS, Roemeling-van Rhijn M, Franquesa M, Strini T, et al. Inactivated mesenchymal stem cells maintain immunomodulatory capacity. Stem Cells Dev. 2016;25(18):1342–54.
92. Howard D, Buttery LD, Shakesheff KM, Roberts SJ. Tissue engineering: strategies, stem cells and scaffolds. J Anat. 2008;213(1):66–72.
93. Petrella F, Spaggiari L, Acocella F, Barberis M, Bellomi M, Brizzola S, et al. Airway fistula closure after stem-cell infusion. N Engl J Med. 2015;372(1):96–7.
94. Luk F, Carreras-Planella L, Korevaar SS, de Witte SFH, Borras FE, Betjes MGH, et al. Inflammatory conditions dictate the effect of mesenchymal stem or stromal cells on B cell function. Front Immunol. 2017;8:1042.
95. Wu Y, Hoogduijn MJ, Baan CC, Korevaar SS, de Kuiper R, Yan L, et al. Adipose tissue-derived mesenchymal stem cells have a heterogenic cytokine secretion profile. Stem Cells Int. 2017;2017:4960831.
96. De Witte SFH, Peters FS, Merino A, Korevaar SS, Van Meurs JBJ, O'Flynn L, et al. Epigenetic changes in umbilical cord mesenchymal stromal cells upon stimulation and culture expansion. Cytotherapy. 2018;20(7):919–29.

97. Melief SM, Geutskens SB, Fibbe WE, Roelofs H. Multipotent stromal cells skew monocytes towards an anti-inflammatory interleukin-10-producing phenotype by production of interleukin-6. Haematologica. 2013;98(6):888–95.
98. Nemeth K, Leelahavanichkul A, Yuen PS, Mayer B, Parmelee A, Doi K, et al. Bone marrow stromal cells attenuate sepsis via prostaglandin E(2)-dependent reprogramming of host macrophages to increase their interleukin-10 production. Nat Med. 2009;15(1):42–9.
99. Ko JH, Lee HJ, Jeong HJ, Kim MK, Wee WR, Yoon SO, et al. Mesenchymal stem/stromal cells precondition lung monocytes/macrophages to produce tolerance against Allo- and autoimmunity in the eye. Proc Natl Acad Sci U S A. 2016;113(1):158–63.
100. Krasnodembskaya A, Samarani G, Song Y, Zhuo H, Su X, Lee JW, et al. Human mesenchymal stem cells reduce mortality and bacteremia in gram-negative sepsis in mice in part by enhancing the phagocytic activity of blood monocytes. Am J Physiol Lung Cell Mol Physiol. 2012;302(10):L1003–13.
101. Braza F, Dirou S, Forest V, Sauzeau V, Hassoun D, Chesne J, et al. Mesenchymal stem cells induce suppressive macrophages through phagocytosis in a mouse model of asthma. Stem Cells. 2016;34(7):1836–45.
102. Ge W, Jiang J, Arp J, Liu W, Garcia B, Wang H. Regulatory T-cell generation and kidney allograft tolerance induced by mesenchymal stem cells associated with indoleamine 2,3-dioxygenase expression. Transplantation. 2010;90(12):1312–20.
103. Miteva K, Pappritz K, El-Shafeey M, Dong F, Ringe J, Tschope C, et al. Mesenchymal stromal cells modulate monocytes trafficking in Coxsackievirus B3-induced myocarditis. Stem Cells Transl Med. 2017;6(4):1249–61.
104. Duffy MM, Ritter T, Ceredig R, Griffin MD. Mesenchymal stem cell effects on T-cell effector pathways. Stem Cell Res Ther. 2011;2(4):34.
105. Sakaguchi S, Sakaguchi N, Asano M, Itoh M, Toda M. Immunologic self-tolerance maintained by activated T cells expressing IL-2 receptor alpha-chains (CD25). Breakdown of a single mechanism of self-tolerance causes various autoimmune diseases. J Immunol. 1995;155(3):1151–64.
106. Khosravi M, Karimi MH, Hossein Aghdaie M, Kalani M, Naserian S, Bidmeshkipour A. Mesenchymal stem cells can induce regulatory T cells via modulating miR-126a but not miR-10a. Gene. 2017;627:327–36.
107. Gieseke F, Bohringer J, Bussolari R, Dominici M, Handgretinger R, Muller I. Human multipotent mesenchymal stromal cells use galectin-1 to inhibit immune effector cells. Blood. 2010;116(19):3770–9.
108. Rosser EC, Mauri C. Regulatory B cells: origin, phenotype, and function. Immunity. 2015;42(4):607–12.
109. Franquesa M, Mensah FK, Huizinga R, Strini T, Boon L, Lombardo E, et al. Human adipose tissue-derived mesenchymal stem cells abrogate plasmablast formation and induce regulatory B cells independently of T helper cells. Stem Cells. 2015;33(3):880–91.
110. Luz-Crawford P, Djouad F, Toupet K, Bony C, Franquesa M, Hoogduijn MJ, et al. Mesenchymal stem cell-derived interleukin 1 receptor antagonist promotes macrophage polarization and inhibits B cell differentiation. Stem Cells. 2016;34(2):483–92.
111. Deng Y, Zhang Y, Ye L, Zhang T, Cheng J, Chen G, et al. Umbilical cord-derived mesenchymal stem cells instruct monocytes towards an IL10-producing phenotype by secreting IL6 and HGF. Sci Rep. 2016;6:37566.
112. Sato K, Ozaki K, Oh I, Meguro A, Hatanaka K, Nagai T, et al. Nitric oxide plays a critical role in suppression of T-cell proliferation by mesenchymal stem cells. Blood. 2007;109(1):228–34.
113. Spaggiari GM, Capobianco A, Abdelrazik H, Becchetti F, Mingari MC, Moretta L. Mesenchymal stem cells inhibit natural killer-cell proliferation, cytotoxicity, and cytokine production: role of indoleamine 2,3-dioxygenase and prostaglandin E2. Blood. 2008;111(3):1327–33.

114. Moll G, Rasmusson-Duprez I, von Bahr L, Connolly-Andersen AM, Elgue G, Funke L, et al. Are therapeutic human mesenchymal stromal cells compatible with human blood? Stem Cells. 2012;30(7):1565–74.

115. Moll G, Ignatowicz L, Catar R, Luecht C, Sadeghi B, Hamad O, et al. Different Procoagulant activity of therapeutic mesenchymal stromal cells derived from bone marrow and placental decidua. Stem Cells Dev. 2015;24(19):2269–79.

116. Christy BA, Herzig MC, Montgomery RK, Delavan C, Bynum JA, Reddoch KM, et al. Procoagulant activity of human mesenchymal stem cells. J Trauma Acute Care Surg. 2017;83(1 Suppl 1):S164–S9.

117. Liao L, Shi B, Chang H, Su X, Zhang L, Bi C, et al. Heparin improves BMSC cell therapy: anticoagulant treatment by heparin improves the safety and therapeutic effect of bone marrow-derived mesenchymal stem cell cytotherapy. Theranostics. 2017;7(1):106–16.

118. Moll G, Ankrum JA, Kamhieh-Milz J, Bieback K, Ringden O, Volk HD, et al. Intravascular mesenchymal stromal/stem cell therapy product diversification: time for new clinical guidelines. Trends Mol Med. 2019;25(2):149–63.

119. Roobrouck VD, Clavel C, Jacobs SA, Ulloa-Montoya F, Crippa S, Sohni A, et al. Differentiation potential of human postnatal mesenchymal stem cells, mesoangioblasts, and multipotent adult progenitor cells reflected in their transcriptome and partially influenced by the culture conditions. Stem Cells. 2011;29(5):871–82.

120. Gruber R, Kandler B, Holzmann P, Vogele-Kadletz M, Losert U, Fischer MB, et al. Bone marrow stromal cells can provide a local environment that favors migration and formation of tubular structures of endothelial cells. Tissue Eng. 2005;11(5–6):896–903.

121. Kinnaird T, Stabile E, Burnett MS, Lee CW, Barr S, Fuchs S, et al. Marrow-derived stromal cells express genes encoding a broad spectrum of arteriogenic cytokines and promote in vitro and in vivo arteriogenesis through paracrine mechanisms. Circ Res. 2004;94(5):678–85.

122. Crisostomo PR, Wang Y, Markel TA, Wang M, Lahm T, Meldrum DR. Human mesenchymal stem cells stimulated by TNF-alpha, LPS, or hypoxia produce growth factors by an NF kappa B- but not JNK-dependent mechanism. Am J Physiol Cell Physiol. 2008;294(3):C675–82.

123. Whyte JL, Ball SG, Shuttleworth CA, Brennan K, Kielty CM. Density of human bone marrow stromal cells regulates commitment to vascular lineages. Stem Cell Res. 2011;6(3):238–50.

124. Takahashi M, Suzuki E, Oba S, Nishimatsu H, Kimura K, Nagano T, et al. Adipose tissue-derived stem cells inhibit neointimal formation in a paracrine fashion in rat femoral artery. Am J Physiol Heart Circ Physiol. 2010;298(2):H415–23.

125. Thum T, Bauersachs J, Poole-Wilson PA, Volk HD, Anker SD. The dying stem cell hypothesis: immune modulation as a novel mechanism for progenitor cell therapy in cardiac muscle. J Am Coll Cardiol. 2005;46(10):1799–802.

126. Weiss ARR, Dahlke MH. Immunomodulation by Mesenchymal Stem Cells (MSCs): mechanisms of action of living, apoptotic, and dead MSCs. Front Immunol. 2019;10:1191.

127. Sung PH, Chang CL, Tsai TH, Chang LT, Leu S, Chen YL, et al. Apoptotic adipose-derived mesenchymal stem cell therapy protects against lung and kidney injury in sepsis syndrome caused by cecal ligation puncture in rats. Stem Cell Res Ther. 2013;4(6):155.

128. Bruno S, Grange C, Deregibus MC, Calogero RA, Saviozzi S, Collino F, et al. Mesenchymal stem cell-derived microvesicles protect against acute tubular injury. J Am Soc Nephrol. 2009;20(5):1053–67.

129. Li T, Yan Y, Wang B, Qian H, Zhang X, Shen L, et al. Exosomes derived from human umbilical cord mesenchymal stem cells alleviate liver fibrosis. Stem Cells Dev. 2013;22(6):845–54.

130. Arslan F, Lai RC, Smeets MB, Akeroyd L, Choo A, Aguor EN, et al. Mesenchymal stem cell-derived exosomes increase ATP levels, decrease oxidative stress and activate PI3K/Akt pathway to enhance myocardial viability and prevent adverse remodeling after myocardial ischemia/reperfusion injury. Stem Cell Res. 2013;10(3):301–12.

131. Xin H, Li Y, Cui Y, Yang JJ, Zhang ZG, Chopp M. Systemic administration of exosomes released from mesenchymal stromal cells promote functional recovery and neurovascular plasticity after stroke in rats. J Cereb Blood Flow Metab. 2013;33(11):1711–5.

132. Rani S, Ryan AE, Griffin MD, Ritter T. Mesenchymal stem cell-derived extracellular vesicles: toward cell-free therapeutic applications. Mol Ther. 2015;23(5):812–23.
133. Wu HH, Zhou Y, Tabata Y, Gao JQ. Mesenchymal stem cell-based drug delivery strategy: from cells to biomimetic. J Control Release. 2019;294:102–13.
134. Coccè V, Farronato D, Brini AT, Masia C, Giannì AB, Piovani G, et al. Drug loaded gingival mesenchymal stromal cells (GinPa-MSCs) inhibit in vitro proliferation of Oral squamous cell carcinoma. Sci Rep. 2017;7(1):9376.
135. Bonomi A, Silini A, Vertua E, Signoroni PB, Coccè V, Cavicchini L, et al. Human amniotic mesenchymal stromal cells (hAMSCs) as potential vehicles for drug delivery in cancer therapy: an in vitro study. Stem Cell Res Ther. 2015;6(1):155.
136. Pessina A, Coccè V, Pascucci L, Bonomi A, Cavicchini L, Sisto F, et al. Mesenchymal stromal cells primed with paclitaxel attract and kill leukaemia cells, inhibit angiogenesis and improve survival of leukaemia-bearing mice. Br J Haematol. 2013;160(6):766–78.
137. Cao B, Yang M, Zhu Y, Qu X, Mao C. Stem cells loaded with nanoparticles as a drug carrier for in vivo breast cancer therapy. Adv Mater. 2014;26(27):4627–31.
138. Huang X, Neretina S, El-Sayed MA. Gold Nanorods: from synthesis and properties to biological and biomedical applications. Adv Mater. 2009;21(48):4880–910.
139. Cheng L, Wang C, Ma X, Wang Q, Cheng Y, Wang H, et al. Multifunctional upconversion nanoparticles for dual-modal imaging-guided stem cell therapy under remote magnetic control. Adv Funct Mater. 2013;23(3):272–80.
140. Boltze J, Arnold A, Walczak P, Jolkkonen J, Cui L, Wagner DC. The dark side of the force – constraints and complications of cell therapies for stroke. Front Neurol. 2015;6:155.
141. Duijvestein M, Vos AC, Roelofs H, Wildenberg ME, Wendrich BB, Verspaget HW, et al. Autologous bone marrow-derived mesenchymal stromal cell treatment for refractory luminal Crohn's disease: results of a phase I study. Gut. 2010;59(12):1662–9.
142. Savolainen H. Encephalopathy, stroke, and myocardial infarction with DMSO use in stem cell transplantation. Neurology. 2007;69(5):494; author reply -5
143. Stolzing A, Jones E, McGonagle D, Scutt A. Age-related changes in human bone marrow-derived mesenchymal stem cells: consequences for cell therapies. Mech Ageing Dev. 2008;129(3):163–73.
144. Turinetto V, Vitale E, Giachino C. Senescence in human mesenchymal stem cells: functional changes and implications in stem cell-based therapy. Int J Mol Sci. 2016;17(7):6–8.
145. Bonab MM, Alimoghaddam K, Talebian F, Ghaffari SH, Ghavamzadeh A, Nikbin B. Aging of mesenchymal stem cell in vitro. BMC Cell Biol. 2006;7:14.
146. von Bahr L, Sundberg B, Lonnies L, Sander B, Karbach H, Hagglund H, et al. Long-term complications, immunologic effects, and role of passage for outcome in mesenchymal stromal cell therapy. Biol Blood Marrow Transplant. 2012;18(4):557–64.
147. Cornelio DA, Tavares JC, Pimentel TV, Cavalcanti GB Jr, Batistuzzo de Medeiros SR. Cytokinesis-block micronucleus assay adapted for analyzing genomic instability of human mesenchymal stem cells. Stem Cells Dev. 2014;23(8):823–38.
148. Wagner J, Kean T, Young R, Dennis JE, Caplan AI. Optimizing mesenchymal stem cell-based therapeutics. Curr Opin Biotechnol. 2009;20(5):531–6.
149. Jung JW, Kwon M, Choi JC, Shin JW, Park IW, Choi BW, et al. Familial occurrence of pulmonary embolism after intravenous, adipose tissue-derived stem cell therapy. Yonsei Med J. 2013;54(5):1293–6.
150. Wu Z, Zhang S, Zhou L, Cai J, Tan J, Gao X, et al. Thromboembolism induced by umbilical cord mesenchymal stem cell infusion: a report of two cases and literature review. Transplant Proc. 2017;49(7):1656–8.
151. Sokal EM, Stéphenne X, Ottolenghi C, Jazouli N, Clapuyt P, Lacaille F, et al. Liver engraftment and repopulation by in vitro expanded adult derived human liver stem cells in a child with ornithine carbamoyltransferase deficiency. JIMD Rep. 2014;13:65–72.
152. Toma C, Wagner WR, Bowry S, Schwartz A, Villanueva F. Fate of culture-expanded mesenchymal stem cells in the microvasculature: in vivo observations of cell kinetics. Circ Res. 2009;104(3):398–402.

153. Gleeson BM, Martin K, Ali MT, Kumar AHS, Pillai MG-K, Kumar SPG, et al. Bone marrow-derived mesenchymal stem cells have innate Procoagulant activity and cause microvascular obstruction following intracoronary delivery: amelioration by Antithrombin therapy. Stem Cells. 2015;33(9):2726–37.

154. Acosta L, Hmadcha A, Escacena N, Perez-Camacho I, de la Cuesta A, Ruiz-Salmeron R, et al. Adipose mesenchymal stromal cells isolated from type 2 diabetic patients display reduced fibrinolytic activity. Diabetes. 2013;62(12):4266–9.

155. Coppin L, Sokal E, Stéphenne X. Thrombogenic risk induced by intravascular mesenchymal stem cell therapy: current status and future perspectives. Cell. 2019;8(10):1160.

156. Melmed GY, Pandak WM, Casey K, Abraham B, Valentine J, Schwartz D, et al. Human placenta-derived cells (PDA-001) for the treatment of moderate-to-severe Crohn's disease: a phase 1b/2a study. Inflamm Bowel Dis. 2015;21(8):1809–16.

157. Baygan A, Aronsson-Kurttilà W, Moretti G, Tibert B, Dahllöf G, Klingspor L, et al. Safety and side effects of using placenta-derived Decidual stromal cells for graft-versus-host disease and hemorrhagic cystitis. Front Immunol. 2017;8:795.

158. Kaipe H, Carlson LM, Erkers T, Nava S, Mollden P, Gustafsson B, et al. Immunogenicity of decidual stromal cells in an epidermolysis bullosa patient and in allogeneic hematopoietic stem cell transplantation patients. Stem Cells Dev. 2015;24(12):1471–82.

159. Lohan P, Treacy O, Griffin MD, Ritter T, Ryan AE. Anti-donor immune responses elicited by allogeneic mesenchymal stem cells and their extracellular vesicles: are we still learning? Front Immunol. 2017;8:1626.

160. Steward O, Sharp KG, Yee KM, Hatch MN, Bonner JF. Characterization of ectopic colonies that form in widespread areas of the nervous system with neural stem cell transplants into the site of a severe spinal cord injury. J Neurosci. 2014;34(42):14013–21.

161. Kawai H, Yamashita T, Ohta Y, Deguchi K, Nagotani S, Zhang X, et al. Tridermal tumorigenesis of induced pluripotent stem cells transplanted in ischemic brain. J Cereb Blood Flow Metab. 2010;30(8):1487–93.

162. Erdo F, Buhrle C, Blunk J, Hoehn M, Xia Y, Fleischmann B, et al. Host-dependent tumorigenesis of embryonic stem cell transplantation in experimental stroke. J Cereb Blood Flow Metab. 2003;23(7):780–5.

163. Minieri V, Saviozzi S, Gambarotta G, Lo Iacono M, Accomasso L, Cibrario Rocchietti E, et al. Persistent DNA damage-induced premature senescence alters the functional features of human bone marrow mesenchymal stem cells. J Cell Mol Med. 2015;19(4):734–43.

164. Schu S, Nosov M, O'Flynn L, Shaw G, Treacy O, Barry F, et al. Immunogenicity of allogeneic mesenchymal stem cells. J Cell Mol Med. 2012;16(9):2094–103.

165. Posel C, Scheibe J, Kranz A, Bothe V, Quente E, Frohlich W, et al. Bone marrow cell transplantation time-dependently abolishes efficacy of granulocyte colony-stimulating factor after stroke in hypertensive rats. Stroke. 2014;45(8):2431–7.

166. Chen X, Gan Y, Li W, Su J, Zhang Y, Huang Y, et al. The interaction between mesenchymal stem cells and steroids during inflammation. Cell Death Dis. 2014;5:e1009.

167. Liu C, Fan Y, Zhou L, Zhu HY, Song YC, Hu L, et al. Pretreatment of mesenchymal stem cells with angiotensin II enhances paracrine effects, angiogenesis, gap junction formation and therapeutic efficacy for myocardial infarction. Int J Cardiol. 2015;188:22–32.

168. Liu J, Zhu P, Song P, Xiong W, Chen H, Peng W, et al. Pretreatment of adipose derived stem cells with curcumin facilitates myocardial recovery via Antiapoptosis and angiogenesis. Stem Cells Int. 2015;2015:638153.

169. Wei ZZ, Zhu YB, Zhang JY, McCrary MR, Wang S, Zhang YB, et al. Priming of the cells: hypoxic preconditioning for stem cell therapy. Chin Med J. 2017;130(19):2361–74.

170. Liu ZJ, Daftarian P, Kovalski L, Wang B, Tian R, Castilla DM, et al. Directing and potentiating stem cell-mediated angiogenesis and tissue repair by cell surface E-selectin coating. PLoS One. 2016;11(4):e0154053.

Chapter 2
Types and Origin of Stem Cells

Lucíola da Silva Barcelos, Pollyana Ribeiro Castro, Elisabeth Tamara Straessler, and Nicolle Kränkel

2.1　Introduction

Stem cells are undifferentiated cells with both self-renewal capacity and the potential to differentiate into specialized cell types according to the microenvironment. They may be referred to as embryonic or adult stem cells according to their presence either in the inner cell mass of the embryo or in specific tissues throughout the fetal and postnatal life, respectively. They may also be distinguished according to their developmental potency, which refers to the range of their potential fates, i.e., their varying ability to give rise to different cell types. In this case, they can be classified as totipotent (a term restricted to the zygote and the two-cell stage blastomeres with the capacity to generate both embryonic and extraembryonic tissues), pluripotent (the stem cells that are capable of forming all specialized tissues that originate from the embryo germ layers), and multipotent or unipotent cells (that are tissue-restricted stem cells and give rise to specific cell types). Besides, they may be obtained from their natural niche (the specific microenvironment in which they reside) or may be engineered in a laboratory by reprogramming somatic cells, as will be discussed later in this chapter.

At all stages of potency, stem cells play essential roles in development as well as in homeostasis and disease pathogenesis. Based on the concept that stem cells are the organizing principle for tissue formation and homeostasis, their use in clinical applications in the field of regenerative medicine, including cell transplantation therapy and tissue engineering, was a matter of time and great hope and expectation

L. da Silva Barcelos (✉) · P. R. Castro
Physiology and Biophysics, Federal University of Minas Gerais (UFMG),
Belo Horizonte, Brazil

E. T. Straessler · N. Kränkel
Department of Cardiology, Campus Benjamin Franklin, Charité – Universitätsmedizin Berlin,
Berlin, Germany

© Springer Nature Switzerland AG 2021　　　　　　　　　　　　　　　　　　33
T. P. Navarro et al. (eds.), *Stem Cell Therapy for Vascular Diseases*,
https://doi.org/10.1007/978-3-030-56954-9_2

has been placed in it. In fact, much effort has been made to identify and test different sources of cells to treat and cure a wide range of diseases, including cardiovascular diseases. In that way, among promising therapies for vascular diseases, the stem cell-based ones are in progress and demand for stem cell specialists.

Virtually, all stem cell types could be used for regenerative purposes. Nevertheless, it is important to keep in mind that, although stem cells have the capability of differentiating into specialized cell types, they may themselves, without the need of differentiating, act as biofactories for producing a wide range of molecules that modulate cells around them by paracrine signaling and likewise are significant for inducing processes central to tissue healing and regeneration.

2.2 Autologous, Syngeneic, Allogeneic, and Xenotransplantation

The procedure in which stem cells are introduced into patients with regenerative and medical purposes is generally referred to as stem cell transplantation. The primary goal of stem cell transplantation is to repopulate injured areas with specific cells so that tissues become functional again. The transplantation procedure may occur by different strategies, including autologous, syngeneic, allogeneic, or xenograft transplants. The type of transplant chosen will depend on the recipient's medical conditions and the availability of a matching donor. The assurance of a sufficient number of donor stem cells must also be offered [36].

2.2.1 Autologous Transplantation

In autologous transplantation, also called autotransplant or autograft, stem cells are extracted from the patient themselves, for example, from the peripheral blood, bone marrow, or adipose tissue, and transplanted back to the patient. This modality of transplantation is readily available, and there is no need for human leukocyte antigen (HLA, i.e., markers used for the immune cells to recognize what is self and nonself) typing and matching. Autologous transplants have a lower risk of rejection, and there is no need for immunosuppressive therapy to prevent graft rejection.

2.2.2 Syngeneic Transplantation

Also known as syngeneic graft or isograft. In this modality of transplantation, cells come from a different but genetically identical donor, such as the identical twin. In this case, individuals must be sufficiently identical and immunologically compatible. Similarly to autologous transplantation, the syngeneic graft has a lower risk of being rejected.

2.2.3 Allogeneic Transplantation

In the allogeneic transplantation, also called allotransplant, allograft, or homograft, stem cells are extracted, for example, from peripheral blood, bone marrow, umbilical cord, or adipose tissue, from a compatible donor and transplanted to the recipient. Therefore, the primary condition for donor selection is HLA compatibility. A close match between HLA markers between patients and donors is essential for a successful transplant; however, less than 30% of patients can find an HLA-matched sibling. To circumvent this, alternative sources, such as HLA-matched adult unrelated donors, umbilical cord blood stem cells, and partially HLA-mismatched (also known as HLA-haploidentical) related donors, are in continuous advance, especially in the hematopoietic stem cells (HSC) transplantation segment [94]. Besides, regenerative medicine researchers have put much effort into studying stem cells either with intrinsic immunomodulatory effects, such as the mesenchymal stromal cells (MSC) [103], or by HLA engineering of donor cells [63, 88, 105, 125]. Nevertheless, although this modality strengthens the possibility of finding a donor, allotransplant shows a higher risk of potentially fatal complications associated with organ toxicity, graft failure, and graft-versus-host disease (GVHD).

2.2.4 Xenotransplantation

In this type of transplant, the donor belongs to a different species than the recipient. This modality has emerged as an alternative to human transplants due to the scarcity of donor cells, tissues, and organs in contrast to rising numbers of potential recipients. Sheep, pigs, and nonhuman primates have been studied as potential sources of human stem cells and organs. Mesenchymal stem cells (MSC) obtained from different animals are of significant potential due to their immunosuppressive effects [108]. Xenograft practices such as blood transfusion from nonhuman species to patients were customary between the seventeenth and twentieth centuries. The first chimpanzee to human organ transplantation was attempted in the early 1960s [44, 69, 144, 153]. However, the high mortality due to vigorous immunogenicity and donor organ failure, combined with concern over viral transmission, has halted xenotransplantation for a time. To circumvent these issues, scientists have recently introduced gene editing (CRISPR/Cas9) and human pluripotent stem cells to create genetically "humanized" animals owning human organs [68, 112]. The idea is to create animals that possess organs, like the heart, lungs, kidney, liver, or even vessels, made up entirely of human cells. Attempts to genetically engineer cells to modify the immune-related genes making xenotransplantable organs compatible with the human immune system have also been studied.

2.3 Embryonic and Induced Pluripotent Stem Cells

When talking about stem cells, very often one either refers to embryonic stem cells (ESC) or induced pluripotent stem cells (iPSC). Both cell types share many similarities: they possess the ability to self-renew indefinitely and can produce cells from all three primal germ layers (endo-, ecto-, and mesoderm). Furthermore, the cells express "stemness" proteins that support distinct stem cell properties (e.g., fast cell division, telomere elongation). Thus, in many aspects, these cells are comparable and may be used interchangeably for many applications. However, their history and the respective isolation procedures vary considerably as described later in the chapter.

In 1981, the first embryonic stem cells were isolated from a mouse embryo [59]. Followed in 1998 by the first established human embryonic stem cell line [175]. Since then, ESC technology was faced with many ethical concerns leading to strict legal regulation in numerous countries.

In 2006, Yamanaka et al. made the breakthrough discovery that through overexpression of four transcription factors (Oct-4, Sox2, Klf4, and c-Myc) in mouse somatic cells the cells could be reprogrammed to an embryonic-like state [172]. These cells were aptly called induced pluripotent stem cells (iPSC). In 2007, the same group successfully applied the reprogramming procedure also to human somatic cells [171].

2.4 Adult Stem Cells: Bone Marrow, Peripheral Blood, Umbilical Cord, and Adipose Tissue

Adult stem cells, the so-called somatic stem cells or tissue-specific stem cells, are undifferentiated cell populations present during both fetal development and postnatal life. They are multipotent, i.e., they can differentiate into a limited number of different cell types of their tissue of origin and according to the microenvironment they are located in. In physiological conditions, these cells are maintained in a quiescent state (a way to avoid the accumulation of genetic damage) and, in response to specific stimuli, they may be activated and proliferate. They may keep up tissue homeostasis and contribute to cell self-renewal, but also support tissue repair. Which way the cell chooses in any situation depends on the information about the state of the tissue the cell receives, i.e., the microenvironmental cues. Although virtually every organ harbors stem cell niches, we will focus on the most ideal and commonly used sources for the therapeutic application of adult stem cells in vascular diseases, that is, the bone marrow, peripheral blood, umbilical cord, and adipose tissue. They have in common the facility of cell harvesting and the higher number of stem cells when compared to other sources.

2.4.1 Bone Marrow

The bone marrow (BM) is a spongy tissue found inside some bones in the body, including the hip and thigh bones. The primary function of the BM is providing signals to support hematopoiesis (i.e., the production of the blood cells) and the quiescence and self-renewability of the resident stem cells. Stem cells contained in the bone marrow mostly belong to two types: hemopoietic (giving rise to blood cells) and stromal (supporting the hematopoietic development and differentiating into other cell types) [114].

The bone marrow stromal cells consist of several populations, including osteo-lineage cells, endothelial cells, perivascular CXCL12-expressing cells, and mesenchymal stem cells (MSC) [7]. The MSC are of particular interest in vascular regenerative medicine and have been widely explored in clinical trials. The term was first coined by Arnold Caplan in 1991 to describe a perivascular BM stromal cell population able to differentiate into cartilage, bone, and fat [30]. After that, there was a plethora of reports not only alleging the presence of those cells in other tissues but also indicating they would be capable of differentiation in several lineages such as adipocytes, chondrocytes, and osteoblasts, cardiomyocytes, skeletal myocytes, fibroblasts, myofibroblasts, endothelial cells, neural cells, hepatic and tubular renal cells, particularly in vitro [74]. However, the term "stem cells" should be restricted to the populations of cells that demonstrate multipotency and self-renewal in vivo. Thus, it has been appealed that the term "Mesenchymal Stem Cells" should be abandoned as MSC can be induced to differentiate in many cell types in vitro, but they do not seem to do it in vivo. In fact, the therapeutic functionality presented by MSC is suggested to be achieved due to paracrine effects [24, 31, 160]. Therefore, despite still lacking a consensus of which term should be used and based on the recommendation of the International Society for Cellular Therapy (ISCT) for its re designation as "stromal," instead of "stem," [52], the MSC initials will be used throughout this chapter.

The hematopoietic stem cells (HSC) microenvironment of the BM is responsible for controlling the self-renewal, proliferation, differentiation, and migration of HSC and progenitor cells under determined stimuli. HSC give rise to blood cells, including white and red blood cells, as well as platelets. Based on mouse studies (and pieces of evidence that adult human BM is highly similar), the BM is composed of, at least, three hematopoietic niches: endosteal, periarteriolar, and perisinusoidal [34]. Although the prevailing hypothesis used to be that long-time repopulating HSC are maintained in a hypoxic niche in the BM, it has now become more evident that the majority of HSC are located in the perivascular well-oxygenated regions. More precisely, an imaging-based study shows that BM nondividing stem cells are mainly perisinusoidal [3]. The endosteal microenvironment seems to harbor only a subset of early lymphoid progenitors, while the bona fide HSC are found in the perivascular niches [51]. Worth mentioning, it has been shown that differences among the endothelium of the perivascular regions regulate the metabolism and reactive oxygen species (ROS) production in HSC in order to keep them quiescent (periarteriolar) or cycling (perisinusoidal) [170]. This characteristic is relevant to regenerative medicine seeing as it is known that the BM-HSC pool expands during aging, but its regenerative potential is reduced, maybe because of an altered capacity of the BM endothelium in regulating HSC metabolism and ROS production.

Of note, the transplantation of BM-derived mononuclear cells (BM-MNC) expressing CD34+ and/or CD133+, usually used in hematological diseases, has also been considered for treating ischemic diseases in humans [5, 84, 121, 155, 166, 189, 192]. The initial rationale was that those cell fractions would be enriched for the envisioned stem cells believed to be the best option for vascular regenerative purposes, the endothelial stem/progenitor cells (EPC) [11]. This premise was based on the close developmental association between hematopoietic and endothelial cell lineages during embryogenesis. However, the origin and identity of truly adult EPC is still a matter of intense debate in the scientific community, and many studies indicate that the BM is not the source of these stem/progenitors in adults. Instead, the BM-MNC fraction is known to be enriched for proangiogenic hematopoietic cells [37, 66, 197, 198].

2.4.2 Peripheral Blood

Peripheral blood stem cells (PBSC) are present in a very limited number under physiological conditions but may be mobilized from BM under certain conditions and with distinct stimuli, such as ischemia. Furthermore, circulating stem cells may also be derived from the vessel wall, especially during endothelial damage. The identification of such a minimally invasive stem cell source has made PBSC interesting for regenerative medicine and clinical applications. Indeed, peripheral blood (PB) has largely replaced BM in autologous stem cell transplants.

Usually, the stem cells used for transplantation in several hematological and neoplastic diseases are isolated from the bloodstream by their expression of the CD34 surface marker. The average percentage of CD34+ cells among total circulating cells is 0.06% in the bloodstream, while in BM, this percentage reaches 1.1% in healthy donors [102]. Strategies such as cytokine treatment are used to mobilize stem cells from BM to the bloodstream, including recombinant human granulocyte colony-stimulating factor (rhG-CSF) administration, which increases CD34+ cell concentration in the peripheral blood by 50–100-fold over baseline, and CXCR4 antagonists, which, in combination with G-CSF, contribute a further two- to threefold increase [90].

The cell composition of unmanipulated PBSC differs significantly from bone marrow stem cells (BMSC). It has been demonstrated, for example, that T cells, monocytes, and natural killer cells contaminants in a PBSC allograft were more than ten times higher than in a BM one [102]. In practice, cells isolated from the bloodstream intended to be used in cellular therapy correspond to the fraction of the mononuclear cells. The so-called peripheral blood mononuclear cells (PBMC) are a mixture of leukocytes and stem/progenitor cells that, when cytokine-mobilized, are enriched for CD34+ cells that also express the VEGF receptor 2 (VEGFR2/KDR) and the leukocyte marker CD45, although only a few of them express CD133 [90, 198]. Besides, some researchers have tried to isolate MSC from PBMC, but their existence in the bloodstream remains controversial [56, 110, 118].

Regarding EPC, the presence of a hierarchy of resident endothelial progenitor cells in the endothelium of blood vessels has been recognized that could account for the presence of EPC in the bloodstream replacing the earlier theory that these cells would come from BM [86, 186]. In the 2010s, there was further progress in understanding the origin and identity of the true EPC in adults and the paradigm shift began to strengthen. It was initially demonstrated that CD117/c-Kit+ cells present in the endothelium, the so-called vascular endothelium-resident stem cells (VESC), display high-clonogenic capacity and can differentiate into endothelial cells [60]. More recently, it was shown that these quiescent endothelial stem/progenitor cells are activated in response to injury [126, 188]. Overall, these studies, along with other recent findings, provide strong support not only for the existence of vascular endothelial stem/progenitor cells but also for the hierarchy of endothelial cell types within the endothelium [80], suggesting they can be used for therapeutic purposes. Further studies, however, are still necessary to better understand the identity of these vessel-derived endothelial stem/progenitor cells and their projected application in vascular regeneration.

2.4.3   Umbilical Cord

The ISBT 128 standard terminology for medical products of human origin [87] classifies the umbilical cord-derived cells into two categories: cord blood (CB)- and umbilical cord tissue (UCT)-derived cells.

The CB is a rich source of HSC and can be used as an alternative to BM- or PB-derived HSC in allogeneic transplants, especially when HLA-matched sibling and unrelated donors are unavailable. Although the CB yields lower numbers of HSC when compared to BM or cytokine-induced PB, it holds the advantage of being less immunogenic, thus requiring less stringent HLA-matching criteria. When compared to BM and PB, the CB-HSC presents a lower risk of graft-versus-host disease, a fatal complication of HSC transplantation. Besides, the CB-CD34+ cells exhibit higher hematopoietic repopulating ability than those from BM and PB. However, with the advent of the transplantation of haploidentical HSC, in addition to the high cost of allogenic CB transplantation, there was a decline in the use of CB for HSC transplantation purposes. On the other hand, the existence of cord blood banks allows its correct frozen maintenance for future use, making CB-derived cells available for, at least, 20 years without loss of their viability and engraftment potential. Noteworthy, beyond its primary use in hematological disorders, recent evidence points toward the potential use of CB cells in nonhematopoietic conditions as a source for regenerative cell therapy and immune modulation, amplifying the perspective for the use of CB-derived cells [48, 152].

UCT is a rich source of MSC and can be used as an alternative to BM- or adipose tissue (AT)-derived MSC. UCT-MSC may be isolated from the placenta, the perivascular space, and the Wharton's jelly present in the umbilical cord stroma and yields higher numbers of MSC when compared to BM or AT. Besides, UCT-MSC have higher proliferative potential than BM- and AT-MSC and express higher amounts of cytokines and hematopoietic growth factors, such as G-CSF, GM-CSF, LIF, IL-1α, IL-6, and IL-8. Of note, its proangiogenic capacity is independent of VEGF-A. As a source of perinatal cells, UCT-MSC express markers of pluripotency higher than postnatal tissue, but lesser than ESC, and are not known to induce tumorigenesis. Its therapeutic effects in preclinical and clinical studies, including vascular diseases, encourage further studies to pursue the clinical use of UCT-MSC [10].

2.4.4   Adipose Tissue

The white adipose tissue is one of the most important adult sources for therapies based on MSC, the so-called adipose-derived MSC (ASC). They are more readily available and yield a higher amount of stem/stromal cells when compared to bone marrow-derived MSC. Therefore, ASC are of great interest for cell therapy and tissue engineering [38]. These cells are obtained from the Stromal Vascular Fraction (SVF) that, besides ASC, typically contains various cell types, such as endothelial cells, smooth muscle cells, pericytes, leukocytes, fibroblasts, and pre-adipocytes. Of note, similar to ASC the freshly isolated SVF can induce new blood vessel formation and may be used directly for therapeutic neovascularization without the need for cell isolation [99, 206]. Compared to BM-MSC, ASC are less osteogenic and more effective in producing collagen. Besides, ASC are more stable in long-term culture with reduced senescence and higher proliferation capacity [165].

The CD34$^+$ ASC subpopulation has been associated with the formation of non-hematopoietic colonies in vitro. They may show endothelial characteristics, such as the expression of the surface markers CD146 and CD31, depending on culture conditions. Pericyte-like subpopulations expressing CD146 but that are CD31$^-$ and may be CD34+ or CD34$^-$, may also be present among ASC. Moreover, the CD146$^-$CD31$^-$CD34$^+$ subpopulation shows a higher potential to form adipocytes [209].

The use of ASC for cellular therapy has advantages regarding its easy access by subcutaneous lipoaspiration, which is a less painful procedure when compared to BMSC collection [70, 130]. In fact, ASC have been employed in many clinical trials for treating conditions that require tissue regeneration, diabetes mellitus, liver disease, corneal lesions, articular, and cutaneous lesions [19, 50, 101, 194, 196, 210, 211].

2.5 Isolation and Cell Culture

2.5.1 Isolation of Embryonic Stem Cells

Embryonic stem cells are obtained by isolation of cells from the inner cell mass (ICM) of a mammalian embryo in the blastocyst stage (Fig. 2.1). This is usually done by the destruction of the trophoblast or by the isolation of ICM cells from the embryo. The cells are then cultured either on a layer of murine or human feeder cells or on culture plates treated with extracellular matrix proteins. After cell culture has been established, adequate quality control is tantamount. First, cells are continuously cultured for at least 6 months to ascertain indefinite proliferation capacity. Furthermore, cells need to be able to form cells from all three primal germ layers: endoderm, ectoderm, and mesoderm. Cells are then tested for NANOG expression, an essential protein for upholding pluripotency.

2.5.2 Isolation of Induced Pluripotent Stem Cells

Induced pluripotent stem cells (iPSC) are obtained through cellular reprogramming of somatic cells. Most commonly, skin fibroblasts, peripheral blood monocytes, or urine-derived cells are used. However, iPSC lines have been established from numerous other cell types. Following the isolation of somatic cells, the overexpression of Yamanaka factors is induced by the use of various vectors (Fig. 2.2).

Early approaches used retroviral vectors [171, 172], while subsequent approaches used adeno-, RNA-virus, or plasmid vectors [137, 158, 207, 208]. In recent years, reprogramming through mRNA vectors has gained traction [33]. This method has the advantage that it lacks the potential for mutagenic DNA insertions and mRNA

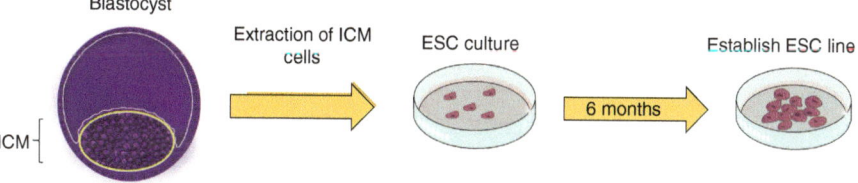

Fig. 2.1 Schematic of embryonic stem cell derivation, ICM = inner cell mass

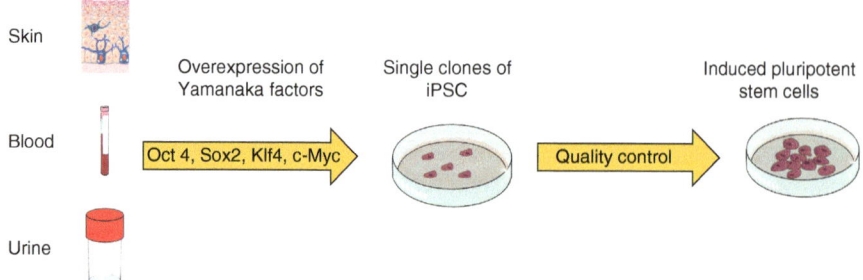

Fig. 2.2 Schematic-induced pluripotent stem cell derivation from somatic cells of different tissue origin

is quickly degraded; however, not all somatic cell types are susceptible to mRNA vectors and in animal experiments mRNA induced iPSC-derived somatic cells demonstrated increased immunogenicity.

About two weeks after induction of overexpression of Yamanaka factors, small colonies appear in the culture dish. These colonies each represent a distinct clone of emerging iPSC. Several of these clones are then picked and propagated separately. Afterward, cells need to undergo quality control and are tested for their pluripotency, ability for indefinite self-renewal as well as expression of at least two of the species-specific stem cell proteins. For human iPSC, these are Oct-4, SSEA-4, NANOG, Sox-2, TRA-1-60, and TRA-1-81 [168]. The gold standard for assessment of pluripotency is the implantation into immunodeficient mice where pluripotent stem cells will form teratomata (tumors consisting of tissues from all three germ layers).

2.5.3   Culture of ESC and iPSC

As previously stated, ESC and iPSC are very similar in many regards and there are few differences in their respective culture methods; thus, they are described together in the following. In the beginning, ESC and iPSC were commonly cultured on a layer of mitomycin-treated or irradiated (to stop any further proliferation) mouse embryonal fibroblasts. This feeder layer not only helps the stem cells attach to the culture dish but also produces essential growth factors. However, in recent years the trend has been going toward GMP (good manufacturing practice) and GTP (good tissue practice) conform culture methods. This includes the use of chemically defined, xeno- and serum-free culture media sans the use of either mouse or human feeder cells. Culture media are widely available from numerous companies, but all contain either bFGF (basic fibroblast growth factor) for human or LIF (leukocyte inhibitory factor) for mouse stem cells to keep the cells in their pluripotent state. Nevertheless, significant variations exist in the composition and concentration of the respective growth factor mixtures between different culture media. This represents a significant hurdle for the broad application of standardized culture conditions and hampers the reproducibility of differentiation protocols between labs.

2.5.4 Isolation and Culture of Adult Stem Cells

2.5.4.1 Bone Marrow Stem Cells (BMSC)

Hematopoietic stem/progenitor cells (HSPC) and BM-MSC are the two main cell populations that can be isolated from the BM. Human BM can be obtained by aspiration from the iliac crest [132], the femoral head [45], and the vertebral body [146].

Regarding the MSC, they are present at a shallow frequency in the BM. Although they can grow in culture and their number is expanded [12], there is still some challenge to use them in cell-based therapies due to the high variability in the culture conditions used for their isolation and expansion. As a result, a range of protocols has been published. Besides, xenogeneic substances for cell expansion may affect the cells properties compromising clinical application. Except for their tissue source, there are no standardized culture methods yet available for culturing and expanding MSC for transplantation purposes. Therefore, although very promising, its approval for clinical use as a feasible treatment modality is still a matter of intense study to define optimal conditions and enable standardization.

BM-MSC show important characteristics that permit their isolation and purification process, such as their physical adherence to plastic cell culture plates [178]. The main techniques used for isolation and BM-MSC enrichment include an antibody-based cell sorting, low- and high-density culture techniques, positive and negative selection methods, frequent medium changes, and enzymatic digestion procedures [13, 57, 58, 159, 162, 185]. Following the ISCT proposed minimal criteria for human MSC identification [52], these cells exhibit (a) plastic adherence, (b) the ability to differentiate in vitro into adipocyte, chondrocyte, and osteoblasts, and (c) can be immunophenotypically characterized by the expression of CD73, CD90, CD105, and the lack of expression of CD14, CD34, CD45, and human leukocyte antigen-DR (HLA-DR). Moreover, the expression of the cell markers CD29 and CD71, as well as the absence of endothelial cell markers, such as CD31, VEGFR2, CD62E, and vWF, is also very often used to characterize these cells better [14].

For MSC isolation, the procedure involves the isolation of the mononuclear (MNC) fraction by density centrifugation [15, 77–79]. The resultant buffy coat is then seeded in culture flasks containing the medium of choice supplemented with 10% of fetal bovine serum (FBS) and maintained at 37 °C in a humidified atmosphere. The MSC-like cells form a single layer and the adherent cells are maintained in culture for 8–12 days. The resultant cells show heterogeneous fibroblastic appearance, distinct colony formation, and high proliferation [14].

In order to perform the functional characterization, known as the ability of the cultured cells to differentiate in osteoblastic- and adipocytic-like cells, alizarin staining is used to show the formation of calcium oxalates for characterizing osteoblastic activity and, for adipocytic activity, the oil red staining is commonly employed [14, 141].

BM-MNC positive for CD34 are selected for HSPC isolation and transplantation. However, it is worth mentioning that this fraction contains cells that vary either in their metabolic or mitotic activities and the CD34$^+$ expression alone does not provide an accurate measure of HSPC in BM. Therefore, it is advised to use cocktails of antibodies to deplete or exclude hematopoietic lineage positive cells to better characterize the BM-HSPC [107, 193]. The isolation methods used to separate these cells include immunomagnetic and fluorescence-activated cell sorting (FACS).

Similar to BM-MSC, BM-HSPC can be stimulated to proliferate in culture for expansion. Different methods have been used, and the composition and biological characteristics depend on the procedure adopted. CD34$^+$ cells may be cultured for several weeks in a medium supplemented with some cytokines such as IL-3, IL-6, SCF, Flt3 ligand, TPO, GM-CSF, and G-CSF [22, 41, 131]. Moreover, HSC may also be co-cultured with MSC that are shown to support their survival and self-renewal [62].

Among human hematopoietic stem/progenitor cells, the CD34 surface marker is known for its unique expression, although recent findings suggest the existence of a population of cells that do not express CD34 (CD34$^-$) but become CD34$^+$ before cell division [2, 53]. Differently, the HSPC expression profile of naïve mice includes Lin$^-$Sca-1$^+$cKit$^+$ (LSK) [8, 167]. Besides, other markers may also be used to identify HSC isolated from BM, such as the absence of expression of CD41 and CD48 and the expression of CD150 [96].

2.5.4.2 Peripheral Blood Stem Cells (PBSC)

Peripheral blood is an alternative and highly envisioned source of stem cells since it can be easily acquired with minimal invasiveness. PBSC includes HSPC and, possibly, endothelial progenitor cells (EPC) and MSC. All of them are present in the mononuclear cell (MNC) fraction [49, 75, 140]. The culture protocols and expansion conditions of PB-MSC, however, are not well defined, and even their presence in the bloodstream has been challenged. Additionally, for PB-EPC, due to the new body of evidence about vessel-derived stem/progenitor endothelial cells, thus far there are no protocols available that ensure their cultivation and expansion in vitro. Nevertheless, what exists are well-defined cultivation protocols of the PB-MNC fraction to enrich for proangiogenic cells, as will be described at the end of this subtopic. Therefore, the use of PBSC cells for transplantation is currently only approved for hematopoietic stem cell transplantation.

Two primary techniques are used to isolate PBMC from the bloodstream: density gradient centrifugation or leukapheresis. In the first one, the PBMC fraction corresponds to the thin white layer at the interface between the plasma and the density medium. The leukapheresis method uses an automated machine to separate the whole blood from the target PBMC fraction through high-speed centrifugation.

The isolated PBMC comprise a heterogeneous mixture of cells. The so-called peripheral blood mononuclear cells (PBMC) fraction contains circulating cells that include lymphocytes – CD3$^+$ T cells (45–70%) and CD19$^+$ B cells (5–15%) – monocytes (10–30%), natural killer cells (5–10%), dendritic cells (1–2%), and HSC (0.1–0.2%). Nevertheless, as mentioned earlier in this chapter, it is possible to increase the percentage of circulating HSPC by the administration of G-CSF to the donor.

After that, readily transplantable cells, mainly used for treating hematological and neoplastic diseases, are isolated based on their positivity for the CD34 surface marker. The cell profile of the PBMC subset may be analyzed by flow cytometry which allows differentiating cell populations based on complexity – side scatter (SSC) and forward scatter proprieties (FSC) – and biomarkers expression [16, 136].

As mentioned above, the PBMC fraction may also be used for the culture-based isolation of proangiogenic cells. The reported assays rely on the adhesion of MNC to specific substrates, such as fibronectin and collagen I, in endothelial-specific culture media. At least two types of circulating angiogenic cells, formerly known as "putative EPC", may be isolated in culture dishes: (1) the so-called early outgrowth endothelial progenitor cells (eEPC or EOC) and (2) the late outgrowth endothelial progenitor cells possessing clonal endothelial colony-forming cells (ECFC) ability [127, 145, 199].

The first one (EOC) appears after 4–7 days in culture, can be spherical or spindle-shaped, and has low proliferative potential (if any). The second one (ECFC) appears after 2–4 weeks in culture, forms a cobblestone-shaped cell monolayer, and has high proliferative potential. Both cell types bind to isolectin, endocyte acetylated LDL, and express CD31. However, only ECFC express the endothelial cell marker von Willebrand Factor (vWF), besides to express more VEGFR2, CD105, and CD146 than EOC. The progenitor cell markers CD34 and CD117/c-Kit are more expressed in ECFC than EOC. In contrast, hematopoietic markers are present in EOC, but not in ECFC, suggesting ECFC are more committed to the endothelial lineage. Finally, in functional assays, ECFC, but not EOC, are much more prone to integrate into endothelial cells network in vitro and in vivo. Overall, although both cell types are interesting candidates for inducing therapeutic angiogenesis, while EOC are undoubtedly hematopoietic cells with paracrine angiogenic capacity, ECFC appear to be programmed to differentiate into endothelium [18].

2.5.4.3 Umbilical Cord Stem Cells (UCSC)

Cord Blood (CB) Collection and Processing for Cell Isolation

The procedure of CB collection is noninvasive, not painful, and relies on a venipuncture and blood drainage to a sterile container, usually with a citrate-based anticoagulant. The most critical steps at the moment of the collection are to avoid contamination during the venipuncture procedure and to clamp and extract the cord blood within a precise timing before umbilical vessels collapse and blood entrapping. Usually, the red blood cells (RBC)-depleted fraction is used for cryopreservation, as it allows volume reduction and lesser RBC-related thawing cytotoxicity. Several methods may be used to isolate CB cells, including density gradient separation of mononuclear (MNC) cells, sedimentation by gelatin, rouleaux formation induced by hydroxyethyl starch and centrifugation, and differential centrifugation with separation of RBC and plasma.

The optimization of recovery procedures for cells from CB is a vital step for its clinical use and, according to FDA recommendations, must achieve a recovery of, at least, 85% of viable nucleated cells after volume reduction and before cryopreservation. Each banked cord blood unit must contain, at least, 5×10^8 total nucleated cells (TNC). The minimum dose acceptable for consistent engraftment of CB is 2.5×10^7 TNC per kilogram of body weight of the prospective recipient. This dose is considered to reflect the MNC content that meets the required CD34$^+$ count of, at least, 0.25% of viable TNC before cryopreservation (approximately 2×10^6 CD34$^+$ cells). A suboptimal dose may result in delayed hematological recovery, graft failure, and a higher risk of infection. Of note, this minimum dose limits the CB transplantation to children and adults of low body weight. For weightier individuals, the double-unit of CB transplantation augments the graft doses, but its clinical benefits are still controversial [61, 152, 190]. Although controversial, the TNC count is mostly used in hematopoietic cell transplantation. However, its advantages (especially when considering the reduction in time of isolation and costs) have been challenged. It has been demonstrated that storing UCB units as MNC fractions instead of TNC fractions would provide more accurate and reliable results concerning the quality and potency of the UCB unit [139].

Although the CB-HSPC isolation for transplantation purposes is primarily based on the CD34 expression in the MNC fraction, further characterization of CB cells is a challenge since it involves the maturation degree of these cells in the UCB. It is known that the phenotype CD34$^+$CD38$^-$ is more primitive than the CD34$^+$CD38$^+$ [176]. Besides, other surface markers can be used to determine the maturity degree of CB cells, among them CD90, CD117 (c-Kit), CD135, CD75 [82, 154].

In an attempt to increase the number of cells, the expansion of CB-HSC in culture is possible as long as supplemental factors are present in the medium. The main factors used for the CB-HSC enrichment and culture are thrombopoietin, Flt3 ligand, IL-6, fibroblast growth factor (FGF), angiopoietin, insulin-like growth factor binding protein 2 (IGFBP2), Notch ligands, Wnts, and insulin-like growth factor 2 (IGF-2) [142, 201, 203, 204]. Besides, co-culture with MSC enhances the process of HSC expansion, as adhesion, proliferation, and differentiation of HSC depend on the production of soluble factors produced by MSC and matrix molecules [147].

Umbilical Cord Tissue (UCT) Isolation and Culture

Two main techniques are used to isolate cells from the umbilical cord tissue: enzymatic digestion and explants [29, 85]. Different lab-made protocols for isolation and expansion have been used. In the method of enzymatic digestion, collagenase and hyaluronidase are used to digest UCT and release cells from the extracellular matrix. The disadvantage of this method is the long duration of tissue incubation with enzymes, which may compromise the biology and the process of cell adhesion. The explant method is cheaper and more straightforward and does not require enzymatic incubation. However, this method depends on the ability of cells to migrate and adhere to the culture vessel [73, 76, 200].

Although there is no standardized protocol for isolation, expansion, or cryo-preservation, UCT-MSC have mainly been isolated by enzymatic digestion of Wharton's jelly and cultured in medium supplemented with human or fetal calf serum. The culture medium may also contain specific growth factors such as bFGF, EGF, PDGF, and VEGF. Besides, the UCT-MSC may be isolated by a nonenzymatic explant culture method. However, some studies show the isolated cells obtained by each method display different characteristics as the cells isolated by the explant culture present a higher proliferative potential (although cells reach arrest earlier) and higher variation of phenotypes, being, therefore, a more heterogeneous population. Overall, independent of enzymatic or nonenzymatic isolation, the UCT-MSC phenotyping follows the minimum criteria of ISCT. Besides, they display higher proliferative potential in culture than MSC from other postnatal or neonatal sources and, under specific conditions, may display pluripotent specific markers that are not present in other postnatal sources. Of note, culture conditions influence the immunomodulatory properties of UCT-MSC as xeno-free or serum-free media and allow a more effective suppression of T-cell proliferation [10].

2.5.4.4 Adipose Tissue Stem Cells (ASC)

Subcutaneous fat deposits are present in high quantities in the human body, and liposuction surgeries are an excellent choice for harvesting adipose tissue. Adipose tissue stem cells (ASC) are isolated from the stromal vascular fraction (SVF). SVF is heterogeneous and contains ASC, endothelial cells, fibroblasts, leukocytes, pericytes, and pre-adipocytes, among others [156, 202].

Despite the high volume of publications in recent years, the procedure for collecting and isolating ASC requires better standardization of the forms of manipulation of the collected tissue in order to optimize and unify the processes [40, 182]. For isolating cells from liposuction, enzymatic and nonenzymatic methods may be used. After centrifugation, the SVF corresponds to the pellet present in the aqueous fraction of the enzymatically digested lipoaspirate or to the nontumescent non-oily fat fraction of the nonenzymatic mechanical disrupted lipoaspirate [47]. The choice of the method may interfere with the phenotype and biology of the isolated cells.

The enzymatic digestion is the method adopted by most research groups and represents a modification of the methods initially described by Rodbell and colleagues [150]. In brief, adipose tissue is minced, digested with collagenase and fractionated by differential centrifugation, and the pelleted SVF cells placed in culture [133, 148–150]. This method is particularly indicated for extracellular matrix (ECM) disruption and separation from binding adipocytes and other cells. Although effective, this method is complex, expensive, time-consuming, and yet more restricted to experimental approaches since the high manipulation of these cells makes their clinical use difficult [156].

As an alternative procedure, nonenzymatic methods that use mechanical (manual or in automated commercially available closed systems) forces appear to be promising for the therapeutic use of cells. The resulting product is a suspension composed of adipose tissue micro fragments, suspended cells, growth factors, and ECM components of the original adipose tissue. The nonenzymatic methods are faster and easier for handling than enzymatic digestion and can be performed inside the operating room, besides guaranteeing the maintenance of structural integrity of the cells [9, 23, 47, 169, 181].

Similar to BM-MSC, ASC are characterized by the expression of a range of surface markers, such as CD29, CD90, CD105, CD73, and CD44, and the absence of the expression of CD45 and CD31 [65]. Besides, according to the joint statement of the International Federation for Adipose Therapeutics and Science (IFATS) and the International Society for Cellular Therapy (ISCT) to establish minimal definitions of stromal cells and avoid confusion in the use of the terms ASC, the culture adherent stromal/stem cells population, and the heterogeneous uncultured SVF (that cannot be called stem cells), ASC can be distinguished from BM-MSC by their positivity for CD36 and negativity for CD106. Moreover, the IFATS/ISCT joint statement recommends the immunophenotype characterization of SVF and ASC as follows: CD13, CD29, CD44, CD73, CD90 (>40%), and CD34 (>20%) as primary positive markers for SVF and CD13, CD29, CD44, CD73, CD90, and CD105 (>80%) for ASC. CD34 is also considered a primary, although unstable, positive marker for ASC, as its expression can be found in freshly isolated cells but disappears when they are expanded in culture. As negative markers CD31 (<20%), and CD45 (<50%) are considered for SVF and, CD31, CD45, and CD235a (<2%) for ASC. Other secondary positive, such as CD36, or negative, such as CD3, CD11b, and CD106, markers may also be considered for ASC [28].

Regarding the cell culture protocols, the employment of commercial media (e.g., DMEM and aMEM), routinely used for ASC expansion, and two supplements, fetal bovine serum (FBS) and human platelet lysate, results in satisfactory conditions. Of note, platelet lysate provides the highest isolation and proliferation rates and commitment for osteogenic lineage. The hematopoietic support is performed through a constant secretion of G-CSF and SCF [134].

Nevertheless, it is important to highlight that most of the described culture settings are not actually xeno-free and are instead research-grade conditions. Therefore, they need to be adapted to attend good manufacturing practice (GMP) or good tissue practice (GTP) conditions following regulations and standards for quality and safety clinical applications.

2.6   Advantages and Disadvantages

The biggest hurdles for stem cell research before the discovery of iPSC have been ethical concerns and legal restrictions for working with stem cells of embryonic origin. Worldwide, the work with ESC is heavily regulated and sometimes excluded from national funding programs. In most cases, it is not allowed to generate embryos solely for research purposes and ESCs have to be obtained from surplus embryos from in vitro fertilization procedures with the consent of the donors. Nonetheless, many ethical concerns remain. The discovery of iPSC has relieved many of these aforementioned problems. Seeing as donors for iPSC can give their informed consent for the generation of iPSC, and there is no longer any need for the destruction of human embryos for the generation of stem cells.

Furthermore, using donor-specific somatic tissue for stem cell manufacturing allows for the application of autologous stem cell-derived tissues and therapies, minimizing the need for post-intervention immunosuppression. One of the major advantages of ESC and iPSC is simultaneously a chief disadvantage of stem cell technology: the inherent self-renewal capacity. By culturing cell lines over long periods, sometimes for multiple decades, not only may cell characteristics change, but there is also the risk of acquired genetic abnormalities and the resulting potential for tumorigenesis in the recipient. Moreover, certain induction vectors carry the risk of genome integration further increasing the risk for genetic aberrations in resulting cells. This is best addressed by building a cell bank with a low passage number as well as regular quality checks of cultured stem cells (e.g., karyotyping, genotyping).

The main advantages of adult stem cells are their ready availability for therapeutic applications and the possibility of autologous transplantation, in addition to lower ethical concerns and risk of oncogenesis. Also, they exert significant paracrine effects that allow their widespread use in several different medical conditions, besides the possibility to be used as biofactories. Most of them are also easily expanded in vitro, besides to be possible to improve their functionality ex vivo before transplantation. This, however, adds a drawback to the cost and increases the possibility of contamination with other products. One significant disadvantage, when compared to ESC or iPSC, is the restricted differentiation potential of adult stem cells. Furthermore, the possibility of impaired cell function, especially concerning donor morbidity, and even disease transmission, represents a hurdle to be overcome as new methods and technologies for cell improvement are being generated.

Finally, despite the considerable advances in our understanding of stem cell biology and the harnessing of their potential as cell therapy, much progress still has to be made in order to standardize protocols for isolation, manipulation, and identification of cells suitable for therapeutical purposes.

2.7   Clinical Applications and Future Perspectives

While ESC- and iPSC-based therapies hold great promise, only a minimal number of clinical trials have been undertaken. Most were targeted toward the treatment of retinal degenerative diseases due to the easy accessibility of the retina and its immunologically privileged status [120, 163]. Some progress has also been made toward cardiovascular stem cell treatments. One animal study in mini pigs tested the survival of human iPSC-derived cardiomyocytes in combination with an omentum flap and could show improved survival of the transplant as well as increased vascular density [93]. After iPSC-CM/omentum transplantation, mini pigs received a triple immunosuppressive therapy consisting of tacrolimus, mycophenolate mofetil, and corticosteroid, due to the procedure constituting xenotransplantation. In another study, mice received a stem cell treatment 48 h after myocardial infarction and were intramyocardially injected either with iPSC or iPSC-derived extracellular vesicles (iPSC-EV) [4]. While both groups demonstrated improved left ventricular function, iPSC-EV was more effective than iPSC alone. This highlights the importance of contributing paracrine effects in stem cell treatments, especially for regenerative therapies. Another study showed similar results using an ESC-based approach [95]. However, ESC-derived cells and ESC-derived extracellular vesicles displayed comparable improvements in left ventricular function. Moreover, in 2018, the first human trial for cardiovascular disease took place. Patients with severe ischemic heart disease undergoing bypass surgery received an epicardial ESC-cardiomyocyte patch with the primary endpoints being feasibility and safety, which were both successfully reached [128].

Even as there have been many fears about the safety profile of ESC- and iPSC-based therapies, no serious adverse reactions have been observed in clinical trials so far. Still, safety concerns need to be taken seriously as showed by the discontinuation of a Japanese iPSC-based clinical trial conducted at the RIKEN institute due to irregularities in the iPSC-derived retinal cells intended for transplantation. This reinforces the need for rigorous and standardized quality control.

While the number of performed trials is still small, they have proven the feasibility of both ESC- and iPSC-derived therapies in multiple fields of medicine. Recently a novel iPSC line has been established which lacks major histocompatibility complex I and II and is thus hypoimmunogenic. Although this is a promising approach, the potential for tumorigenesis is increased and this issue needs to be addressed, e.g., by adding a "suicide switch" to the cells.

Regarding adult stem cells, most studies in which those cells are used as strategies for therapies focused on vascular diseases use the fraction of MNC in autologous transplants from BM and PB after stimulation of G-CSF mobilization [143]. Currently, new sources of SCs have been proposed, in addition to cell populations with different immunophenotypic characteristics, including CD34$^+$ cells, tissue repair-associated monocytes (CD14$^+$CD45$^+$), high aldehyde dehydrogenase (ALDH)-activity progenitors, and expanded MSC [143]. However, the challenges in this area hinder advances related to vascular therapy focused on vascular diseases, among them lack of standardization of isolation and culture protocols that prevent comparisons between research groups, and the necessity of an effective immunophenotypic characterization of cells used in therapies.

In this section, we will discuss the advances associated with the use of stem cells for the clinical treatment of vascular diseases, as well as the challenges and perspectives for this field. We hope that the information will foster discussions aimed at improving processes that allow advances in the field of vascular regenerative medicine associated with better understanding and use of stem cells.

2.7.1 *Peripheral Arterial Disease (PAD)*

Peripheral arterial disease (PAD) is a term often used to refer to the lower extremity arterial disease secondary to atherosclerotic narrowing or occlusion of the arteries, which results in a decline in blood supply to the limbs. This disease is the third leading cause of cardiovascular morbidity related to atherosclerotic disease after coronary diseases and stroke and is associated with life and limb-threatening complications. Patients with PAD may be asymptomatic or may have symptoms such as intermittent claudication (pain in the lower limbs during walking) or pain at rest with or without ulcers or gangrene.

In the worst scenario, when available therapies (whether pharmacological, endovascular or surgical) are not effective or are not indicated, amputations of digits and limbs are common. Angiogenic therapies haves been considered as novel attempts to direct stimulate the revascularization of the affected limb. Among the possible approaches, cell therapy has been evaluated experimentally [25].

MNC derived either from BM or PB have been used in models of hindlimb ischemia and in patients with PAD. Although the injection of autologous BM-MNC in the gastrocnemius of patients with ischemic limbs have reduced rest pain and increased transcutaneous oxygen pressure, there was no significant effect of the cell therapy on amputation rate [173]. The selection of MNC subsets with angiogenic or cytoprotective properties could be an interesting approach for further development of cell therapy strategies in PAD patients [64].

In a double-blind study, autologous BM-derived aldehyde dehydrogenase bright (ALDH[br]) cells were injected in the leg of patients with symptom-limiting intermittent claudication. ALDH[br] administration did not improve peak walking time (PWT) or capillary perfusion measured by magnetic resonance imaging (MRI) outcomes. The benefits of cell therapy were more apparent in patients with completely occluded femoral arteries, which showed an increased number of collateral arteries [138]. The selection of higher doses or treatment of patients with different clinical characteristics remains to be investigated.

Despite some benefits of cell therapy in PAD treatment, the efficacy of these cells on all endpoints was no longer significant in placebo-controlled studies, and the current knowledge does not support the effectiveness of cell therapy in patients with PAD. However, treatments that bring improvement in symptoms and that benefit, even temporarily, patients with PAD should be encouraged. For this, refinement of isolation techniques, administration routes, parameters to be evaluated, testing different doses, and selection of the source and phenotypic profile of the cells to be used may help in the improvement and response of the treatment.

Chronic limb-threatening ischemia (CLTI) is the end stage of PAD and shows higher rates of limb amputation, mortality, and impaired quality of life. CLTI is a clinical syndrome characterized by rest pain, gangrene, and/or lower limb ulcerations longer than 2 weeks. Venous, traumatic, embolic, and nonatherosclerotic etiologies are excluded. Since 2013, by the time of the launch of the Global Vascular Guidelines initiative, CLTI is considered the first priority disease area of focus for vascular specialists [42].

Treatment options for patients with CLTI are limited to surgical procedures that include arterial reconstruction, endovascular therapy, and limb amputation. Moreover, patients with severe comorbidities and limb gangrene/sepsis are often not eligible for surgical revascularization procedures. Stem cell-based therapies for limb amputation prevention in these patients have been encouraged [6, 46]. Indeed, in the above mentioned guidelines [42], stem cell therapy was identified as one of the key research priorities to advances the management of CLTI.

Although promising clinical results based on cell therapy still show more discreet results when compared to preclinical studies, a meta-analysis indicates that cell therapy in CLTI is associated with a reduction of the risk of a major amputation, identifying it as a promising strategy in the management of the disease [39, 43, 109]. Strategies such as the search for new sources of stem cells and the possibility of allogeneic transplants and cell enrichment may lead to the increase and success of cell therapy aimed at treating patients with CLTI. Besides, the ability of pluripotent stem cells in differentiating into endothelial cells should be assessed in the clinic since neovascularization processes are essential to the CLTI prognostic [115].

The intramuscular transplantation of autologous BM-MNC or G-CSF-mobilized PB-MNC in CLTI patients has shown promising results associated with the improvement of the ankle-brachial index (ABI) and tissue oxygenation compared to cells administrated in the contralateral leg [83, 173]. Besides, pain and ulcer reduction in the follow-up of intramuscular BM-MNC transplantation has been reported [124]. Adverse effects related to intramuscular injection include the only transient presence of the graft after intramuscular injection, with poor survival and retention of the cells in the ischemic tissue and poor integration into the host vasculature [32, 183].

Intra-arterial administration of BM-MNC arose on the premise that stem cell delivery with hematopoietic potential would bring benefits to ischemic tissue since cell delivery would occur more effectively through well-vascularized areas potentiating their angiogenic effects [143]. Studies using this approache have shown improvement in clinical parameters related to resting pain and ulcer pattern compared to the placebo group [184, 189]. However, cell therapy did not reduce the incidence of limb amputation when compared to control groups in two independently performed studies [184]. Strategies that could optimize the efficacy of cell delivery are required to improve the efficiency of cell therapy in vascular disease. Alternatives combining intramuscular and intra-arterial modes of delivery could improve cell graft survival along with more refined techniques with more specific and guided microinjections.

The transplantation of a more homogenous cell population has been suggested to improve cell survival. Additionally, a better definition and characterization of transplanted cells should be encouraged for comparisons and replicability in other studies. Furthermore, the development of strategies seeking to minimize and treating comorbidities to CLTI should be emphasized and is central to improving the success of cell therapy [143].

Another question to be considered concerns the so-called stem cell exhaustion in case of autologous transplantation. Meaning that in end-stage CLTI patients, the functions of stem cells and their progenitors could be compromised or in some cases, these cells could be barely present. Thus, the continuous search for new methods of cell enrichment and enhancement of functionality, for alternative stem cells sources and for improvements in allogeneic and xenotransplantation are crucial [89, 174].

One example of a promising alternative to cell therapy is the use of extracellular vesicles (EV) containing potent proangiogenic agents, exosomes, and microvesicles in the management of CLTI. These strategies aim to promote a microenvironment where cell-to-cell communication is most effective in promoting the development, growth, and maturation of new blood vessels [177]. The injection of CD34+ cell-derived exosomes into the ischemic hindlimb in a preclinical model showed enhanced limb perfusion via the upregulation of important proangiogenic molecules such as VEGF, ANGF1, ANG2 and MMP9 [123]. Also, MSC-derived EV increased blood reperfusion and stimulated the formation of new blood vessels in a preclinical murine model of hindlimb ischemia via overexpression of VEGFR1 and VEGFR2 in endothelial cells [67].

Other shortcomings to be addressed concern the delivery systems and stem cell survival after administration. Both intramuscular and intra-arterial injections may be inefficient because they do not deliver cells to the target site due to inefficient host vasculature [39]. Moreover, studies on the microenvironment at the injection site, as well as dosage and frequency of cell therapy, should be conducted. Complementary approaches using biocompatible scaffolds may also represent interesting experimental strategies.

2.7.2 Diabetic Foot Ulcers (DFU)

Diabetic foot ulcers develop as a result of the progressive and cumulative effects of longstanding diabetes that significantly disturbs the wound healing process [26]. The pathophysiology of DFU is complex and multifactorial and requires interventions able to accelerate and improve healing. In this sense, cell therapy emerges as a promising strategy to ameliorate the severity of foot ulcers in diabetic patients.

Many authors have demonstrated the benefits of stem cell therapy to ischemic and wounded tissues by secretion of growth factors and chemokines that promoting neovascularization and tissue remodeling [91, 195]. In a study comparing the effects of BM-MNC and PB-derived progenitor cell therapies in patients with diabetic foot disease and CLTI unresponsive to revascularization, for example, a lower rate of amputation and improved oxygenation and blood flow at the ulcer site have been observed [54]. These results are comparable to percutaneous transluminal angioplasty (PTA) and prove that cell therapy is safe and may constitute a new therapeutic approach for the treatment of diabetic ulcers [55]. In another study, autologous CD90+ BM-derived cells were used in the treatment of diabetic ulcers. Parameters such as ABI, TcPO$_2$, reactive hyperemia, and angiographic imaging before and after therapy were taken. Improved microvascularization and complete wound closure in most of the patients who received cell therapy were observed [98].

A meta-analysis conducted by Zhang et al. [205], including randomized controlled clinical trials, suggested that cellular therapy could accelerate the healing of DFU, associated with a higher ankle-branchial index, higher transcutaneous oxygen pressure, higher ulcer healing rate, the lower reported pain levels and higher amputation-free survival. However, the authors draw attention to the limitations of the study that includes only a small number of papers and a lack of standardization in the execution and evaluation in the underlying trials, possibly limiting the conclusions drawn by the meta-analysis.

Therefore, although preclinical and clinical studies indicate the benefits of cell therapy on DFU treatment, the meta-analysis highlights the lack of a consensus regarding the optimal type of stem cell to be used, therapy regimen, and protocols to deliver cells properly. More effective delivery methods would improve the rates of success [113].

2.7.3   Venous Leg Ulcer (VLU)

Venous leg ulcers (VLU) arise from chronic venous insufficiency in the lower limbs and are widespread and debilitating, with high morbidity and associated costs, straining healthcare budgets and negatively impacting quality of life. The treatment of VLU can be conservative or surgical, but they are quite resistant to healing with standard care compression therapy and have high recurrence rates often leading to chronicity [92, 164].

The use of stem cells in VLU has been based on their capacity to stimulate wound healing through two mechanisms: attenuating the general inflammatory response and differentiating into cells involved in tissue repair, such as fibroblasts, myofibroblasts, and antigen-presenting cells [157].

In recent years, the use of adipose tissue as a source for cell therapy has been explored. The variety of cell types found in SVF represents a potential advantage for wound healing compared to cultured stem cells. Although the current clinical trials are significantly different in terms of study design and included subjects, most of them demonstrate the safety of ASC and SVF, as well as the improvement of chronic ulcers and reduction of pain [81]. A study involving 31 patients who had undergone surgery for an underlying venous pathology where venous ulcers had not healed post-surgery were treated with adipose-derived autologous stem cell injection at the ulcer site. Cell injection induced ulcer contraction and epithelization, even though no full closure was observed. In the follow-up, only three patients exhibited a recurrent ulcer. No adverse events were reported [92].

The ability of autologous SVF in treating chronic ulcers of venous (VLU) and arterial-venous (AVLU) origin were studied by Konstantinow et al. [100]. The patients received a single topical treatment with noncultured $9–15 \times 10^6$ cells isolated from abdominal lipoaspirates by enzymatic digestion. All VLU and four of nine AVLU patients who received the cells showed complete epithelization of the ulcers within 71–174 days. A considerable reduction in the intensity of pain and no severe side effects were observed. The authors emphasize, however, that one-time application may not be sufficient in patients with larger predominantly ischemic AVLU and comorbidities.

2.7.4 Lymphedema

Lymphedema represents a debilitating condition manifesting as an excess of lymphatic fluid and swelling of subcutaneous tissue due to obstruction, destruction, or hypoplasia of lymphatic vessels [179]. Besides, lymphedema is a common complication with breast cancer treatment and does not have a definitive cure despite several microsurgical techniques and conservative management used in clinical practice [117].

Lymphedema treatment requires restoration lymphatic vessels from the capillary to the collector level and stem cell therapy could be an effective strategy to induce a complex regenerative response in patients affected by disorders of the lymphatic system. The transplantation of BM-derived cells in a murine skin flap wound model, for example, promoted the growth of blood vessels and lymphatic capillaries at the injury site and restored lymphatic drainage. The xenotransplantation of human cells into mice was also able to improve survival and functional reconnection of lymph nodes transplanted to the host lymphatic network, enhancing lymphatic vascular supply [20]. Given this evidence, cell therapy may be promising for improving lymphatic circulation and treating lymphedema in the clinical setting.

In another example, autologous G-CSF-mobilized CD34$^+$ cells were used for the treatment of lymphedema secondary to mastectomy and axillary lymphadenectomy. The cells were administered via microinjections in the affected arm, followed by a 12-week follow-up. Volume reduction of lymphedema compared to standard therapy (compression sleeves) was observed as well as pain reduction and improved sensitivity [117]. In contrast, a more recent study using autologous adipose-derived regenerative cells for treating breast cancer-related lymphedema reported no improvement in lymphoscintigraphy, despite patients requiring less conservative management after transplantation. No serious adverse effects were observed [180]. The authors conclude that more refined, randomized studies should be conducted to confirm findings and propose improvements in cell therapy applicable to lymphedema.

2.7.5 Thromboangiitis Obliterans (TAO): Buerger Disease

Thromboangiitis obliterans (TAO) or Buerger's disease is a nonatherosclerotic, segmental inflammatory disease affecting small- and medium-sized arteries and veins in the upper and lower extremities [187]. The pharmacological treatment of TAO focuses on anticoagulation, vasodilators, systemic anti-inflammatory drugs, and analgesics. Besides, surgical options are limited in efficacy and the absence of distal vascular targets makes surgical revascularization complicated. Cellular therapy represents a potential alternative treatment for TAO patients since benefits associated with this modality include more rapid angiogenesis, reduced inflammation, increased temperature and perfusion of ischemic limbs and healing rates of wounds size [122].

The use of adult human BM-derived, cultured, pooled, allogeneic MSC is safe when injected via intramuscular (i.m.) route in TAO patients [71]. In a phase II, prospective, nonrandomized, open-label, multicentric, dose-ranging study, the same authors also tested the efficacy and safety of i.m. injection of adult human BM-derived MSC as a treatment of TAO disease. Reduction in rest pain and improved ulcer healing were demonstrated in the group receiving cell therapy compared to the control group. Few adverse effects were reported, indicating the possible use of cell therapy in TAO treatment [72].

When G-CSF-mobilized PB cells were subcutaneously injected close to the tibia bone, 26 out of 34 treated TAO patients showed a moderately improved outcome. Among them, 13 out of 17 limb ulcers healed. The development of new collaterals was also observed, indicating that autologous cells could be used safely and effectively for therapeutic angiogenesis in patients with TAO [97]. Corroborating these findings, a study involving 67 patients with symptomatic TAO that received autologous whole BM cells into the limb by intramuscular injections, showed clinical and angiographic improvements in almost half of the patients evaluated. Reduction in the amputation rate in symptomatic TAO patients was also a critical prognostic factor considered in this study [106].

Intravenous allogeneic MSC administration has also been explored since it could exert a systemic anti-inflammatory effect in the vasculature and modulate the immune response in TAO. In the case of a single male patient at risk of amputation, four sequential intravenous infusions of BM-MSC from a healthy donor induced significant regression of foot ulcers and improvements in rest pain, walking impairment, and quality of life. 16 months after infusion, the patient had no requirement for further amputation, indicating a potential for sequential infusions as an effective schedule treatment for TAO [122].

2.7.6 Myocardial Infarction (MI)

Cardiovascular events as a consequence of ischemic heart disease represent the leading cause of morbidity and mortality worldwide. Although medical and surgical treatments can improve patient outcomes, no treatment currently available can generate new contractile tissue or reverse ischemia in the myocardium [116]. In this context, the use of stem cells has emerged as a promising and potential therapeutic strategy to regenerate damaged heart tissue as an option for myocardial infarction (MI) treatment.

The use of BM-derived cells, adipose tissue-derived stem cells, skeletal myoblasts, as well as embryonic stem cell-derived cardiomyocytes had been proposed as cardiac cell therapy substrates [104]. An ideal cell therapy applicable to MI should regenerate the vascular network and stimulate the formation of new contractile tissue that can align and synchronize with the existing heart tissue. Also, stem cells should be able to differentiate into other cardiac cell types such as myocytes and vascular endothelial cells or, at least, act via paracrine effects to promote the regenerative process [116].

Pericardial adipose-derived stem cells, for example, were shown to be superior in inducing reparative activities, including myogenesis, vasculogenesis, and expression of cardiogenic transcription factors compared to subcutaneous stem cells, indicating that cell origin is also essential to the outcome in cell therapy applicable to MI [191].

On the other hand, early clinical trials using BM-derived cells only show modest or marginal benefits when cellular therapy was used in acute or chronic MI patients [1, 111]. However, more recent studies have shown promising results with patients experiencing beneficial cardiac effects such as enhanced perfusion, improved left ventricular ejection fraction, and reduced left ventricular end-systolic volume [135]. The differences in outcomes from studies using BM-MNC could be explained by the inter-individual heterogeneity of this cell population. Of note, a clinical trial using an intramyocardial injection of cardiopoietic BM-MSC in post-MI ischemic heart failure patients showed a favorable effect on left ventricular ejection fraction (LVEF), remodeling and overall patient wellness compared to unstimulated BM-MSC or standard clinical care. The cardiopoietic BM-MSC were generated by priming BM-MSC using a combination of cardiogenic factors to transform these cells into cardiac progenitors able to differentiate in functional cardiomyocytes [17, 21].

Cardiac stem cells (CSC) might be more appropriate to promote heart tissue repair since these cells are residing in the heart itself. They are considered a heterogeneous cell population isolated from atrial appendages, pericardial adipose tissue, or epi-/endomyocardial biopsies that represent a purer source of cells with the capacity to differentiate into cardiomyocytes [27]. CSC have been shown to more efficiently express cardiac markers and more effectively differentiate into cardiomyocytes in vitro and in MI murine in vivo models, emerging as the most effective cell source for cell therapy in MI [151]. The challenges of using these cells, however, concern their low availability, the invasive isolation, and the need for costly ex vivo expansion to obtain adequate cell numbers for injection.

Likewise, cardiosphere-derived cells (CDC) constitute a cardiac progenitor cell population isolated from atrial or ventricular biopsy specimens of patients undergoing heart surgery. After tissue processing and culturing, a fibroblast-like cell layer forms and can be further purified and cultured to form cardiospheres. Most of the expanded cells are CD105$^+$, and also express CD117/c-Kit, CD90, CD34, and CD31. These cells were also negative for the MDR1, CD133, and CD45 [129, 161]. Autologous and allogeneic intracoronary CDC transplantation induces myocardial regeneration with a decrease in scar size and an increase in viable and functional tissue in patients with MI, and ischemic left ventricular dysfunction [35, 119]. Despite promising findings, the challenge of obtaining cardiac stem cells should be considered and standardization of isolation, and culturing protocols should be addressed.

2.8   Final Remarks

Although no ideal stem cell source is yet established for treating vascular diseases, there is an expected interest in clinical research using the transplantation of endothelial progenitor cells (EPC) as a potential approach to regenerate endothelial cells and blood vessels and to induce therapeutic angiogenesis. Even though very promising, the clinical trials have shown moderate to low improvements in humans when compared to animal preclinical studies. The clinical effectiveness may vary among patients, in part, due to different genetic and physiologic status and medical conditions. It is also important to highlight that what has been termed as "putative EPC" and used in clinical trials are, actually, a heterogeneous population of hematopoietic cells that may take part in neovascularization processes by paracrine supportive mechanisms. Nonetheless, the scientific community is getting closer to reaching a consensus on the bonafide endothelial stem/progenitor cells' identity. Additionaly, many efforts are being made using the differentiation of induced pluripotent cells into vascular progenitors for therapeutic purposes.

Beyond the efforts to identify actual EPC, the majority of clinical trials on cell-based transplantation for vascular diseases concentrates on using MSC with paracrine activity derived mainly from BM and AT. As discussed earlier in this chapter, MSC is a generic term for a variety of cell types derived from bone marrow and connective tissue that meet the minimum criteria formulated by the ISCT. The high interest in using these cells for therapeutic purposes relies on their angiogenic and immunosuppressive properties and tissue repair capabilities, besides the easy accessibility from BM, AT, or even UC. This makes them not only an attractive therapeutical option in autologous but also in allogeneic transplants. Furthermore, the already completed trials have shown that MSC are safe and seem to cause no significant side effects to the patients.

Finally, it is also important to keep in mind that even if the best cells are transplanted into a patient, arriving in a hostile environment, they are susceptible to fail. Therefore, the parallel modulation of the host environments also appears to be important in order to achieve long-term effects. Taken together, the fast-growing field of regenerative medicine is progressively paving the road for the future use of cell-based bioproducts for vascular diseases. These bioproducts may originate not only from cells and known modalities of transplantation as discussed in this chapter but also from bioengineering of cells and tissues and their use as an "off-the-shelf" medical product. Given the significant advances made in adult stem cell research in conjunction with the, as of now, tentative entry of both ESC- and iPSC-based therapies into clinical practice, the future seems very promising. The ground is fertile, and much remains to come.

References

1. Abdel-Latif A, Bolli R, Tleyjeh IM, et al. Adult bone marrow-derived cells for cardiac repair: a systematic review and meta-analysis. Arch Intern Med. 2007;167:989–97.
2. AbuSamra DB, Aleisa FA, Al-Amoodi AS, et al. Not just a marker: CD34 on human hematopoietic stem/progenitor cells dominates vascular selectin binding along with CD44. Blood Adv. 2017;(27):2799–816.
3. Acar M, Kocherlakota KS, Murphy MM, et al. Deep imaging of bone marrows shows nondividing stem cells are mainly perisinusoidal. Nature. 2015;526:16–130.
4. Adamiak M, Cheng G, Bobis-Wozowicz S, et al. Induced pluripotent stem cell (iPSC)–derived extracellular vesicles are safer and more effective for cardiac repair than iPSCs. Circ Res. 2018;122:296–309.
5. Adler DS, Lazarus H, Nair R, et al. Safety and efficacy of bone marrow-derived autologous CD133 stem cell therapy. Front Biosci. 2011;3:506–14.
6. Anderson JL, Halperin JL, Albert NM, et al. Management of patients with peripheral artery disease (compilation of 2005 and 2011 ACCF/AHA guideline recommendations): a report of the American College of Cardiology Foundation/American Heart Association task force on practice guidelines. Circulation. 2013;127:1425–43.
7. Anthony B, Link DC. Regulation of hematopoietic stem cells by bone marrow stromal cells. Trends Immunol. 2013;35:32–7.
8. Arai F, Hirao A, Ohmura M, et al. Tie2/ angiopoietin-1 signaling regulates hematopoietic stem cell quiescence in the bone marrow niche. Cell. 2004;118:149–61.
9. Aronowitz JA, Lockhart RA, Hakakian CS. Mechanical versus enzymatic isolation of stromal vascular fraction cells from adipose tissue. Springerplus. 2015;4:713.
10. Arutyunyan I, Elchaninov A, Makarov A, et al. Umbilical cord as prospective source for mesenchymal stem cell-based therapy. Stem Cells Int. 2016;2016:ID 6901286. 17 pages
11. Asahara T, Murohara T, Sullivan A, et al. Isolation of putative progenitor endothelial cells for angiogenesis. Science. 1997;275:964–7.
12. Ashton B, Eaglesom C, Bab I, et al. Distribution of fibroblastic colony forming cells in rabbit bone marrow and assay of their osteogenic potential by an *in vivo* diffusion chamber method. Calc Tissue Int. 1984;36:83–6.
13. Baddoo M, Hill K, Wilkinson R, et al. Characterization of mesenchymal stem cells isolated from murine bone marrow by negative selection. J Cell Biochem. 2003;89:1235–49.
14. Baghaei K, Hashemi SM, Tokhanbiglil S, et al. Isolation, differentiation, and characterization of mesenchymal stem cells from human bone marrow. Gastroenterol Hepatol Bed Bench. 2017;10:208–13.
15. Bara JJ, Herrmann M, Menzel U, et al. Three-dimensional culture and characterization of mononuclear cells from human bone marrow. Cytotherapy. 2015;17:458–72.
16. Baran J, Kowalczyk D, Ozog M, et al. Three-color flow cytometry detection of intracellular cytokines in peripheral blood mononuclear cells: comparative analysis of phorbol myristate acetate-ionomycin and phytohemagglutinin stimulation. Cell Immunol. 2001;8:303–13.
17. Bartunek J, Behfar A, Dolatabadi D, et al. Cardiopoietic stem cell therapy in heart failure. The C-CURE (Cardiopoietic stem cell therapy in heart failURE) multicenter randomized trial with lineage-specified biologics. J Am Coll Cardiol. 2013;61:2329–38.
18. Basile DP, Yoder MC. Circulating and tissue resident endothelial progenitor cells. J Cell Physiol. 2014;229:10–6.
19. Beane OS, Fonseca VC, Cooper LL, et al. Impact of aging on the regenerative properties of bone marrow-, muscle-, and adipose-derived mesenchymal stem/stromal cells. PLoS One. 2014;9:e115963.
20. Beerens M, Aranguren XL, Hendrickx B, et al. Multipotent adult progenitor cells support lymphatic regeneration at multiple anatomical levels during wound healing and lymphedema. Sci Rep. 2018;8:3852.

21. Behfar A, Terzic A. Derivation of a cardiopoietic population from human mesenchymal stem cells yields cardiac progeny. Nat Clin Pract Cardiovasc Med. 2006;3:S78–82.
22. Bhatia M, Bonnet D, Kapp U, et al. Quantitative analysis reveals expansion of human hematopoietic repopulating cells after short-term *ex vivo* culture. J Exp Med. 1997;186(4):619–24.
23. Bianchi F, Maioli F, Leonardi E, et al. A new nonenzymatic method and device to obtain a fat tissue derivative highly enriched in pericyte-like elements by mild mechanical forces from human lipoaspirates. Cell Transplant. 2012;22:2063–77.
24. Bianco P, Cao X, Frenette PS, et al. The meaning, the sense and the significance: translating the science of mesenchymal stem cells into medicine. Nat Med. 2013;19:35–42.
25. Biscetti F, Bonadia N, Nardella E, et al. The role of the stem cells therapy in the peripheral artery disease. Int J Mol Sci. 2019;20:2233.
26. Blumberg SN, Berger A, Hwang L, et al. The role of stem cells in the treatment of diabetic foot ulcer. Diabetes Res Clin Pract. 2012;96:1–9.
27. Bolli R, Chugh AR, D'Amario D, et al. Cardiac stem cells in patients with ischaemic cardiomyopathy (Scipio): initial results of a randomized phase 1 trial. Lancet. 2011;378:1847–57.
28. Bourin P, Bunnell BA, Casteilla L, et al. Stromal cells from the adipose tissue-derived stromal vascular fraction and culture expanded adipose tissue-derived stromal/stem cells: a joint statement of the International Federation for Adipose Therapeutics and Science (IFATS) and the International Society for Cellular Therapy (ISCT). Cytotherapy. 2013;15:641–8.
29. Can A, Karahuseyinoglu S. Concise review: human umbilical cord stroma with regard to the source of fetus-derived stem cells. Stem Cells. 2007;25:2886–95.
30. Caplan AI. Mesenchymal stem cells. J Orthop Res. 1991;9:641–50.
31. Caplan AI. What's in a name? Tissue Eng Part A. 2010;16:2415–7.
32. Capoccia BJ, Robson DL, Levac KD, et al. Revascularization of ischemic limbs after transplantation of human bone marrow cells with high aldehyde dehydrogenase activity. Blood. 2009;113:5340–51.
33. Castro A, León M, del Furió V, et al. Generation of a human iPSC line by mRNA reprogramming. Stem Cell Res. 2018;28:157–60.
34. Ceafalan LC, Enciu AM, Fertig TEM, et al. Heterocellular molecular contacts in the mammalian stem cell niche. Eur J Cell Biol. 2018;97:442–61.
35. Chakravarty T, Makkar RR, Ascheim DD, et al. ALLogeneic heart STem cells to achieve myocardial regeneration (ALLSTAR) trial: rationale and design. Cell Transplant. 2017;26:205–14.
36. Champlin R. Chapter 69: Hematopoietic cellular transplantation. In: Kufe DW, Pollock RR, Weichselbaum RR, Bast RC, Gansler TS, Holland JF, Frei E, editors. Holland-Frei cancer medicine. 6th ed; 2003. ISBN-10:1-55009-213-8.
37. Chopra H, Hung MK, Kwong DL, et al. Insights into endothelial progenitor cells: origin, classification, potentials, and prospects. Stem Cells International ID9847015. 2018. 24p.
38. Chu DT, Phuong TNT, Tien NLB, et al. Adipose tissue stem cells for therapy: an update on the Progress of isolation, culture, storage, and clinical application. J Clin Med. 2019;8:917.
39. Compagna R, Amato B, Massa S, et al. Cell therapy in patients with critical limb ischemia. Stem Cells Int. 2015;2015:931420.
40. Condé-Green A, de Amorim NF, Pitanguy I. Influence of decantation, washing and centrifugation on adipocyte and mesenchymal stem cell content of aspirated adipose tissue: a comparative study. J Plast Sreconstr Aesthet Surg. 2010;63:1375–81.
41. Conneally E, Cashman J, Petzer A, et al. Expansion *in vitro* of transplantable human cord blood stem cells demonstrated using q quantitative assay of their lympho-myeloid repopulating activity in nonobese diabetic- scid/scid mice. PNAS. 1997;94:9836–41.
42. Conte MS, Bradbury AW, Kolh P, et al. Global vascular guidelines on the management of chronic limb-threatening ischemia. Eur J Vasc Endovasc Surg. 2019;58(1S):S1–S109.e33.
43. Cooke JP, Losordo DW. Modulating the vascular response to limb ischemia: angiogenic and cell therapies. Circ Res. 2015;116:1561–78.
44. Cooper DKC, Ekser B, Tector AJ. A brief history of clinical xenotransplantation. Int J Surg. 2015;23:205–10.

45. Davies BM, Snelling SJB, Quek L, et al. Identifying the optimum source of mesenchymal stem cells for use in knee surgery. J Orthop Res O Publ Orthop Res Soc. 2017;35:1868–75.
46. Davies MG. Critical limb ischemia: cell and molecular therapies for limb salvage. Methodist Debakey Cardiovasc J. 2012;8:20–7.
47. De Francesco F, Mannucci S, Conti G, et al. A non-enzymatic method to obtain a fat tissue derivative highly enriched in adipose stem cells (ASCs) from human Lipoaspirates: preliminary results. Int J Mol Sci. 2018;19:2061.
48. Dessels LC, Alessandrini M, Pepper MS. Factors influencing the umbilical cord blood stem cell industry: an evolving treatment landscape. Stem Cells Transl Med. 2018;7:643–50.
49. Dhar M, Neilsen N, Beatty K, et al. Equine peripheral blood-derived mesenchymal stem cells: isolation, identification, trilineage differentiation and effect of hyperbaric oxygen treatment. Equine Vet J. 2012;44:600–5.
50. Digirolamo CM, Stokes D, Colter D, et al. Propagation and senescence of human marrow stromal cells in culture: a simple colony-forming assay identifies samples with the greatest potential to propagate and differentiate. Br J Haematol. 1999;107:275–81.
51. Ding L, Morrison SJ. Haematopoietic stem cells and early lymphoid progenitors occupy distinct bone marrow niches. Nature. 2013;14:231–5.
52. Dominici M, Le Blanc K, Mueller I, et al. Minimal criteria for defining multipotent mesenchymal stromal cells. The International Society for Cellular Therapy position statement. Cytotherapy. 2006;8:315–7.
53. Dooley DC, Oppenlander BK, Xiao M. Analysis of primitive CD34- and CD34+ hematopoietic cells from adults: gain and loss of CD34 antigen by undifferentiated cells are closely linked to proliferative status in culture. Stem Cells. 2004;22:556–69.
54. Dubsky M, Jirkovska A, Bem R, et al. Both autologous bone marrow mononuclear cell and peripheral blood progenitor cell therapies similarly improve ischaemia in patients with diabetic foot in comparison with control treatment. Diabetes Metab Res Rev. 2013;29:369–76.
55. Dubsky M, Jirkovská A, Bem R, et al. Comparison of the effect of stem cell therapy and percutaneous transluminal angioplasty on diabetic foot disease in patients with critical limb ischemia. Cytotherapy. 2014;16:1733e–1738.
56. Egusa H, Sonoyama W, Nishimura M, et al. Stem cells in dentistry part I: stem cell sources. J Prosthodont Res. 2012;56:151–65.
57. Eslaminejad MB, Nadri S. Murine mesenchymal stem cell isolated and expanded in low- and high-density culture system: surface antigen expression and osteogenic culture mineralization. In Vitro Cell Dev Biol Anim. 2009;45:451–9.
58. Eslaminejad MB, Nikmahzar A, Taghiyar L, et al. Murine mesenchymal stem cells isolated by low density primary culture system. Develop Growth Differ. 2006;48:361–70.
59. Evans MJ, Kaufman MH. Establishment in culture of pluripotential cells from mouse embryos. Nature. 1981;292:154–6.
60. Fang S, Wei J, Pentinmikko N, et al. Generation of functional vessels from a single ckit+ adult vascular endothelial stem cell. PLoS Biol. 2012;10:e1001407.
61. FDA U.S. Food and Drug Administration (FDA). Guidance for Industry. Biologics license applications for minimally manipulated unrelated allogeneic placenta/umbilical cord blood intended for hematopoietic and immunologic reconstitution in patients with disorders affecting the hematopoietic system. 2014. Available from: http://www.fda.gov/downloads/BiologicsBloodVaccines/GuidanceComplianceRegulatoryInformation/Guidances/CellularandGeneTherapy/UCM357135.pdf.
62. Fei X, Wu Y, Chang K, et al. Co-culture of cord blood CD34+ cells with human BM mesenchymal stromal cells enhances short-term engraftment of cord blood cells in NOD/SCID mice. Cytotherapy. 2007;9:338–47.
63. Figueiredo C, Blasczyk R. A future with less HLA: potential clinical applications of HLA-universal cells. Tissue Antigens. 2015;85:443–9.
64. Frangogiannis NG. Cell therapy for peripheral artery disease. Curr Opin Pharmacol. 2018;39:27–34.

65. Frese L, Dijkman PE, Hoerstrup SP. Adipose tissue-derived stem cells in regenerative medicine. Transfus Med Hemother. 2016;43:268–74.
66. Fujisawa T, Tura-Ceide O, Hunter A, et al. Endothelial progenitor cells do not originate from the bone marrow. Circulation. 2019;14:1524–6.
67. Gangadaran P, Rajendran RL, Lee HW, et al. Extracellular vesicles from mesenchymal stem cells activates VEGF receptors and accelerates recovery of hindlimb ischemia. J Control Release. 2017;264:112–26.
68. Garry DJ, Garry MG. Interspecies chimeras and the generation of humanizes organs. Circ Res. 2019;124:23–5.
69. Gibson T. Zoografting: a curious chapter in the history of plastic surgery. Br J Plast Surg. 1955;8:234–42.
70. Gimble J, Katz A, Bunnell B. Adipose-derived stem cells for regenerative medicine. Circ Res. 2007;100:1249–60.
71. Gupta PK, Chullikana A, Parakh R, et al. A double blind randomized placebo-controlled phase I/II study assessing the safety and efficacy of allogeneic bone marrow derived mesenchymal stem cell in critical limb ischemia. J Transl Med. 2013;11:143.
72. Gupta PK, Krishna A, Chullikana A, et al. Administration of adult human bone marrow-derived, cultured, pooled, allogeneic mesenchymal stromal cells in critical limb ischemia due to Buerger's disease: phase II study report suggests clinical efficacy. Stem Cells Transl Med. 2017;5:1–11.
73. Hassan G, Kasem I, Soukkarieh C, et al. A simple method to isolate and expand human umbilical cord derived mesenchymal stem cells: using explant method and umbilical cord blood serum. Int J Stem Cells. 2017;10:184–92.
74. Hassan HT, El-Sheemy M. Adult bone-marrow stem cells and their potential in medicine. J R Soc Med. 2004;97:465–71.
75. He QL, Wan C, Li G. Concise review: multipotent mesenchymal stromal cells in blood. Stem Cells. 2007;25:69e77.
76. Hendijani F, Sadeghi-Aliabadi H, Haghjooy Javanmard S. Comparison of human mesenchymal stem cells isolated by explant culture method from entire umbilical cord and Wharton's jelly matrix. Cell Tissue Bank. 2014;15:555–65.
77. Herrmann M, Bara JJ, Sprecher CM, et al. Pericyte plasticity-comparative investigation of the angiogenic and multilineage potential of pericytes from different human tissues. Eur Cells Mater. 2016;31:236–49.
78. Herrmann M, Binder A, Menzel U, et al. CD34/CD133 enriched bone marrow progenitor cells promote neovascularization of tissue engineered constructs in vivo. Stem Cell Res. 2014;13:465–77.
79. Herrmann M, Hildebrand M, Menzel U, et al. Phenotypic characterization of bone marrow mononuclear cells and derived stromal cell populations from iliac crest, vertebral body and femoral head. Int J Mol Sci. 2019;20:piiE3454.
80. Hirschi K, Dejana E. Resident endothelial progenitors make themselves at home. Cell Stem Cell. 2018;23:153–5.
81. Holm JS, Toyserkani NM, Sorensen JA. Adipose-derived stem cells for treatment of chronic ulcers: current status. Stem Cell Res Ther. 2018;9:142.
82. Hordviewska A, Popiotek T, Horecka A. Characteristics of hematopoietic stem cells of umbilical cord blood. Cytotechnology. 2015;67:387–96.
83. Huang P, Li S, Han M, et al. Autologous transplantation of granulocyte colony stimulating factor-mobilized peripheral blood mononuclear cells improves critical limb ischemia in diabetes. Diabetes Care. 2005;28:2155–60.
84. Idei N, Soga J, Hata T, et al. Autologous bone-marrow mononuclear cell implantation reduces long-term major amputation risk in patients with limb ischemia: a comparison of atherosclerotic peripheral arterial disease and Buerger disease. Circ Cardiovasc Interv. 2011;4:15–25.
85. Iftimia-Mander A, Hourd P, Dainty R, et al. Mesenchymal stem cell isolation from human umbilical cord tissue: understanding and minimizing variability in cell yield for process optimization. Biopreserv Biobank. 2013;11:291–8.

86. Ingram DA, Caplice NM, Yoder MC. Unresolved questions, changing definitions, and novel paradigms for defining endothelial progenitor cells. Blood. 2015;106:1525–31.
87. International Council for Commonality in Blood Banking Automation: B Rice, editors. ISBT 128 standard, standard terminology for medical products of human origin. Version 7.32. San Bernardino, CA: 2020. Available from: http://www.iccbba.org/tech-library/iccbba-documents/standard-terminology. Accessed in 28/01/2020.
88. Jang Y, Choi J, Park N, et al. Development of immunocompatible pluripotent stem cells via CRISPR-based human leukocyte antigen engineering. Exp Mol Med. 2019;51(3)
89. Jialal I, Devaraj S, Singh U, et al. Decreased number and impaired functionality of endothelial progenitor cells in subjects with metabolic syndrome: implications for increased cardiovascular risk. Atherosclerosis. 2010;211:297–302.
90. Karpova D, Rettig MP, DiPersio JF. Mobilized peripheral blood: an updated perspective. F1000Res. 2019;8:2125.
91. Kataoka K, Medina RJ, Kageyama T, et al. Participation of adult mouse bone marrow cells in reconstitution of skin. Am J Pathol. 2003;163:1227–31.
92. Kavala AA, Turkyilmaz S. Autogenously derived regenerative cell therapy for venous leg ulcers. Arch Med Sci Atheroscler Dis. 2018;3:e156–63.
93. Kawamura M, Miyagawa S, Fukushima S, et al. Enhanced survival of transplanted human induced pluripotent stem cell–derived cardiomyocytes by the combination of cell sheets with the pedicled omental flap technique in a porcine heart. Circulation. 2013;128:S87–94.
94. Kekre N, Antin JH. Hematopoietic stem cell transplantation donor sources in the 21st century: choosing the ideal donor when a perfect match does not exist. Blood. 2014;124:334–43.
95. Kervadec A, Bellamy V, El Harane N, et al. Cardiovascular progenitor–derived extracellular vesicles recapitulate the beneficial effects of their parent cells in the treatment of chronic heart failure. J Hear Lung Transpl. 2016;35:795–807.
96. Kiel MJ, Yilmaz OH, Iwashita T, et al. SLAM family receptors distinguish hematopoietic stem and progenitor cell and reveal endothelial niches for stem cells. Cell. 2005;1217:1109–21.
97. Kim D, Kim AM, Joh DJ, et al. Angiogenesis facilitated by autologous whole bone marrow stem cell transplantation for Buerger's disease. Stem Cells. 2006;24:1194–200.
98. Kirana S, Stratmann B, Prante C, et al. Autologous stem cell therapy in the treatment of limb ischaemia induced chronic tissue ulcers of diabetic foot patients. Int J Clin Pract. 2012;66:384–93.
99. Koh YJ, Koh BI, Kim H, et al. Stromal vascular fraction from adipose tissue forms profound vascular network through the dynamic reassembly of blood endothelial cells. Arterioscler Thromb Vasc Biol. 2011;31:1141–50.
100. Konstantinow A, Arnold A, Djabali K, et al. Therapy of ulcus cruris of venous and mixed venous arterial origin with autologous, adult, native progenitor cells from subcutaneous adipose tissue: a prospective clinical pilot study. J Eur Acad Dermatol Venereol. 2017;31:2104–18.
101. Koobatian MT, Liang MS, Swartz DD, et al. Differential effects of culture senescence and mechanical stimulation on the proliferation and leiomyogenic differentiation of MSC from different sources: implications for engineering vascular grafts. Tissue Eng Part A. 2015;1:1364–75.
102. Körbling M, Anderlini P. Peripheral blood stem cell versus bone marrow allotransplantation: does the source of hematopietic stem cells matter? Blood. 2001;98:2900–8.
103. Kot M, Baj-Krzyworzek M, Szatanek R, et al. The importance of HLA in "off-the-shelf" allogeneic mesenchymal stem cells based-therapies. Int J Mol Sci. 2019;20:5680.
104. Kwon YW, Yang HM, Cho HJ. Cell therapy for myocardial infarction. Int J Stem Cells. 2010;3:8–15.
105. Lau S, Eicke D, Oliveira MC, et al. Low immunogenic endothelial cells maintain morphological and functional properties required for vascular tissue engineering. Tissue Eng A. 2018;24:432–47.
106. Lee KB, Kang ES, Kim AK, et al. Stem cell therapy in patients with thromboangiitis obliterans: assessment of the long-term clinical outcome and analysis of the prognostic factors. Int J Stem Cells. 2011;4:2.

107. Leemhuis T, Yoder MC, Grigsby S, et al. Isolation of primitive human bone marrow hematopoietic progenitor cells using Hoechst 33342 and rhodamine 123. Exp Hematol. 1996;24:1215–24.
108. Li J, Ezzelarab MB, Cooper DKC. Do mesenchymal stem cells function across species barriers? Relevance for xenotransplantation. Xenotransplantation. 2012;19:273–85.
109. Liew A, Bhattacharya V, Shaw J, et al. Cell therapy for critical limb ischemia: a meta-analysis of randomized controlled trials. Angiology. 2016;67:444–55.
110. Lin TC, Lee OK. Stem cells: a primer. Chin J Physiol. 2008;51:197–207.
111. Lipinski MJ, Biondi-Zoccai GG, Abbate A, et al. Impact of intracoronary cell therapy on left ventricular function in the setting of acute myocardial infarction: a collaborative systematic review and meta-analysis of controlled clinical trials. J Am Coll Cardiol. 2007;50:1761–7.
112. Loike JD, Kadish A. Ethical rejections of xenotransplantation? EMBO Rep. 2018;9:e46337.
113. Lopes L, Setia O, Aurshina A, et al. Stem cell therapy for diabetic foot ulcers: a review of preclinical and clinical research. Stem Cell Res Ther. 2018;9:188.
114. Lucas D. The bone marrow microenvironment for hematopoietic stem cells. In: Birbrair A, editor. Stem cell microenvironments and beyond, Advances in experimental medicine and biology, vol. 1041: Springer Nature Switzerland; 2017.
115. MacAskill MG, Saif J, Jansen MA, et al. Robust revascularization in models of limb ischemia using a clinically translatable human stem cell-derived endothelial cell product. Mol Ther. 2018;26:7.
116. Madigan M, Atoui R. Therapeutic use of stem cells for myocardial infarction. Bioengineering. 2018;5:28.
117. Maldonado GEM, Alvarez CA, Rez PE, et al. Autologous stem cells for the treatment of post-mastectomy lymphedema: a pilot study. Cytotherapy. 2011;13:1249–55.
118. Maleki M, Ghanbarvand F, Mohammad RBME, et al. Comparison of mesenchymal stem cell markers in multiple human adult stem cells. Int J Stem Cells. 2014;7:118–26.
119. Malliaras K, Makkar RR, Smith RR, et al. Intracoronary cardiosphere-derived cells after myocardial infarction: evidence of therapeutic regeneration in the final 1-year results of the CADUCEUS trial (Cardiosphere- derived autologous stem cells to reverse ventricular dysfunction). J Am Coll Cardiol. 2007;63:110–22.
120. Mandai M, Watanabe A, Kurimoto Y, et al. Autologous induced stem-cell–derived retinal cells for macular degeneration. New Engl J Med. 2017;376:1038–46.
121. Martin-Rendon E, Brunskill S, Dore'e C, et al. Stem cell treatment for acute myocardial infarction. Cochrane Database Syst Rev. 2008;9:CD006536.
122. Martin-Rufino JD, Lozano FS, Redondo AM, et al. Sequential intravenous allogeneic mesenchymal stromal cells as a potential treatment for thromboangiitis obliterans (Buerger's disease). Stem Cell Res Ther. 2018;9:150.
123. Mathiyalagan P, Liang Y, Kim D, et al. Angiogenic mechanisms of human CD341 stem cell exosomes in the repair of ischemic hindlimb. Circ Res. 2017;120:1466–76.
124. Matoba S, Tatsumi T, Murohara T, et al. Long-term clinical outcome after intramuscular implantation of bone marrow mononuclear cells (therapeutic angiogenesis by cell transplantation [TACT] trial) in patients with chronic limb ischemia. Am Heart J. 2008;156:1010–8.
125. Mattapally S, Pawlik KM, Fast VG, et al. Human leukocyte antigen class I and II knockout human induced pluripotent stem cell-derived cells: universal donor for cell therapy. J Am Heart Assoc. 2018;7:e010239.
126. McDonald AI, Shirali AS, Aragón R, et al. Endothelial regeneration of large vessels is a biphasic process driven by local cells with distinct proliferative capacities. Cell Stem Cell. 2018;23:210–25.
127. Medina RJ, O'Neill CL, Humphreys MW, et al. Outgrowth endothelial cells: characterization and their potential for reversing ischemic retinopathy. Invest Ophthalmol Vis Sci. 2010;51:5906–13.
128. Menasché P, Vanneaux V, Hagège A, et al. Transplantation of human embryonic stem cell–derived cardiovascular progenitors for severe ischemic left ventricular dysfunction. J Am Coll Cardiol. 2018;71:429–38.

129. Messina E, De Angelis L, Frati G, et al. Isolation and expansion of adult cardiac stem cells from human and murine heart. Circ Res. 2004;29:911–21.
130. Miana VV, González EAP. Adipose tissue stem cells in regenerative medicine. eCancer. 2018;12:822.
131. Miller CL, Eaves CJ. Expansion *in vitro* of adult murine hematopoietic stem cells with transplantable lympho-myeloid reconstituting ability. PNAS. 1997;94:13648–53.
132. Min WK, Bae JS, Park BC, et al. Proliferation and osteoblastic differentiation of bone marrow stem cells: comparison of vertebral body and iliac crest. Eur Spine J O Publ Eur Spine Soc Eur Spinal Deform Soc Eur Sect Cerv Spine Res Soc. 2010;19:1753–60.
133. Mitchell JB, Mcintosh K, Zvonic S, et al. Immunophenotype of human adipose-derived cells: temporal changes in stromal-associated and stem cell–associated markers. Stem Cells. 2006;24:376–85.
134. Montelatici E, Baluce B, Ragni E, et al. Defining the identity of human adipose-derived mesenchymal stem cells. Biochem Cell Biol. 2014;93:1–9.
135. Nigro P, Bassetti B, Cavallotti L, et al. Cell therapy for heart disease after 15 years: unmet expectations. Pharmacol Res. 2018;127:77–91.
136. O'Donnell EA, Ernst DN, Hingorani R. Multiparameter flow cytometry: advances in high resolution analysis. Immune Netw. 2013;13:43–54.
137. Okita K, Nakagawa M, Hyenjong H, et al. Generation of mouse induced pluripotent stem cells without viral vectors. Sci New York N Y. 2008;322:949–53.
138. Perin EC, Murphy MP, March KL, et al. Evaluation of cell therapy on exercise performance and limb perfusion in peripheral artery disease: the CCTRN patients with intermittent claudication injected with ALDH bright cells (PACE) trial. Circulation. 2017;11:1417–28.
139. Petterson J, Moore CH, Palser E, et al. Detecting primitive hematopoietic stem cells in total nucleated and mononuclear cell fractions from umbilical cord blood segments and units. J Transl Med. 2015;13:94.
140. Pignolo RJ, Kassem M. Circulating osteogenic cells: implications for injury, repair, and regeneration. J Bone Miner Res. 2011;26:1685e93.
141. Pittenger MF, Mackay AM, Beck SC, et al. Multilineage potential of adult human mesenchymal stem cells. Science. 1999;284:143–7.
142. Pranke P, Hendrikx J, Debnath G, et al. Immunophenotype of hematopoietic stem cells from placental/umbilical cord blood after culture placental/umbilical cord blood. Braz J Med Biol Res. 2005;38:1775–89.
143. Qadura M, Terenzi DC, Verma S, et al. Concise review: cell therapy for critical limb ischemia: an integrated review of preclinical and clinical studies. Stem Cells. 2018;36:161–71.
144. Reemtsma K, McCracken BH, Schlegel JU, et al. Renal heterotransplantation in man. Ann Surg. 1964;160:384–410.
145. Reinisch A, Hofmann NA, Obenauf AC, et al. Humanized large-scale expanded endothelial colony-forming cells function *in vitro* and *in vivo*. Blood. 2009;113:6716–25.
146. Risbud MV, Shapiro IM, Guttapalli A, et al. Osteogenic potential of adult human stem cells of the lumbar vertebral body and the iliac crest. Spine. 2006;31:83–9.
147. Robinson SN, Ng J, Niu T, et al. Adult and embryonic stem cells. Bone Marrow Transplant. 2006;37:359–66.
148. Rodbell M. The metabolism of isolated fat cells, IV: regulation of release of protein by lipolytic hormones and insulin. J Biol Chem. 1966b;241:3909–17.
149. Rodbell M, Jones AB. Metabolism of isolated fat cells, 3: the similar inhibitory action of phospholipase C (Clostridium perfringens alpha toxin) and of insulin on lipolysis stimulated by lipolytic hormones and theophylline. J Biol Chem. 1966;241:140–2.
150. Rodbell M. Metabolism of isolated fat cells, II: the similar effects of phospholipase C (Clostridium perfringens alpha toxin) and of insulin on glucose and amino acid metabolism. J Biol Chem. 1966a;241:130–9.
151. Rossini A, Frati C, Lagrasta C, et al. Human cardiac and bone marrow stromal cells exhibit distinctive properties related to their origin. Cardiovasc Res. 2011;89:650–60.

152. Roura S, Pujal JM, Montón CG, et al. The role and potential of umbilical cord blood in an era of news therapies: a review. Stem Cell Res Ther. 2015;6:123.
153. Roux FA, Sai P, Deschamps JY. Xenotransfusions, past and present. Xenotransplantation. 2007;14:208–16.
154. Ruzicka K, Grskovic B, Pavlovic V, et al. Differentiation of human umbilical cord blood CD133 stem cells towards myelo-monocytic lineage. Clin Chim Acta. 2004;343:85–92.
155. Schächinger V, Erbs S, Elsässer A, et al. Intracoronary bone marrow-derived progenitor cells in acute myocardical infarction. N Engl J Med. 2006;355:1210–21.
156. Senesi L, De Francesco F, Farinelli L, et al. Mechanical and enzymatic procedures to isolate the stromal vascular fraction from adipose tissue: preliminar results. Front Cell Dev Biol. 2019;7:88.
157. Sharma RK, John JR. Role of stem cells in the management of chronic wounds. Indian J Plast Surg. 2012;45:237–43.
158. Shi Y, Desponts C, Do JT, et al. Induction of pluripotent stem cells from mouse embryonic fibroblasts by Oct4 and Klf4 with small-molecule compounds. Cell Stem Cell. 2008;6:568–74.
159. Siclari VA, Zhu J, Akiyama K, et al. Mesenchymal progenitors residing close to the bone surface are functionally distinct from those in the central bone marrow. Bone. 2013;53:575–86.
160. Sipp D, Robey PG, Turner L. Clear up this stem-cell mess. Nature. 2018;561:455–7.
161. Smith RR, Barile L, Cho HC, et al. Regenerative potential of cardiosphere-derived cells expanded from percutaneous endomyocardial biopsy specimens. Circulation. 2007;20:896–908.
162. Soleimani M, Nadri S. A protocol for isolation and culture of mesenchymal stem cells from mouse bone marrow. Nat Protoc. 2009;4:102–6.
163. Song WK, Park KM, Kim HJ, et al. Treatment of macular degeneration using embryonic stem cell-derived retinal pigment epithelium: preliminary results in Asian patients. Stem Cell Rep. 2015;4:860–72.
164. Stone RC, Stojadinovic O, Rosa AM, et al. A bioengineered living cell construct activates an acute wound healing response in venous leg ulcers. Sci Transl Med. 2017;04:371.
165. Strioga M, Viswanathan S, Darinskas A, et al. Same or not the same? Comparison of adipose tissue-derived versus bone marrow-derived mesenchymal stem and stromal cells. Stem Cells Dev. 2012;21:2724–52.
166. Suarez LJ, Herrera C, Pan M, et al. Regenerative therapy in patients with a revascularized acute anterior myocardial infarction and depressed ventricular function. Rev Esp Cardiol. 2007;60:357–65.
167. Sugiyama T, Kohara H, Noda M, et al. Maintenance of the hematopoietic stem cell pool by CXCL12-CXCR4 chemokine signaling in bone marrow stromal cell niches. Immunity. 2006;256:977–88.
168. Sullivan S, Stacey GN, Akazawa C, et al. Quality control guidelines for clinical-grade human induced pluripotent stem cell lines. Regen Med. 2018;13:859–66.
169. Svolacchia F, De Francesco F, Trovato L, et al. An innovative regenerative treatment of scars with dermal micrografts. J Cosmet Dermatol. 2016;1–9.
170. Szade K, Gulati GS, Chan CKF, et al. Where hematopoietic stem cells live: the bone marrow niche. Antioxid Redox Signal. 2018;29:191–204.
171. Takahashi K, Tanabe K, Ohnuki M, et al. Induction of pluripotent stem cells from adult human fibroblasts by defined factors. Cell. 2007;131:861–72.
172. Takahashi K, Yamanaka S. Induction of pluripotent stem cells from mouse embryonic and adult fibroblasts cultures by defined factors. Cell. 2006;126:663–76.
173. Tateishi-Yuyama E, Matsubara H, Murohara T, et al. Therapeutic angiogenesis using cell transplantation study I. therapeutic angiogenesis for patients with limb ischaemia by autologous transplantation of bone-marrow cells: a pilot study and a randomised controlled trial. Lancet. 2002;360:427–35.
174. Tepper OM, Carr J, Allen RJ, et al. Decreased circulating progenitor cell number and failed mechanisms of stromal cell derived factor-1alpha mediated bone marrow mobilization impair diabetic tissue repair. Diabetes. 2010;59:1974–83.

175. Thomson JA, Itskovitz-Eldor J, Shapiro SS, et al. Embryonic stem cell lines derived from human blastocysts. Science. 1998;282:1145–7.
176. Tian H, Huang S, Gong F, et al. Karyotyping, immunophenotyping, and apoptosis analyses on human hematopoietic precursor cells derived from umbilical cord blood following long-term *ex vivo* expansion. Cancer Genet Cytogenet. 2005;157:33–6.
177. Todorova D, Simoncini S, Lacroix R, et al. Extracellular vesicles in angiogenesis. Circ Res. 2017;120:1658–73.
178. Tondreau T, Lagneaux L, Dejeneffe M, et al. Isolation of BM mesenchymal stem cells by plastic adhesion or negative selection: phenotype, proliferation kinetics and differentiation potential. Cytotherapy. 2004;6:372–9.
179. Toyserkani NM, Christensen ML, Sheikh SP, et al. Stem cells show promising results for lymphoedema treatment – a literature review. J Plast Surg Hand Surg. 2014;49:65–71.
180. Toyserkani NM, Jensen CII, Tabatabaeifar S, et al. Adipose-derived regenerative cells and fat grafting for treating breast cancer-related lymphedema: lymphoscintigraphic evaluation with 1 year of follow-up. J Plast Reconstr Aesthet Surg. 2019;72:71–7.
181. Tremolada C. Mesenchymal stem cells and regenerative medicine: how Lipogems technology make them easy, safe and more effective to use. Mol Biol Med. 2017;2:223–6.
182. Tuin AJ, Domerchie PN, Schepers RH, et al. What is the current optimal fat grafting processing technique? A systematic review. J Craniomaxillofac Surg. 2016;44:45–55.
183. Urbich C, Heeschen C, Aicher A, et al. Relevance of monocytic features for neovascularization capacity of circulating endothelial progenitor cells. Circulation. 2003;108:2511–6.
184. van Tongeren RB, Hamming JF, Fibbe WE, et al. Intramuscular or combined intramuscular/intra-arterial administration of bone marrow mononuclear cells: a clinical trial in patients with advanced limb ischemia. J Cardiovasc Surg. 2008;49:51–8.
185. van Vlasselaer P, Falla N, Snoeck H, et al. Characterization and purification of osteogenic cells from murine bone marrow by two-color cell sorting using anti-Sca1 monoclonal antibody and wheat germ agglutinin. Blood. 1994;84:753–63.
186. Vanlandewijck M, He L, Mäe MA, et al. A molecular atlas of cell types and zonation in the brain vasculature. Nature. 2018;14:1–34.
187. Vijayakumar A, Tiwari R, Kumar PV. Thromboangiitis obliterans (Buerger's disease)-current practices. Int J Inflamm. 2013;2013:156905.
188. Wakabayashi T, Naito H, Suehiro JI, et al. CD157 marks tissue-resident endothelial stem cells with homeostatic and regenerative properties. Cell Stem Cell. 2018;22:384–397.e6.
189. Walter DH, Krankenberg H, Balzer JO, et al. Intraarterial administration of bone marrow mononuclear cells in patients with critical limb ischemia: a randomized-start, placebo-controlled pilot trial (PROVASA). Circ Cardiovasc Interv. 2011;4:26–37.
190. Wang L, Gu ZY, Liu SF, et al. Single-versus double- unit umbilical cord blood transplantation for hematologic diseases: a systematic review. Transfus Med Rev. 2019;33:51–60.
191. Wang X, Zhang H, Nie L, et al. Myogenic differentiation and reparative activity of stromal cells derived from pericardial adipose in comparison to subcutaneous origin. Stem Cell Res Ther. 2014;5:1–11.
192. Williams AR, Trachtenberg B, Velazquez DL, et al. Intramyocardial stem cell injection in patients with ischemic cardiomyopathy: functional recovery and reverse remodeling. Circ Res. 2011;108:792–6.
193. Wognum AW, Eaves AC, Thomas TE. Identification and isolation of hematopietic stem cells. Arch Med Res. 2003;34:461–75.
194. Woo DH, Hwang HS, Shim JH. Comparison of adult stem cells derived from multiple stem cell niches. Biotechnol Lett. 2016;16:751–9.
195. Wu Y, Wang J, Scott PG, et al. Bone marrow-derived stem cells in wound healing: a review. Wound Repair Regen. 2007;15(Suppl. 1):S18–26.
196. Xu H, Barnes GT, Yang Q, et al. Chronic inflammation in fat plays a crucial role in the development of obesity-related insulin resistance. J Clin Invest. 2003;112:1821–30.
197. Yoder M. Human endothelial progenitor cells. Cold Spring Harb Perspect Med. 2012;2:a006692.

198. Yoder M. Endothelial progenitor cell: a blood cell by many other names may serve similar functions. J Mol Med. 2013;91:285–95.
199. Yoder MC, Mead LE, Prater D, et al. Redefinig endothelial progenitor cells via clonal analysis and hematopoietic stem/ progenitor cell principals. Blood. 2007;109:1801–9.
200. Yoon JH, Roh EY, Shin S, et al. Comparison of explant-derived and enzymatic digestion-derived MSCs and the growth factors from Wharton's jelly. Biomed Res Int. 2013;2013:428726.
201. Yoshida M, Tsuji K, Ebihara Y, et al. Thrombopoietin alone stimulates the early proliferation and survival of human erythroid, myeloid and multipotential progenitors in serum-free culture. Br J Haematol. 1997;98:254–64.
202. Yoshimura K, Shigeura T, Matsumoto D, et al. Characterization of freshly isolated and cultured cells derived from the fatty and fluid portions of liposuction aspirates. J Cell Physiol. 2006;208:64–76.
203. Zhang CC, Kaba M, Iizuka S, et al. Angiopoietin-like 5 and IGFBP2 stimulate *ex vivo* expansion of human cord blood hematopoietic stem cells as assayed by NOD/SCID transplantation. Blood. 2008;111:3415–23.
204. Zhang CC, Lodish HF. Cytokines regulating hematopoietic stem cell function. Curr Opin Hematol. 2008;15:307–11.
205. Zhang Y, Deng H, Tang Z. Efficacy of cellular therapy for diabetic foot ulcer: a meta-analysis of randomized controlled clinical trials. Cell Transplant. 2017;26:12.
206. Zhao L, Johnson T, Liu D. Therapeutic angiogenesis of adipose derived stem cells for ischemic diseases. Stem Cell Res Ther. 2017;8:125.
207. Zhou H, Wu S, Joo JY, et al. Generation of induced pluripotent stem cells using recombinant proteins. Cell Stem Cell. 2009;4:381–4.
208. Zhou W, Freed CR. Adenoviral gene delivery can reprogram human fibroblasts to induced pluripotent stem cells. Stem Cells. 2009;27:2667–74.
209. Zimmerlin L, Donnenberg VS, Rubin JP, et al. Mesenchymal markers on human adipose stem/progenitor cells. Cytometry A. 2013;83:134–40.
210. Zuk PA, Zhu M, Ashjian P, et al. Human adipose tissue is a source of multipotent stem cells. Mol Biol Cell. 2002;13:4279–95.
211. Zuk PA, Zhu M, Mizuno H, et al. Multilineage cells from human adipose tissue: implications for cell-based therapies. Tissue Eng. 2001;7:211–28.

Chapter 3
Stem Cell Delivery Techniques for Stroke and Peripheral Artery Disease

Shin-Rong Lee, Arash Fereydooni, and Alan Dardik

3.1 Introduction

Vascular diseases are fundamentally characterized by end-organ hypoperfusion leading to a vicious cycle of tissue ischemia, cell death, maladaptive remodeling, and organ dysfunction. The promise of stem cells as therapy for vascular diseases arises from their potential to interrupt this cycle by (a) reducing hypoxia through increased angiogenesis [1, 2]; (b) improving native cell survival and regeneration, as well as guiding beneficial remodeling through secretion of growth factors [3, 4]; and ultimately (c) replacing lost tissue to recover organ function [5]. While the dream of regenerative organ replacement remains elusive for most applications of cell therapy—except for the notable success of bone marrow transplantation [6]—the more modest goals of improving end-organ function via locoregional modulation have been suggested in some clinical studies of several vascular diseases. These investigations include ischemic heart disease, critical limb ischemia, and ischemic stroke, where modest improvements in the left ventricular ejection fraction, amputation-free survival, or neurologic outcomes have, respectively, been demonstrated following cell therapy [7–11]. Unfortunately, there have also been a number of clinical trials that have failed to show benefit after stem cell implantation [12], highlighting the multiple challenges still facing this burgeoning and innovative field.

S.-R. Lee · A. Fereydooni
Yale School of Medicine, New Haven, CT, USA
e-mail: shinrong.lee@yale.edu; arash.fereydooni@yale.edu

A. Dardik (✉)
Vascular Biology and Therapeutics Program and the Departments of Surgery and Cellular and Molecular Physiology, Yale University School of Medicine, New Haven, CT, USA
e-mail: alan.dardik@yale.edu

© Springer Nature Switzerland AG 2021
T. P. Navarro et al. (eds.), *Stem Cell Therapy for Vascular Diseases*,
https://doi.org/10.1007/978-3-030-56954-9_3

An important challenge in stem cell therapy, and the focus of this chapter, lies in the determination of the optimal method of delivering stem cells to the injured organ. The best delivery method should be the least invasive procedure that achieves the highest fraction of engrafted, viable, stem cells within the targeted area. This critically depends on patient-specific, disease-specific, and stem cell-specific factors, which themselves are also important determinants of success in cell therapy. For example, careful examination of patients and consideration of their comorbidities and functional status are necessary not only to determine which patients can benefit from stem cell therapy—many trials exclude, for instance, patients with advanced infections, cancers, or life-threatening illnesses—but also what type of invasive procedure they might be able to tolerate to receive cell therapy. Similarly, the disease for which stem cell therapy is indicated is also important, as this influences the type of stem cell used, the timing, and dose of cell therapy. Anatomical considerations also dictate the available delivery routes. Finally, stem cell factors such as providing sufficient numbers and quality of the right type of stem cell to a receptive environment are crucial in any successful cell therapy, with the route of administration playing an important modulatory role in each of these variables.

Stem cells can be delivered locally, regionally, or systemically (Fig. 3.1). This chapter considers the different techniques for stem cell delivery from these viewpoints for two vascular diseases—stroke and peripheral artery disease. Relevant preclinical and clinical studies for each area are reviewed and general concepts fundamental to each delivery technique analyzed and summarized.

3.2 Stroke

A stroke occurs when there is an interruption of cerebral blood flow due to cerebrovascular thrombosis, embolism, or hemorrhage, leading to a neurological deficit due to ischemic neuronal cell death. According to the 2016 Global Burden of Disease Stroke Collaborators, stroke is a leading cause of death and disability-adjusted life years worldwide [13]. Early preclinical studies investigating stem cell therapy in rodent models of ischemic stroke garnered much enthusiasm when it was shown that implanted stem cells differentiated into neurons, formed connections, and engendered functional recovery [14–18]. To provide therapeutic benefit, stem cells must first be delivered into the appropriate region of injury. However, the brain is an anatomically difficult organ to access—encapsulated by the skull exteriorly and the blood-brain barrier internally, delivering therapeutics to the central nervous system is a difficult task that has frustrated many pharmaceuticals. This section summarizes approaches for stem cell delivery implemented in recent clinical trials, highlighting the unique challenges and opportunities in delivering cell therapy to the brain.

Fig. 3.1 Stem cell delivery approaches in stroke and peripheral artery disease

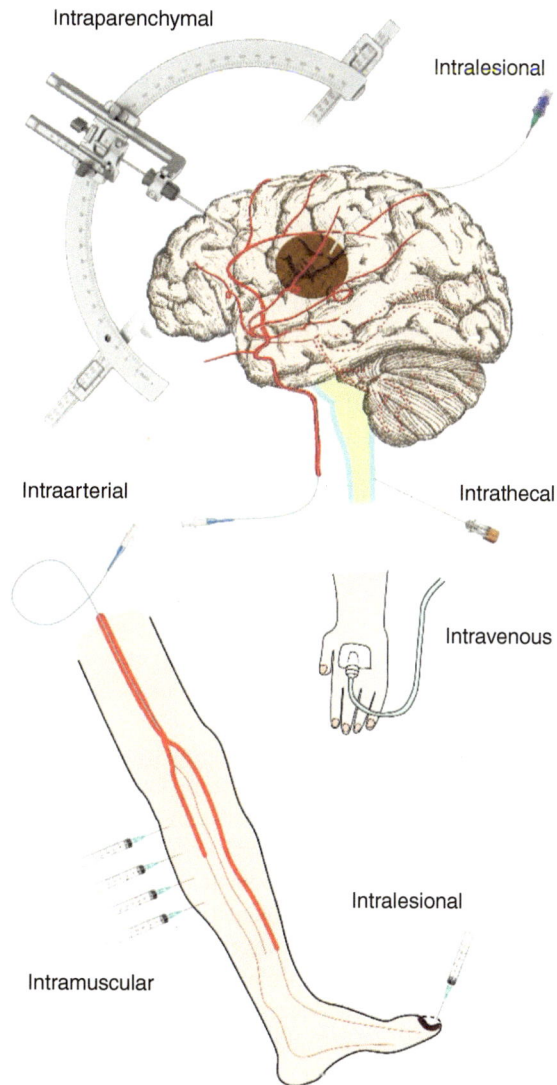

3.2.1   *Local*

3.2.1.1   Intraparenchymal

One of the earliest cell therapy trials for stroke in human patients was performed by intraparenchymal injection of cultured human neuronal cells into the brain. This is the most invasive approach of cell delivery but is the only approach that guarantees that the desired dose of cells is delivered to the region of interest. Pioneering and influential studies within the field of intracerebral delivery were studies sponsored by Layton Biosciences [19, 20], with many of their study methods replicated by subsequent investigators.

In the Layton studies [19, 20], patients with stable, chronic (1–5 years) ischemic, or hemorrhagic strokes were recruited, and these patients had human cultured human neuronal cells (LBS-Neurons; Layton BioScience, Inc.) stereotactically implanted into the peri-infact region. Twelve patients received 2–6 million cells each in the phase 1 study, and 14 patients received 5–10 million cells in the phase 2 study. Their methodology was as follows: patients were fitted with a stereotactic frame, and a Burr hole was created through the skull. A needle with an outer diameter (OD) of 0.9 mm and inner diameter (ID) of 0.25 mm was then advanced under image guidance to a target inferior to the stroke region. In phase 1, either 1 or 3 needle tracts were used to deliver 2 or 6 million cells via 3 boluses of 20 µl per tract, while in phase 2, the cell dosage of 5 or 10 million cells was divided into a total of 25 implants through 5 needle tracts with 5 boluses of 10 µl per tract at a rate of 5 µl per min. These studies demonstrated acceptable safety of the procedures, with few procedure-related serious complications. Out of 26 surgeries, 1 patient had an asymptomatic chronic subdural hematoma 1 month after surgery that was drained without sequelae. However, although there were improvements in some indices of neurologic functions, these studies failed to show improvement in the primary outcome measure (European Stroke Scale motor score). There was a suggestion that patients with hemorrhagic strokes may not have responded as well to cell therapy compared to patients with ischemic strokes, but this finding did not reach statistical significance.

Although the primary outcome measure was not achieved, these studies were nevertheless important in establishing the safety and feasibility of intraparenchymal cell injections, and their experience identified several important considerations. For example, the requirement of delivering a small volume (10s of microliters) of cells in a stereotactic fashion necessitated the development of an injection cannula—this led to the Pittsburgh Cell Implantation Cannula, which is a stainless steel-constructed rigid cannula that is 19 cm in length with a 0.9 mm outer diameter and an internal volume of 20 ul, and a special hub designed to eliminate dead space between the cannula and an attached syringe [21]. The authors demonstrated that injecting cells through the cannula at 5 µl per min did not affect cell viability. They also noted that the slow rate of injection could result in cell sedimentation, and so the syringe was frequently rotated to maintain a uniform cell suspension. Bolus volumes were kept low to minimize the possibility of axonal disruption, and needle tracts, which are needed to distribute the cells around the infarct but can result in hyperintensities on T2 MRI of undetermined clinical significance [22], were kept to a minimum.

Subsequent studies (Table 3.1) utilizing intraparenchymal cell delivery focused on patients with chronic ischemic strokes, perhaps in response to the trend of decreased efficacy with hemorrhagic strokes observed in the Layton studies. Methodologically, these studies were similar, utilizing stereotactic surgery to implant different types and doses of stem cells in the (peri)-infarct region. There were variations in the cell type and dosage used, needle type, number of needle tracts, number and size of boluses, and infusion rate, which are summarized in

Table 3.1 Local delivery of stem cells for stroke

Study	Treated/control	Stroke	Timing	Cell type (Dose x10^6)	Needle size (OD)	Bolus size, ul (rate, ul/min)	# tracts (# bolus per tract)	Follow-up (months)	Serious adverse events
Intraparenchymal									
Kondziolka 2000 (1)	12/0	Ischemic	6–60 months	hNT (2 or 6)	0.9 mm	20 ul (5 ul/min)	3 (1 or 3)	18	None
Kondziolka 2005 (2)	14/4	Ischemic/hemorrhagic	12–72 months	hNT (5 or 10)	0.9 mm	10 ul (5 ul/min)	5 (5)	24	1 post-op seizure, 1 asymp. SDH that was drained
Chen 2014 (3)	15/15	Ischemic	6–60 months	CD34+ PBSC (3–8)	N/A	83 ul (N/A)	3 (3)	12	None
Kalladka 2016 (4)	13/0	Ischemic	6–60 months	hNSC (2–20)	0.9 mm	20 ul (5 ul/min)	5 (1, 2 or 4)	24	2 Burr hole bleeding, 1 SDH, 1 extradural hematoma
Steinberg 2016 (5)	18/0	Ischemic	6–60 months	SB623 (2.5–10)	0.9 mm	20 ul (10 ul/min)	3 (5)	12	1 SDH, 1 seizure
Zhang 2019 (6)	9/0	Ischemic	5–24 months	NSI-566 (12–72)	0.9 mm	20–40 ul (10 ul/min)	5 or 15 (3)	24	1 microcerebral hemorrhage, 2 mild seizures

(continued)

Table 3.1 (continued)

Study	Treated/ control	Stroke	Timing	Cell type (Dose x10⁶)	Needle size (OD)	Bolus size, ul (rate, ul/min)	# tracts (# bolus per tract)	Follow-up (months)	Serious adverse events
Intralesional									
Li (2013) (7)	60/40	Cerebral hemorrhage	5.9 days	BMMNC (13.3)	N/A	3.5 ml(N/A)	N/A	6	New lung cancer
Chang (2016) (8)	7, 9/8	Cerebral hemorrhage	2 weeks poststroke	BMMNC (180); UCMSC (N/A)	N/A	N/A(N/A)	N/A	60	None

References

1. Kondziolka D, Wechsler L, Goldstein S, Meltzer C, Thulborn KR, Gebel J, et al. Transplantation of cultured human neuronal cells for patients with stroke. Neurology. 2000;55(4):565–9. PubMed PMID: 10953194
2. Bang OY, Lee JS, Lee PH, Lee G. Autologous mesenchymal stem cell transplantation in stroke patients. Ann Neurol. 2005;57(6):874–82. PubMed PMID: 15929052
3. Chen DC, Lin SZ, Fan JR, Lin CH, Lee W, Lin CC, et al. Intracerebral implantation of autologous peripheral blood stem cells in stroke patients: a randomized phase II study. Cell Transpl. 2014;23(12):1599–612. PubMed PMID: 24480430
4. Kalladka D, Sinden J, Pollock K, Haig C, McLean J, Smith W, et al. Human neural stem cells in patients with chronic ischaemic stroke (PISCES): a phase 1, first-in-man study. Lancet. 2016;388(10046):787–96. PubMed PMID: 27497862
5. Steinberg GK, Kondziolka D, Wechsler LR, Lunsford LD, Kim AS, Johnson JN, et al. Two-year safety and clinical outcomes in chronic ischemic stroke patients after implantation of modified bone marrow–derived mesenchymal stem cells (SB623): a phase 1/2a study. J Neurosurg. 2018:1–11. PubMed PMID: 30497166
6. Zhang G, Li Y, Reuss JL, Liu N, Wu C, Li J, et al. Stable intracerebral transplantation of neural stem cells for the treatment of paralysis due to ischemic stroke. Stem Cells Transl Med. 2019;8(10):999–1007. PubMed PMID: 31241246. Pubmed Central PMCID: 6766600
7. Li ZM, Zhang ZT, Guo CJ, Geng FY, Qiang F, Wang LX. Autologous bone marrow mononuclear cell implantation for intracerebral hemorrhage-a prospective clinical observation. Clinical neurology and neurosurgery. 2013;115(1):72–6. PubMed PMID: 22657095
8. Chang Z, Mao G, Sun L, Ao Q, Gu Y, Liu Y. Cell therapy for cerebral hemorrhage: five year follow-up report. Exp Therap Med. 2016;12(6):3535–40. PubMed PMID: 28101148. Pubmed Central PMCID: 5228203

hNT clonal human neural grafts, *PBSC* peripheral blood stem cells, *hNSC* human neural stem cells, *SB623* modified bone marrow–derived mesenchymal stem cells, *NSI-566* human neural stem cells, *BMMNC* bone marrow mononuclear cells, *UCMSC* umbilical cord mesenchymal stem cells

Table 3.1. Consistent with the experience of the Layton reports, these studies showed acceptable safety profiles with no cell-related adverse effects and only a few procedural-related complications such as surgical site bleeding and chronic subdural hematomas. However, while most studies demonstrated modest improvements in function, many of these were small single-arm studies. Thus, efficacy of this method of cell therapy still needs to be established with larger phase 2/3 studies, some of which are currently in progress [23].

3.2.1.2 Intralesional

The intralesional approach is another local method of stem cell delivery to the brain, whereby cells are delivered into the lesion by infusion through a catheter. Li et al. [24] utilized this approach in patients with acute hemorrhagic stroke. Their study included 100 patients (60 treatment, 40 control) who had cerebral hemorrhage that required surgical evacuation either by craniotomy or Burr hole. During the hematoma evacuation, patients had a tube placed into the hematoma cavity for drainage. Approximately 5 days after surgery, patients underwent bone marrow aspiration and extraction of mononuclear cells, 3.5 ml of which were subsequently infused via the drainage tube into the peripheral area of the hematoma cavity (average of 13.3 million cells). Patients in the control group received 3.5 ml of saline. Relevant adverse events included low-grade fever in five patients (5.3%) within 24 hours of cell implantation (compared to one patient, 2.5% in control), and one patient in the cell therapy group was diagnosed with lung cancer 4 months postimplantation. Patients treated with stem cells had significantly improved neurological function (NIHSS, BI) compared to control at 6 months post-op.

Chang et al. [25] utilized a similar approach also in patients with cerebral hemorrhages. Their study included patients (16 treatment, 8 control) with acute cerebral hemorrhages that required surgical hematoma evacuation, but they tested autologous BMMNC (180 million, n = 7) and allogeneic umbilical cord MSCs (unknown dose, n = 9). During the hematoma evacuation, patients in the treatment groups also had a tube placed into the hematoma cavity, but this tube was sutured subcutaneously and the overlying skin closed. Two weeks after hemorrhage, the tube was accessed surgically, and stem cells were infused into the hematoma cavity. Patients received a second dose in a similar fashion 1 week after. No adverse events were noted, and patients receiving both types of cell therapy had improved NIHSS compared to control from 3 months–5 years poststroke, with the UCMSC group faring slightly better than the BMMNC group.

These studies (Table 3.1) illustrate the feasibility and long-term safety of the intralesional approach for hemorrhagic stroke. This approach is attractive as administering cell therapy coincidentally with existing lifesaving therapies which allow delivery of stem cells locally with minimal additional procedural risk. However, further studies are needed not only to establish efficacy but to also determine the time after hemorrhage, stem cell type, and cell dose that can confer the most benefit.

3.2.2   Regional

3.2.2.1   Intra-arterial

One of the earliest examples of intra-arterial stem cell therapy for stroke was a case report from Brazil by Mendonca et al. in 2006 [26]. A 54-year-old woman had acute-onset right hemiparesis and global aphasia and presented to the emergency department 6 hours after symptom onset, beyond the therapeutic window for IV thrombolytics. Subsequent workup showed an ischemic stroke in the left MCA territory, but her intracranial and extracranial vessels as assessed by transcranial doppler (TCD) and carotid/vertebral ultrasounds were patent. She was enrolled into a phase I trial assessing the safety and feasibility of autologous transplantation of bone marrow mononuclear cells in stroke. Four days after her stroke, bone marrow mononuclear cells (BMMNCs) were aspirated and isolated from her iliac crest. She was taken into the interventional lab where endovascular access was obtained and cerebral arteriography demonstrated patency of the left MCA and its tributaries. A catheter was then advanced into the left MCA, and 3 ml containing 100 million BMMNCs were infused over 10 minutes. Monitoring was performed throughout with EEG and TCD, which showed no significant changes during the procedure. The patient was followed for 2 months post-procedure, where she continued to exhibit functional neurologic recovery.

The above case illustrates the essential features of intra-arterial delivery of stem cells, a regional approach whereby cells are transplanted into the area of injury via an endovascular catheter placed into the artery supplying that area. This method has intuitive appeal as it can achieve a more targeted delivery of cells than intravenous approaches without the invasiveness of stereotactic injections. Furthermore, with the rise of endovascular thrombectomy for ischemic stroke [27], the ability to coincidently deliver cell therapy with other intra-arterial interventions has further increased the attractiveness of this method. However, caution is necessary as some preclinical studies implementing intra-arterial infusion of stem cells in stroke have demonstrated that this method can cause harm by worsening cerebral ischemia [28–34]. This is thought to be due to catheter-induced reductions in cerebral blood flow and/or microembolic strokes from stem cell plugging of capillaries. From these experiences, factors important for preserving safety of intra-arterial delivery were identified, which include stem cell type, dose, location and rate of infusion, and acuity of cell therapy after stroke [35]. These considerations are discussed further below in relation to existing stem cell trials performed in human patients (Table 3.2).

Cell Type

Cells used for transplantation can vary widely in size, from an average diameter of 7 μm for bone marrow mononuclear cells (BMMNC) to over 25 μm for mesenchymal stem cells (MSC) [35]. Since cerebral capillaries are 5–10 μm in diameter, one

Table 3.2 Regional delivery of stem cells for stroke

Study	Treated/control	Stroke	Timing (days)	Location	Stem cell type	Dose (×10⁶)	Infusion rate (ml/min)	Follow-up	Serious adverse events
Intra-arterial									
Mendonca 2006 (9)	1	Ischemic	4	MCA	BMMNC	100	0.3	3 months	None
Correa 2007 (10)	1	Ischemic	9	MCA	BMMNC	30	Unknown	8 hours	None
Barbosa de Fonseca 2009 (11)	1	Ischemic	67	MCA	BMMNC	500	1	48 hours	None
Barbosa de Fonseca 2010 (12)	6/0	Ischemic	59–82	MCA	BMMNC	125–500	1	120 days	None
Battistella 2011 (13)	6/0	Ischemic	<90	MCA	BMMNC	100–500	1	180 days	None
Friedrich 2012 (14)	20/0	Ischemic	3–7	MCA	BMMNC	50–600	0.5	180 days	None
Moniche 2012 (15)	10/10	Ischemic	5–9	MCA	BMMNC	159	0.5–1	180 days	None
Jiang 2013 (16)	4/0	Ischemic	11–50	MCA	UCMSC	20	1	180 days	None
Banerjee 2014 (17)	5/0	Ischemic	<7	MCA	CD34+ HSC	1.2–2.8	Unknown	180 days	None

(continued)

Table 3.2 (continued)

Study	Treated/control	Stroke	Timing (days)	Location	Stem cell type	Dose (×10⁶)	Infusion rate (ml/min)	Follow-up	Serious adverse events
Ghali 2016 (18)	21/18	Ischemic	12–32	MCA	BMMNC	1	Unknown	1 year	None
Intrathecal									
Sharma (2014) (19)	24/0	Ischemic/hemorrhagic	40.5 months	Variable	BMMNC	N/A	N/A	0.5–4.5 years	None
Pan (2019) (20)	12*/0	Ischemic	0.4–36 months	Variable	BMMNC (1/kg weekly x 4 weeks)	N/A	N/A	9–42 months	None

References

9. Mendonca ML, Freitas GR, Silva SA, Manfrim A, Falcao CH, Gonzales C, et al. [Safety of intra-arterial autologous bone marrow mononuclear cell transplantation for acute ischemic stroke]. Arquivos Brasileiros de Cardiologia. 2006;86(1):52–5. PubMed PMID: 16491209. Seguranca do transplante autologo, intra-arterial, de celulas mononucleares da medula ossea na fase aguda do acidente vascular cerebral isquemico

10. Correa PL, Mesquita CT, Felix RM, Azevedo JC, Barbirato GB, Falcao CH, et al. Assessment of intra-arterial injected autologous bone marrow mononuclear cell distribution by radioactive labeling in acute ischemic stroke. Clin Nucl Med. 2007;32(11):839–41. PubMed PMID: 18075415

11. Barbosa da Fonseca LM, Battistella V, de Freitas GR, Gutfilen B, Dos Santos Goldenberg RC, Maiolino A, et al. Early tissue distribution of bone marrow mononuclear cells after intra-arterial delivery in a patient with chronic stroke. Circulation. 2009;120(6):539–41. PubMed PMID: 19667245

12. Barbosa da Fonseca LM, Gutfilen B, Rosado de Castro PH, Battistella V, Goldenberg RC, Kasai-Brunswick T, et al. Migration and homing of bone-marrow mononuclear cells in chronic ischemic stroke after intra-arterial injection. Exp Neurol. 2010;221(1):122–8. PubMed PMID: 19853605

13. Battistella V, de Freitas GR, da Fonseca LM, Mercante D, Gutfilen B, Goldenberg RC, et al. Safety of autologous bone marrow mononuclear cell transplantation in patients with nonacute ischemic stroke. Regenerat Med. 2011;6(1):45–52. PubMed PMID: 21175286

14. Friedrich MA, Martins MP, Araujo MD, Klamt C, Vedolin L, Garicochea B, et al. Intra-arterial infusion of autologous bone marrow mononuclear cells in patients with moderate to severe middle cerebral artery acute ischemic stroke. Cell Transpl. 2012;21(Suppl 1):S13–21. PubMed PMID: 22507676

15. Moniche F, Gonzalez A, Gonzalez-Marcos JR, Carmona M, Pinero P, Espigado I, et al. Intra-arterial bone marrow mononuclear cells in ischemic stroke: a pilot clinical trial. Stroke. 2012;43(8):2242–4. PubMed PMID: 22764211

16. Jiang Y, Zhu W, Zhu J, Wu L, Xu G, Liu X. Feasibility of delivering mesenchymal stem cells via catheter to the proximal end of the lesion artery in patients with stroke in the territory of the middle cerebral artery. Cell Transpl. 2013;22(12):2291–8. PubMed PMID: 23127560

17. Banerjee S, Bentley P, Hamady M, Marley S, Davis J, Shlebak A, et al. Intra-Arterial Immunoselected CD34+ Stem Cells for Acute Ischemic Stroke. Stem Cells Transl Med. 2014;3(11):1322–30. PubMed PMID: 25107583. Pubmed Central PMCID: 4214837

18. Ghali AA, Yousef MK, Ragab OA, ElZamarany EA. Intra-arterial infusion of autologous bone marrow mononuclear stem cells in subacute ischemic stroke patients. Front Neurol. 2016;7:228. PubMed PMID: 28018286. Pubmed Central PMCID: 5159483

19. Sharma A, Sane H, Gokulchandran N, Khopkar D, Paranjape A, Sundaram J, et al. Autologous bone marrow mononuclear cells intrathecal transplantation in chronic stroke. Stroke Res Treat. 2014;2014:234095. PubMed PMID: 25126443. Pubmed Central PMCID: 4121152

20. Pan K, Deng L, Chen P, Peng Q, Pan J, Wu Y, et al. Safety and feasibility of repeated intrathecal allogeneic bone marrow-derived mesenchymal stromal cells in patients with neurological diseases. Stem Cells Int. 2019;2019:8421281. PubMed PMID: 31428161. Pubmed Central PMCID: 6683773 publication of this article

MCA middle cerebral artery, *BMMNC* bone marrow mononuclear cells, *UCMSC* umbilical cord mesenchymal stem cells, *HSC* hematopoeitic stem cells. *37 patients total, 12 with ischemic stroke

might expect that a large influx of large cells, which have a slower rate of extravasation than smaller cells, would carry a higher risk of vessel occlusion. Indeed, it has been observed that cell size correlates with observed complications in a number of preclinical studies. For example, Guzman et al. [35] noted that while 0 of 19 (0%) studies using small cells (bone marrow or cord blood mononuclear cells) reported any complications, 2 of 7 (29%) studies using neural stem cells (13–15 µm) and 11 of 29 (38%) studies using MSCs reported adverse events such as reduced cerebral blood flow, increased mortality, or neurological impairment. Reflecting these concerns, most of the clinical trials performed in humans to date implementing intra-arterial stem cell therapy have used BMMNCs (Table 3.3). Nevertheless, one study that utilized umbilical cord MSCs [36], infusing them into the M1 branch of MCA in four patients, reported no safety events during a follow-up period of 6 months.

Table 3.3 Intravenous delivery of stem cells for stroke

Study	Treated/control	Stroke	Timing (days)	Location	Stem cell type	Dose (x10^6)	Follow-up duration	Serious adverse events
Bang (2005) (2)	5/25	Ischemic	30	MCA	Autologous MSC	100	1 year	None
Savitz (2011) (21)	10	Ischemic	1–3	MCA	Autologous BMMNC	7–10 / kg	6 months	None
Prasad 2014 (22)	60/60	Ischemic	18.5	MCA/ACA	Autologous BMMNC	280.75	1 year	None
Hess 2017 (23)	65/61	Ischemic	1–2	MCA/ACA	Allogeneic MAPC	1200	1 year	None

References
2. Bang OY, Lee JS, Lee PH, Lee G. Autologous mesenchymal stem cell transplantation in stroke patients. Ann Neurol. 2005;57(6):874–82. PubMed PMID: 15929052
21. Savitz SI, Misra V, Kasam M, Juneja H, Cox CS, Jr., Alderman S, et al. Intravenous autologous bone marrow mononuclear cells for ischemic stroke. Ann Neurol. 2011;70(1):59–69. PubMed PMID: 21786299
22. Prasad K, Sharma A, Garg A, Mohanty S, Bhatnagar S, Johri S, et al. Intravenous autologous bone marrow mononuclear stem cell therapy for ischemic stroke: a multicentric, randomized trial. Stroke. 2014;45(12):3618–24. PubMed PMID: 25378424
23. Hess DC, Wechsler LR, Clark WM, Savitz SI, Ford GA, Chiu D, et al. Safety and efficacy of multipotent adult progenitor cells in acute ischaemic stroke (MASTERS): a randomised, double-blind, placebo-controlled, phase 2 trial. Lancet Neurol. 2017;16(5):360–8. PubMed PMID: 28320635
MCA middle cerebral artery, *ACA* anterior cerebral artery, *MSC* mesenchymal stem cells, *BMMNC* bone marrow mononuclear cells, *MAPC* multipotent adult progenitor cells

Cell Dose

The number of cells infused is also an important risk factor for cerebral ischemia [30]. When too many cells are infused at once, capillary lumens can be clogged when the rate of cell clearance or extravasation is overwhelmed by their influx. Thus, a critical objective of clinical studies is to determine the therapeutic window whereby sufficient cell engraftment to provide clinical benefit is achieved without compromising perfusion. A wide range of cell doses (5000–15,000,000 cells/g) have been tested in the mouse, rat, and dog, with cell doses normalized based on average brain mass (0.4 g, 2 g, 72 g, and 1350 g for mouse, rat, dog, and human, respectively) to facilitate comparison across species [35]. These studies find evidence of ischemia when cell doses exceed 40,000–100,000 cells/g for MSCs and 750,000 cells/g for NSCs [35]. Interestingly, no adverse events were reported using BMMNCs even at very high doses (10–15 million cells/g). Studies in humans have chosen cell doses ranging from 1 to 600 million cells (740–450,000 cells/g), with all but 1 study utilizing BMMNCs (Table 3.3). The 1 study that utilized umbilical cord MSCs used a relatively small dose of 20 million cells, or ~15,000 cells/g, without any adverse events.

Infusion Rate

Preclinical studies have also identified high infusion rates as risk factors for stroke [28, 30]. In the rat, while infusion of phosphate-buffered saline through the common carotid artery at rates of 3 mL/min resulted in a drop in cerebral blood flow and lacunar strokes, reducing the infusion rate to 0.2 mL/min eliminated these adverse findings [28]. However, these concerns may not readily apply to human patients, where there is extensive experience delivering contrast during cerebral angiography with low complication rates [37]. Nevertheless, to prevent excessive hemodynamic alterations and pressure-induced endothelial injury, stem cell studies in human patients to date have implemented slow infusion rates of 0.3–1 ml/min, without any reports of adverse events.

Infusion Location

Susceptibility to microemboli differs across anatomic regions within the brain, with white matter being more sensitive to ischemia than gray matter [38]. In addition, microinfarcts in less dense regions of the brain (i.e., cortex) are more likely to be clinically silent compared to denser regions (brainstem). As a result, given the increased likelihood of iatrogenic microembolism with the intra-arterial method when compared to intravenous, intraparenchymal, or intraventricular approaches, intra-arterial cell therapy for brainstem lesions might have higher rates of complications. To date, existing stroke trials in humans using intra-arterial delivery methods have largely targeted cortical MCA strokes.

In summary, preclinical studies of intra-arterial cell therapy for stroke have raised important safety concerns that have led to identification of a number of technical factors that can modulate the risk of complications. Fortunately, existing human stem cell trials for stroke implementing the intra-arterial method have all demonstrated excellent safety profiles, though randomized trials to demonstrate efficacy remain elusive. Because increasing stem cell engraftment might come at the expense of higher rates of microemboli, maintaining a delicate balance between safety and efficacy will doubtless be a critical element of subsequent trials. Finally, while concurrent cell therapy with thrombectomy remains an important theoretical appeal of the intra-arterial route, it is worth noting that no human trial to date examines intra-arterial stem cell therapy in the hyperacute phase (<24 hours), when thrombectomy is more likely to be indicated.

3.2.2.2 Intrathecal

The intrathecal approach is a regional mode of delivery that is occasionally employed in stroke. Sharma et al. [39] recruited 24 patients with chronic ischemic and hemorrhagic stroke for implantation of autologous BMMNC intrathecally. After harvest of bone marrow cells, the intrathecal space was accessed via standard lumbar puncture using a spinal needle at the L4–L5 lumbar level. Stem cells were then infused intrathecally, and patients were followed for 6 months to 4.5 years. Some patients exhibited neurological function improvement (ambulation, 12 in 24; hand function, 10 in 24; standing balance, 6 in 24; walking balance, 9 in 24). Authors noted that younger patients, ischemic stroke, and stem cell delivery within 2 years of stroke were associated with improved outcomes. Pan et al. [40] also used the intrathecal approach, transplanting autologous BMMNC in a number of neurological diseases, including 12 patients with ischemic stroke. This study did not report functional outcomes, but found no major safety events, with pain at the puncture site being the most common adverse event. These studies showed the feasibility and safety of intrathecal delivery, but efficacy of this approach is difficult to ascertain in this heterogenous population without suitable controls.

3.2.3 Systemic Therapy

The least invasive method of cell therapy for stroke is by intravenous delivery, whereby one or several doses of stem cells are infused through a peripheral venous catheter, relying on signals exuded from the ischemic brain for targeting. This mode of cell therapy for stroke is the best studied to date, with two phase 2 randomized controlled trials completed and one in process.

One of the earliest reports of intravenous delivery of stem cells for stroke came from South Korea, where Bang et al. [41] presented results of a randomized trial whereby patients with MCA infarcts were allocated to intravenous infusions of autologous MSCs ($n = 5$) or control ($n = 25$). Patients with severe and sustained symptoms from acute MCA territory infarcts randomized to the MSC group underwent bone marrow aspiration at 1-week post-infarct. MSCs were then isolated and expanded to 100 million cells over the course of approximately 1 month. 50 million cells were then infused over 15–20 minutes via a peripheral intravenous catheter, once at 4–5 weeks post-infarct, and a second dose 7–9 weeks post-infarct. Patients received close follow-up until 1 year after their initial stroke. No adverse reactions to stem cell therapy were noted, and some functional improvement was seen in the MSC group compared to control with statistically significantly improved Barthel Index scores from 3 months and trend toward decreased modified Rankin scores from 3 months onward. Moreover, MRI at 1 year showed less prominent atrophy in peri-infarct regions in the MSC group. This pioneering work was important in demonstrating that IV transplantation of autologous stem cells for stroke was both safe and feasible and even suggested possible efficacy. Subsequent trials have expanded upon this initial trial, examining different types and doses of stem cells used and the timing of therapy. Unfortunately, the two larger phase 2 trials of intravenous stem cells for acute ischemic stroke failed to show any benefit in their primary outcome measure [42, 43], though subgroup analysis of Hess et al. [43] suggested benefit when stem cells were delivered less than 36 hours poststroke.

A limitation of IV modes of delivery relates to the large numbers of cells needed to provide therapeutic effect, due to a significant first pass effect where cells are sequestered within the pulmonary capillaries [44]. The large number of cells needed presents some financial and logistical challenges and restricts the types of cells available for therapy, especially when therapy during the hyperacute/acute phases is desired. For instance, in the study by Bang et al. [41] where autologous MSCs were used, culture expansion for 2–3 weeks was required in order to obtain their desired stem cell dose of 100 million cells. Thus, trials that offered cell therapy in the 1–3 day window either used autologously harvested BMMNC without culture expansion [45] or took advantage of previously prepared allogeneic stem cells [42, 43]. In fact, the MASTERS trial [43], which used allogeneic multipotent arterial progenitor cells, had to expand their treatment window from the initially designed 18–36 hour window to include patients 36–48 hours after symptom onset due to logistical issues surrounding the provision of adequate quantity and quality of clinical grade allogeneic stem cells within the initial time window. This is an important concern, as subgroup analysis of the MASTERS trial had suggested that cell therapy 18–36 hours after stroke was more efficacious than the 36–48 hour window.

There is also concern that intravenously delivered stem cells would not achieve sufficient engraftment within the brain to provide benefit [46], especially when used to treat chronic ischemic stroke. During the acute phase of stroke, there is disruption of the blood-brain barrier that increases its permeability [47], potentially allowing for increased stem cell penetration and engraftment, compared to more delayed therapy. However, it is increasingly recognized that intravenously delivered stem cell therapy might confer clinical benefit through its systemic effects on modulating inflammation, rather than by providing local trophic support, thus obviating the need to engraft within the brain. Indeed, immunomodulation by stem cells is thought to have marked effects on brain repair processes in animal models, by decreasing neuronal cell death, enhancing brain plasticity, and increasing angiogenesis [48].

Thus, these studies (Table 3.3) show that while intravenous delivery of stem cells is safe, it is yet unclear whether they result in clinical benefit. Fortunately, the logistical issues causing delays in cell therapy in the MASTERS trial were identified and resolved, enabling the currently accruing phase 3 MASTERS-2 trial [49] to test the hypothesis that earlier therapy (18–36 hours after symptom onset) is better.

3.2.4 Combinatorial Therapy

One study explored the use of combinatorial cell therapy by delivering multiple cell types through different approaches. Chen et al. [50] recruited 10 adults with chronic stroke (6 ischemic, 4 hemorrhagic) for whom the following allogeneic cells were implanted—olfactory ensheathing cells (OEC, 1–2 million), neural progenitor cells (NPC, 2–5 million), Schwann cells (SC, 2 million), and umbilical cord mesenchymal stromal cells (UCMSC, 10–23 million). All patients received intracerebral transplant of OEC (±NPC) into the perilesion area via stereotactic surgery. In addition, some patients also received intrathecal transplant (via cerebellar cistern puncture) of NPC (±SC), and two patients received intracerebral and intrathecal cell transplants, as well as UCMSC intravenously. During a follow-up period of 6 months to 2 years, no adverse events were reported. All patients had improvement in neurological function, as measured by a decrease in Clinical Neurologic Impairment Scale and an increase in the Barthel Index score. This ambitious study demonstrated that delivery of cell therapy via simultaneous routes is possible and associated with adequate safety. However, the investigation of multiple cell transplantations through different routes for stroke is likely still premature at this time given that efficacy of a single cell type and dose through one route of administration has yet to be demonstrated.

3.2.5 Summary

Much progress has been made in the last three decades in translating stem cell therapy from the bench to the bedside. A number of clinical trials, mostly demonstrating feasibility and safety, have been completed using an innovative variety of approaches ranging from local to systemic delivery methods. While further phase 2 and 3 studies are needed to show efficacy of each approach, these studies were also important in illustrating the advantages and disadvantages of each method and the patients for whom each method might be best suited for. For example, while patients with acute ischemic stroke might benefit more from intravenous or intra-arterial delivery, chronic stroke patients might gain better recovery from intraparenchymal injections. Taking advantage of coincident therapy, patients who are candidates for endovascular thrombectomy, or who require surgery for cerebral hemorrhage, might be best suited for intra-arterial or intralesional cell therapy, respectively. Looking ahead, one can envision a rationally designed cell therapy program incorporating these various modes of delivery for the different phases of stroke. For ischemic stroke, for instance, one approach might be to provide intravenous MSC hyper-acutely to modulate the systemic immune response, then intra-arterial infusion of bone marrow mononuclear cells acutely for local trophic support of injured neurons, and finally with intraparenchymal injections of neural stem cells chronically to stimulate repair and regeneration.

In conclusion, a number of approaches for delivering stem cells to the brain have been trialed for the treatment of stroke in a diverse patient population, many of which show promise. It is with excitement that we await further studies on efficacy to determine whether cell therapy will provide a new armamentarium for the battle against stroke.

3.3 Peripheral Artery Disease

Peripheral artery disease (PAD) results from the atherosclerotic narrowing and occlusion of medium and large arteries that supply the body outside of the heart and brain. PAD afflicts over 200 million people worldwide and typically manifests as lower extremity symptoms such as pain with walking [51]. A subset of patients with PAD develop critical limb ischemia (CLI) due to severe compromise of blood flow in that limb, resulting in pain at rest, tissue loss, and a markedly increased risk of amputation [52]. The standard of care for patients with CLI, in addition to best medical therapy, is to restore blood flow to the afflicted limb by revascularization, either with endovascular therapy with angioplasty and stenting or surgical bypass with vascular conduits. For a variety of reasons, some patients with CLI are not candidates for revascularization—pessimistically referred to as no-option CLI—and would typically require amputation [53]. These unfortunate patients have poor quality of life due to chronic pain, highlighting the need for novel therapies [54]. It is in this space that the therapeutic potential of stem cell therapy for PAD has been explored. Stem cells in PAD are thought to provide benefit by stimulating angiogenesis, vasculogenesis, and ideally arteriogenesis, thus improving collateral flow to ischemic muscles [9]. Many clinical trials for stem cells in human patients with CLI have now been completed, with many witnessing modest symptomatic improvements [55, 56]. In contrast to the brain, the lower extremities are more readily accessible, and the chosen methods for stem cell delivery used in clinical trials for PAD reflect this, being largely local and regional. This section reviews current approaches to delivering stem cells for PAD and discusses the merits and challenges of each method.

3.3.1 Local

3.3.1.1 Intramuscular

To date, the most common route of cell therapy administration has been intramuscular (Table 3.4). This is illustrated by the first landmark trial in cell therapy for PAD performed in 2002 [57]. Patients suffering from advanced critical limb ischemia (CLI) with failed or impossible endovascular or surgical revascularization were randomized to treatment with a mixed population of bone marrow-derived CD34+ and CD34- cells or placebo [57]. Without any in vitro expansion, these cells were sorted and concentrated before delivery. The cells were implanted about 3 h after marrow aspiration by intramuscular injection into the gastrocnemius of ischemic legs (2.7×10^9 to 0.7×10^9 cells in group A and 2.8×10^9 to 0.88×10^9 cells in group B) [57]. Total injection volume was about 30 mL, with 0.75 mL of bone marrow mononuclear cells implanted into each injection site, spread over 40 sites (3 cm apart, 1.5 cm deep) with a 26-gauge needle. This treatment resulted in a small increase in ABI values (+0.1) and a larger increase in TcPO2 (+12.00 mm) in targeted limbs compared with saline-treated limbs [57]. In the treatment group, 16 out of 20 patients had complete resolution of rest pain, whereas in the control group only 3 out of 20 did [57]. Magnetic resonance angiography (MRA) demonstrated an increase in collateral vessels in the treatment group compared with the control group, suggesting that stem cells are stimulating small vessel neo-angiogenesis without affecting large vessel patency [58].

Those findings were reproduced in a study of patients with CLI and diabetes in 2005, except with peripheral blood mononuclear cells (PBMNCs) [59]. The treatment group received subcutaneous injections of recombinant human granulocyte colony-stimulating factor (G-CSF) (600 μg/day) for 5 days to mobilize stem/progenitor cells, and their PBMNCs were collected and transplanted by multiple intramuscular injections into ischemic limbs (40 sites, ~3 × 3 cm distance, 1–1.5 cm deep) into thigh and leg [59]. The control patients received an intravenous injection of 90–200 μg/day prostaglandin E1. Meanwhile, a perfusion of 10,000 units/day heparin for 5 days by intravenous drip was used to avoid the possible risks of thromboembolism due to concern for G-CSF-induced increase of circulating blood cells [60, 61]. At 3 months follow-up, there were significantly different increases in laser Doppler blood perfusion, angiographic scores, and mean ABI of the treatment group. A total of 14 of 18 limb ulcers in the treatment group were completely healed after cell transplantation; however, only 7 of 18 limb ulcers were healed in the control group [59]. No major amputations were observed in the treatment group, whereas five control patients had a major amputation of treated legs [59].

As illustrated by the two cases above, the intramuscular delivery approach relies on multiple intramuscular injections to spread the stem cells over a broad ischemic area. Injection locations are based on the major muscle compartments of the leg, with most clinical trials using 30–40 points of injection into the calf muscles in the vicinity of the native anterior and posterior tibial and peroneal arteries (Table 3.1)

Table 3.4 Local delivery of stem cells for peripheral artery disease

Study	Treated/control	Disease	Stem cell type	Dose (x10⁶)	Injection location	# sites	Spacing/ depth (cm)	Duration	Significant adverse events
Intramuscular									
Huang 2005 (24)	14/14	CLTI	PBMNC	3000	Thigh and leg	40	3/1–1.5	Twice 40 days apart	None
Arai 2006 (25)	13/12	CLTI	BMMNC	1000–3000	Gastrocnemius	10	2/N/A	Daily for 10 days	1 patient with ventricular fibrillation after G-CSF treatment
Prochazka 2010 (26)	42/54	CLTI	BMMNC	N/A	Along posterior and anterior tibial artery	40	N/A	Single treatment	None
Benoit 2011 (27)	34/14	CLTI	BMMSC	N/A	N/A	40	N/A	Single treatment	Asymptomatic mean drop of hematocrit of 2.6%
Li 2012 (28)	25/29	CLTI	BMMNC	N/A	N/A	6 rows	1/1–1.5	Single treatment	No difference between treatment and control
Losordo 2012 (29)	16/12	CLTI TAO	PB CD34+	0.1/kg (LD) 1/ kg (HD)	N/A	8	N/A	Single treatment	None
Mohammadzadeh 2012 (30)	7/ 4	CLTI	PBMNC	900–1200	N/A	60	3/1–1.5	Single treatment	None

(continued)

Table 3.4 (continued)

Study	Treated/control	Disease	Stem cell type	Dose (x10⁶)	Injection location	# sites	Spacing/depth (cm)	Duration	Significant adverse events
Powell 2012 (31)	48/24	CLTI	Ixmyelocel-T	35–295	Lower thigh and calf	20	2/1–1.5	Single treatment	No difference between treatment and control
Gupta 2013 (32)	10/10	CLTI	BMMSC	200	Gastrocnemius	40–60	1/1–1.5	Single treatment	No difference between treatment and control
Szabo 2013 (33)	10/10	CLTI	PBMNC	66.4	Gastrocnemius	30	1.5/N/A	Single treatment	None
Raval 2014 (34)	7/3	CLTI	PB CD133+	50–400	Anterior and posterior compartments of lower leg	10	N/A/1–5	Single treatment	No difference between treatment and control
Skora 2015 (35)	16/16	CLTI	BMMNC	770–3830	N/A	80	N/A/2	Single treatment	Short-term injection site pain in 2 patients
Intralesional									
Marino 2013 (36)	10/10	CLTI	ADSC	N/A	Ulcer edges	N/A	N/A	Single treatment	
Ismail 2014 (37)	20	CLTI	BMMNC	100	Ulcer bed and edges	N/A	N/A	Single treatment	
Intramuscular and intralesional									
Dash 2009 (38)	12/12	CLTI TAO	BMMSC	N/A	Soleus, gastrocnemius, ulcer	N/A	N/A	Single treatment	None

(continued)

Table 3.4 (continued)

Study	Treated/control	Disease	Stem cell type	Dose (x10⁶)	Injection location	# sites	Spacing/ depth (cm)	Duration	Significant adverse events
Lu 2011 (39)	37/4	CLTI	BMMSC (20) BMMNC (21)	930 (BMMSC)960 (BMMNC)	Lower limb, and ulcer	20	3/1–1.5	Single treatment	2 patients bled at iliac crest; 5 patients had short-term pain after cell implantation
De Angelis 2015 (40)	43;43	CLTI	PBMNC	125.6	Perilesion intramuscular and ulcer bed	N/A	1–2 /1.5–2	Single treatment	None
Carstens 2017 (41)	10	CLTI	ADSVF	71.83	Gastrocnemius and intralesional	22	1.5–2 /N/A	Single treatment	None

References

24. Huang P, Li S, Han M, Xiao Z, Yang R, Han ZC. Autologous transplantation of granulocyte colony-stimulating factor-mobilized peripheral blood mononuclear cells improves critical limb ischemia in diabetes. Diabetes Care. 2005;28(9):2155–60. PubMed PMID: 16123483

25. Arai M, Misao Y, Nagai H, Kawasaki M, Nagashima K, Suzuki K, et al. Granulocyte colony-stimulating factor: a noninvasive regeneration therapy for treating atherosclerotic peripheral artery disease. Circul J. 2006;70(9):1093–8. PubMed PMID: 16936417

26. Prochazka V, Gumulec J, Jaluvka F, Salounova D, Jonszta T, Czerny D, et al. Cell therapy, a new standard in management of chronic critical limb ischemia and foot ulcer. Cell Transpl. 2010;19(11):1413–24. PubMed PMID: 20529449. Pubmed Central PMCID: 5478382

27. Benoit E, O'Donnell TF, Jr., Iafrati MD, Asher E, Bandyk DF, Hallett JW, et al. The role of amputation as an outcome measure in cellular therapy for critical limb ischemia: implications for clinical trial design. J Transl Med. 2011;9:165. PubMed PMID: 21951607. Pubmed Central PMCID: 3191337

28. Li M, Zhou H, Jin X, Wang M, Zharg S, Xu L. Autologous bone marrow mononuclear cells transplant in patients with critical leg ischemia: preliminary clinical results. Exp Clin Transpl. 2013;11(5):435–9. PubMed PMID: 23477421

29. Losordo DW, Kibbe MR, Mendelsohn F, Marston W, Driver VR, Sharafuddin M, et al. A randomized, controlled pilot study of autologous CD34+ cell therapy for critical limb ischemia. Circul Cardiovasc Intervent. 2012;5(6):821–30. PubMed PMID: 23192920. Pubmed Central PMCID: 3549397

30. Mohammadzadeh L, Samedanifard SH, Keshavarzi A, Alimoghaddam K, Larijani B, Ghavamzadeh A, et al. Therapeutic outcomes of transplanting autologous granulocyte colony-stimulating factor-mobilised peripheral mononuclear cells in diabetic patients with critical limb ischaemia. Exp Clin Endocrinol Diab. 2013;121(1):48–53. PubMed PMID: 23329572

Table 3.4 (continued)

31. Powell RJ, Marston WA, Berceli SA, Guzman R, Henry TD, Longcore AT, et al. Cellular therapy with Ixmyelocel-T to treat critical limb ischemia: the randomized, double-blind, placebo-controlled RESTORE-CLI trial. Mol Ther. 2012;20(6):1280–6. Pubmed Central PMCID: 3369291

32. Gupta PK, Chullikana A, Parakh R, Desai S, Das A, Gottipamula S, et al. A double blind randomized placebo controlled phase I/II study assessing the safety and efficacy of allogeneic bone marrow derived mesenchymal stem cell in critical limb ischemia. J Transl Med. 2013;11:143. PubMed PMID: 23758736. Pubmed Central PMCID: 3688296

33. Szabo GV, Kovesd Z, Cserepes J, Daroczy J, Belkin M, Acsady G. Peripheral blood-derived autologous stem cell therapy for the treatment of patients with late-stage peripheral artery disease-results of the short- and long-term follow-up. Cytotherapy. 2013;15(10):1245–52. PubMed PMID: 23993298

34. Raval AN, Schmuck EG, Tefera G, Leitzke C, Ark CV, Hei D, et al. Bilateral administration of autologous CD133+ cells in ambulatory patients with refractory critical limb ischemia: lessons learned from a pilot randomized, double-blind, placebo-controlled trial. Cytotherapy. 2014;16(12):1720–32. PubMed PMID: 25239491. Pubmed Central PMCID: 4253573

35. Skora J, Pupka A, Janczak D, Barc P, Dawiskiba T, Korta K, et al. Combined autologous bone marrow mononuclear cell and gene therapy as the last resort for patients with critical limb ischemia. Arch Med Sci. 2015;11(2):325–31. PubMed PMID: 25995748. Pubmed Central PMCID: 4424239

36. Marino G, Moraci M, Armenia E, Orabona C, Sergio R, De Sena G, et al. Therapy with autologous adipose-derived regenerative cells for the care of chronic ulcer of lower limbs in patients with peripheral arterial disease. J Surg Res. 2013;185(1):36–44. PubMed PMID: 23773718

37. Ismail AM, Abdou SM, Aty HA, Kamhawy AH, Elhinedy M, Elwageh M, et al. Autologous transplantation of CD34(+) bone marrow derived mononuclear cells in management of non-reconstructable critical lower limb ischemia. Cytotechnology. 2016;68(4):771–81. PubMed PMID: 25511801. Pubmed Central PMCID: 4960127

38. Dash NR, Dash SN, Routray P, Mohapatra S, Mohapatra PC. Targeting nonhealing ulcers of lower extremity in human through autologous bone marrow-derived mesenchymal stem cells. Rejuvenat Res. 2009;12(5):359–66. PubMed PMID: 19929258

39. Lu D, Chen B, Liang Z, Deng W, Jiang Y, Li S, et al. Comparison of bone marrow mesenchymal stem cells with bone marrow-derived mononuclear cells for treatment of diabetic critical limb ischemia and foot ulcer: a double-blind, randomized, controlled trial. Diab Res Clin Pract. 2011;92(1):26–36. PubMed PMID: 21216483

40. De Angelis B, Gentile P, Orlandi F, Bocchini I, Di Pasquali C, Agovino A, et al. Limb rescue: a new autologous-peripheral blood mononuclear cells technology in critical limb ischemia and chronic ulcers. Tissue Eng Part C Meth. 2015;21(5):423–35. PubMed PMID: 25341088

41. Carstens MH, Gomez A, Cortes R, Turner E, Perez C, Ocon M, et al. Non-reconstructable peripheral vascular disease of the lower extremity in ten patients treated with adipose-derived stromal vascular fraction cells. Stem Cell Res. 2017;18:14–21. PubMed PMID: 27984756

CLTI chronic limb threatening ischemia, *TAO* thromboangiitis obliterans, *PBMNC* peripheral blood mononuclear cell, *BMMNC* bone marrow mononuclear cell, *BMMSC* bone marrow mesenchymal stem cell, *ADSC* adipose-derived stem cells, *ADSVF* adipose-derived stromal vascular fraction

[62]. Usually a symmetric grid is used to deliver a fixed number of injections along the crural arteries [63–65]. The injection target is approximately in the center of the muscle bundle at 1–1.5 cm depth. Injections are placed as near as possible (±1 cm) to the original albeit occluded arteries because the density of preformed collateral arteries is highest in the vicinity of the original arteries [63], maximizing the chances of graft survival. In contrast to other protocols, one study did not inject into the proximal gastrocnemius muscle, to have an optimal concentration at the site where it was needed [66]. Instead, the pattern of injection was linear, overlying the areas of critical limitation to arterial flow (tibial or pedal arteries) and as distal as possible [66]. Injection sites may also be determined based on findings from magnetic resonance imaging, magnetic resonance angiography, angiograms, or Doppler ultrasound to identify sites of occluded arteries (Table 3.1) [67].

Injections are usually well-tolerated and adverse effects are few. Intramuscular implantations are commonly performed under conscious sedation with midazolam and fentanyl, but spinal/epidural anesthesia and general anesthesia are also utilized [68]. Some studies have also reported local injection of 100 mg tramadol hydrochloride intramuscularly to relieve pain prior to stem cell delivery [69]. Patients are typically observed for injection-related reactions for 2 hours postinjections and followed up with a phone call at day 3 and clinic visits on day 7 and at months 3, 6, 9, and 12 for safety and efficacy assessments [70]. In CD34+-based therapies, fundus oculi examination is performed at week 52 as well as baseline, week 4 and 12 in all patients to assess pathogenic retinal angiogenesis post CD34+ cell therapy [71]. To evaluate the incidence of malignant tumor post cell therapy, fecal human hemoglobin test, urine cytology, and chest and abdominal computed tomography are performed at week 52 [72].

3.3.1.2 Intralesional

The intralesional approach is another local method for stem cell delivery in patients with poorly healing wounds from PAD. The general approach is illustrated by Ismail et al. [73], whereby 20 patients with no-option CLI and ischemic wounds received implantation of autologous BMMNCs into the ulcer. These patients underwent bone marrow stimulation with G CSF for 3–5 days prior to bone marrow aspiration, where CD34+ BMMNCs were extracted, isolated, and purified. Patients were then brought to the OR where their ulcers were surgically debrided down to a clean and viable wound bed, whereby stem cells were then injected into the ulcer bed and ulcer edges using a 19Ga needle. The wound was protected with a wet-to-dry dressing comprising Betadine (povidone-iodine) for 24 hours, after which the wound was washed with saline and a new dressing applied. Adverse events after procedure were few and included injection site pain (25%), mild edema (15%), fever (10%), and small hematoma (5%). While four patients (20%) developed worsening necrosis and gangrene and required amputation, the majority witnessed symptomatic improvements after stem cell therapy, with 80% citing improvements in rest pain and increased pain-free walking distances at 3 years postimplantation.

This approach is also used by other groups, sometimes in combination with intramuscular delivery (Table 3.4). One theoretical concern with the intralesional approach is whether stem cells can survive and engraft when implanted into the inhospitable hypoxic environment that characterizes an ischemic ulcer. Nevertheless, it is possible that even a transient presence of stem cells accelerates wound healing sufficiently to provide clinical benefit. Clearly, more randomized and controlled studies are necessary to validate the efficacy of this approach.

3.3.2 Regional

3.3.2.1 Intra-arterial

The intra-arterial approach is a regional approach to stem cell delivery that has also been trialed for PAD. This method is illustrated by the double-blinded randomized controlled trial JUVENTAS (Rejuvenating Endothelial Progenitor Cells via Transcutaneous Intra-arterial Supplementation), which allocated 160 patients with severe no-option CLI to repetitive intra-arterial infusions of BMMNC or placebo [74]. Bone marrow aspirates (100 mL) were obtained from the right iliac crest of all patients, from which BMMNCs were isolated. These cells (657 million total, on average) were then infused into the common femoral artery of the affected limb by hand injection three times with 3-week intervals. Safety outcomes (all-cause mortality, malignancy, or hospitalization due to infection) were not significantly different between groups. However, the primary outcome of this trial, major amputation, was also not significantly different between stem cell and placebo. Secondary outcomes such as quality of life, rest pain, ABI, and TcPO2 were all improved during follow-up, but were again not significantly different between groups.

To date, a number of trials have investigated the intra-arterial approach for cell therapy in PAD patients (Table 3.5). Their general approach is similar to that taken by the JUVENTAS trial briefly outlined above. Routine angiography is performed before or during the procedure to identify the specific location of stenosis or occlusion [75]. Most commonly, the contralateral common femoral artery is punctured and accessed, through which a delivery catheter is placed proximal to the targeted artery. Typically, artery selection is determined by occlusion location; the popliteal artery is used for tibial occlusions, and the common femoral artery is used for superficial femoral artery occlusions [75]. The infusion is usually then performed over 3 minutes or at 800 or 900 ml/h [76, 77]. In order to enhance cell delivery, some have used a balloon catheter, whereby a balloon proximal to the catheter tip is inflated during infusion to prevent retrograde flow of cells [78].

Conceptually, intra-arterial stem cell delivery is appealing because stem cells can be broadly delivered to a target vessel's tributaries without the discomfort of multiple intramuscular injections. Furthermore, since cells will be deposited in tissues where vessels are still patent (and thus have higher oxygen content), they have a greater chance for survival and regeneration [79]. This rationale is also a cause for

Table 3.5 Intra-arterial delivery of stem cells for peripheral artery disease

Study	Treated/control	Disease	Cell type	Cell dose (×10⁶)	Infusion rate (ml/h)	Injection location	Duration	Serious adverse events
Cobellis 2008 (42)	10/9	CLTI	BMMNC	1000	120	Femoral	Twice, 45 days apart	None
Napoli 2008 (43)	18/18	CLTI	BMC	1310–6030	100	Femoral	Twice, 45 days apart	.N/A
Chochola 2008 (44)	24	CLTI (21) TAO (3)	BMMNC	53,100	900	Femoral	Single treatment	None
Walter 2011 (45)	19/21	CLTI (32) TAO (8)	BMMNC	153	N/A	SFA or PFA	Single treatment	1 in-stent thrombus, 1 groin hematoma, 1 pseudoaneurysm
Ruiz-Salmeron 2011 (46)	20	CLTI	BMMNC	266.2	N/A	SFA or popliteal	Single treatment	None
Schiavetta 2012 (47)	34	CLTI	BMMNC	903	150	Femoral	Twice, 45 days apart	None
Das 2013 (48)	8	CLTI	BMMSC	2/kg	N/A	Femoral	Single treatment	None
Teraa 2015 (49)	81/79	CLTI	BMMNC	657	N/A	CFA	3× every 3 weeks	No difference between treatment and control

References

42. Cobellis G, Silvestroni A, Lillo S, Sica G, Botti C, Maione C, et al. Long-term effects of repeated autologous transplantation of bone marrow cells in patients affected by peripheral arterial disease. Bone Marr Transpl. 2008;42(10):667–72. PubMed PMID: 18695661
43. Napoli C, Farzati B, Sica V, Iannuzzi E, Coppola G, Silvestroni A, et al. Beneficial effects of autologous bone marrow cell infusion and antioxidants/L-arginine in patients with chronic critical limb ischemia. Eur J Cardiovasc Prev Rehabil. 2008;15(6):709–18. PubMed PMID: 19050436

44. Chochola M, Pytlik R, Kobylka P, Skalicka L, Kideryova L, Beran S, et al. Autologous intra-arterial infusion of bone marrow mononuclear cells in patients with critical leg ischemia. Int Angiol. 2008;27(4):281–90. PubMed PMID: 18677289

45. Walter DH, Krankenberg H, Balzer JO, Kalka C, Baumgartner I, Schluter M, et al. Intraarterial administration of bone marrow mononuclear cells in patients with critical limb ischemia: a randomized-start, placebo-controlled pilot trial (PROVASA). Circul Cardiovasc Intervent. 2011;4(1):26–37. PubMed PMID: 21205939

46. Ruiz-Salmeron R, de la Cuesta-Diaz A, Constantino-Bermejo M, Perez-Camacho I, Marcos-Sanchez F, Hmadcha A, et al. Angiographic demonstration of neoangiogenesis after intra-arterial infusion of autologous bone marrow mononuclear cells in diabetic patients with critical limb ischemia. Cell Transpl. 2011;20(10):1629–39. PubMed PMID: 22289660. Epub 2012/02/01. eng

47 Schiavetta A, Maione C, Botti C, Marino G, Lillo S, Garrone A, et al. A phase II trial of autologous transplantation of bone marrow stem cells for critical limb ischemia: results of the Naples and Pietra Ligure Evaluation of Stem Cells study. Stem Cells Transl Med. 2012;1(7):572–8. PubMed PMID: 23197862. Pubmed Central PMCID: PMC3659723. Epub 2012/12/01. eng

48. Das AK, Bin Abdullah BJ, Dhillon SS, Vijanari A, Anoop CH, Gupta PK. Intra-arterial allogeneic mesenchymal stem cells for critical limb ischemia are safe and efficacious: report of a phase I study. World J Surg. 2013;37(4):915–22. PubMed PMID: 23307180

49. Teraa M, Sprengers RW, Schutgens RE, Slaper-Cortenbach IC, van der Graaf Y, Algra A, et al. Effect of repetitive intra-arterial infusion of bone marrow mononuclear cells in patients with no-option limb ischemia: the randomized, double-blind, placebo-controlled Rejuvenating Endothelial Progenitor Cells via Transcutaneous Intra-arterial Supplementation (JUVENTAS) trial. Circulation. 2015;131(10):851–60. PubMed PMID: 25567765

CLTI chronic limb threatening ischemia, *TAO* thromboangiitis obliterans, *BMMNC* bone marrow mononuclear cell, *BMC* bone marrow cells, *BMMSC* bone marrow mesenchymal stem cells, *SFA* superficial femoral artery, *PFA* profunda femoral artery, *CFA* common femoral artery

criticism however, as poorly perfused regions—areas that might benefit most from cell therapy—are also least likely to receive the stem cells.

3.3.2.2 Intramuscular vs Intra-arterial

Only a few small studies have compared intra-arterial to intramuscular routes of stem cell delivery for PAD. Klepanec et al. randomly assigned 41 patients with CLI to intramuscular or intra-arterial delivery of BMMNCs and found that intramuscular and intra-arterial methods of delivery are equally effective in limb salvage and wound healing, with no significant differences in various functional surrogate end points between the techniques [77]. These observations are consistent with a study by Van Tongeren et al. which showed no differences in amputation rate or the extent of perfusion improvement after intramuscular administration or combined intramuscular and intra-arterial administration in 21 randomized patients with CLI [80].

However, in a recent meta-analysis comparing intramuscular and intra-arterial delivery, while rest pain score was significantly improved with either route, only intramuscular administration was associated with a significant improvement in amputation rate, amputation-free survival, complete wound healing, ABI, and TcO2 [81]. This analysis suggests that intramuscular implantation may be preferable to intra-arterial infusion.

3.3.2.3 Combined Intra-Arterial and Intramuscular

Some authors have obviated the need to decide between intramuscular and intra-arterial routes by using both approaches in each patient (Table 3.6). For instance, Bartsch et al. performed stem cell transplantation of autologous BMMNCs using both intra-arterial and intramuscular routes in 13 patients with chronic ischemic limbs [82]. They even utilized a unique four-stage protocol whereby transient ischemia is generated within the muscle groups to enhance honing of stem cells to ischemic regions [83]. In the first stage, they first had patients exercise on a bicycle until ischemic pain was induced. Then, a second ischemic stimulus was introduced by inflating a thigh blood pressure cuff to suprasystolic pressure for a few minutes. The cuff pressure was then released, the femoral artery punctured, and 10 ml of stem cell suspension was infused intra-arterially. The third stage immediately followed the infusion, whereby the blood pressure cuff was reinflated to suprasystolic pressures for a few minutes to stop flow. After releasing the pressure, stem cell suspension was injected intramuscularly in fractions of 1 mL at five different sites of the quadriceps and gastrocnemius muscles. This was finally followed by exercise on a bicycle. No side effects or complications were noted, and patients who received cells had significant improvements in walking distance 2 and 13 months following therapy [82]. Although this was a small non-randomized study, it offers an example of a rationally designed approach to enhance cell therapy by taking advantage of each of the benefits of the intramuscular and intra-arterial methods, optimizing delivery both to the afflicted muscles and ischemic border zones.

Table 3.6 Intra-arterial and intramuscular delivery for peripheral artery disease

Study	Treated/control	Disease	Cell type	Cell dose (×10⁶)	Duration	IM location (# sites)	IA location (infusion rate, ml/hr)	Serious adverse events
Bartsch 2007 (50)	13/12	CLTI	BMMNC	N/A	Single treatment	Quadriceps (5) gastrocnemius (5)	Femoral (N/A)	None
Malyar 2014 (51)	16	CLTI (14) TAO (2)	BMMNC	420	Single treatment	Thigh and calf muscles (80)	Proximal to occlusion (N/A)	1 thrombosis of bypass graft; asymptomatic hemoglobin drop of 1.1 g/dl
Franz 2015 (52)	49	CLTI (47) TAO (2)	BMMNC	N/A	Single treatment	Ischemic muscles (6)	Proximal to occlusion (N/A)	None
*Klepanec 2012 (53)	40	CLTI	BMMNC	N/A	Single treatment	*Affected muscles along crural arteries (N/A)	*Proximal to occlusion (800)	None

References

50. Bartsch T, Brehm M, Zeus T, Kogler G, Wernet P, Strauer BE. Transplantation of autologous mononuclear bone marrow stem cells in patients with peripheral arterial disease (the TAM-PAD study). Clin Res Cardiol. 2007;96(12):891–9. PubMed PMID: 17694378. Epub 2007/08/19. eng
51. Malyar NM, Radtke S, Malyar K, Arjumand J, Horn PA, Kroger K, et al. Autologous bone marrow mononuclear cell therapy improves symptoms in patients with end-stage peripheral arterial disease and reduces inflammation-associated parameters. Cytotherapy. 2014;16(9):1270–9. PubMed PMID: 24972744
52. Franz RW, Shah KJ, Pin RH, Hankins T, Hartman JF, Wright ML. Autologous bone marrow mononuclear cell implantation therapy is an effective limb salvage strategy for patients with severe peripheral arterial disease. J Vasc Surg. 2015 Sep;62(3):673–80. PubMed PMID: 26304481
53. Klepanec A, Mistrik M, Altaner C, Valachovicova M, Olejarova I, Slysko R, et al. No difference in intra-arterial and intramuscular delivery of autologous bone marrow cells in patients with advanced critical limb ischemia. Cell Transpl. 2012;21(9):1909–18. PubMed PMID: 22472173. Epub 2012/04/05. eng
IM intramuscular, *IA*: intra-arterial, *CLTI* chronic limb threatening ischemia, *TAO* thromboangiitis obliterans, *BMMNC* bone marrow mononuclear cells.
*Patients received either intra-arterial or intramuscular, not both

3.3.3 Summary

Stem cell trials for PAD have demonstrated that stem cell therapy is a viable option for "no-option" critical limb ischemia. In fact, in their meta-analysis of autologous stem cells for PAD in 2017, Rigato et al. concluded that "autologous cell therapy may be considered as a new standard of care" and opined that since "there is no alternative to amputation in patients with intractable CLI, but cell therapy has the potential to modify the natural history of this life threatening condition…one can argue that further RCTs [comparing cell therapy to placebo] may not be ethical, and these patients should receive cell therapy, where available" [84]. Nonetheless, important details on how to increase the efficacy of stem cell therapy with optimal patient selection, cell type, dose, and delivery approach(es) still remain to be worked out.

3.4 Conclusions

This chapter summarizes stem cell delivery approaches for stroke and severe PAD. Commensurate with the elevated risk of a novel therapeutic, stem cells have been trialed in severe diseases where few other therapeutic options exist. Even so, the Hippocratic "do no harm" imperative appropriately mandates high standards of safety for any therapy, and these trials have importantly demonstrated both feasibility and adequate safety using a variety of local, regional, and systemic delivery approaches. Local methods are more invasive and harbor greater procedural risk, especially in stroke, but carry the advantage of guaranteed deposition of cells within the desired area and a smaller cell dose requirement. On the other hand, a systemic delivery of cells intravenously is procedurally safe and may have systemically beneficial effects with immunomodulatory effects and potential effects on other organs (e.g., concurrent therapy for ischemic cardiomyopathy) but requires large numbers of cells and may have low rates of engraftment within target organs. Regional delivery methods have intermediate procedural risk associated with vascular/spinal access and, in addition for stroke, risk of microembolism. However, regional delivery requires an intermediate dose of cells, can dovetail with other endovascular interventions, and can provide both local and systemic effects. For stroke patients, the best method for stem cell delivery can vary depending on patient factors such as the type and phase of stroke and other planned therapies. On the other hand, it is yet unclear whether patient factors should influence the best cell delivery approach for patients with CLI. Clearly, a lot of work remains to be done before stem cell therapy can be used routinely in the clinical setting, with the first priority now in establishing the efficacy and confirming the long-term safety of existing stem cell therapies with larger phase 2 and 3 trials. In addition, further research and innovation in improving cell therapy, such as the development of the next generation of engineered stem cells [85–87], and improved cell retention devices employing scaffolds, stents, or bioreactors [88–90] are underway and whose results are eagerly anticipated by providers and patients alike.

References

1. Hou L, Kim JJ, Woo YJ, Huang NF. Stem cell-based therapies to promote angiogenesis in ischemic cardiovascular disease. Am J Phys Heart Circ Phys. 2016;310(4):H455–65. PubMed PMID: 26683902. Pubmed Central PMCID: 4796616.
2. Zhao L, Johnson T, Liu D. Therapeutic angiogenesis of adipose-derived stem cells for ischemic diseases. Stem Cell Res Ther. 2017;8(1):125. PubMed PMID: 28583178. Pubmed Central PMCID: 5460534.
3. Chau M, Zhang J, Wei L, Yu SP. Regeneration after stroke: stem cell transplantation and trophic factors. Brain Circul. 2016;2(2):86–94. PubMed PMID: 30276278. Pubmed Central PMCID: 6126254.
4. Marsh SE, Blurton-Jones M. Neural stem cell therapy for neurodegenerative disorders: the role of neurotrophic support. Neurochem Int. 2017;106:94–100. PubMed PMID: 28219641. Pubmed Central PMCID: 5446923.
5. Baraniak PR, McDevitt TC. Stem cell paracrine actions and tissue regeneration. Regenerat Med. 2010 Jan;5(1):121–43. PubMed PMID: 20017699. Pubmed Central PMCID: 2833273.
6. Singh AK, McGuirk JP. Allogeneic Stem cell transplantation: a historical and scientific overview. Cancer Res. 2016;76(22):6445–51. PubMed PMID: 27784742
7. Katarzyna R. Adult stem cell therapy for cardiac repair in patients after acute myocardial infarction leading to ischemic heart failure: an overview of evidence from the recent clinical trials. Curr Cardiol Rev. 2017;13(3):223–31. PubMed PMID: 28464769. Pubmed Central PMCID: 5633717.
8. Madonna R, Van Laake LW, Davidson SM, Engel FB, Hausenloy DJ, Lecour S, et al. Position Paper of the European Society of Cardiology Working Group Cellular Biology of the Heart: cell-based therapies for myocardial repair and regeneration in ischemic heart disease and heart failure. Eur Heart J. 2016;37(23):1789–98. PubMed PMID: 27055812. Pubmed Central PMCID: 4912026.
9. Qadura M, Terenzi DC, Verma S, Al-Omran M, Hess DA. Concise review: cell therapy for critical limb ischemia: an integrated review of preclinical and clinical studies. Stem Cells. 2018;36(2):161–71. PubMed PMID: 29226477
10. Wahid FSA, Ismail NA, Wan Jamaludin WF, Muhamad NA, Mohamad Idris MA, Lai NM. Efficacy and safety of Autologous cell-based therapy in patients with no-option critical limb Ischaemia: a meta-analysis. Curr Stem Cell Res Ther. 2018;13(4):265–83. PubMed PMID: 29532760
11. Zheng H, Zhang B, Chhatbar PY, Dong Y, Alawieh A, Lowe F, et al. Mesenchymal stem cell therapy in stroke: a systematic review of literature in pre-clinical and clinical research. Cell Transpl. 2018;27(12):1723–30. PubMed PMID: 30343609. Pubmed Central PMCID: 6300779.
12. Steele AN, MacArthur JW, Woo YJ. Stem cell therapy: healing or hype? Why stem cell delivery doesn't work. Circulat Res. 2017;120(12):1868–70. PubMed PMID: 28596172. Pubmed Central PMCID: 5947316.
13. Collaborators GBDS. Global, regional, and national burden of stroke, 1990–2016: a systematic analysis for the Global Burden of Disease Study 2016. Lancet Neurol. 2019;18(5):439–58. PubMed PMID: 30871944. Pubmed Central PMCID: 6494974.
14. Mampalam TJ, Gonzalez MF, Weinstein P, Sharp FR. Neuronal changes in fetal cortex transplanted to ischemic adult rat cortex. J Neurosurg. 1988;69(6):904–12. PubMed PMID: 3193196
15. Grabowski M, Brundin P, Johansson BB. Fetal neocortical grafts implanted in adult hypertensive rats with cortical infarcts following a middle cerebral artery occlusion: ingrowth of afferent fibers from the host brain. Exp Neurol. 1992;116(2):105–21. PubMed PMID: 1577119
16. Grabowski M, Christofferson RH, Brundin P, Johansson BB. Vascularization of fetal neocortical grafts implanted in brain infarcts in spontaneously hypertensive rats. Neuroscience. 1992;51(3):673–82. PubMed PMID: 1488117

17. Grabowski M, Brundin P, Johansson BB. Functional integration of cortical grafts placed in brain infarcts of rats. Ann Neurol. 1993;34(3):362–8. PubMed PMID: 8363353
18. Nishino H, Aihara N, Czurko A, Hashitani T, Isobe Y, Ichikawa O, et al. Reconstruction of GABAergic transmission and behavior by striatal cell grafts in rats with ischemic infarcts in the middle cerebral artery. J Neural Transpl Plast. 1993;4(2):147–55. PubMed PMID: 8110865. Pubmed Central PMCID: 2565254.
19. Kondziolka D, Wechsler L, Goldstein S, Meltzer C, Thulborn KR, Gebel J, et al. Transplantation of cultured human neuronal cells for patients with stroke. Neurology. 2000;55(4):565–9. PubMed PMID: 10953194
20. Kondziolka D, Steinberg GK, Wechsler L, Meltzer CC, Elder E, Gebel J, et al. Neurotransplantation for patients with subcortical motor stroke: a phase 2 randomized trial. J Neurosurg. 2005;103(1):38–45. PubMed PMID: 16121971
21. Kondziolka D, Steinberg GK, Cullen SB, McGrogan M. Evaluation of surgical techniques for neuronal cell transplantation used in patients with stroke. Cell Transplant. 2004;13(7–8):749–54. PubMed PMID: 15690976
22. Kalladka D, Sinden J, Pollock K, Haig C, McLean J, Smith W, et al. Human neural stem cells in patients with chronic ischaemic stroke (PISCES): a phase 1, first-in-man study. Lancet. 2016;388(10046):787–96. PubMed PMID: 27497862
23. Investigation of Neural Stem Cells in Ischemic Stroke. https://ClinicalTrials.gov/show/NCT03629275.
24. Li ZM, Zhang ZT, Guo CJ, Geng FY, Qiang F, Wang LX. Autologous bone marrow mononuclear cell implantation for intracerebral hemorrhage-a prospective clinical observation. Clin Neurol Neurosurg. 2013;115(1):72–6. PubMed PMID: 22657095
25. Chang Z, Mao G, Sun L, Ao Q, Gu Y, Liu Y. Cell therapy for cerebral hemorrhage: Five year follow-up report. Exp Therap Med. 2016;12(6):3535–40. PubMed PMID: 28101148. Pubmed Central PMCID: 5228203.
26. Mendonca ML, Freitas GR, Silva SA, Manfrim A, Falcao CH, Gonzales C, et al. [Safety of intra-arterial autologous bone marrow mononuclear cell transplantation for acute ischemic stroke]. Arquivos Brasileiros de Cardiologia. 2006;86(1):52–5. PubMed PMID: 16491209. Seguranca do transplante autologo, intra-arterial, de celulas mononucleares da medula ossea na fase aguda do acidente vascular cerebral isquemico.
27. Papanagiotou P, Ntaios G. Endovascular Thrombectomy in acute ischemic stroke. Circ Cardiovasc Interv. 2018;11(1):e005362. PubMed PMID: 29311286
28. Janowski M, Lyczek A, Engels C, Xu J, Lukomska B, Bulte JW, et al. Cell size and velocity of injection are major determinants of the safety of intracarotid stem cell transplantation. Journal of cerebral blood flow and metabolism: official journal of the International Society of Cerebral Blood Flow and Metabolism. 2013;33(6):921–7. PubMed PMID: 23486296. Pubmed Central PMCID: 3677113.
29. Ge J, Guo L, Wang S, Zhang Y, Cai T, Zhao RC, et al. The size of mesenchymal stem cells is a significant cause of vascular obstructions and stroke. Stem Cell Rev Rep. 2014;10(2):295–303. PubMed PMID: 24390934
30. Cui LL, Kerkela E, Bakreen A, Nitzsche F, Andrzejewska A, Nowakowski A, et al. The cerebral embolism evoked by intra-arterial delivery of allogeneic bone marrow mesenchymal stem cells in rats is related to cell dose and infusion velocity. Stem Cell Res Ther 2015;6:11. PubMed PMID: 25971703. Pubmed Central PMCID: 4429328.
31. Mitkari B, Kerkela E, Nystedt J, Korhonen M, Jolkkonen J. Unexpected complication in a rat stroke model: exacerbation of secondary pathology in the thalamus by subacute intraarterial administration of human bone marrow-derived mesenchymal stem cells. J Cerebral Blood Flow Metab. 2015;35(3):363–6. PubMed PMID: 25564231. Pubmed Central PMCID: 4348397.
32. Argibay B, Trekker J, Himmelreich U, Beiras A, Topete A, Taboada P, et al. Intraarterial route increases the risk of cerebral lesions after mesenchymal cell administration in animal model

of ischemia. Sci Rep. 2017;7:40758. PubMed PMID: 28091591. Pubmed Central PMCID: 5238501.

33. Li L, Jiang Q, Ding G, Zhang L, Zhang ZG, Li Q, et al. Effects of administration route on migration and distribution of neural progenitor cells transplanted into rats with focal cerebral ischemia, an MRI study. J Cerebral Blood Flow Metab. 2010;30(3):653–62. PubMed PMID: 19888287. Pubmed Central PMCID: 2844252.

34. Walczak P, Zhang J, Gilad AA, Kedziorek DA, Ruiz-Cabello J, Young RG, et al. Dual-modality monitoring of targeted intraarterial delivery of mesenchymal stem cells after transient ischemia. Stroke. 2008;39(5):1569–74. PubMed PMID: 18323495. Pubmed Central PMCID: 2857730.

35. Guzman R, Janowski M, Walczak P. Intra-arterial delivery of cell therapies for stroke. Stroke. 2018;49(5):1075–82. PubMed PMID: 29669876. Pubmed Central PMCID: 6027638.

36. Jiang Y, Zhu W, Zhu J, Wu L, Xu G, Liu X. Feasibility of delivering mesenchymal stem cells via catheter to the proximal end of the lesion artery in patients with stroke in the territory of the middle cerebral artery. Cell Transplant. 2013;22(12):2291–8. PubMed PMID: 23127560

37. Kaufmann TJ, Huston J 3rd, Mandrekar JN, Schleck CD, Thielen KR, Kallmes DF. Complications of diagnostic cerebral angiography: evaluation of 19,826 consecutive patients. Radiology. 2007;243(3):812–9. PubMed PMID: 17517935

38. Meng S, Qiao M, Foniok T, Tuor UI. White matter damage precedes that in gray matter despite similar magnetic resonance imaging changes following cerebral hypoxia-ischemia in neonatal rats. Exp Brain Res. 2005;166(1):56–60. PubMed PMID: 15968456

39. Sharma A, Sane H, Gokulchandran N, Khopkar D, Paranjape A, Sundaram J, et al. Autologous bone marrow mononuclear cells intrathecal transplantation in chronic stroke. Stroke Res Treat. 2014;2014:234095. PubMed PMID: 25126443. Pubmed Central PMCID: 4121152.

40. Pan K, Deng L, Chen P, Peng Q, Pan J, Wu Y, et al. Safety and feasibility of repeated intrathecal allogeneic bone marrow-derived mesenchymal stromal cells in patients with neurological diseases. Stem Cells Int. 2019;2019:8421281. PubMed PMID: 31428161. Pubmed Central PMCID: 6683773 publication of this article.

41. Bang OY, Lee JS, Lee PH, Lee G. Autologous mesenchymal stem cell transplantation in stroke patients. Ann Neurol. 2005;57(6):874–82. PubMed PMID: 15929052

42. Prasad K, Sharma A, Garg A, Mohanty S, Bhatnagar S, Johri S, et al. Intravenous autologous bone marrow mononuclear stem cell therapy for ischemic stroke: a multicentric, randomized trial. Stroke. 2014;45(12):3618–24. PubMed PMID: 25378424

43. Hess DC, Wechsler LR, Clark WM, Savitz SI, Ford GA, Chiu D, et al. Safety and efficacy of multipotent adult progenitor cells in acute ischaemic stroke (MASTERS): a randomised, double-blind, placebo-controlled, phase 2 trial. Lancet Neurol. 2017;16(5):360–8. PubMed PMID: 28320635

44. Fischer UM, Harting MT, Jimenez F, Monzon-Posadas WO, Xue H, Savitz SI, et al. Pulmonary passage is a major obstacle for intravenous stem cell delivery: the pulmonary first-pass effect. Stem Cells Develop. 2009;18(5):683–92. PubMed PMID: 19099374. Pubmed Central PMCID: 3190292.

45. Savitz SI, Misra V, Kasam M, Juneja H, Cox CS Jr, Alderman S, et al. Intravenous autologous bone marrow mononuclear cells for ischemic stroke. Ann Neurol. 2011;70(1):59–69. PubMed PMID: 21786299

46. Misra V, Ritchie MM, Stone LL, Low WC, Janardhan V. Stem cell therapy in ischemic stroke: role of IV and intra-arterial therapy. Neurology. 2012;79(13 Suppl 1):S207–12. PubMed PMID: 23008400. Pubmed Central PMCID: 4109232.

47. Kassner A, Merali Z. Assessment of blood-brain barrier disruption in stroke. Stroke. 2015;46(11):3310–5. PubMed PMID: 26463696

48. Boshuizen MCS, Steinberg GK. Stem cell-based immunomodulation after stroke: effects on brain repair processes. Stroke. 2018;49(6):1563–70. PubMed PMID: 29724892. Pubmed Central PMCID: 6063361.

49. MultiStem® Administration for Stroke Treatment and Enhanced Recovery Study. https://ClinicalTrials.gov/show/NCT03545607.
50. Chen L, Xi H, Huang H, Zhang F, Liu Y, Chen D, et al. Multiple cell transplantation based on an intraparenchymal approach for patients with chronic phase stroke. Cell Transplant. 2013;22(Suppl 1):S83–91. PubMed PMID: 23992950
51. Shu J, Santulli G. Update on peripheral artery disease: epidemiology and evidence-based facts. Atherosclerosis. 2018;275:379–81. PubMed PMID: 29843915. Pubmed Central PMCID: 6113064.
52. Varu VN, Hogg ME, Kibbe MR. Critical limb ischemia. J Vasc Surg. 2010;51(1):230–41. PubMed PMID: 20117502
53. Uccioli L, Meloni M, Izzo V, Giurato L, Merolla S, Gandini R. Critical limb ischemia: current challenges and future prospects. Vasc Health Risk Manag. 2018;14:63–74. PubMed PMID: 29731636. Pubmed Central PMCID: 5927064.
54. Sprengers RW, Teraa M, Moll FL, de Wit GA, van der Graaf Y, Verhaar MC, et al. Quality of life in patients with no-option critical limb ischemia underlines the need for new effective treatment. J Vasc Surg. 2010;52(4):843–9, 9.e1. PubMed PMID: 20598482
55. Xie B, Luo H, Zhang Y, Wang Q, Zhou C, Xu D. Autologous stem cell therapy in critical limb ischemia: a meta-analysis of randomized controlled trials. Stem Cells Int. 2018;2018:7528464. PubMed PMID: 29977308. Pubmed Central PMCID: 5994285.
56. Gao W, Chen D, Liu G, Ran X. Autologous stem cell therapy for peripheral arterial disease: a systematic review and meta-analysis of randomized controlled trials. Stem Cell Res Therap. 2019;10(1):140. PubMed PMID: 31113463. Pubmed Central PMCID: 6528204.
57. Tateishi-Yuyama E, Matsubara H, Murohara T, Ikeda U, Shintani S, Masaki H, et al. Therapeutic angiogenesis for patients with limb ischaemia by autologous transplantation of bone-marrow cells: a pilot study and a randomised controlled trial. Lancet. 2002;360(9331):427–35. PubMed PMID: 12241713. Epub 2002/09/21. eng
58. Biscetti F, Bonadia N, Nardella E, Cecchini AL, Landolfi R, Flex A. The role of the stem cells therapy in the peripheral artery disease. Int J Mol Sci. 2019;20(9):2233. PubMed PMID: 31067647. eng
59. Huang P, Li S, Han M, Xiao Z, Yang R, Han ZC. Autologous transplantation of granulocyte colony-stimulating factor-mobilized peripheral blood mononuclear cells improves critical limb ischemia in diabetes. Diabetes Care. 2005;28(9):2155–60. PubMed PMID: 16123483. Epub 2005/08/27. eng.
60. Fukumoto Y, Miyamoto T, Okamura T, Gondo H, Iwasaki H, Horiuchi T, et al. Angina pectoris occurring during granulocyte colony-stimulating factor-combined preparatory regimen for autologous peripheral blood stem cell transplantation in a patient with acute myelogenous leukaemia. Br J Haematol. 1997;97(3):666–8. PubMed PMID: 9207419. Epub 1997/06/01. eng.
61. Kawachi Y, Watanabe A, Uchida T, Yoshizawa K, Kurooka N, Setsu K. Acute arterial thrombosis due to platelet aggregation in a patient receiving granulocyte colony-stimulating factor. Br J Haematol. 1996;94(2):413–6. PubMed PMID: 8759907. Epub 1996/08/01. eng.
62. Heo S-H, Park Y-S, Kang E-S, Park K-B, Do Y-S, Kang K-S, et al. Early results of clinical application of Autologous whole bone marrow Stem cell transplantation for critical limb ischemia with Buerger's disease. Sci Rep. 2016;6(1):19690.
63. Amann B, Luedemann C, Ratei R, Schmidt-Lucke JA. Autologous bone marrow cell transplantation increases leg perfusion and reduces amputations in patients with advanced critical limb ischemia due to peripheral artery disease. Cell Transplant. 2009;18(3):371–80. PubMed PMID: 19500466. Epub 2009/06/09. eng
64. Prochazka V, Gumulec J, Jaluvka F, Salounova D, Jonszta T, Czerny D, et al. Cell therapy, a new standard in management of chronic critical limb ischemia and foot ulcer. Cell Transplant. 2010;19(11):1413–24. PubMed PMID: 20529449. Pubmed Central PMCID: PMC5478382. Epub 2010/06/10. eng
65. Madaric J, Klepanec A. Cell therapy in peripheral artery disease. In: Lanzer P, editor. PanVascular medicine. Berlin, Heidelberg: Springer Berlin Heidelberg; 2015. p. 3227–52.

66. Kolvenbach R, Kreissig C, Cagiannos C, Afifi R, Schmaltz E. Intraoperative adjunctive stem cell treatment in patients with critical limb ischemia using a novel point-of-care device. Ann Vasc Surg. 2010;24(3):367–72. PubMed PMID: 19896796. Epub 2009/11/10. eng

67. Burt RK, Testori A, Oyama Y, Rodriguez HE, Yaung K, Villa M, et al. Autologous peripheral blood CD133+ cell implantation for limb salvage in patients with critical limb ischemia. Bone Marrow Transplant. 2010;45(1):111–6. PubMed PMID: 19448678. Pubmed Central PMCID: PMC3951860. Epub 2009/05/19. eng

68. Szabo GV, Kovesd Z, Cserepes J, Daroczy J, Belkin M, Acsady G. Peripheral blood-derived autologous stem cell therapy for the treatment of patients with late-stage peripheral artery disease-results of the short- and long-term follow-up. Cytotherapy. 2013;15(10):1245–52. PubMed PMID: 23993298. Epub 2013/09/03. eng

69. Lu D, Chen B, Liang Z, Deng W, Jiang Y, Li S, et al. Comparison of bone marrow mesenchymal stem cells with bone marrow-derived mononuclear cells for treatment of diabetic critical limb ischemia and foot ulcer: a double-blind, randomized, controlled trial. Diabetes Res Clin Pract. 2011;92(1):26–36. PubMed PMID: 21216483. Epub 2011/01/11. eng

70. Powell RJ, Marston WA, Berceli SA, Guzman R, Henry TD, Longcore AT, et al. Cellular therapy with Ixmyelocel-T to treat critical limb ischemia: the randomized, double-blind, placebo-controlled RESTORE-CLI trial. Mol Ther. 2012;20(6):1280–6. PubMed PMID: 22453769. Pubmed Central PMCID: PMC3369291. Epub 2012/03/29. eng

71. Kinoshita M, Fujita Y, Katayama M, Baba R, Shibakawa M, Yoshikawa K, et al. Long-term clinical outcome after intramuscular transplantation of granulocyte colony stimulating factor-mobilized CD34 positive cells in patients with critical limb ischemia. Atherosclerosis. 2012;224(2):440–5. PubMed PMID: 22877866. Epub 2012/08/11. eng

72. Napoli C, Farzati B, Sica V, Iannuzzi E, Coppola G, Silvestroni A, et al. Beneficial effects of autologous bone marrow cell infusion and antioxidants/L-arginine in patients with chronic critical limb ischemia. Eur J Cardiovasc Prev Rehabil. 2008;15(6):709–18. PubMed PMID: 19050436. Epub 2008/12/04. eng

73. Ismail AM, Abdou SM, Aty HA, Kamhawy AH, Elhinedy M, Elwageh M, et al. Autologous transplantation of CD34(+) bone marrow derived mononuclear cells in management of non-reconstructable critical lower limb ischemia. Cytotechnology. 2016;68(4):771–81. PubMed PMID: 25511801. Pubmed Central PMCID: 4960127.

74. Teraa M, Sprengers RW, Schutgens RE, Slaper-Cortenbach IC, van der Graaf Y, Algra A, et al. Effect of repetitive intra-arterial infusion of bone marrow mononuclear cells in patients with no-option limb ischemia: the randomized, double-blind, placebo-controlled rejuvenating endothelial progenitor cells via transcutaneous intra-arterial supplementation (JUVENTAS) trial. Circulation. 2015;131(10):851–60. PubMed PMID: 25567765

75. Franz RW, Shah KJ, Pin RH, Hankins T, Hartman JF, Wright ML. Autologous bone marrow mononuclear cell implantation therapy is an effective limb salvage strategy for patients with severe peripheral arterial disease. J Vasc Surg. 2015;62(3):673–80. PubMed PMID: 26304481. Epub 2015/08/26. eng

76. Chochola M, Pytlik R, Kobylka P, Skalicka L, Kideryova L, Beran S, et al. Autologous intra-arterial infusion of bone marrow mononuclear cells in patients with critical leg ischemia. Int Angiol. 2008;27(4):281–90. PubMed PMID: 18677289. Epub 2008/08/05. eng.

77. Klepanec A, Mistrik M, Altaner C, Valachovicova M, Olejarova I, Slysko R, et al. No difference in intra-arterial and intramuscular delivery of autologous bone marrow cells in patients with advanced critical limb ischemia. Cell Transpl. 2012;21(9):1909–18. PubMed PMID: 22472173. Epub 2012/04/05. eng.

78. Ruiz-Salmeron R, de la Cuesta-Diaz A, Constantino-Bermejo M, Perez-Camacho I, Marcos-Sanchez F, Hmadcha A, et al. Angiographic demonstration of neoangiogenesis after intra-arterial infusion of autologous bone marrow mononuclear cells in diabetic patients with critical limb ischemia. Cell Transplant. 2011;20(10):1629–39. PubMed PMID: 22289660. Epub 2012/02/01. eng.

79. Sprengers RW, Moll FL, Verhaar MC. Stem cell therapy in PAD. Eur J Vasc Endovasc Surg. 2010;39:S38–43.
80. Van Tongeren RB, Hamming JF, Fibbe WE, Van Weel V, Frerichs SJ, Stiggelbout AM, et al. Intramuscular or combined intramuscular/intra-arterial administration of bone marrow mononuclear cells: a clinical trial in patients with advanced limb ischemia. J Cardiovasc Surg. 2008;49(1):51–8. PubMed PMID: 18212687. Epub 2008/01/24. eng
81. Rigato M, Monami M, Fadini GP. Autologous cell therapy for peripheral arterial disease. Circ Res. 2017;120(8):1326–40.
82. Bartsch T, Brehm M, Zeus T, Kogler G, Wernet P, Strauer BE. Transplantation of autologous mononuclear bone marrow stem cells in patients with peripheral arterial disease (the TAM-PAD study). Clin Res Cardiol. 2007;96(12):891–9. PubMed PMID: 17694378. Epub 2007/08/19. eng.
83. Takahashi T, Kalka C, Masuda H, Chen D, Silver M, Kearney M, et al. Ischemia- and cytokine-induced mobilization of bone marrow-derived endothelial progenitor cells for neovascularization. Nat Med. 1999;5(4):434–8. PubMed PMID: 10202935
84. Rigato M, Monami M, Fadini GP. Autologous cell therapy for peripheral arterial disease: systematic review and meta-analysis of randomized, nonrandomized, and noncontrolled studies. Circ Res. 2017;120(8):1326–40. PubMed PMID: 28096194
85. Chen Z, Chen L, Zeng C, Wang WE. Functionally improved mesenchymal stem cells to better treat myocardial infarction. Stem Cells Int. 2018;2018:7045245. PubMed PMID: 30622568. Pubmed Central PMCID: 6286742.
86. Shafei AE, Ali MA, Ghanem HG, Shehata AI, Abdelgawad AA, Handal HR, et al. Mesenchymal stem cell therapy: a promising cell-based therapy for treatment of myocardial infarction. J Gene Med. 2017;19(12) PubMed PMID: 29044850
87. Ocansey DKW, Pei B, Yan Y, Qian H, Zhang X, Xu W, et al. Improved therapeutics of modified mesenchymal stem cells: an update. J Transl Med. 2020;18(1):42. PubMed PMID: 32000804. Pubmed Central PMCID: 6993499.
88. Hwang CW, Johnston PV, Gerstenblith G, Weiss RG, Tomaselli GF, Bogdan VE, et al. Stem cell impregnated nanofiber stent sleeve for on-stent production and intravascular delivery of paracrine factors. Biomaterials. 2015;52:318–26. PubMed PMID: 25818438
89. Johnston PV, Hwang CW, Bogdan V, Mills KJ, Eggan ER, Leszczynska A, et al. Intravascular stem cell bioreactor for prevention of adverse remodeling after myocardial infarction. J Am Heart Assoc. 2019;8(15):e012351. PubMed PMID: 31340693. Pubmed Central PMCID: 6761667.
90. Carotenuto F, Teodori L, Maccari AM, Delbono L, Orlando G, Di Nardo P. Turning regenerative technologies into treatment to repair myocardial injuries. J Cell Mol Med. 2020;24(5):2704–16. PubMed PMID: 31568640. Pubmed Central PMCID: 7077550.

Chapter 4
The Ethical Challenges of Stem Cell Therapy in Vascular Disorders

Ramesh K. Batra

4.1 Introduction

Stem cell-based therapeutics were initially used for bone marrow transplantation but further advancements, reprogramming and thus transformation has paved the way for a modern era of therapeutic applications targeting differing principles and modes of treatment. Stem cell therapy in vascular disorders, including cardiovascular disease, largely provides an angiogenic and vascular regenerative microenvironment for tissue remodeling and repair.

The advancements in stem cell therapy, although promising, are scientifically complex and ethically challenging both at the bench and bedside. The landscape of ethical challenges with stem cells ranges from the disputes regarding the onset of life and reproduction, to allowable practices for donation of embryos and creation of embryos from donated oocytes. Needless to say, each stem cell therapy poses a unique scientific and technical challenge including ethical and political issues that require thoughtful deliberation as the field progresses.

4.2 Embryonic Stem Cell (ESC)

ESCs are derived from the inner cell mass of the blastocyst, and their pluripotent potential to differentiate into any cell type is of particular use in therapeutics. Pluripotent ESCs have been directed to differentiate into vascular endothelial cells, smooth muscle cells, and cardiac myocytes [1, 2]. This is the foundation for therapeutic applications of ESCs in vascular regeneration and angiogenesis for vascular

R. K. Batra (✉)
Yale School of Medicine, Yale University, Yale New Haven Transplant Center,
New Haven, CT, USA
e-mail: Ramesh.batra@yale.edu

© Springer Nature Switzerland AG 2021
T. P. Navarro et al. (eds.), *Stem Cell Therapy for Vascular Diseases*,
https://doi.org/10.1007/978-3-030-56954-9_4

compromised ischemic limb or ischemic myocardial injury. However, besides the immunological barrier with the use of ESCs, there is a significant ethical challenge to its pluripotential and highly proliferative capability. The ethical challenge and hence the debate on ESCs revolve around the moral state of an embryo and the arbitrary nature of the initiation of "personhood" for the embryo.

4.2.1 The Moral State of the Embryo

The embryonal development starts with fertilization between a sperm and an oocyte, resulting in a blastocyst, which then implants itself onto the uterine wall for further differentiation and development, to form a fetus. Within these multiple stages of the pre-fetal developmental period, to pinpoint the exact time when life begins is arbitrary and thus debatable. Some hold a strong opinion that life begins at conception and therefore an embryo holds the same moral status as another human being, albeit with a developing and intermediate moral worth, carries full potential to grow into one and hence deserves full rights of "personhood." Besides the moral equality, they further claim that the biological existence of an embryo is similar to a human being, because it envelops within it the genetic code to human species. Similar views are also upheld by the President's Council on Bioethics who also support the claim to recognize an embryo as a member of the human family [3]. People with similar pro-life views also state that terminating an embryo's programmed course is not different than committing murder of a human being, wherein the future existence and relationships of an embryo or human are abruptly terminated.

Others, who are reluctant to grant the human being status to an embryo, do so due to various beliefs. Some agree that although the embryos belong to the human species, i.e., contains the human genetic code, the species membership alone is insufficient to grant the moral status of personhood [4]. But to define personhood is equally controversial, and the different capabilities defining personhood, i.e., sentience, consciousness, and mental capacity for intentional behavior, have all had their advocates [4, 5]. Yet the question remains, as to which behavioral or mental capacities will be eligible for the honorific term "person"; and whether the definition of personhood is maximalist or minimalist in nature [5]. With the indecision to define eligibility criterion for "personhood," the embryo finds itself simply nonexistent for the lack of all those qualities. While denying the moral status claim of an embryo as a human being, an interesting opinion states that the claim is based on potentiality rather than grounded in actual, whereby once the embryo becomes a person, its claim to personhood will be of relevance, but not until it stays an embryo [4, 6].

The third variation of thought is somewhere in the middle, i.e., the intermediate moral status of an embryo. This group does not regard human embryo to be a full human with its honorific "personhood," yet not a mere human tissue to be discarded at will either and deserves serious moral respect [3]. In a survey of 2,212 Americans by the Johns Hopkins University, majority of respondents (42%) accorded embryos an intermediate moral status [7]. Given the indecision and debate halting embryonic stem cell research from exploring its true potential, in 2001, President Bush, despite his pro-life views, approved the allowance of federal funding for stem cell research using ESC lines already in existence at the time, but prohibited creating additional ESC lines for that purpose. Also, the allowed funding was restricted to some existing cell lines only. In response, in 2009, President Obama lifted the controversial restraints for federal funding for ESC research to expand beyond the 60 extant cell lines, restricted by President Bush [8].

4.2.2   Donation of a Frozen Embryo for New ESC Lines

Ethical issues surrounding donation of frozen embryos for research present an additional set of hurdles. Infertility patients often freeze their remaining embryos after they have completed infertility treatment. The fate, i.e., the disposition of these remaining embryos has three paths to follow: be discarded, be donated to another couple for reproductive purposes, and lastly, be donated for research. Interestingly, since these embryos were created primarily for reproduction purposes and not research, it falls outside the restrictions imposed on stem cell research on new ESC lines by both the Obama and Bush administrations, hence minimizing the political controversies. In a survey of 2,210 infertility patients in the United States, majority of them expressed their willingness to donate their cryopreserved embryos for research [9], but the survey also revealed that the unwillingness to donate was due to the lack of trust on infertility clinics and clinicians, for the concern that their cryopreserved embryos could be used without consent [10]. This is because, in the United States, federal research regulations permit waiver of informed consent if the de-identified biological material cannot be linked back to the donor [11]. Such a waiver is perceived as breach of trust, as people often choose to place personal emotional and moral significance on their reproductive biological materials, and de-identifying ESC lines may not always be desirable. Because to use these cell lines for human transplantation in future, FDA may require linkage to donors to ascertain and minimize infectious and genetic disease transmission [12].

So, an informed consent ethically upholds the autonomy of the donors, and the consent also serves as the token of donor's participation in the research process which in turn ethically supports their willingness to donate. But to uphold autonomy, the integral component of informed consent, is not always feasible, especially in cases where frozen embryos were created from donated sperms or oocytes, i.e., gamete donors. Some may argue that consents from gamete donors are not needed, since they ceded their right to direct further usage of their gametes to the patients undergoing artificial reproductive treatment (ART) [13]. However, the rescinding of consent and usage rights of the gamete donors directly violates their autonomy, especially when in a study, 25% women who donated oocytes for ART patients did not want the resulting embryos to be used for research [14]. As for the sperm donors, little information exists about their wishes concerning research, because ART clinics often obtain donor sperm from sperm banks, therefore unable to have direct contact with the sperm donors, unlike oocyte donors. Moreover, sperms donated to sperm banks are done so with strict anonymity and confidentiality provisions, further limiting linkage of their opinions about research on the resulting embryo. Thereby, in the United States, National Academy of Sciences recommends specific guidelines to consent for stem cell research from embryo and also gamete donors [15].

4.3   Somatic Cell Nuclear Transfer (SCNT)

SCNT, as the name implies, is a technique to transfer nuclear material from a somatic cell to an enucleated cell. After the transference of nucleus, the somatic nucleus is then reprogrammed to eventually become a zygote, which is further allowed to develop into an embryo, a technique successfully used in creating "Dolly" the cloned sheep. Alternative to this is, allowing the zygote to reach blastocyst stage, after which embryonic stem cells are created from the inner cell mass of a blastocyst. The stem cells created through this technique have a similar potential to differentiate into vascular endothelial cells or cardiac myocytes, like ESCs, and be used in vascular regeneration models described earlier.

4.3.1   Human Oocytes for SCNT

Hwang et al. infamously claimed to successfully clone a human embryo through SCNT from donated oocytes and derive 11 ESC lines [16]. The research was groundbreaking but not only was it fraudulent with fabricated results but also included unethical procurement of donor oocytes. Investigations by the South Korean National Bioethics Committee in this case [17] revealed four different types of oocyte donations, three of which raised red flags due to payments to donors (approximately $1,400); benefit in kind, i.e., discount on IVF treatments ($2,134 approximately); and lastly, coerced unethical donation from his own laboratory's researchers, one of whom was the co-author on the paper [18].

Oocyte donation in general, be it research or ART purposes, is not a risk-free undertaking by the donor, and historically donated during and by patients undergoing IVF treatment, and lately also includes healthy volunteer donation. It requires ovarian stimulation by daily injections, and is associated with a plethora of side effects such as mood swings, nausea, pelvic bloating, and ovarian hyperstimulation syndrome (OHSS), the risk of which is 5–10% [19, 20]. In severe cases it may even cause renal failure, stroke, pulmonary embolism, and although rare but can be life-threatening [21, 22]. Therefore, it is unethical to knowingly subject voluntary egg donors through the risks of ovarian stimulation including the life-threatening risks, especially wherein other donation options exist, i.e., infertile women undergoing

IVF treatment. But, is it ethical and safe to unjustly lay the entire burden of donor oocytes on infertile women? The unethical Nazi experiments on prisoners or the Willowbrook study in the 1960s [23, 24] established the tenet of research ethics in the Declaration of Helsinki and the Belmont report to eliminate unjust participant selection, whereby participants of a research need to stand to benefit from the proposed research [25]. Therefore on the principle of just participant selection, it is unethical to exclusively recruit infertile women to donate eggs for stem cell research when that research would answer generic questions, fertility related stem cell research would, however, be an exception to this [26]. Furthermore, the evaluation and thence comparison of the safety threshold for women donating "spare" eggs for research while undergoing ART versus the healthy volunteer donor is based on the assumption that the risks and discomfort of egg donation is subsumed in the process of infertility treatment. However, the assumption is false, and the term "spare" egg is a misnomer. Since patients undergoing ART could very well fertilize all the eggs and have the extra embryos frozen for any future ART if the initial embryos were to fail, instead of undergoing additional cycles for egg retrieval [26] . Additionally, not only do we lack data about long-term risks of drugs for ovulation stimulation, we also lack the relative risks of repeated rounds of ovulation stimulatory drugs [27] and the risk of OHSS from recurrent stimulation. Therefore, as the focus of oocyte donation expands to healthy volunteer donation, it is only reasonable to have a fairer compensation model for the discomfort and other risks of oocyte donation that they would be consenting to accept.

4.3.2 Direct and Indirect Compensation for Human Oocyte Donation

Direct compensation is openly allowed in most countries including United States to oocyte donors for ART purposes and oocyte sharing for ART. But direct compensation to oocyte donors for stem cell research is an area of hot debate in several countries including the United States, Canada, Australia, and the United Kingdom. Oocyte donors for stem cell research are only allowed compensation for incurred expenses [28]. In the United States, the National Academy of Sciences has stated that gamete donors for stem cell research should not receive compensation beyond reimbursement for time and travel, i.e., indirect costs [29–31]. This has been adopted by some states like Massachusetts and California [32], whereas others leave the final decision onto the local Embryonic Stem Cell Research Oversight (ESCRO) Committees. In the United Kingdom, Human Fertilization and Embryology Authority (HEFA) permits egg sharing of extra donated eggs for research by women undergoing IVF treatment and receive the treatment for free or reduced rates, but still prohibits payment to any other egg donors, like healthy volunteer research donors [28]. This may not seem fair, but it is necessary to put some restrictions on compensation models for protection of vulnerable groups. Otherwise, commoditization of donated oocytes for stem cell research will expose the vulnerable at-risk population and open doors to foul practices of black market, e.g., human trafficking for oocytes in Romania for stem cell research [33] and removal of eggs from babies postmortem in Ukraine without parental consent [34].

4.3.3   Nonhuman Oocytes for SCNT: Solution or Problem?

Given the shortage of human oocytes and the several safety and ethical concerns it raises from both voluntary oocyte donors and also donors who are undergoing ART, some scientists propose to use nonhuman oocytes to derive stem cell lines by using human nuclear DNA through SCNT. The interspecies somatic cell nuclear transfer (iSCNT) has the potential to be a powerful research tool to promote advances in human biology, in vivo disease modeling and drug discoveries. But besides the highest technical, immunological advancement iSCNT required, there is a rather imaginatively disturbing ethical hiccup that needs attention. The ethical debate on iSCNT is in the creation of cytoplasmic hybrid embryos, also called "cybrids." The concern, however, is more of an instinctive moral repugnance of the idea rather than a rational argument [35], because such an embryo will not grow into a fully or partially grown entity on uterine transfer [36]. As it is, iSCNT has seen limited success and that too only in the closely related species that would crossbreed [37], therefore its current application in humans seems a farfetched idea.

4.4   Induced Pluripotent Stem Cell (iPSC)

Even though the ESC and SCNT carries a strong research potential, the heated political, religious, and ethical debate has slowed the wheels of stem cell research and wide landscape of patients and diseases it could benefit. The unlocked potential, and hence the unmet need has pushed scientists to think of alternate options, iPSC lines being one. In this, somatic cells are reprogrammed to form pluripotent stem cells, and since they are derived from the somatic cells of the donor, it is better accepted immunologically for allogenic use when compared to ESCs. Furthermore, since they can be derived in plentiful amounts from less invasive and easily accessible sites like skin, hair, fat, etc., they minimize the safety concerns [38] and do not compromise the non-maleficence principle in cases of oocyte stimulation and donation from both infertile women and healthy volunteer donors.

In cardiovascular medicine, iPSCs have been able to differentiate into functional cardiac myocytes [2] and also vascular endothelial cells [39]; and as there is previous successful work with ESCs in incorporating endothelial cells for both angiogenesis and vascular regeneration in ischemic heart disease and also in limb ischemia [40, 41], iPSC carries a great future potential. iPSCs have also proven to facilitate vascular and neural regenerative environment in a mouse model with diabetic polyneuropathy by differentiation into Schwann cell-like cells and vascular smooth muscle cells [42].

iPSCs although quite similar to ESCs in functionality, thus application, is labeled "ethically unproblematic" by the President's council on bioethics [43], making for a promising time for iPSC research. Although iPSC is beginning to show its true capability and potential, there are few ethical concerns with the future of iPSC: (A) iPSC in experimental models have raised concerns about the tumorigenicity, by alteration of the nature of some latent and undetectable tumor cells into a more aggressive form, hence clinical applications need to be cautioned for its use [44]. (B) Pluripotency of iPSC has been used to successfully create animal clones [45], and similar cloning principles have the potential to be applied in creating genetically identical human offspring, which raises the ethical and religious debate about human cloning. The possibility of cloning humans, challenges the deeply held beliefs about creation and mankind's relationship with God [46]. The Catholic Church, therefore strongly condemns human cloning of any kind, and some strongly believe that no one should have the power to predetermine another person's complete genetic composition [47]. Few consider human cloning to be fundamentally wrong by allowing the ability and choice to create children of a kind, i.e., treating children as projects of our will than a Gift. However, one shouldn't concern themselves of the aforementioned "slippery slope" examples as long as cloning is performed for biomedical research only, with highest medical, moral standards and the strictest of the regulations and licensing requirements.

4.5 Conclusion

Stem cell research has an immense potential of groundbreaking research in understanding human development/differentiation, disease modeling, newer drug discoveries and innovative therapeutic options for complex and chronic medical problems. It provides a cellular approach for therapeutic options by altering the microenvironment and diverting the course of disease *from ground up,* potentially providing a more definitive treatment option. However, the progress in stem cell therapy has been slower than it could be, therefore yet to unlock its true potential and application, because it violates the deep seated religious beliefs and cultural values that are considered unique and thus important to one's identity and thus ignite political and ethical debate. It also challenges human morality and whether personhood is a maximalist or minimalist paradigm. It seems disappointing for stem cell researchers that the expansive landscape of stem cell therapy which includes the capacity to form human clones is perceived as the "slippery slope" extension; and the instinctive moral abhorrence associated with the words *chimera, cybrids, clones, and hybrids* does not allow science to be able to put a convincing argument in its support. However, these emotional visceral reactions need a rational balance, so as not to become moral prejudices and give science, religion, and ethics an opportunity to work with each other, than be in conflict.

References

1. Adams B, Xiao Q, Xu Q. Stem cell therapy for vascular disease. Trends Cardiovasc Med. 2007;17(7):246–51.
2. Mauritz C, Schwanke K, Reppel M, Neef S, Katsirntaki K, Maier LS, et al. Generation of functional murine cardiac myocytes from induced pluripotent stem cells. Circulation. 2008;118(5):507–17.
3. The President's Council on Bioethics Human cloning and human dignity: an ethical inquiry. Washington, DC. US Government Printing Office, 2002.
4. Brock DW. Is a consensus possible on stem cell research? Moral and political obstacles. J Med Ethics. 2006;32(1):36–42.
5. Warren M. Moral Status: Obligations to Persons and Other Living Things. Oxford University Press (2000). Retrieved 22 Nov 2019, from https://www.oxfordscholarship.com/view/10.1093/acprof:oso/9780198250401.001.0001/acprof-9780198250401.
6. Orr R. The moral status of the embryonal stem cell: inherent or imputed? Am J Bioethics 2002;2(1):57–9.
7. Hudson K, Scott J, Faden R. Values in conflict: Public attitudes on embryonic stem cell research: Genetic and Public Policy Center, 2005.
8. Wolinsky H. The pendulum swung. President Barack Obama removes restrictions on stem-cell research, but are expectations now too high? EMBO Rep. 2009;10(5):436–9.
9. Lyerly AD, Faden RR. Willingness to donate frozen embryos for stem cell research. Science. 2007;317(5834):46–7.
10. Lyerly AD, Steinhauser K, Namey E, Tulsky JA, Cook-Deegan R, Sugarman J, et al. Factors that affect infertility patients' decisions about disposition of frozen embryos. Fertil Steril. 2006;85(6):1623–30.
11. National Bioethics Advisory Commission. Research involving human biological materials: ethical issues and policy guidance vRMNBAC. 1999.
12. Lo B, Chou V, Cedars MI, Gates E, Taylor RN, Wagner RM, et al. Informed consent in human oocyte, embryo, and embryonic stem cell research. Fertil Steril. 2004;82(3):559–63.
13. Lo B, Parham L. Ethical issues in stem cell research. Endocr Rev. 2009;30(3):204–13.
14. Kalfoglou AL, Geller G. A follow-up study with oocyte donors exploring their experiences, knowledge, and attitudes about the use of their oocytes and the outcome of the donation. Fertil Steril. 2000;74(4):660–7.
15. National Research Council and Institute of Medicine. Guidelines for human embryonic stem cell research. Washington DCNAP. 2005.
16. Hwang WS, Roh SI, Lee BC, Kang SK, Kwon DK, Kim S, et al. Patient-specific embryonic stem cells derived from human SCNT blastocysts. Science. 2005;308(5729):1777–83.
17. National Bioethics Committee, Republic of Korea. The National Bioethics Committee's report on bioethical problems in Hwang Woo-Suk research, Seoul: Bioethics Policy and Research Center, 2006.
18. Clay AS. Hwang Woo-suk's Use of Human Eggs for Research 2002–2005. Embryo Project Encyclopedia (2014-08-12) ISSN: 1940–5030. http://www.embryo.asu.edu/handle/10776/8145.
19. Golan A, Ron-el R, Herman A, Soffer Y, Weinraub Z, Caspi E. Ovarian hyperstimulation syndrome: an update review. Obstet Gynecol Surv. 1989;44(6):430–40.
20. Schenker JG, Weinstein D. Ovarian hyperstimulation syndrome: a current survey. Fertil Steril. 1978;30(3):255–68.
21. Cluroe AD, Synek BJ. A fatal case of ovarian hyperstimulation syndrome with cerebral infarction. Pathology. 1995;27(4):344–6.
22. Semba S, Moriya T, Youssef EM, Sasano H. An autopsy case of ovarian hyperstimulation syndrome with massive pulmonary edema and pleural effusion. Pathol Int. 2000;50(7):549–52.
23. Ward R, Krugman S, Giles JP, Jacobs AM, Bodansky O. Infectious hepatitis; studies of its natural history and prevention. N Engl J Med. 1958;258(9):407–16.
24. Krugman S, Ward R, Giles JP, Bodansky O, Jacobs AM. Infectious hepatitis: detection of virus during the incubation period and in clinically inapparent infection. N Engl J Med. 1959;261:729–34.

25. World Medical Association (WMA). 1964 Declaration of Helsinki. Amended by the WMA 52nd General Assembly 2000, Edinburgh.
26. Ballantyne A, de Lacey S. Wanted—egg donors for research: a research ethics approach to donor recruitment and compensation. Int J Feminist Appr Bioeth. 2008;1(2):145–64.
27. Pearson H. Health effects of egg donation may take decades to emerge. Nature. 2006;442(7103):607–8.
28. Klitzman R, Sauer MV. Payment of egg donors in stem cell research in the USA. Reprod Biomed Online. 2009;18(5):603–8.
29. National Academy of Sciences. The National Academies' guidelines for human embryonic stem cell research. The National Academies Press; Washington, DC: 2005 Available at: http://www.nap.edu/catalog/11278.html.
30. National Academy of Sciences. Amendments to the National Academies' guidelines for human embryonic stem cell research. The National Academies Press; Washington, DC: 2007 Available at: http://www.books.nap.edu/catalog.php?record_id=11871#toc.
31. National Academy of Sciences. Amendments to the National Academies' guidelines for human embryonic stem cell research. The National Academies Press; Washington, DC: 2008 Available at http://www.nap.edu/catalogphp?record_id=12260.
32. California Institute for Regenerative Medicine. Guidance for CIRM medical and ethical standards regulations governing donation of oocytes for CIRM-funded research. 2008. Available at: http://www.cirm.ca.gov/workgroups/pdf/Guidance_Donation_Oocytes.pdf.
33. Beeson D, Lippman A. Egg harvesting for stem cell research: medical risks and ethical problems. Reprod Biomed Online. 2006;13(4):573–9.
34. BBC News 2006. Available at: http://www.news.bbc.co.uk/2/hi/europe/6171083.stm.
35. Camporesi S, Boniolo G. Fearing a non-existing Minotaur? The ethical challenges of research on cytoplasmic hybrid embryos. J Med Ethics. 2008;34(11):821–5.
36. Milliez J. Ethical guidelines concerning cytoplasmic animal–human hybrid embryos. Int J Gynecol Obstet. 2009;107(2):167.
37. Beyhan Z, Iager AE, Cibelli JB. Interspecies nuclear transfer: implications for embryonic stem cell biology. Cell Stem Cell. 2007;1(5):502–12.
38. Leeper NJ, Hunter AL, Cooke JP. Stem cell therapy for vascular regeneration: adult, embryonic, and induced pluripotent stem cells. Circulation. 2010;122(5):517–26.
39. Narazaki G, Uosaki H, Teranishi M, Okita K, Kim B, Matsuoka S, et al. Directed and systematic differentiation of cardiovascular cells from mouse induced pluripotent stem cells. Circulation. 2008;118(5):498–506.
40. Yamahara K, Sone M, Itoh H, Yamashita JK, Yurugi-Kobayashi T, Homma K, et al. Augmentation of neovascularization [corrected] in hindlimb ischemia by combined transplantation of human embryonic stem cells-derived endothelial and mural cells. PLoS One. 2008;3(2):e1666.
41. Li Z, Wu JC, Sheikh AY, Kraft D, Cao F, Xie X, et al. Differentiation, survival, and function of embryonic stem cell derived endothelial cells for ischemic heart disease. Circulation. 2007;116(11 Suppl):146–54.
42. Okawa T, Kamiya H, Himeno T, Kato J, Seino Y, Fujiya A, et al. Transplantation of neural crest-like cells derived from induced pluripotent stem cells improves diabetic polyneuropathy in mice. Cell Transplant. 2013;22(10):1767–83.
43. President's Council on Bioethics (US). Alternative sources of human pluripotent stem cells: a white paper of the President's Council on Bioethics. President's Council on Bioethics, 2005.
44. Chen L, Mizutani A, Kasai T, Yan T, Jin G, Vaidyanath A, et al. Mouse induced pluripotent stem cell microenvironment generates epithelial-mesenchymal transition in mouse Lewis lung cancer cells. Am J Cancer Res. 2014;4(1):80–8.
45. Kou Z, Kang L, Yuan Y, Tao Y, Zhang Y, Wu T, et al. Mice cloned from induced pluripotent stem cells (iPSCs). Biol Reprod. 2010;83(2):238–43.
46. Frazzetto G. Embryos, cells and god. EMBO Rep. 2004;5(6):553–5.
47. Bruce DM. Stem cells, embryos and cloning–unravelling the ethics of a knotty debate. J Mol Biol. 2002;319(4):917–25.

Chapter 5
Bone Marrow-Derived Cells: From the Laboratory to the Clinic

Justin R. King, Jie Xie, and Michael P. Murphy

5.1 Isolation and Characterization of Bone Marrow Mononuclear Cells

5.1.1 Definition and Composition of BMMNC

The bone marrow mononuclear cell (BMMNC) component of bone marrow (BM) is defined as all cells with unilobed or round nuclei and without granules. This cell population includes hematopoietic stem and progenitor cells (HSC/HPC), lymphocytes, monocytes, and mesenchymal stromal cells (MSC). Myeloid derivatives, including erythrocytes and granulocytes, are excluded by the process of separating BMMNC from the BM.

Within the BMMNC fraction, further characterization of specific subsets of angiogenic populations can be made. Asahara et al. have shown that circulating mononuclear cells expressing CD34 or Flk-1 could differentiate into endothelial cells in vitro and contribute to vasculogenesis in vivo in adult animals and thus were identified as putative endothelial progenitor cells (EPC) [1]. Kamihata et al. demonstrated that BMMNC contain EPC in the CD34+ hematopoietic stem and progenitor

J. R. King · M. P. Murphy (✉)
Indiana Center for Vascular Biology and Medicine, Indiana University School of Medicine, Indianapolis, IN, USA

Department of Surgery, Indiana University School of Medicine, Indianapolis, IN, USA

Center for Regenerative Medicine, Richard L. Roudebush Veterans Administration Medical Center, Indianapolis, IN, USA
e-mail: mipmurph@iupui.edu

J. Xie
Indiana Center for Vascular Biology and Medicine, Indiana University School of Medicine, Indianapolis, IN, USA

Department of Surgery, Indiana University School of Medicine, Indianapolis, IN, USA

© Springer Nature Switzerland AG 2021
T. P. Navarro et al. (eds.), *Stem Cell Therapy for Vascular Diseases*,
https://doi.org/10.1007/978-3-030-56954-9_5

cell fraction, as well as pro-angiogenic factor-producing cells in the CD34− cell fraction. The CD34+ BMMNC actively form cord-like structures by co-culture with CD34- BMMNC, suggesting a synergy between these two fractions to enhance the angiogenesis process [2]. These CD34+ cells can then be mobilized to peripheral blood by systemic injection of granulocyte colony-stimulating factor (G-CSF), allowing for harvesting of these CD34+ peripheral blood mononuclear cells (PBMNC) for therapeutic angiogenesis.

As we have expanded our ability to harvest EPC, our categorization of them has expanded well. Different groups have used different terms to describe "EPC"-like cells by different identification and isolation methods, thus raising some controversy on naming convention. These terms include but are not limited to colony-forming unit of endothelial cells (CFU-EC) [3, 4], circulating angiogenic cells (CAC) [5], culture-expanded endothelial progenitor cells (CE-EPC) [6], culture-modified mono-nuclear cells (CMMC) [7], endothelial outgrowth cells (EOC) [8], endothelial pro-genitor-derived cells (EPDC) [9], circulating endothelial cells (CEC) [10], circulating endothelial progenitors (CEP) [11], and endothelial colony-forming cells (ECFC) [12]. Additionally, markers previously attributed to EPC alone, including CD34, CD 117, and CD 133, are shared by myeloid cells of various stages of differentiation, this further blurring the boundary between EPC and myeloid derivatives [13–15].

Aldehyde dehydrogenase (ALDH) is an enzyme responsible for oxidizing a variety of aldehydes within the cytosol [16]. ALDH exists at high levels in hematopoietic stem and progenitor cells (HSC/HPC) and is responsible for the resistance of HSC/HPC to the inhibitory effects of alkylating agents such as cyclophosphamide and 4-hydroxyperoxycyclophosphamide on cell proliferation [17–19]. Using the ALDH fluorescent substrate BODIPY aminoacetaldehyde (BAAA), HSC/HPC can be fluo-rescently labelled and enriched through flow cytometry [20]. Capoccia et al. purified primitive HSC/HPC from human BM by selection of cells with high aldehyde dehydrogenase (ALDH) activity. An immune-deficient murine hindlimb ischemia model that demonstrated that intravenous injection of these cells resulted in increased recovery of blood perfusion and capillary density in the ischemic limb. This is in part due to the high concentration of CD34 + CD133 + CD14 + CD117 (c-Kit) + cells in ALDH activity-high cells compared to those with low ALDH activity [21].

MSC are another critical subset of BMMNC. MSC are characterized by their ability to adhere to plastic surfaces, to self-renew, and, in permissive cultures, to differentiate into osteocytes, chondrocytes, and adipocytes [22]. These cells are rare in the BM, representing 1 in every 100,000 total BM cells, though it can be expanded ex vivo to larger quantities to achieve desirable dosage for therapeutic use [23]. A dedicated chapter with more thorough introduction of BMMSC in the context of peripheral arterial disease is also included in this book.

5.1.2   Isolation of BMMNC

Multiple clinical trials utilize BMMNC sample for patients with peripheral artery disease (PAD). In order to obtain these samples, aspiration occurs from the ileum under local anesthetic. The sample is then purified and concentrated to a final volume of 40–50 mL, before being delivered back to patients intra-arterially or intramuscularly at the site of interest, most commonly the gastrocnemius [24, 25].

To purify the BMMNC sample, traditionally a Ficoll™ density-gradient centrifugation system is used, though different laboratories use unique variations [26, 27]. In order to use these samples in clinical trials, both a good clinical practice (GCP)-certified facility and sterile cell biology laboratory are required for BM processing and cell culture expansion.

The ability to completely purify the BMMNC does seem to play a role in their efficacy. In a study using BMMNC for the treatment of ST-elevation myocardial infarction, the amount of contaminated RBC in the BMMNC exceeding $0.4 \times 10^9/200$ million BMMNC was inversely correlated with the recovery of left ventricular ejection fraction (LVEF) [28]. Despite the use of standard density-gradient centrifugation method with Lymphocyte Separation Medium (Lonza), nearly 0.2×10^9 residual RBC were still present in the 200 million BMMNC, and 36% of the BMMNC were neutrophils. No significant association was detected for the number of contaminating neutrophils.

In preclinical studies, primarily in rodents, BMMNC harvest requires sacrificing the donor and flushing long bones (i.e., femur and tibia) to obtain total BM cells. Further purification of BMMNC is achieved by lysis of red blood cells and density-gradient centrifugation with Ficoll™ solution.

For use in clinical practice, multiple point-of-care systems have been developed to expedite the process from BM aspiration to final cell product generation. Examples of these devices include MarrowStim™ system from Biomet Inc. and SmartPrep system from Harvest Technologies. These new isolation techniques were able to achieve similar yield of progenitor cells compared to conventional density-gradient-based method while decreasing both time and cost of laboratory resources previously required for cell processing [29, 30]. These bedside tools have demonstrated equivalent angiogenic potency in murine models [31].

5.2   Preclinical Evidence for BMMNC Benefits in PAD

Multiple animal models of hindlimb ischemia (HLI) have been described, including rodent, rabbit, porcine, canine, and primate [32–35]. Rodent models are most commonly used due to their inherent advantages of larger sample size, lower cost, and modifiable genetic background. If use of larger animals is feasible, they do offer the benefits of closer resemblance of human vascular wall structure and hemodynamics and easier access to individual blood vessels [36]. In vivo studies using BMMNC in these animal models have demonstrated promotion of blood perfusion, increased capillary density and homing of EPC, upregulation of local vascular endothelial growth factor (VEGF) and basic fibroblast growth factor (bFGF) levels, and decreased auto-amputation rate and muscle atrophy [37].

Laser Doppler perfusion imaging (LDPI) is one common method of measuring improvements in blood flow in the distal limb. In order to ascertain if improvements in LDPI measurements are the result of enhanced angiogenesis, immunohistochemical (IHC) staining for endothelial cell markers such as CD31 can be used to quantify capillary density within the gastrocnemius or soleus muscles. Finally, imaging modalities, including arterial flow probes, microspheres, contrast-enhanced direct injection X-ray, MRI angiography, micro-CT, and contrast-enhanced ultrasound sonography (CEUS), can be used to assess limb perfusion but is beyond the scope of this review and summarized in great details by Lotfi et al. [38]

Clinical outcomes are other endpoints in the animal models of CLI to evaluate the efficacy of progenitor cells. These include exercise tolerance, tissue necrosis, and functional recovery from claudication [39, 40]. Tissue necrosis is the most reproducible measure of therapeutic intervention in CLI. In the immunocompromised BALB/c mice, for instance, the degree of distal limb necrosis after femoral artery ligation could be scored from 1 to 5 to allow quantitative comparisons between individual animals. Responses may vary greatly between different strains of mice or even within the same strain, believed to be due to the inter- and intrastrain differences in collateralization; thus larger size of treatment groups is often necessary in the experimental design to assure sufficient statistical power [41].

Although the use of HLI models as an in vivo angiogenesis assay is common practice, its value as a preclinical model to represent the pathogenesis of PAD is still controversial. The practice of murine femoral arterial ligation with or without excision is acute, as compared to the chronic atherosclerotic changes seen in human PAD. Additionally, mice used for HLI models are often young and healthy, differing from the comorbidities most commonly seen in PAD patients. Possibly due to these differences, there have been some different outcomes in murine and human studies. VEGF, FGF, and hepatocyte growth factor (HGF) have each consistently demonstrated promising effects in rodent models of HLI, though yield mixed results in human clinical trials. HGF has shown the most promising effects on improving rest pain and quality-of-life scores in a randomized, double-blind, placebo-controlled clinical trial, while VEGF and FGF have failed to improve the primary endpoints of amputation rate or time to amputation and death [42–45].

5.3 Potential Mechanisms of BMMNC in PAD

5.3.1 Reconstruction of Vascular Endothelial Architecture

The primary theory behind BMMNC use is neovascularization at the site of ischemia following cell replacement and regeneration by the various adult stem and progenitor cells found in BMMNC. Using multiple physiological and pathological neovascularization models, Asahara et al. demonstrated that progenitor cells can be mobilized from BM to incorporate into newly formed capillaries [46, 47]. CD34+ mononuclear cells have been characterized as putative endothelial progenitor cells given their ability to differentiate into endothelial cells producing nitric oxide in response to the EC-dependent agonist acetylcholine and the EC-specific mitogen VEGF [1]. This is consistent with the well-described ability of BM-derived cells to incorporate into the vascular architecture of tumor vessels [48].

The extent to which BM-derived HSC incorporate into the neovasculature remains controversial, however. This is because some studies have demonstrated a lack of the endothelial cell marker von Willebrand factor. Additionally, other studies using GFP-labeled BM-derived cells were unable to detect this label in newly formed blood vessels.

5.3.2 Stabilization of Neovasculature via Pericyte Differentiation

Pericytes are polymorphic, multibranched cells located within the basement membrane of capillary and postcapillary venules that surround endothelial cells to support blood vessel structure. They are responsible for multiple functions but most critically help to stabilize the vascular wall, control endothelial cell proliferation, and regulate microvascular blood flow [49]. During neovascularization, pericytes provide both pro-survival signaling and mechanical support to maintain the newly formed endothelium [50]. Pericytes can be identified in studies by their expression of nerve/glial antigen-2 (NG2) and platelet-derived growth factor receptor β (PDGF-β).

Studies by Rajantie et al. utilizing BM GFP+ chimeric mice demonstrated that BM-derived pericytes were persistently detected at sites of tumor- or VEGF-induced angiogenesis, as opposed to BM-derived endothelial cells which were not consistently found [51]. Similarly, Ziegelhoeffer et al. also used GFP+ chimeric mice to investigate the involvement of BM-derived GFP+ cells in the postischemic angiogenesis process in a mouse CLI model. They were not able to colocalize GFP signals with endothelial or smooth muscle cell markers but instead found ample GFP+ cells in the perivascular space resembling fibroblasts and pericytes based on their shape and distribution [52]. This phenomenon of recruitment of BM-derived pericyte precursors has also been described in the process of corneal vasculogenesis [53]. Notably, over 90% of BM-derived pericytes also express CD45 and CD11b, suggesting a hematopoietic origin.

5.3.3 Secretion of Proangiogenic Factors

BMMNC also exhibit potent paracrine signaling activity, specifically via secretion of proangiogenic factors [54]. The ability to be proangiogenic is shared by almost all subsets of BMMNC, including HSC and EPC, although the specific cytokines being secreted may vary between cell types [5, 55]. This mutual complementation may explain the synergy between different subsets of BMMNC. For example, Kamihata et al. demonstrated that CD34-positive cells from peripheral or cord blood may be induced to form cord-like structures after coculturing with the CD34-negative fraction of BMMNC that secretes bFGF, VEGF, and angiopoietin 1 (Ang1) [2].

It is worth noting that more mature cellular components are also critical parts of the BMMNC, including T lymphocytes, megakaryocytes, platelets, and monocytes [56–59]. Murine models with CD4-deficient mice have seen reduced collateral flow induction, diminished VEGF levels, increased muscle atrophy and fibrosis, and delayed recovery of hindlimb function compared to wild-type mice; however, these effects are diminished following infusion of purified CD4+ T cells [56].

MSC may represent the most interesting component of BMMNC. This unique population of cells is capable of secreting a broad spectrum of chemokines, cytokines, and proangiogenic factors [60]. Their paracrine functions are highly adaptive to the microenvironment signals, as demonstrated by their ability to change the level and composition of trophic factors secreted [61, 62]. In vitro studies have demonstrated a conditioned medium generated from MSC has the ability to promote proliferation and migration of endothelial cells and vascular smooth muscle cells [39, 60, 63, 64]. As evidence for the use of these cells improves, more stringent quality control procedures and larger-scale manufacturing may allow for use of "off-the-shelf" cellular products for multiple indications.

5.4 Clinical Trials Using BMMNC for CLI Patients

5.4.1 Overview of BMMNC in CLI

In 2002, Tateishi-Yuyama et al. published the results of the Therapeutic Angiogenesis using Cell Transplantation (TACT) study, the first large clinical trial using autologous BMMNC for patients with CLI [24]. In part one of this study, 25 patients with unilateral limb ischemia, as defined by ankle-brachial index (ABI) < 0.6, received an intramuscular injection of autologous BMMNC ($1.6 \pm 0.6 \times 10^9$ cells) into the gastrocnemius of the ischemic limb. The contralateral less ischemic limb (ABI > 0.6) received intramuscular saline injection as a control. No adverse events related to treatment were reported. BMMNC administration improved subjects' ABI, transcutaneous oxygen pressure ($TcPO_2$), rest pain, and pain-free walking distance at 4 and 24 weeks [24]. In part two of this study, an additional 22 patients with bilateral limb ischemia were recruited. Each subject randomly received intramuscular BMMNC injection into one limb as active treatment and PBMNC into the other limb as a control. Compared to PBMNC, BMMNC significantly improved ABI, $TcPO_2$, rest pain, and pain-free walking time at 4 and 24 weeks [24].

The results of the TACT study provided the first piece of clinical evidence for the use of BMMNC in patients with CLI and thus inspired more clinical trials internationally. The first phase I/II clinical trial approved by FDA was conducted by our group in the United States [65]. In this open-label trial, 29 patients with CLI defined as symptoms of rest pain and/or ulceration with an ABI ≤ 0.55 and/or toe-brachial index (TBI) ≤ 0.40 were enrolled. Among these patients, 30 limbs were treated. As determined by appropriate imaging, patients had no patent artery below the knee that was continuous to the foot and thus no options for bypass or endovascular therapies to improve perfusion. Patients underwent single intramuscular injection in the gastrocnemius. Ficoll density centrifugation (FC) was used to isolate BMMNC for the first 14 patients, and MarrowStim™ (MS) closed centrifugation system was used for the other 15 patients. The average number of cells injected was $1.3 \pm 0.7 \times 10^9$ using FC method and $2.0 \pm 1.6 \times 10^9$ using MS method. Amputation-free survival (AFS) at 1 year was 86.3%, higher than the reported 1-year AFS of 59–66.7% in similar studies [30, 66]. There was a significant increase from baseline in first toe pressure (FTP) by 10.2 ± 6.2 mmHg ($P = 0.02$) and in TBI by $0.10 + 0.05$ ($P = 0.02$) at week 12. Rest pain decreased significantly at 12 weeks from baseline. The VascuQol total score increased in all categories, especially in the domains of emotion (2.5 ± 0.3 to 4.3 ± 0.5) and pain (2.5 ± 0.4 to 4.0 ± 0.7). Three of nine ulcers (33%) healed completely by week 12. There were two procedure-related serious adverse events (SAEs): anemia-related myocardial ischemia and entrapment of a guidewire during contrast arteriography, which was initially used to assess efficacy of cell therapy. Similar CLI studies have also reported anemia in patients after large volume BM aspiration; however, it was transient and well tolerated without any need for interventions [67].

Since the TACT study in 2002, clinical studies on BMMNC therapy in PAD patients have advanced from early small-scale, uncontrolled phase I trials to randomized, controlled, phase III clinical trials. A meta-analysis published in 2013 selected studies that are randomized and controlled, involve BM-derived cells, have a comparator group, and have endpoints such as major amputation, survival, ABI, $PTcO_2$, pain score, and pain-free walking distance. The exclusion criteria include animal studies, studies performed in children or neonates, reviews or case series ($n < 10$), no CLI or diabetic foot, not published in English, Dutch, or German, gene therapy, and diagnostic, prognostic, or etiologic studies. The meta-analysis identified 12 RCT using BM-derived cells, including BMMNC, BMMSC, PBMNC, and Ixmyelocel-T cells [68]. Six out of these 12 RCT used only BMMNC and were summarized in Table 5.1.

5.4.2 Safety of BMMNC in CLI

Use of BMMNC requires both BM aspiration and either intramuscular or intra-arterial injection. Both procedures have generally demonstrated safety in patients with CLI. Acute anemia can occur with BM aspiration, with a mean decrease in hematocrit of 2.6% compared to controls [67]. Though generally well-tolerated, this may cause problems for patients with underlying anemia or coronary artery disease. In our experience, we have addressed this issue by adjusting the volume of BM aspirated for patients with preexisting cardiovascular conditions to minimize risk of ischemic events [65].

Intramuscular injection of BMMNC has not demonstrated muscular damage, vascular malformation, or acute renal injury. In cases of intra-arterial injection, three procedure-related adverse events have been reported, including stent thrombosis, groin hematoma, and arterial pseudoaneurysm, each of which resolved [25].

Table 5.1 Randomized controlled trials of BMMNC for CLI

Reference	Sample size	Cell number (10^9)	Route	Follow-up (months)	Outcome
Arai et al. (2006) [82]	13/12	1–3	IM	4	Improved ABI, TcPO$_2$, rest pain, pain-free walking distance, ulcer healing
Benoit et al. [67]	34/14	240 ml	IM	24	No change in ABI or AFS
Lu et al. [76]	21/41 limbs	0.93	IM	24	Improved ABI, TcPO$_2$, pain-free walking time, ulcer healing
Prochazka et al. (2010)	42/54	240 ml	IM	16	Decreased amputation rate
Tateishi-Yuyama et al. [24]	22/22 limbs	0.88-2.8	IM	24	Improved ABI, TcPO$_2$, rest pain, pain-free walking time
Walter et al. [25]	19/21	0.15	IA	72	Improved pain score, ulcer healing

Sample size, treatment group/control group; *ABI* ankle brachial index; *TcPO$_2$*, transcutaneous O$_2$ pressure; *AFS* amputation-free survival; *IM* intramuscular; *IA*, intra-arterial

To assess the long-term safety of BMMNC therapy, Matoba et al. followed patients from the TACT study for 3 years. Patients with atherosclerotic PAD demonstrated 3-year overall survival rates of 80%, while a smaller group with thromboangiitis obliterans demonstrated 100% survival [69]. Another study followed 51 patients for 3.2 years and reported limb salvage rate of 59% at 6 months and 53% at last follow-up. No unexpected long-term adverse events were reported [30].

5.4.3 Primary Endpoints for BMMNC in CLI

The most widely accepted primary outcomes to evaluate the efficacy of therapeutic agents for CLI patients are major amputation rates and AFS, a composite of major amputation, and all-cause mortality [70]. Benoit et al. conducted a double-blinded RCT evaluating the efficacy of concentrated bone marrow cells (BMAC) in 48 no-option CLI patients. At 6 months, patients treated with BMAC demonstrated a lower amputation rate than placebo (39.1% vs. 71.4%, $p = 0.1337$). The Kaplan-Meier time to amputation was longer in the BMAC group than in the placebo group ($p = 0.067$). Based on a bootstrap simulation model, in order to detect significant difference in AFS between BMAC and placebo with a power of 95%, a sample size of 210 patients would be required, which would be difficult to achieve in a single-site clinical trial [67].

One meta-analysis analyzed the results from 9 RCTs to achieve an aggregate therapeutic group with 259 limbs and control group with 232 limbs [68]. The results showed that BM-derived cell therapy significantly reduced major amputation rates compared with the placebo control, with a RR of 0.58 (95%CI, 0.40–0.84; $P = 0.004$).

Conventional surgical revascularization options, such as prosthetic femorotibial bypass, achieve limb salvage rates of 72.5% at 1 year and 61.9% at 5 years [71]. Although the reduction in limb salvage seen with cell therapy is inferior to outcomes of surgical revascularization, it still remains a promising treatments modality for CLI patients. It has proven to be safe and minimally invasive. It is assuredly a possibility for patients without surgical or endovascular revascularization options or with poor options including prosthetic or composite grafts. The higher morbidity, longer hospital stay, and increased utilization of intensive care resources associated with surgery all must be considered.

5.4.4 Secondary Endpoints for BMMNC in CLI

Common secondary endpoints include functional outcomes such as pain-free walking distance and time, pain score, ulcer healing, and quality of life. These have demonstrated consistency and significantly improved after BMMNC therapy across numerous studies. A meta-analysis of 8 RCTs with 237 limbs showed an overall odds ratio (OR) of complete ulcer healing of 1.87 (95% CI, 1.49–2.36; $p < 0.00001$) in the BM cell treatment group, as well as a decrease in pain score of 1.10 (95% CI, -1.37 to -0.83) based on 8 RCT [72]. Additionally, pain-free walking distance was substantially longer in the therapeutic arm based on three RCTs. Although these functional endpoints may represent clinically significant outcomes, the subjective nature of the patient and investigator must be considered.

Physiological measurements, such as ABI, TBI, FTP, and TcPO$_2$, make up the remainder of secondary outcomes. Meta-analysis of 7 RCTs showed that ABI was significantly improved by 0.12 (95% CI, 0.09–0.15, $P < 0.00001$) and TcPO$_2$ was significantly increased by 14.28 mmHg (95%CI, 8.54–20.02; $P < 0.00001$) following BM-derived cell treatment [72]. These improvements may not completely reflect the mechanistic changes seen with BMMNC therapy, specifically considering the expected microvascular formation rather than improvements in large vessel blood flow.

5.5 Clinical Trials Using Subsets of BMMNC for CLI Patients

Rather than using the entire BMMNC, recent clinical trials have explored using bone marrow-derived subsets. In particular, PBMNC is a commonly used substitute to avoid BM aspiration. This can be mobilized by a 6-day treatment with granulocyte colony-stimulating factor (G-CSF), after which the PBMNC can be harvested by apheresis. Patients treated with PBMNC have demonstrated consistently improved primary and secondary endpoints. Huang et al. reported significant improvement in limb pain, ulcer healing, and ABI, in patients receiving PBMNC at 3-month follow-up compared to those receiving the placebo control [73]. Ozturk et al. reported improved ABI and pain score [74]. Mohammadzadeh et al. reported improved ABI and decreased amputation rates [75].

Bone marrow mesenchymal stromal cells (BMMSC) are another promising subpopulation of BM cells. This cell population offers multiple advantages. Primarily, their ability to be expanded ex vivo to larger quantities allows for smaller volume BM aspiration. Second, BMMSC demonstrate immunomodulatory properties, which may allow for allogeneic transplantation of cells from young healthy donors, as well as industrial manufacturing of "off-the-shelf" cellular products. Finally, they are a more defined cell population than BMMNC and thus can be tested in preclinical models for potency before applying to patients. Lu et al. conducted a RCT to compare BMMSC with BMMNC in CLI patients with bilateral limb ischemia [76]. Within the BMMSC group, only 30 mL of BM was aspirated before isolating and expanding the BMMSC population in vitro to reach the target dose. Conversely, the BMMNC group required aspiration of 300 mL of BM. By 24 weeks, BMMSC and BMMNC both significantly improved ABI, $TcPO_2$, and pain-free walking time, compared to placebo control. MRA-based collateral blood vessel scores were significantly higher, and the ulcer healing was faster in the BMMSC group. Gupta et al. tested safety and efficacy of allogeneic BMMSC in 20 CLI patients. At 6-month follow-up, ABI was improved significantly in the BMMSC by an average of 0.22 ($p = 0.0018$). No adverse events were associated with BMMSC treatment [77].

In addition to PBMNC and BMMSC, a variety of other cell types have been or are still under active investigation for treatment of CLI. These include CD34 + PBMNC, ALDH+ BMMNC, and Ixmyelocel-T [78–81]. Most of these studies are still in phase I/II stage, and as such, their efficacy for CLI patients remains untested in larger phase III clinical trials.

5.6   Conclusions and Future Directions

BMMNC are comprised of a mixture of angiogenic stem and progenitor cells and mature hematopoietic cells that function synergistically to promote neovascularization. The use of BMMNC cell therapy in preclinical animal models has demonstrated significant revascularization of ischemic tissue. Numerous clinical trials in PAD patients have helped to establish the safety of BMMNC and have shown promising results in improving ischemic pain, ulceration, pain-free walking distance, and physiological parameters such as ABI and $TcPO_2$. These studies are largely limited to phase I and II clinical trials, thus limiting out ability to determine the efficacy of BMMNC on major amputation rates, AFS, and all-cause mortality. Other limiting factors toward meaningful results include disparity in cell doses used, method of delivery, and a heterogenous CLI patient population. The ideal patient population has yet to be determined.

Large, placebo-controlled RCT are clearly required before BMMNC therapy can be considered standard care. Our institution continues with our own phase III trial to help further determine efficacy of BMMNC therapy.

In addition, this work will provide a demographic and genomic signature of patients who best respond to BMMNC treatment. Of equally critical importance are clinical studies designed to optimize the BMMNC therapy through multi-dosing comparisons, enhancing BMMNC survival with adjunctive biomatrices, and pre-conditioning cells with treatment such as hypoxia to maximize the performance of cells in vivo.

References

1. Asahara T, et al. Isolation of putative progenitor endothelial cells for angiogenesis. Science. 1997;275:964–7.
2. Kamihata H, et al. Implantation of bone marrow mononuclear cells into ischemic myocardium enhances collateral perfusion and regional function via side supply of angioblasts, angiogenic ligands, and cytokines. Circulation. 2001;104:1046–52.
3. Gehling UM, et al. In vitro differentiation of endothelial cells from AC133-positive progenitor cells. Blood. 2000;95:3106–12.
4. Hill JM, et al. Circulating endothelial progenitor cells, vascular function, and cardiovascular risk. N Engl J Med. 2003;348:593–600.
5. Rehman J, Li J, Orschell CM, March KL. Peripheral blood "endothelial progenitor cells" are derived from monocyte/macrophages and secrete angiogenic growth factors. Circulation. 2003;107:1164–9.
6. Sharpe EE 3rd, et al. The origin and in vivo significance of murine and human culture-expanded endothelial progenitor cells. Am J Pathol. 2006;168:1710–21.
7. Gulati R, et al. Autologous culture-modified mononuclear cells confer vascular protection after arterial injury. Circulation. 2003;108:1520–6.
8. Lin Y, Weisdorf DJ, Solovey A, Hebbel RP. Origins of circulating endothelial cells and endothelial outgrowth from blood. J Clin Invest. 2000;105:71–7.
9. Bompais H, et al. Human endothelial cells derived from circulating progenitors display specific functional properties compared with mature vessel wall endothelial cells. Blood. 2004;103:2577–84.
10. Lin Y, et al. Use of blood outgrowth endothelial cells for gene therapy for hemophilia A. Blood. 2002;99:457–62.
11. Romagnani P, et al. CD14+CD34low cells with stem cell phenotypic and functional features are the major source of circulating endothelial progenitors. Circ Res. 2005,97.314–22.
12. Ingram DA, et al. Identification of a novel hierarchy of endothelial progenitor cells using human peripheral and umbilical cord blood. Blood. 2004;104:2752–60.
13. Fadini GP, Losordo D, Dimmeler S. Critical reevaluation of endothelial progenitor cell phenotypes for therapeutic and diagnostic use. Circ Res. 2012;110:624–37.
14. Yoder MC. Human endothelial progenitor cells. Cold Spring Harb Perspect Med. 2012;2:a006692.
15. Yoder MC. Endothelial progenitor cell: a blood cell by many other names may serve similar functions. J Mol Med (Berl). 2013;91:285–95.

16. Labrecque J, Bhat PV, Lacroix A. Purification and partial characterization of a rat kidney aldehyde dehydrogenase that oxidizes retinal to retinoic acid. Biochem Cell Biol (Biochimie et biologie cellulaire). 1993;71:85–9.

17. Gordon MY, Goldman JM, Gordon-Smith EC. 4-Hydroperoxycyclophosphamide inhibits proliferation by human granulocyte-macrophage colony-forming cells (GM-CFC) but spares more primitive progenitor cells. Leuk Res. 1985;9:1017–21.

18. Sahovic EA, Colvin M, Hilton J, Ogawa M. Role for aldehyde dehydrogenase in survival of pro-genitors for murine blast cell colonies after treatment with 4-hydroperoxycyclophosphamide in vitro. Cancer Res. 1988;48:1223–6.

19. Smith C, et al. Purification and partial characterization of a human hematopoietic precursor population. Blood. 1991;77:2122–8.

20. Storms RW, et al. Isolation of primitive human hematopoietic progenitors on the basis of alde-hyde dehydrogenase activity. Proc Natl Acad Sci U S A. 1999;96:9118–23.

21. Capoccia BJ, et al. Revascularization of ischemic limbs after transplantation of human bone marrow cells with high aldehyde dehydrogenase activity. Blood. 2009;113:5340–51.

22. Pittenger MF, et al. Multilineage potential of adult human mesenchymal stem cells. Science. 1999;284:143–7.

23. Thirumala S, Goebel WS, Woods EJ. Manufacturing and banking of mesenchymal stem cells. Expert Opin Biol Ther. 2013;13:673–91.

24. Tateishi-Yuyama E, et al. Therapeutic angiogenesis for patients with limb ischaemia by autolo-gous transplantation of bone-marrow cells: a pilot study and a randomised controlled trial. Lancet. 2002;360:427–35.

25. Walter DH, et al. Intraarterial administration of bone marrow mononuclear cells in patients with critical limb ischemia: a randomized-start, placebo-controlled pilot trial (PROVASA). Circ Cardiovasc Interv. 2011;4:26–37.

26. Boyum A. Separation of lymphocytes, lymphocyte subgroups and monocytes: a review. Lymphology. 1977;10:71–6.

27. Boyum A, Brincker Fjerdingstad H, Martinsen I, Lea T, Lovhaug D. Separation of human lymphocytes from citrated blood by density gradient (NycoPrep) centrifugation: monocyte depletion depending upon activation of membrane potassium channels. Scand J Immunol. 2002;56:76–84.

28. Assmus B, et al. Red blood cell contamination of the final cell product impairs the efficacy of autologous bone marrow mononuclear cell therapy. J Am Coll Cardiol. 2010;55:1385–94.

29. Prochazka V, et al. Autologous bone marrow stem cell transplantation in patients with end-stage chronical critical limb ischemia and diabetic foot. Vnitrni lekarstvi. 2009;55:173–8. https://pubmed.ncbi.nlm.nih.gov/19378841/.

30. Amann B, Luedemann C, Ratei R, Schmidt-Lucke JA. Autologous bone marrow cell trans-plantation increases leg perfusion and reduces amputations in patients with advanced critical limb ischemia due to peripheral artery disease. Cell Transplant. 2009;18:371–80.

31. Hermann PC, et al. Concentration of bone marrow total nucleated cells by a point-of-care device provides a high yield and preserves their functional activity. Cell Transplant. 2008;16:1059–69.

32. Burkhardt GE, et al. A large animal survival model (Sus scrofa) of extremity ischemia/reper-fusion and neuromuscular outcomes assessment: a pilot study. J Trauma. 2010;69(Suppl 1):S146–53.

33. Nakada MT, et al. Clot lysis in a primate model of peripheral arterial occlusive disease with use of systemic or intraarterial reteplase: addition of abciximab results in improved vessel reperfu-sion. J Vascu Intervent Radiol. 2004;15:169–76.

34. Arras M, et al. Monocyte activation in angiogenesis and collateral growth in the rabbit hindlimb. J Clin Invest. 1998;101:40–50.

35. Rosenthal SL, Guyton AC. Hemodynamics of collateral vasodilatation following femoral artery occlusion in anesthetized dogs. Circ Res. 1968;23:239–48.

36. Madeddu P, et al. Murine models of myocardial and limb ischemia: diagnostic end-points and relevance to clinical problems. Vasc Pharmacol. 2006;45:281–301.

37. Lawall H, Bramlage P, Amann B. Stem cell and progenitor cell therapy in peripheral artery disease. A critical appraisal. Thromb Haemost. 2010;103:696–709.
38. Lotfi S, et al. Towards a more relevant hind limb model of muscle ischaemia. Atherosclerosis. 2013;227:1–8.
39. Kinnaird T, et al. Local delivery of marrow-derived stromal cells augments collateral perfusion through paracrine mechanisms. Circulation. 2004;109:1543–9.
40. Helisch A, et al. Impact of mouse strain differences in innate hindlimb collateral vasculature. Arterioscler Thromb Vasc Biol. 2006;26:520–6.
41. Dokun AO, et al. A quantitative trait locus (LSq-1) on mouse chromosome 7 is linked to the absence of tissue loss after surgical hindlimb ischemia. Circulation. 2008;117:1207–15.
42. Becit N, et al. The effect of vascular endothelial growth factor on angiogenesis: an experimental study. Eur J Vasc Endovasc Surg. 2001;22:310–6.
43. Mac Gabhann F, Qutub AA, Annex BH, Popel AS. Systems biology of pro-angiogenic therapies targeting the VEGF system. Wiley Interdiscip Rev Syst Biol Med. 2010;2:694–707.
44. Belch J, et al. Effect of fibroblast growth factor NV1FGF on amputation and death: a randomised placebo-controlled trial of gene therapy in critical limb ischaemia. Lancet. 2011;377:1929–37.
45. Shigematsu H, et al. Randomized, double-blind, placebo-controlled clinical trial of hepatocyte growth factor plasmid for critical limb ischemia. Gene Ther. 2010;17:1152–61.
46. Asahara T, et al. Bone marrow origin of endothelial progenitor cells responsible for postnatal vasculogenesis in physiological and pathological neovascularization. Circ Res. 1999;85:221–8.
47. Takahashi T, et al. Ischemia- and cytokine-induced mobilization of bone marrow-derived endothelial progenitor cells for neovascularization. Nat Med. 1999;5:434–8.
48. Santarelli JG, et al. Incorporation of bone marrow-derived Flk-1-expressing CD34+ cells in the endothelium of tumor vessels in the mouse brain. Neurosurgery. 2006;59:374–82; discussion 374–82.
49. Ribatti D, Nico B, Crivellato E. The role of pericytes in angiogenesis. Int J Dev Biol. 2011;55:261–8.
50. Hall AP. Review of the pericyte during angiogenesis and its role in cancer and diabetic retinopathy. Toxicol Pathol. 2006;34:763–75.
51. Rajantie I, et al. Adult bone marrow-derived cells recruited during angiogenesis comprise precursors for periendothelial vascular mural cells. Blood. 2004;104:2084–6.
52. Ziegelhoeffer T, et al. Bone marrow-derived cells do not incorporate into the adult growing vasculature. Circ Res. 2004;94:230–8.
53. Ozerdem U, Alitalo K, Salven P, Li A. Contribution of bone marrow-derived pericyte precursor cells to corneal vasculogenesis. Invest Ophthalmol Vis Sci. 2005;46:3502–6.
54. Fuchs S, et al. Transendocardial delivery of autologous bone marrow enhances collateral perfusion and regional function in pigs with chronic experimental myocardial ischemia. J Am Coll Cardiol. 2001;37:1726–32.
55. Jackson KA, et al. Regeneration of ischemic cardiac muscle and vascular endothelium by adult stem cells. J Clin Invest. 2001;107:1395–402.
56. Stabile E, et al. Impaired arteriogenic response to acute hindlimb ischemia in CD4-knockout mice. Circulation. 2003;108:205–10.
57. Mohle R, Green D, Moore MA, Nachman RL, Rafii S. Constitutive production and thrombin-induced release of vascular endothelial growth factor by human megakaryocytes and platelets. Proc Natl Acad Sci U S A. 1997;94:663–8.
58. Blotnick S, Peoples GE, Freeman MR, Eberlein TJ, Klagsbrun M. T lymphocytes synthesize and export heparin-binding epidermal growth factor-like growth factor and basic fibroblast growth factor, mitogens for vascular cells and fibroblasts: differential production and release by CD4+ and CD8+ T cells. Proc Natl Acad Sci U S A. 1994;91:2890–4.
59. Melter M, et al. Ligation of CD40 induces the expression of vascular endothelial growth factor by endothelial cells and monocytes and promotes angiogenesis in vivo. Blood. 2000;96:3801–8.
60. Kinnaird T, et al. Marrow-derived stromal cells express genes encoding a broad spectrum of arteriogenic cytokines and promote in vitro and in vivo arteriogenesis through paracrine mechanisms. Circ Res. 2004;94:678–85.

61. Bernardo ME, Fibbe WE. Mesenchymal stromal cells: sensors and switchers of inflammation. Cell Stem Cell. 2013;13:392–402.
62. Prockop DJ, Oh JY. Mesenchymal stem/stromal cells (MSCs): role as guardians of inflammation. Mol Therap. 2012;20:14–20.
63. Timmermans F, De Sutter J, Gillebert TC. Stem cells for the heart, are we there yet? Cardiology. 2003;100:176–85.
64. Kinnaird T, Stabile E, Burnett MS, Epstein SE. Bone-marrow-derived cells for enhancing collateral development: mechanisms, animal data, and initial clinical experiences. Circ Res. 2004;95:354–63.
65. Murphy MP, et al. Autologous bone marrow mononuclear cell therapy is safe and promotes amputation-free survival in patients with critical limb ischemia. J Vasc Surg. 2011;53:1565–1574 e1561.
66. Franz RW, et al. Use of autologous bone marrow mononuclear cell implantation therapy as a limb salvage procedure in patients with severe peripheral arterial disease. J Vasc Surg. 2009;50:1378–90.
67. Benoit E, et al. The role of amputation as an outcome measure in cellular therapy for critical limb ischemia: implications for clinical trial design. J Transl Med. 2011;9:165.
68. Teraa M, et al. Autologous bone marrow-derived cell therapy in patients with critical limb ischemia: a meta-analysis of randomized controlled clinical trials. Ann Surg. 2013;258:922–9.
69. Matoba S, et al. Long-term clinical outcome after intramuscular implantation of bone marrow mononuclear cells (therapeutic angiogenesis by cell transplantation [TACT] trial) in patients with chronic limb ischemia. Am Heart J. 2008;156:1010–8.
70. Norgren L, et al. Inter-society consensus for the management of peripheral arterial disease (TASC II). J Vasc Surg. 2007;45(Suppl S):S5–67.
71. Klinkert P, van Dijk PJ, Breslau PJ. Polytetrafluoroethylene femorotibial bypass grafting: 5-year patency and limb salvage. Ann Vasc Surg. 2003;17:486–91.
72. Wen Y, Meng L, Gao Q. Autologous bone marrow cell therapy for patients with peripheral arterial disease: a meta-analysis of randomized controlled trials. Expert Opin Biol Ther. 2011;11:1581–9.
73. Huang P, et al. Autologous transplantation of granulocyte colony-stimulating factor-mobilized peripheral blood mononuclear cells improves critical limb ischemia in diabetes. Diabetes Care. 2005;28:2155–60.
74. Ozturk A, et al. Therapeutical potential of autologous peripheral blood mononuclear cell transplantation in patients with type 2 diabetic critical limb ischemia. J Diabetes Complicat. 2012;26:29–33.
75. Mohammadzadeh L, et al. Therapeutic outcomes of transplanting autologous granulocyte colony-stimulating factor-mobilised peripheral mononuclear cells in diabetic patients with critical limb ischaemia. Exp Clin Endocrinol Diab. 2013;121:48–53.
76. Lu D, et al. Comparison of bone marrow mesenchymal stem cells with bone marrow-derived mononuclear cells for treatment of diabetic critical limb ischemia and foot ulcer: a double-blind, randomized, controlled trial. Diabetes Res Clin Pract. 2011;92:26–36.
77. Gupta PK, et al. A double blind randomized placebo controlled phase I/II study assessing the safety and efficacy of allogeneic bone marrow derived mesenchymal stem cell in critical limb ischemia. J Transl Med. 2013;11:143.
78. Fujita Y, et al. Phase II clinical trial of CD34+ cell therapy to explore endpoint selection and timing in patients with critical limb ischemia. Circ J. 2014;78:490–501.
79. Losordo DW, et al. A randomized, controlled pilot study of autologous CD34+ cell therapy for critical limb ischemia. Circ Cardiovasc Interv. 2012;5:821–30.
80. Perin EC, et al. A randomized, controlled study of autologous therapy with bone marrow-derived aldehyde dehydrogenase bright cells in patients with critical limb ischemia. Catheteriz Cardiovasc Intervent. 2011;78:1060–7.
81. Powell RJ, et al. Cellular therapy with Ixmyelocel-T to treat critical limb ischemia: the randomized, double-blind, placebo-controlled RESTORE-CLI trial. Mol Therap. 2012;20:1280–6.
82. Arai M, Misao Y, Nagai H, Kawasaki M, Nagashima K, Suzuki K, Tsuchiya K, Otsuka S, Uno Y, Takemura G, Nishigaki K, Minatoguchi S, Fujiwara H. Granulocyte colony-stimulating factor: a noninvasive regeneration therapy for treating atherosclerotic peripheral artery disease. Circ J. 2006;70:1093–8. https://pubmed.ncbi.nlm.nih.gov/16936417/.

Chapter 6
Angiogenesis: Perspectives from Therapeutic Angiogenesis

Monique Bethel, Vishal Arora, and Brian H. Annex

6.1 Introduction

Systemic atherosclerosis remains the number one cause of morbidity and mortality worldwide. Peripheral arterial disease (PAD) is one form of systemic atherosclerosis, and PAD alone is estimated to affect over 200 million people worldwide [1]. PAD is defined as reduced ankle-brachial blood pressure index (ABI). Smoking and diabetes are the major risk factors for PAD, and the prevalence of PAD rises sharply with advancing age [2]. PAD is a systemic disease, and its presence raises the risk of disease in other vascular beds including the coronary arteries and renovascular and cerebrovascular system [2]. Thus, PAD affects both legs and life. In patients with PAD, symptoms may manifest as intermittent claudication, which is defined as exertional pain in the lower extremity, typically in the calf, that is relieved with rest. However, many patients with significant vascular obstruction do not have classic symptoms or even any symptoms at all. In such patients with PAD, the initial clinical manifestation of the disease may be critical limb ischemia (CLI) where patients are at a very high risk for amputation and stroke. Mainstays of medical therapy for PAD include antiplatelet therapy and optimal control of other risk factors for PAD including hypertension, diabetes, and hyperlipidemia [3]. Tobacco use is a stronger risk factor for PAD than for coronary artery disease [4]. Patients that are smokers should be aggressively encouraged to quit. Currently, there are few proven medical therapies that treat symptoms of PAD and improve exercise capacity. Cilostazol is a phosphodiesterase-3 inhibitor that has weak antiplatelet and arterial dilating properties and is one of the few medications shown to improve symptoms and functional capacity in patients with PAD [3]. Unfortunately, the side effect profile of the medication leads to discontinuation in a substantial number of patients, and studies of cilastazol were conducted when

M. Bethel · V. Arora · B. H. Annex (✉)
Division of Cardiology and Department of Medicine, Medical College of Georgia at Augusta University, Augusta, GA, USA
e-mail: BANNEX@augusta.edu

© Springer Nature Switzerland AG 2021
T. P. Navarro et al. (eds.), *Stem Cell Therapy for Vascular Diseases*,
https://doi.org/10.1007/978-3-030-56954-9_6

baseline medical therapies for patients with PAD were limited [3]. A structured exercise program, involving repeated exercise to submaximal claudication, has also been shown to improve exercise capacity [3]. For patients who are symptomatic despite optimal medical therapy, or those that have progression to symptoms at rest, non-healing ulcers, or gangrene, the treatment options are endovascular therapies or bypass surgery [5]. The development of critical limb ischemia is a poor prognostic indicator, both for the affected limb and overall mortality. Dormandy et al. found yearly all-cause mortality rates of 10–20% in this population [6], and Fridh et al. showed 3-year combined incidence of death or amputation in patients with critical limb ischemia was 48.8% [7]. The large public health burden and limited treatment options for PAD have spurred research into alternative therapies, one of which is stem cell therapy.

The hope of stem cell therapy was enormous: what if stem cells could be taken from a patient and put into an ischemic limb to promote revascularization? This would be an attractive option, as there would be no problems with rejection and the cells could potentially integrate and function for long periods. Despite promising findings in numerous small studies, the results of large studies have been largely disappointing. This chapter will review the background of stem cell therapy in PAD, important research studies, and the current status of this therapy as a treatment option for PAD.

6.2   Embryologic Origins

As the human embryo grows, one of the first organ systems to develop is a circulatory system to support necessary biological functions [8]. This occurs via two processes: vasculogenesis, which is the development of new blood vessels de novo, and the other is angiogenesis, which is the formation of new blood vessels from those already in existence [9]. In vasculogenesis, hemangioblasts, which are precursors to hematopoietic stem cells and endothelial cells, form conglomerations of cells called blood islands under the influence of fibroblastic growth factor. The hemangioblasts in the center of these islands differentiate into hematopoietic cells, and the cells on the periphery differentiate into angioblasts [9]. The angioblasts on the periphery form vacuoles that coalesce, undergo liquefaction, and ultimately form the lumen of the blood vessel. Eventually, these peripheral angioblasts terminally differentiate into endothelial cells [9].

Subsequent development of the circulatory system proceeds as angioblasts migrate and then fuse to form new vessels or merge with small capillaries to form branches or a capillary network [8]. The primitive capillary network then forms into larger arteries and veins, a complex process that is due to hemodynamic and local influences [10]. The big picture of embryonic circulatory development is that an initial vascular plexus is formed and remodeled many times over [8]. A more fixed adult pattern emerges, and endothelial cell proliferation, which is active in the fetus and infant, becomes quiescent in the adult [8]. However, the adult still maintains a population of cells with the ability to form new blood vessels, which might be required during wound healing or may be pathologically involved in the development of tumors or malignancies. Importantly, the skeletal muscle has satellite cells which have the capacity to form myocytes and endothelial cells [11].

6.3   Bone Marrow Mesenchymal Cells

As a topic, stem cell therapy is inclusive of a host of distinct cells. For example, the bone marrow contains two main categories of stem cells: hematopoietic stem cells and mesenchymal stem cells (also known as stromal cells, MSCs) [12]. Hematopoietic stem cells give rise to the cellular components of blood, i.e., erythrocytes, lymphocytes, platelets, etc. MSCs are a multipotent cell line that can differentiate into the bone, fat, muscle, and also blood vessels. In adults, these cells can be extracted from the bone marrow or peripheral blood. Whole blood or bone marrow is placed into a solution, and after several minutes of centrifugation at high speeds, red blood cells and platelets fall to the bottom, and a mononuclear cell layer rises to the top [13]. Bone marrow MSCs (BM-MSCs) or peripheral blood MSCs (PB-MSCs) can be found in the monocyte fraction of cells separated by a density gradient. This layer can easily be extracted and put into culture or injected into a patient as a means of therapy. In cell culture, the cells may be driven down a certain differentiation pathway based on exposure to cytokines or growth factors, or potentially modified. Oswald et al. were able to grow endothelial-like cells in culture after exposing BM-MSCs to vascular endothelial growth factor (VEGF) [14]. Beyond the potential of BM-MSCs to differentiate into endothelial cells, there is evidence that these cells also secrete vascular growth factors such as VEGF [15], fibroblast growth factor, and hepatocyte growth factor [16]. These characteristics made BM-MSCs an appealing option for study in the treatment of PAD.

While attractive for study, there are limitations to this approach. First, there is patient-to-patient and preparation-to-preparation variation in the cells and their characteristics. The manner in which the cell is delivered is another variable. The major limitation of this approach is that the fate of the cells after delivery is unknown [17].

6.4   Vascular Endothelial Growth Factor

The direct delivery of cytokines as protein or gene has been studied in PAD. Vascular endothelial growth factor (VEGF), perhaps the most extensively studied angiogenic agent, is a cytokine first described by Senger in 1983 [18]. It was found to markedly increase vascular permeability, promoting ascites formation in rodent species with cancer. Over time, several unique VEGF proteins have been discovered, including VEGF-A through E and placental growth factor. Each of these genes are encoded from different chromosomes, and within each gene, splice variations are also found [19]. The different VEGF proteins preferentially activate receptors VEGFR-1 and VEGFR-2 which promote angiogenesis or VEGFR-3 which promotes lymphangiogenesis [19]. VEGFR-2 is considered the dominant VEGFR in post-natal angiogenesis, and activation of VEGFR-2 increases signaling through the PLCγ-PKC-MAPK pathway to cause endothelial cell proliferation [19]. VEGFR activation has been exploited to promote angiogenesis in animal models of PAD. Most studies of gene therapy for PAD have involved different isoforms of VEGF [20], and many were small Phase I trials studying safety and Phase II trials looking at efficacy. As will be shown with stem cell therapy, progress in gene therapy has been limited by many small studies that show benefit in some outcomes, but large, randomized, placebo-controlled studies with positive findings are rare. In the RAVE trial, patients were randomized in a double-blind, placebo-controlled study of VEGF gene therapy in patients with severe, life-limiting intermittent claudication in a single limb, and it represented one of the first larger trials of this experimental therapy [21]. Patients were randomized to receive a low-dose intramuscular (IM)) injection of adenoviral VEGF121 (n = 32), a high dose of adenoviral VEGF121 (n = 40), or placebo (n = 33). The primary endpoint of this trial – change in pain-free walking time – was not met. Similarly, secondary outcomes, including change in ABI and claudication onset time, were not different between the three groups at 12 and 26 weeks. Amputations occurred rarely during the period of observation, with one occurring in the placebo group at day 114 and in the low-dose group at day 293. Over the ensuing years, different vector constructs for delivery, different isoforms of VEGF, or different routes of administration would be tested (Table 6.1).

Table 6.1 Comparison of two of the major clinical classifications of PAD

Fontaine Classification		Rutherford Classification			
Grade	Symptoms	Grade	Category	Clinical Symptoms	Objective Criteria
Stage I	Asymptomatic	0	0	No symptoms	Normal treadmill or hyperemia test
Stage II	Mild claudication		1	Mild claudication	Can complete standard treadmill exercise test. Ankle pressure after exercise >50 mmHg but at least 20 mmHg lower than resting value
Stage IIA	Claudication at a distance >200 m	I	2	Moderate claudication	Between categories 1 and 3
Stage IIB	Claudication at a distance <200 m		3	Severe claudication	Cannot complete standard treadmill testing. Ankle pressure <50 mmHg
Stage III	Rest pain	II	4	Rest pain	Resting ankle pressure <40 mmHg, toe pressure <30 mmHg, flat ankle or metatarsal pulse volume recording
Stage IV	Necrosis and/or gangrene	III	5	Minor tissue loss-focal gangrene, non-healing wound	Resting ankle pressure <60 mmHg, toe pressure <40 mmHg, flat ankle or metatarsal pulse volume recording
			6	Major tissue loss extending above the transmetatarsal level; foot not salvageable	Same as category 5

6.5 Fibroblastic Growth Factor

When compared to the VEGF systems, the FGF system is far more complicated with more than 20 different ligands and receptors [22]. Moreover, the FGF systems acts in concert with VEGF and platelet-derived growth factor (PDGF). Specifically, FGF has been shown to activate VEFG pathways, and murine endothelial cells lacking FGF signaling have been shown to become unresponsive to VEGF [23]. FGF also increases expression of the PDGF receptor on vascular smooth muscle cells, which plays a role in physiologic angiogenesis as well as pathophysiologic atherosclerosis [24]. Due to these complex interactions, the precise role of FGF in angiogenesis has yet to be elucidated. Several trials evaluated the safety and efficacy of FGF gene therapy in the treatment of PAD. There was some evidence of benefit, such as in the TRAFFIC trial, a randomized, placebo-controlled trial of recombinant FGF-2 administered intra-arterially (IA) in a single dose or two divided doses [25]. The administered dose was 30 µg/kg, which was the highest dose injected into the coronary arteries before causing hypotension in other studies. At 90 days, there were significant increases in pain-free walking time (PWT) in both treatment groups with no significant increase in PWT in the placebo group. ABI also significantly increased in the treatment groups compared to placebo. However, at 180 days, PWT increased in the placebo group to levels similar to the treatment groups. Other FGF studies (using gene based delivery) have shown a significant decrease in rest pain [26], but inconsistent findings on reduction of amputations [27, 28], and there was no mortality benefit shown [27, 28].

6.6 Hypoxia-Inducible Factor 1-Alpha (HIF-1α)

HIF-1α is a "master" transcription factor that is highly conserved across species [29] and is expressed on numerous cell types. HIF-1α is responsive to states of cell injury and exerts this effect by regulating cell metabolism and survival of cells in conditions of hypoxia [30] by transcriptional regulation of many proteins, including erythropoeitin [31] and other genes involved in glucose metabolism [29]. It has been called a master regulator because its expression leads to upregulation of a host of other cytokines including VEGF, PDGF, angiopoietin, and SDF-1 [32]. It is expressed in BM-MSCs, and in addition to the roles described above, HIF-1α appears to regulate the migration of BM-MSCs to areas of ischemia or tissue damage through expression of SDF-1 [33]. This led to trials of HIF-1α as a therapy in patients with PAD, especially after the lackluster results in prior trials focusing on VEGF gene therapy. Creager et al. studied adenovirus supplemented with the herpes virus transactivator to locally overexpress HIF-1α in ischemic muscle tissue of patients with intermittent claudication [32]. There was no increase in pain-free walking time (PWT), which was the primary outcome in this study.

6.7   Hepatocyte Growth Factor (HGF)

Despite its name, this cytokine was chosen for study in PAD due to its potent angiogenic properties. In the early 1990s, it was shown to induce endothelial cells in culture to form tube-like structures [34], to stimulate endothelial cell proliferation and migration [34], and to release pro-angiogenic factors [35]. This cytokine is expressed by adult BM-MSCs [36] and also has anti-thrombotic and anti-fibrotic properties [37]. There were several clinical trials with HGF delivered intramuscularly via plasmid. All were Phase II trials, and most were small; the largest trial included 79 participants. Depending on the outcome studied, each trial had some positive outcome and often in the primary endpoint, but no outcome was consistent across all the trials. Only one study showed significant improvement in the ABI [38]; others showed improvement in rest pain [38, 39], ulcer size [38, 39], and QoL [39]. For the more concrete outcomes such as amputations, the data were more discouraging, with one study showing no difference between the groups [39, 40]. In other studies, rates of amputations were not reported [38].

6.8   Early Studies of Stem Cell Therapy

In a landmark study in 1997, Asahara et al. isolated human angioblasts from peripheral blood [41]. Using the cell surface marker CD34 to isolate the progenitor cells, the isolates were grown in culture for several weeks. CD34 is a cell surface marker that identifies a progenitor cell that may differentiate into several different cell types, including hematopoietic cells and endothelial cells [42]. With time, the cells were observed to form networks and tube-like structures in culture. The investigators took these findings one step further and injected these human cells into athymic mice with hind-limb ischemia induced by femoral artery ligation. Histological examination of the tissue several weeks later showed the human cells had been incorporated into the capillary walls of the affected limb. The human cells did not appear in the normal limb. In an additional experiment using rabbits [41], CD34+ cells were isolated from the peripheral blood of the animals, grown in culture, labeled, and then given back to the animals after hind-limb ischemia induction. Again, the labeled cells were found in areas of active revascularization.

Further work has shown that in addition to CD34 expression, expression of AC133 [43] and the VEGF-2 receptor more specifically identifies an endothelial cell precursor [43, 44]. As the progenitor cell terminally differentiates, expression of AC133 diminishes, and the cells begin to express adhesion molecules and to produce nitric oxide [45].

Other investigators isolated endothelial progenitor cells from bone marrow in animals [46]. Shi et al. used a bone marrow transplantation model in dogs, where bone marrow cells from a donor animal were injected into a recipient animal [47]. The endothelial progenitors were identified by possessing cell surface markers for

CD34, von Willebrand factor, and low-density lipoprotein. The bone marrow cells were then injected into another dog treated with immunosuppressant therapy to prevent graft-versus-host disease. Further, an impervious Dacron graft was placed in the descending thoracic aorta. As the graft was impervious, there could be no ingrowth of native capillaries from the surrounding tissue. After 12 weeks, the graft was stained for endothelial cells, and it was observed that only donor cells were identified in the graft material, signifying that these endothelial progenitors were able to migrate from the bone marrow to the peripheral circulation and incorporate into sites of vascular tissue.

Preclinical cell therapy studies such as these paved the way for clinical trials in humans with the goal that if an isolation and production process could be replicated, then stem cells derived in this fashion could represent a novel therapeutic approach to the treatment of PAD. As the cells would be derived from the patient (i.e., autologous), there would be no immunological phenomena which would result in rejection and destruction of the cells. Theoretically, the advantage to this strategy over gene therapy would be the potential of the cells to maintain local levels of angiogenic factors and to be incorporated into new vessels. Still, to this day, direct evidence for this effect is lacking.

6.9   Trials of Stem Cell Therapy in Humans

6.9.1   Bone Marrow Mesenchymal Stem Cells (BM-MSCs)

One of the first human studies of stem cell implantation for treatment of PAD was the TACT trial conducted by Tateishi-Yuyama et al. in 2002 [48]. The TACT trial included two groups of patients: Group A had unilateral limb ischemia, and Group B had bilateral limb ischemia. Both groups required an ABI less than 0.6 in the affected limb, rest pain, and/or, a non-healing ulcer and were deemed not amenable to surgical treatment. Group A received an injection of BM-MNCs in the affected limb, and the contralateral limb was injected with normal saline. In the second group with bilateral ischemia, half of the limbs were randomized to receive BM-MNCs, and the other half received an injection of peripheral blood mononuclear cells (PB-MNCs), which had been noted to contain only 1/500th the concentration of endothelial cell precursors [48]. Outcomes were measured at 4 and 24 weeks following the injections. There were three primary clinical outcomes of this trial including change in ABI, transcutaneous oxygen saturation (TcO_2), and resolution of rest pain. All of the primary outcomes in this trial were met with significant increases in ABI and TcO_2 and reduction in rest pain. The secondary outcomes assessed included new collateral vessel formation which was measured with digital subtraction angiography (DSA) and pain-free walking time (PWT). Collateral vessel formation was described on a scale from 0 to 3, with 0 being no collateral vessel formation and 3+ being "rich" collateral vessel formation. On average, new collateral vessel formation in group A was graded 1 and 1.1 in group B. For those in group B who received PB-MNCs in one limb, there was less robust formation of collateral vessels in that limb compared to the limb injected with BM-MSCs.

Safety was a critical focus of study. There were two deaths in Group A with unilateral ischemia. The cause of death was determined to be myocardial infarction in both patients and was considered unrelated to the treatment. There were no reports of edema or pain at the injection sites for up to 72 hours following the procedure. The safety outcomes of these trials will be discussed later in the chapter.

The TACT trial provided evidence of the safety and efficacy of this strategy for treatment of critical limb ischemia in patients who were not candidates for surgical revascularization and opened the door for a multitude of studies further examining this method. This line of investigation started with several studies that examined intra-arterial (IA) and/or intra-muscular (IM) administration of BM-MSCs.

In another small pilot trial, seven patients with CLI were treated with BM-MSC using the same technique described by Tateisi-Yuyama [49]. The primary outcomes of this trial included change in the ABI, PWT, TCO_2, and leg blood flow (LBF), measured at 4 and 24 weeks after the injection. LBF was measured by plethysmography, a noninvasive technique that measures changes in volume in a segment of the body [50]. There were significant increases in TcO_2, pain-free walking time, and LBF at 4 weeks. ABI increased as well, but this change did not quite meet statistical significance. At 24 weeks, there was no significant difference in the measured variables compared to baseline with the exception of PWT, which was still significantly increased at 24 weeks compared to baseline measures at 24 weeks. Endothelial dependent vasodilatory response to acetylcholine was enhanced in the group that received the bone marrow cells, compared to a control group of patients with leg ischemia that did not. This indicated that BM-MSCs may also improve endothelial function in this patient population.

Cobellis et al. studied 19 individuals with critical limb ischemia as defined by the Fontaine classification system [51]. Fontaine stage III or IV PAD includes the presence of rest pain or ulceration and/or gangrene (Table 6.1) [52]. The control group consisted of nine patients who were clinically similar to the treatment group but did not undergo the experimental treatment for "personal reasons." The treatment group received two infusions of BM cells that were filtered for large particles but were otherwise non-selective. A second infusion was given 45 days later. Outcomes were measured at 6 and 12 months and included perfusion as measured by laser Doppler flowmetry assessed under several conditions as well as capillary density and neoangiogenesis (new capillary formation). Perfusion was significantly increased at 6 months with the exception of perfusion measured with the leg in a lowered position. These changes largely persisted at 12 months. There were no significant changes in capillary density or enlargement, but there were significant increases in neoangiogenesis at 6 months in the tibia, foot, and toe. Only neoangiogenesis at the toe remained significant at 12 months. The majority of patients, 80%, also had clinical improvement with increases in the pain-free walking distance.

Several years later, a study of diabetic patients with severe limb ischemia with BM-MSCs administered once intra-arterially was undertaken [53]. These patients showed improvement in ABI, wound healing, and symptoms. This study also included an angiographic evaluation at 3 months with novel findings of two patterns of neovascularization: one pattern consisted of increased branching of the existing vessels, and the other pattern showed an increase in the diameter of the existing vessels. Though unrelated to the experimental therapy, mortality remained high in this small cohort, with 4 of the 20 patients dying in 1 year. The overall amputation rate was high, with seven patients having minor amputations, though most occurred before the BM injection.

So far, the studies described to this point have demonstrated efficacy on multiple fronts as well as an acceptable safety profile. However, the sample sizes remained small and the target patient population highly selected. Additionally, outcome measures were inconsistent.

Franz et al. conducted a study of patients with severe PAD in whom the only viable treatment option remaining was amputation [54]. Patients received BM-MSCs intramuscularly and intra-arterially and were followed for 3 months. Though the study was small, the patient sample was interesting in that the sample was high risk, not only in terms of the ischemic limb but also in the presence of comorbidities: eight of the nine patients were smokers, seven were diabetics, four had previously suffered strokes, four had concomitant coronary artery disease, and all had hypertension. The primary outcomes were ABI measurements, major or minor amputations, symptoms (rest pain), wound healing, and amputations.

There were no significant differences in ABI at 3 months compared to baseline. Minor amputations occurred in two patients, and three patients ultimately needed major amputations; however, the authors cite three examples in which the patients required a less extensive amputation after treatment than would have been done without treatment. Of the six patients who did not require major amputation, five did not have rest pain at follow-up. There was complete ulcer healing in three patients. Overall, eight of the nine patients derived some benefit from the experimental therapy. This was one of the first trials of this particular therapy in the United States. These investigators continued recruiting additional patients and published additional data on a total of 20 patients (21 limbs) [55]. In this larger cohort, there were four major and two minor amputations, and of the 18 limbs with a 3-month follow-up, only 1 limb did not demonstrate any of the criteria defining success.

Many of the early trials of stem cell therapy for PAD involved IM injections of stem cells, but there were questions about the best route for delivery, and the potential benefits of IA versus IM administration need to be considered. Bartsch et al. were the first to report results on the administration of BM-MSCs both IM and IA [56]. This study involved patients with moderate PAD, Fontaine class 2b disease [52]. Patients were deemed not to be surgical candidates. A control group ($n = 12$) was comprised of patients with similar clinical characteristics that could not or were unwilling to undergo the stem cell therapy. Following the treatment, patients were assessed at 2 and 13 months. Primary outcomes included walking distance and parameters of perfusion, including venous occlusion plethysmography and capillary venous oxygen saturation via transcutaneous oximetry. Importantly, before the administration of the BM-MSCs, the patients in the treatment group ($n = 13$) had ischemic pre-conditioning which was achieved by having the patients exercise to claudication, followed by compression of the thigh above systolic pressure. After this, IA injection was given and was followed by a second compression of the thigh. In the final step, BM-MSCs were administered via IM administration. This maneuver was designed with the intention to increase the contact time of the stem cells with the target ischemic tissue. At both 2 and 13 months following the injections, there was a significant increase in total walking distance, while there was no change in the control group. Additionally, the ABI and measures of oxygen saturations and flow significantly increased in the treatment group. These changes were sustained at the 13-month mark. In contrast, the control group showed significant decreases in ABI and flow when assessed at an average of 4 months. There were no other significant changes in the other outcomes measured other than what was expected, but this does give some idea of the natural history of moderate PAD in this patient population.

In the OPTIPEC trial, Smadja et al. quantified the levels of "endothelial precursor cells" circulating in the peripheral blood of patients with CLIPAD who had received BM-MNC as therapy [57]. Additionally, BM-MSCs were grown in culture, and cell marker expression was measured. Importantly, this study also quantified the levels of neo-angiogenesis that had occurred histologically by comparing amputated limbs of individuals who received treatment compared to age- and gender-matched controls with CLI that did not receive therapy and also had amputations. In this study, 11 patients received BM-MNCs injected multiple times in the ischemic gastrocnemius muscle. These patients had significantly fewer circulating early and late endothelial cell precursors compared to controls free of cardiovascular disease and cancer. Most of the patients (8 of 11, 73%) went on to have amputations. Histological studies of the amputated limbs were conducted to quantify the levels of neoangiogenesis that had occurred. These were then compared to amputated limbs of age- and gender-matched individuals who did not receive BM-MSC. In the patients who demonstrated new vessel formation in the anatomic specimen, there were higher levels of colony-forming units endothelial cells (CFU-EC) grown in cultures. CFU-EC are groups of cells in culture that have differentiated down the pathway to the endothelial cell lineage but are not terminally differentiated and typically grow in close association with T-lymphocytes [58]. New vessel formation was defined as vessels observed in unusual locations; vessels identified in this manner were subjected to immunohistochemical staining to confirm the endothelial origin of the cell. This study also showed that patients with PAD had fewer circulating early and late endothelial cell precursors compared to control patients free of cardiovascular disease and cancer.

Hur et al. had shown that "early" EPCs isolated from peripheral blood, i.e., cells with peak growth in culture at approximately 3 weeks followed by death at 4 weeks, secreted larger amounts of angiogenic cytokines [58]. This is compared to late EPC, whose first appearance in culture was at 2–3 weeks, with peak growth at 4–8 weeks, and persisted for up to 12 weeks. These late EPC cells better incorporated into a cell culture of human umbilical vein endothelial cells, produced more nitric oxide, and formed capillary tubes better than early EPC [58].

Van Tongeren et al. also attempted to address the question of optimal method of delivery for BM-MSCs in a small (n = 27), randomized but un-blinded trial [59]. The study subjects had CLI, or persistent claudication (at least 12 months) with maximal walking distance of <100 m. The subjects had no options for surgical or percutaneous revascularization and had a life expectancy of at least 1 year. Subjects were randomized to IM (n = 12) or IA + IM (n = 15) administration of BM-MSCs isolated by the typical protocol. Primary endpoints were pain-free walking distance, complete healing of any ulcers, and avoidance of amputation at 1, 6, and 12 months. Secondary outcomes included changes in ABI and a pain levels. New vessel formation was measured via digital subtraction angiography (DSA) at 6 months following the procedure and compared to baseline anatomy established by DSA 1–2 weeks prior to the procedure. Subjects were followed for a mean of 24 months. Of the original 24 patients, one died from pneumonia prior to the 6-month time point, and the other became extremely ill so as not to be able to participate in the final outcome measures; these two patients were excluded from the final analysis. Therefore, 25 patients were included in the final analysis. Of these, nine had major amputations within 3 months of the BM-MSC infusion and were also excluded from the final analysis.

Overall, in the remaining cohort that did not undergo amputation, there was significant improvement in pain-free walking distance at 6 and 12 months (81 ± 56 m vs 257 ± 126 m vs 282 ± 139, at baseline, 6 months, and 12 months, respectively). Similarly, there were significant increases in the ABI compared to baseline at both 6 months and 12 months. There was no difference in these outcomes based on the method of administration. Most interesting were the results of the DSA, which showed increase in collateral vessel formation in seven patients, no difference compared to baseline in four patients, and deterioration of vessels in four patients. For one patient, DSA values were not able to be compared. Based on the findings of the DSA, "responders" were compared to "non-responders" in terms of the overall number of BMCs received, the number of CD34+ cells, and the number of CFU grown in culture, and there was no significant difference in any of these measures. This led to a quandary to explain the positive clinical benefit with no definite anatomical explanation. The authors proffered an explanation that there may have been undersized collateral vessels unable to be visualized by DSA. The smallest vessel that can be imaged via DSA is approximately 200 microns in diameter [60], a parameter that has not changed significantly over the years [61].

The RESTORE-CLI trial was a novel Phase II, randomized, double-blind, placebo-controlled trial. The novelty of this trial was that in the treatment arm, BM-MSCs were expanded to include a higher concentration of CD90+ cells (mesenchymal stem cells) and CD14+ cells of the monocyte/macrophage lineage [62]. Outcomes in this study included time to first treatment failure, defined as major amputation in the treated limb, all-cause death, and/or new tissue necrosis. This endpoint occurred significantly later in the treatment group compared to the control group. A Cox proportional hazard ratio analysis was included and illustrated that the time-to-event curves separated early and maintained distance throughout the observation period. A post hoc analysis of patients with existing wounds found an even greater treatment effect in this subset of patients. There was a trend toward longer amputation-free survival in the treatment group, but this did not meet statistical significance. Another highlight of this study was a much smaller volume injected due to the proprietary processing of the BM-MSCs that resulted in higher concentration of the target cells, a process that took approximately 2 weeks. However, this and future studies that thought to use this approach also introduced an important limitation to the study, as several patients did not have enough aspirate to create the final injection product.

In 2010, Iafrati et al. published another randomized, double-blind, placebo-controlled pilot trial of BM-MSCs used for therapy of CLI in patients deemed not to be candidates for surgical revascularization [63]. In this trial, a rapid, point-of-care system was used to process the BM-MSCs and have them ready for reinjection in less than 15 minutes. Control patients received an injection of diluted peripheral blood. Both the treatment and control groups underwent iliac crest puncture, but the treatment group ($n = 34$) had 240 mL of bone marrow removed, while the control group ($n = 14$) had only 2 mL removed. A total volume of 40 mL of the BM-MSCs was injected under ultrasound guidance in small aliquots into the affected limb. Patients had follow-up at 1, 4, 8, and 12 weeks after the procedure for amputation, ABI, TCO_2, Rutherford class, pain, walking distance, and quality of life (QoL). The study was not sufficiently powered to determine statistical significance, but there was a trend for lower amputation rates in the treatment group (17.6% vs 28.6%), a finding that did not meet statistical significance. There was also a trend for greater improvement in pain. A composite endpoint that the patient was (1) alive, (2) did not have a major amputation in the treated limb, (3) had an improvement in the Rutherford class, and (4) did not have worsening of pain was also measured. More patients in the treatment group met these criteria for success compared to the placebo group, 17/34 (50%) vs 3/14 (21.4%), though this too did not meet statistical significance. In the QoL assessment, again, there were trends favoring the treatment arm, though none met significance. With the exception of mental health, the treatment group showed greater improvement or less decline in all factors related to QoL. Similar findings were observed with the ABI and TCO_2, with trends in improvement in both in the treatment groups. Beyond the small size of the study that hampered statistical analysis of the findings, this study also had difficulties with collecting some of the follow-up data, particularly walking distance, ABI, and TCO_2 measurements.

This was also one of the few studies to quantify the level of blinding. The patients and investigators were questioned on the treatment day about which group they thought the patients were assigned. The blinding index is the percentage of incorrect guesses added to the percentage of undecided answers; if this is greater than 50%, the study is appropriately blinded [64].

As time progressed, larger trials testing the efficacy of BM-MSCs were conducted. The PROVASA trial was performed in Germany and randomized patients to receive IA BM-MSCs or placebo as a first treatment [65]. This next part of the trial was also double-blinded. However, all patients ultimately received IA BM-MSCs after 3 months in the trial in an open-label fashion. The primary outcome was improvement in ABI, and this outcome was not met in this trial. The investigators did observe positive outcomes including improved wound healing and reduced rest pain. However, for other outcomes, such as amputation-free survival and limb salvage, there was no difference between the treatment and placebo groups. Median follow-up time was 28 months. Notably, patients with the most advanced CLI, Rutherford 5 or 6 [52], had the worse outcomes. All patients with category 6 went on to have an amputation. Wound healing was a strong positive outcome in this study, as ulcer area significantly declined at 3 months in the group randomized to receive BM-MSC treatment initially ($p = 0.014$). A dose-response effect was shown in this study with regard to ulcer healing, and additional doses of BM-MSCs showed greater decrease in wound area. A similar dose response was noted for pain relief. TCO_2 levels generally increased in the BM-MSC treatment group. The TCO_2 trend in the placebo group was an initial decrease followed by an increase seen after the placebo group crossed over.

The largest randomized stem cell trial to date, JUVENTAS, was published in 2015 [66]. Conducted in the Netherlands, this study included the typical patient population of patients with CLI that was not amenable to revascularization. An additional strength of this study was the randomized, double-blind, placebo-controlled design. Study recruits were randomized to receive multiple IA injections of BM-MSCs via the femoral artery or matching peripheral blood, processed to have the same appearance as the bone marrow aspirate. All subjects underwent bone marrow aspiration. The original sample was divided into three aliquots, with 2/3 cryopreserved for future administration. The cryopreservation consisted of addition of 10% dimethyl sulfoxide followed by freezing in liquid nitrogen. Subjects received additional doses at 3-week intervals.

The primary outcome was major amputation, defined as any amputation occurring above the ankle joint up to 6 months after receiving therapy. Other outcomes included the following: combined major amputation or death, minor amputations, ulcer size, rest pain, pain-free walking distance, ABI, transcutaneous O2 pressure, clinic status, and quality of life. This trial included a large number of outcomes which were measured at 2 months and 6 months. The cell counts injected were the highest for the initial injection and were smaller on subsequent injections. The same was true for the number of CD34+ cell and CFU, suggesting a loss of cells with time and cryopreservation. There was no significant difference in the isolates obtained from the treatment and placebo groups.

There was little positive data in this trial. There was no difference in amputations at either time point or overall. There was no difference in the composite end point of death or major amputation. The study also included composite endpoints fashioned after previously published studies [62, 63], and no significant difference was observed. There was also no difference in any of the secondary endpoints, including ABI, TcO2, QoL, or ulcer area. The investigators also conducted a meta-analysis of the previous trials (including their own) and found a very small benefit to the cell-based therapies that disappeared when only properly blinded and placebo-controlled studies were included.

6.9.2 Peripheral Blood Mononuclear Cells (PB-MNCs)

As another method of stem cell therapy, peripheral blood MNCs (PB-MNCs) were also studied. The obvious advantage of this approach is the ease of material acquisition. Lenk et al. administered an average of 39×10^6 PB-MNCs to seven patients with CLI not amenable to surgical revascularization [67]. The patients were given granulocyte colony-stimulating factor (G-CSF) as a stimulus for production/mobilization of PB-MNCs for 4 days prior to harvesting the cells. Isolation of PB-MNCs from the blood involved a gradient separation system similar to the protocols using BM-MNCs: the cells were grown in culture for 4 days and then administered IA to the patients. A small sample of the cells from culture was tested by flow cytometry to determine the expression of CD34. Outcomes assessed included ABI, TCO_2, PWT, and endothelial function. There were significant improvements in all of these outcomes at 12 weeks after the procedure. Flow cytometry analysis showed that approximately 50% of the cells were positive for CD34, as well as markers of endothelial cells lineage [67].

Larger trials of IM injections of PB-MNCs were conducted by Lara-Hernandez et al. [68]. The patient population ($n = 28$) included severe CLI with no options for surgery. The cells were obtained by apheresis after stimulation with G-CSF for 5 days. The investigators reported "high" levels of EPCs as determined by the expression of CD34 and CD133. There was no control arm. There were significant improvements in ABI and pain. The limb salvage rate was 74.4% after 1 year.

Another promising study was conducted in diabetics with CLI [69]. In this randomized controlled trial, patients received two IM injections 40 days apart of unselected PB-MNCs after granulocyte colony-stimulating factor (G-CSF) stimulation. Control group received IM prostaglandin E1. Compared to the control group, the treatment group showed significant improvements in rest pain, wound healing (Huang et al.), and amputations. PWT was also higher in the treatment group, but this narrowly missed statistical significance.

Losordo et al. studied low and high doses of enriched CD34+ PB-MNCs administered IM in a double-blind, placebo-controlled pilot trial [70]. Amputations occurred more frequently in the control arm (66.7%) compared to the low-dose (42.9%) and in the high-dose (22.2%) group though the difference did not meet statistical significance ($p = 0.137$). Other outcomes studied, including wound healing, PWT, rest pain, and QoL, also did not show differences between the treatment and control groups. The study was small and not powered to detect statistical differences.

Next, trials were conducted comparing PB-MNCs to BM-MNCs. There were mixed results. The TACT trial described above favored BM-MSCs, as did an extension of the TACT trial examining long-term outcomes [71]. One trial favored PB-MNCs [69] but also found improvements in the patients treated with BM-MSCs.

Table 6.2 summarizes the trials discussed. The trials were small Phase I or II trials with few participants. Most of the trials included individuals with advanced PAD; however, two trials included individuals with less severe disease, and both

Table 6.2 A summary of human BM-MSC therapeutic angiogenesis clinical trials

Author/trial	Phase/year	Disease	Treatment	Cell number	Subject (n) Treatment/Control	Findings
TACT	Phase II 2002	Rutherford grade III, category 5	Intramuscular Unselected BM-MNCs and PB-MNCs	2.7–2.8×10^9	25 unilateral 22 bilateral Diabetes excluded	Improved ABI, TcO2 Improved rest and pain-free walking Evidence of increased collateral vessels
Higashi et al.	Phase I 2004	Rutherford grade III, category 5	Intramuscular BM-MNCs	1.6×10^9 CD34+ 3.8×10^7	7/0 Diabetes, CAD excluded	Improved ABI, pain-free walking, TcPO2 Increased vasodilation dependent leg blood flow by plethysmography
Bartsch et al.	Phase II 2007	Fontaine class 2b	Intra-arterial + intramuscular BM-MNC	83×10^6	13/12	Improved pain-free walking, ABI Increased oxygen saturation and both rest and peak blood flow
OPTIPEC	Phase I 2008	Rutherford grade III, category 5	Intramuscular BM-MNCs	Not reported	11/0	Evidence of endothelial cell proliferation in distal amputated limb
Van Tongeren et al.	Phase II 2008	Fontaine IIB or greater	Intra-arterial + intramuscular vs intramuscular alone BM-MNCs grown in culture	1.23×10^9 total CD34+ 3.07×10^6	12/15	Both groups improved pain-free walking and ABI
Cobellis et al.	Phase II 2008	Fontaine III (21%) Fontaine IV (79%)	Intra-arterial Unselected BM-MSCs	10^9	10/9	Increased perfusion and neoangiogenesis Increased PWT

(continued)

Table 6.2 (continued)

Author/trial	Phase/year	Disease	Treatment	Cell number	Subject (n) Treatment/Control	Findings
Franz et al.	Phase I 2009	Rutherford grade II, category 4 $n = 1$ Rutherford grade III, category 5, $n = 6$; category $6 = 2$	Intramuscular Intra-arterial	Not reported	9/0	8/9 patients had improvement 6/9 patients avoided amputation
Ruiz-Salmeron et al.	Phase I-IIa 2011	Rutherford grade III Category 4 $n = 3$ Category 5 $n = 11$ Category 6 $n = 6$	Intra-arterial Unselected BM-MSCs	266.2×10^6 CD34+ 4.37×10^6	20/0	Improved wound healing, ABI and symptoms
Iafrati et al.	Phase II 2011	Rutherford grade IV or V	Intramuscular BM-MSCs rapidly prepared for injection	3.23×10^9	34/14	Decreased amputations Improved pain, QoL and Rutherford class Improved ABI
PROVASA	Phase II 2011	Rutherford grade II, category 4 or greater Fontaine stage III or greater	Intramuscular BM-MNCs	1st tx: 153×10^6 Second tx: 155×10^6 Third tx: 165×10^6 CD34+ First tx: 3.6×10^6 Second tx: 2.5×10^6 Third tx: 2.4×10^6	19/21	Improved ulcer size, rest pain No difference in ABI, amputation, death

(continued)

Table 6.2 (continued)

Author/trial	Phase/year	Disease	Treatment	Cell number	Subject (n) Treatment/Control	Findings
RESTORE-CLI	Phase II 2012	Rutherford grade II, category 4	Intramuscular BM-MSCs	136×10^6 total CD90+ 25×10^6	48/24	Longer time to treatment failure Increased amputation-free survival (32%, NS)
JUVENTAS	Phase II 2015	Rutherford category 3 or greater	Intra-arterial BM-MNCs	1st tx: 199×10^6 Second tx: 144×10^6 Third tx: 144×10^6	81/79	No difference in amputation, death, ABI, ulcer size, quality of life, rest pain, TcPO2

Abbreviations: TCO$_2$ transcutaneous partial pressure of oxygen, *PWT* peak walking time, *BM-MNC* bone marrow mononuclear cells, *NS* not significant

were positive trials. The mode of delivery for therapy was mostly IM injection, with only two studies exclusively administering cells intra-arterially. There were several studies that compared IM and IA injections, and there was little evidence that one method was superior to the other. An IA injection would call for cannulation of an artery, which requires special equipment and carries risks of bleeding and arterial injury, though there were few reports of these events occurring. In many of the trials, unselected BM-MSCs were administered as treatment, with cell counts on the order of 10^9; however, several of the trials administered substantially fewer cells, on the order of 10^6. The RESTORE-CLI trial used a proprietary process to isolate higher concentrations of MSCs and HSCs and was a positive trial. Some, but not all of the studies, quantified the types of cells being injected. There was also some heterogeneity among the primary outcomes, which makes direct comparison of the trials difficult.

6.10 Safety Outcomes

All medical therapies must be assessed as a balance of benefit vs. risk. In the von Tongeren trial [59], two patients developed heart failure following the BM-MSC extraction and injection. The procedure took place under general anesthesia, and this was implicated as the cause of the complication versus the volume of BM-MSCs received or any other aspect of the bone marrow extraction. In the PROVASA trial, three adverse events were associated with the treatment procedure: thrombus formation in a previously placed stent after inflation of a low-pressure balloon, one hematoma, and one pseudoaneurysm associated with the IA administration of the BM-MSCs [65]. The JUVENTAS trial reported a large number of adverse events at 213, but only one, a femoral hematoma, was directly attributed to the procedure [66]. The RESTORE-CLI trial also reported a high number of adverse events, though there was no significant difference in the number of adverse events in the treatment and control arms; many of the adverse events reported were also sequelae of the disease process, including pain, wound infection, and necrosis. In this trial, an event of wound infection in the hallux of the infected limb was thought to be possibly due to the treatment [62]. Other safety outcomes that were anticipated but not observed included rhabdomyolysis, kidney injury, or proliferative retinopathy [63]. A small drop in hematocrit was noted but did not require any therapy [63].

The studies involving PB-MNCs were also generally safe. Losordo reported 60 serious adverse events, with no differences in incidence of events between the treatment and control arms [70]. While the vast majority was felt not to be related to the procedure, one patient developed hypotension with G-CSF treatment, and another had worsening of rest pain after the injection that required hospitalization. Huang et al. documented one patient with bone pain and malaise during treatment with G-CSF [69]. No deaths that occurred in these trials were attributed to the procedure or the treatments received.

6.11   Perspectives on Stem Cell Therapy

Despite the grave nature of CLI, owing to the lack of positive data, stem cell therapy has not emerged as a proven strategy for the treatment of PAD. In the most recent AHA/ACC [72] and ESC [73] clinical guidelines on the treatment of PAD, there are no recommendations supporting the use of stem cell therapy. There are several potential reasons for the overall lack of success. Several studies have called into question the quality of stem cells from a population of patients with PAD, unfortunately the patients most in need of treatment. Imanishi et al. found that endothelial progenitor cells (EPCs) from patients with hypertension reached senescence and had decreased telomerase activity compared to age-matched control patients without hypertension [74]. Similarly, EPCs isolated from the peripheral blood of healthy smokers were found to have impaired migratory and proliferative response and decreased ability to form precapillary structures in cell culture [75]. Patients with type I diabetes have also been noted to have fewer EPCs with reduced function in culture, even when the cells were grown in culture with normal glucose levels [76]. Hypercholesterolemia has also been associated with lower EPC numbers and dysfunction [77]. Taken together, it is likely that stem cells from patients with PAD are dysfunctional at baseline when compared to similar cells from a non-PAD population.

It has also been shown that the established cell markers used to identify EPCs in bone marrow cells may lead to contamination of the product with cells of the hematopoietic lineage [78]. This raises questions about the actual mechanisms involved in the effects of BM-MSCs in the treatment of PAD: it may be that other mechanisms besides EPC-mediated angiogenesis are involved. Along the same lines, one study in mice with induced hind-limb ischemia found that BM-MSCs did not incorporate into developing blood vessels and that there has been false-positive identification of EPCs from surrounding cells [79]. There is also the question of whether EPCs, also called endothelial colony-forming cells (ECFCs) [80], exist in the general population of BM-MSCs; true EPCs may actually be found in the peripheral blood [81]. The majority of studies highlighted in this chapter used BM-MSCs as compared to PB-MSCs. Evidence is emerging that ECFCs and BM-MSCs may act in concert to support angiogenesis [82](Lin et al); therefore, a strategy using BM-MSCs alone may be inadequate to produce a clinical effect.

Other considerations include the severity of disease in the patient population. These trials included patients with the most severe PAD who were not candidates for surgery. Some have argued that the time to try such therapies may be at an earlier stage of disease.

6.12   Future Directions

Has stem cell therapy for PAD reached a dead end? In a meta-analysis of the trials published in 2019, Gao et al. demonstrated that the cumulative evidence shows a clear benefit for stem cell therapy in terms of improving rest pain and pain-free walking distance [83]. The evidence for ulcer healing and ABI were less certain, but the preponderance of the studies included in the analysis favored stem cell therapy. Conversely, the data for amputations favored placebo, and this analysis also highlighted the high potential for bias in a large proportion of the studies, particularly related to blinding.

It can, however, be argued that further studies may reveal the true benefit of stem cells. As nearly every study examined patients with the most severe PAD, stem cell therapy considered at an earlier time point in the natural history may prove beneficial. Furthermore, there may be a specific cell population that would provide a benefit.

There may also be benefit from stem cells derived from adipose tissue. Bura et al. conducted a Phase I trial of MSCs obtained from adipose tissue as stem cell therapy in patients with CLI [84]. This small trial of seven patients demonstrated the safety of this technique, as no adverse events were reported. In terms of efficacy, there were overall decreases in wound area and increases in TCO_2 ($p < 0.05$).

Unfortunately, the proportion of studies examining treatment for PAD is low: according to a study published in 2014, 1.7% of all active trials registered in ClinicalTrials.gov from October of 2007 to September 2010 were devoted to examining interventions for PAD [85]. More recently, Biscetti et al., in their review of stem cell therapy in PAD, noted a lack of well-designed Phase III trials [86]. Taken together, this suggests that there are few studies on the horizon.

6.13 Conclusions

PAD remains at epidemic proportions. Current medical therapy is limited, and the jury is still out on the true benefit of novel therapies such as stem cell therapy. Before abandoning the option of stem cell therapy, future studies should focus on well-designed trials that limit bias and explore the optimal population of patients with PAD who may benefit from such therapy.

References

1. Hirsch AT, Duval S. The global pandemic of peripheral artery disease. Lancet. 2013;382(9901):1312–4.
2. Criqui MH, Aboyans V. Epidemiology of peripheral artery disease. Circ Res. 2015;116(9):1509–26.
3. Gerhard-Herman MD, Gornik HL, Barrett C, Barshes NR, Corriere MA, Drachman DE, et al. 2016 AHA/ACC guideline on the management of patients with lower extremity peripheral artery disease: executive summary: a report of the American College of Cardiology/ American Heart Association Task Force on Clinical Practice Guidelines. J Am Coll Cardiol. 2017;69(11):1465–508.

4. Price J, Mowbray P, Lee A, Rumley A, Lowe G, Fowkes F. Relationship between smoking and cardiovascular risk factors in the development of peripheral arterial disease and coronary artery disease; Edinburgh artery study: Edinburgh artery study. Eur Heart J. 1999;20(5):344–53.
5. Vartanian SM, Conte MS. Surgical intervention for peripheral arterial disease. Circ Res. 2015;116(9):1614–28.
6. Dormandy J, Heeck L, Vig S. Semin Vasc Surg. 1999;12(2):142–7. PMID: 10777241.
7. Fridh EB, Andersson M, Thuresson M, Sigvant B, Kragsterman B, Johansson S, et al. Amputation rates, mortality, and pre-operative comorbidities in patients revascularised for intermittent claudication or critical limb ischaemia: a population based study. Eur J Vasc Endovasc Surg. 2017;54(4):480–6.
8. Risau W. Differentiation of endothelium. FASEB J. 1995;9(10):926–33.
9. Raval Z, Losordo DW. Cell therapy of peripheral arterial disease: from experimental findings to clinical trials. Circ Res. 2013;112(9):1288–302.
10. Eichmann A, Yuan L, Moyon D, Lenoble F, Pardanaud L, Breant C. Vascular development: from precursor cells to branched arterial and venous networks. Int J Dev Biol. 2003;49(2–3):259–67.
11. Ceafalan LC, Popescu BO, Hinescu ME.Biomed Res Int. 2014;2014:957014. https://doi.org/10.1155/2014/957014. Epub 2014 Mar 23.
12. Majumdar MK, Thiede MA, Mosca JD, Moorman M, Gerson SL. Phenotypic and functional comparison of cultures of marrow-derived mesenchymal stem cells (MSCs) and stromal cells. JcCellcPhysiol. 1998;176(1):57–66.
13. Fuss IJ, Kanof ME, Smith PD, Zola H. Isolation of whole mononuclear cells from peripheral blood and cord blood. Curr Protoc Immunol. 2009;85(1):7.1–7.1. 8.
14. Oswald J, Boxberger S, Jørgensen B, Feldmann S, Ehninger G, Bornhäuser M, et al. Mesenchymal stem cells can be differentiated into endothelial cells in vitro. Stem Cells. 2004;22(3):377–84.
15. Kaigler D, Krebsbach PH, Polverini PJ, Mooney DJ. Role of vascular endothelial growth factor in bone marrow stromal cell modulation of endothelial cells. Tissue Eng. 2003;9(1):95–103.
16. Wu L, Leijten J, van Blitterswijk CA, Karperien M. Fibroblast growth factor-1 is a mesenchymal stromal cell-secreted factor stimulating proliferation of osteoarthritic chondrocytes in co-culture. Stem Cells Dev. 2013;22(17):2356–67.
17. Eggenhofer E, Luk F, Dahlke MH, Hoogduijn MJ. The life and fate of mesenchymal stem cells. Front Immunol. 2014;5:148.
18. Senger DR, Galli SJ, Dvorak AM, Perruzzi CA, Harvey VS, Dvorak HF. Tumor cells secrete a vascular permeability factor that promotes accumulation of ascites fluid. Science. 1983;219(4587):983–5.
19. Shibuya M. Vascular endothelial growth factor (VEGF) and its receptor (VEGFR) signaling in angiogenesis: a crucial target for anti-and pro-angiogenic therapies. Genes Cancer. 2011;2(12):1097–105.
20. Forster R, Liew A, Bhattacharya V, Shaw J, Stansby G. Gene therapy for peripheral arterial disease. Cochrane Database Syst Rev. 2018;2018(10):CD012058.
21. Rajagopalan S, Mohler ER III, Lederman RJ, Mendelsohn FO, Saucedo JF, Goldman CK, et al. Regional angiogenesis with vascular endothelial growth factor in peripheral arterial disease: a phase II randomized, double-blind, controlled study of adenoviral delivery of vascular endothelial growth factor 121 in patients with disabling intermittent claudication. Circulation. 2003;108(16):1933–8.
22. Eswarakumar V, Lax I, Schlessinger J. Cellular signaling by fibroblast growth factor receptors. Cytokine Growth Factor Rev. 2005;16(2):139–49.
23. Murakami M, Nguyen LT, Hatanaka K, Schachterle W, Chen P-Y, Zhuang ZW, et al. FGF-dependent regulation of VEGF receptor 2 expression in mice. J Clin Invest. 2011;121(7):2668–78.
24. Chen P-Y, Simons M, Friesel R. FRS2 via fibroblast growth factor receptor 1 is required for platelet-derived growth factor receptor β-mediated regulation of vascular smooth muscle marker gene expression. J Biol Chem. 2009;284(23):15980–92.

25. Lederman RJ, Mendelsohn FO, Anderson RD, Saucedo JF, Tenaglia AN, Hermiller JB, et al. Therapeutic angiogenesis with recombinant fibroblast growth factor-2 for intermittent claudication (the TRAFFIC study): a randomised trial. Lancet. 2002;359(9323):2053–8.
26. Comerota AJ, Throm RC, Miller KA, Henry T, Chronos N, Laird J, et al. Naked plasmid DNA encoding fibroblast growth factor type 1 for the treatment of end-stage unreconstructible lower extremity ischemia: preliminary results of a phase I trial. J Vasc Surg. 2002;35(5):930–6.
27. Nikol S, Baumgartner I, Van Belle E, Diehm C, Visoná A, Capogrossi MC, et al. Therapeutic angiogenesis with intramuscular NV1FGF improves amputation-free survival in patients with critical limb ischemia. Mol Ther. 2008;16(5):972–8.
28. Fowkes FGR, Price JF. Gene therapy for critical limb ischaemia: the TAMARIS trial. Lancet. 2011;377(9781):1894–6.
29. Semenza GL. Hypoxia-inducible factors in physiology and medicine. Cell. 2012;148(3):399–408.
30. Gupta N, Nizet V. Stabilization of hypoxia-inducible factor-1 alpha augments the therapeutic capacity of bone marrow-derived mesenchymal stem cells in experimental pneumonia. Front Med. 2018;5:131.
31. Haase VH. Regulation of erythropoiesis by hypoxia-inducible factors. Blood Rev. 2013;27(1):41–53.
32. Creager MA, Olin JW, Belch JJ, Moneta GL, Henry TD, Rajagopalan S, et al. Effect of hypoxia-inducible factor-1α gene therapy on walking performance in patients with intermittent claudication. Circulation. 2011;124(16):1765–73.
33. Das R, Jahr H, van Osch GJ, Farrell E. The role of hypoxia in bone marrow–derived mesenchymal stem cells: considerations for regenerative medicine approaches. Tissue Eng Part B Rev. 2009;16(2):159–68.
34. Morimoto A, Okamura K, Hamanaka R, Sato Y, Shima N, Higashio K, et al. Hepatocyte growth factor modulates migration and proliferation of human microvascular endothelial cells in culture. Biochem Biophys Res Commun. 1991;179(2):1042–9.
35. Grant DS, Kleinman HK, Goldberg ID, Bhargava MM, Nickoloff BJ, Kinsella JL, et al. Scatter factor induces blood vessel formation in vivo. Proc Natl Acad Sci. 1993;90(5):1937–41.
36. Nita I, Hostettler K, Tamo L, Medová M, Bombaci G, Zhong J, et al. Hepatocyte growth factor secreted by bone marrow stem cell reduce ER stress and improves repair in alveolar epithelial II cells. Sci Rep. 2017;7:41901.
37. Nakamura T, Mizuno S. The discovery of hepatocyte growth factor (HGF) and its significance for cell biology, life sciences and clinical medicine. Proc Japan Acad Ser B. 2010;86(6):588–610.
38. Morishita R, Aoki M, Hashiya N, Makino H, Yamasaki K, Azuma J, et al. Safety evaluation of clinical gene therapy using hepatocyte growth factor to treat peripheral arterial disease. Hypertension. 2004;44(2):203–9.
39. Shigematsu H, Yasuda K, Iwai T, Sasajima T, Ishimaru S, Ohashi Y, et al. Randomized, double-blind, placebo-controlled clinical trial of hepatocyte growth factor plasmid for critical limb ischemia. Gene Ther. 2010;17(9):1152.
40. Powell RJ, Goodney P, Mendelsohn FO, Moen EK, Annex BH, Investigators H-T. Safety and efficacy of patient specific intramuscular injection of HGF plasmid gene therapy on limb perfusion and wound healing in patients with ischemic lower extremity ulceration: results of the HGF-0205 trial. J Vasc Surg. 2010;52(6):1525–30.
41. Asahara T, Murohara T, Sullivan A, Silver M, van der Zee R, Li T, et al. Isolation of putative progenitor endothelial cells for angiogenesis. Science. 1997;275(5302):964–6.
42. Sidney LE, Branch MJ, Dunphy SE, Dua HS, Hopkinson A. Concise review: evidence for CD34 as a common marker for diverse progenitors. Stem Cells. 2014;32(6):1380–9.
43. Gehling UM, Ergün S, Schumacher U, Wagener C, Pantel K, Otte M, et al. In vitro differentiation of endothelial cells from AC133-positive progenitor cells. Blood. 2000;95(10):3106–12.
44. Peichev M, Naiyer AJ, Pereira D, Zhu Z, Lane WJ, Williams M, et al. Expression of VEGFR-2 and AC133 by circulating human CD34+ cells identifies a population of functional endothelial precursors. Blood. 2000;95(3):952–8.

45. Garlanda C, Dejana E. Heterogeneity of endothelial cells: specific markers. Arterioscler Thromb Vasc Biol. 1997;17(7):1193–202.
46. Masek LC, Sweetenham JW. Isolation and culture of endothelial cells from human bone marrow. Br J Haematol. 1994;88(4):855–65.
47. Shi Q, Rafii S, Hong-De Wu M, Wijelath ES, Yu C, Ishida A, et al. Evidence for circulating bone marrow-derived endothelial cells. Blood. 1998;92(2):362–7.
48. Tateishi-Yuyama E, Matsubara H, Murohara T, Ikeda U, Shintani S, Masaki H, et al. Therapeutic angiogenesis for patients with limb ischaemia by autologous transplantation of bone-marrow cells: a pilot study and a randomised controlled trial. Lancet. 2002;360(9331):427–35.
49. Higashi Y, Kimura M, Hara K, Noma K, Jitsuiki D, Nakagawa K, et al. Autologous bone-marrow mononuclear cell implantation improves endothelium-dependent vasodilation in patients with limb ischemia. Circulation. 2004;109(10):1215–8.
50. Forconi S, Jageneau A, Guerrini M, Pecchi S, Cappelli R. Strain gauge plethysmography in the study of circulation of the limbs. Angiology. 1979;30(7):487–97.
51. Cobellis G, Silvestroni A, Lillo S, Sica G, Botti C, Maione C, et al. Long-term effects of repeated autologous transplantation of bone marrow cells in patients affected by peripheral arterial disease. Bone Marrow Transplant. 2008;42(10):667.
52. Hardman RL, Jazaeri O, Yi J, Smith M, Gupta R, editors. Overview of classification systems in peripheral artery disease. Seminars in interventional radiology. Thieme Medical Publishers; Semin Intervent Radiol. 2014;31:378–88.
53. Ruiz-Salmeron R, De La Cuesta-Diaz A, Constantino-Bermejo M, Pérez-Camacho I, Marcos-Sánchez F, Hmadcha A, et al. Angiographic demonstration of neoangiogenesis after intra-arterial infusion of autologous bone marrow mononuclear cells in diabetic patients with critical limb ischemia. Cell Transplant. 2011;20(10):1629–39.
54. Franz RW, Parks A, Shah KJ, Hankins T, Hartman JF, Wright ML. Use of autologous bone marrow mononuclear cell implantation therapy as a limb salvage procedure in patients with severe peripheral arterial disease. J Vasc Surg. 2009;50(6):1378–90.
55. Franz RW, Shah KJ, Johnson JD, Pin RH, Parks AM, Hankins T, et al. Short-to mid-term results using autologous bone-marrow mononuclear cell implantation therapy as a limb salvage procedure in patients with severe peripheral arterial disease. Vasc Endovasc Surg. 2011;45(5):398–406.
56. Bartsch T, Brehm M, Zeus T, Kögler G, Wernet P, Strauer BE. Transplantation of autologous mononuclear bone marrow stem cells in patients with peripheral arterial disease (the TAM-PAD study). Clin Res Cardiol. 2007;96(12):891–9.
57. Smadja DM, Duong-van-Huyen J-P, Dal Cortivo L, Blanchard A, Bruneval P, Emmerich J, et al. Early endothelial progenitor cells in bone marrow are a biomarker of cell therapy success in patients with critical limb ischemia. Cytotherapy. 2012;14(2):232–9.
58. Hur J, Yoon C-H, Kim H-S, Choi J-H, Kang H-J, Hwang K-K, et al. Characterization of two types of endothelial progenitor cells and their different contributions to neovasculogenesis. Arterioscler Thromb Vasc Biol. 2004;24(2):288–93.
59. Van Tongeren R, Hamming J, Fibbe W, Van Weel V, Frerichs S, Stiggelbout A, et al. Intramuscular or combined intramuscular/intra-arterial administration of bone marrow mono-nuclear cells: a clinical trial in patients with advanced limb ischemia. J Cardiovasc Surg. 2008;49(1):51.
60. Brant-Zawadzki M, Gould R, Norman D, Newton T, Lane B. Digital subtraction cerebral angiography by intraarterial injection: comparison with conventional angiography. Am J Roentgenol. 1983;140(2):347–53.
61. Meijer FJ, Schuijf JD, de Vries J, Boogaarts HD, van der Woude W-J, Prokop M. Ultra-high-resolution subtraction CT angiography in the follow-up of treated intracranial aneurysms. Insights Imaging. 2019;10(1):2.
62. Powell RJ, Marston WA, Berceli SA, Guzman R, Henry TD, Longcore AT, et al. Cellular therapy with Ixmyelocel-T to treat critical limb ischemia: the randomized, double-blind, placebo-controlled RESTORE-CLI trial. Mol Ther. 2012;20(6):1280–6.

63. Iafrati MD, Hallett JW, Geils G, Pearl G, Lumsden A, Peden E, et al. Early results and lessons learned from a multicenter, randomized, double-blind trial of bone marrow aspirate concentrate in critical limb ischemia. J Vasc Surg. 2011;54(6):1650–8.
64. James KE, Bloch DA, Lee KK, Kraemer HC, Fuller RK. An index for assessing blindness in a multi-centre clinical trial: disulfiram for alcohol cessation—a VA cooperative study. Stat Med. 1996;15(13):1421–34.
65. Walter DH, Krankenberg H, Balzer JO, Kalka C, Baumgartner I, Schlüter M, et al. Intraarterial administration of bone marrow mononuclear cells in patients with critical limb ischemia: a randomized-start, placebo-controlled pilot trial (PROVASA). Circ Cardiovasc Interv. 2011;4(1):26–37.
66. Teraa M, Sprengers RW, Schutgens RE, Slaper-Cortenbach IC, Van Der Graaf Y, Algra A, et al. Effect of repetitive intra-arterial infusion of bone marrow mononuclear cells in patients with no-option limb ischemia: the randomized, double-blind, placebo-controlled rejuvenating endothelial progenitor cells via transcutaneous intra-arterial supplementation (JUVENTAS) trial. Circulation. 2015;131(10):851–60.
67. Lenk K, Adams V, Lurz P, Erbs S, Linke A, Gielen S, et al. Therapeutical potential of blood-derived progenitor cells in patients with peripheral arterial occlusive disease and critical limb ischaemia. Eur Heart J. 2005;26(18):1903–9.
68. Lara-Hernandez R, Lozano-Vilardell P, Blanes P, Torreguitart-Mirada N, Galmes A, Besalduch J. Safety and efficacy of therapeutic angiogenesis as a novel treatment in patients with critical limb ischemia. Ann Vasc Surg. 2010;24(2):287–94.
69. Huang PP, Yang XF, Li SZ, Wen JC, Zhang Y, Han ZC. Randomised comparison of G-CSF-mobilized peripheral blood mononuclear cells versus bone marrow-mononuclear cells for the treatment of patients with lower limb arteriosclerosis obliterans. Thromb Haemost. 2007;98(12):1335–42.
70. Losordo DW, Kibbe MR, Mendelsohn F, Marston W, Driver VR, Sharafuddin M, et al. A randomized, controlled pilot study of autologous CD34+ cell therapy for critical limb ischemia. Circ Cardiovasc Interv. 2012;5(6):821–30.
71. Matoba S, Tatsumi T, Murohara T, Imaizumi T, Katsuda Y, Ito M, et al. Long-term clinical outcome after intramuscular implantation of bone marrow mononuclear cells (therapeutic angiogenesis by cell transplantation [TACT] trial) in patients with chronic limb ischemia. Am Heart J. 2008;156(5):1010–8.
72. Gerhard-Herman MD, Gornik HL, Barrett C, Barshes NR, Corriere MA, Drachman DE, et al. 2016 AHA/ACC guideline on the management of patients with lower extremity peripheral artery disease: a report of the American College of Cardiology/American Heart Association task force on clinical practice guidelines. J Am Coll Cardiol. 2017;69(11):e71–e126.
73. Aboyans V, Ricco J-B, Bartelink M-LE, Björck M, Brodmann M, Cohnert T, et al. 2017 ESC guidelines on the diagnosis and treatment of peripheral arterial diseases, in collaboration with the European Society for Vascular Surgery (ESVS) document covering atherosclerotic disease of extracranial carotid and vertebral, mesenteric, renal, upper and lower extremity arteries endorsed by: the European stroke organization (ESO) the task force for the diagnosis and treatment of peripheral arterial diseases of the European Society of Cardiology (ESC) and of the European Society for Vascular Surgery (ESVS). Eur Heart J. 2017;39(9):763–816.
74. Imanishi T, Moriwaki C, Hano T, Nishio I. Endothelial progenitor cell senescence is accelerated in both experimental hypertensive rats and patients with essential hypertension. J Hypertens. 2005;23(10):1831–7.
75. Michaud SÉ, Dussault S, Haddad P, Groleau J, Rivard A. Circulating endothelial progenitor cells from healthy smokers exhibit impaired functional activities. Atherosclerosis. 2006;187(2):423–32.
76. Loomans CJ, de Koning EJ, Staal FJ, Rookmaaker MB, Verseyden C, de Boer HC, et al. Endothelial progenitor cell dysfunction: a novel concept in the pathogenesis of vascular complications of type 1 diabetes. Diabetes. 2004;53(1):195–9.

77. Chen JZ, Zhang FR, Tao QM, Wang XX, Zhu JH, Zhu JH. Number and activity of endothelial progenitor cells from peripheral blood in patients with hypercholesterolaemia. Clin Sci. 2004;107(3):273–80.
78. Prokopi M, Pula G, Mayr U, Devue C, Gallagher J, Xiao Q, et al. Proteomic analysis reveals presence of platelet microparticles in endothelial progenitor cell cultures. Blood. 2009;114(3):723–32.
79. Ziegelhoeffer T, Fernandez B, Kostin S, Heil M, Voswinckel R, Helisch A, et al. Bone marrow-derived cells do not incorporate into the adult growing vasculature. Circ Res. 2004;94(2):230–8.
80. Medina RJ, Barber CL, Sabatier F, Dignat-George F, Melero-Martin JM, Khosrotehrani K, et al. Endothelial progenitors: a consensus statement on nomenclature. Stem Cells Transl Med. 2017;6(5):1316–20.
81. Ingram DA, Mead LE, Tanaka H, Meade V, Fenoglio A, Mortell K, et al. Identification of a novel hierarchy of endothelial progenitor cells using human peripheral and umbilical cord blood. Blood. 2004;104(9):2752–60.
82. Lin R-Z, Moreno-Luna R, Li D, Jaminet S-C, Greene AK, Melero-Martin JM. Human endothelial colony-forming cells serve as trophic mediators for mesenchymal stem cell engraftment via paracrine signaling. Proc Natl Acad Sci. 2014;111(28):10137–42.
83. Gao W, Chen D, Liu G, Ran X. Autologous stem cell therapy for peripheral arterial disease: a systematic review and meta-analysis of randomized controlled trials. Stem Cell Res Ther. 2019;10(1):140.
84. Bura A, Planat-Benard V, Bourin P, Silvestre J-S, Gross F, Grolleau J-L, et al. Phase I trial: the use of autologous cultured adipose-derived stroma/stem cells to treat patients with non-revascularizable critical limb ischemia. Cytotherapy. 2014;16(2):245–57.
85. Subherwal S, Patel MR, Chiswell K, Tidemann-Miller BA, Jones WS, Conte MS, et al. Clinical trials in peripheral vascular disease: pipeline and trial designs: an evaluation of the ClinicalTrials.gov database. Circulation. 2014;130(20):1812–9.
86. Biscetti F, Bonadia N, Nardella E, Cecchini AL, Landolfi R, Flex A. The role of the stem cells therapy in the peripheral artery disease. Int J Mol Sci. 2019;20(9):2233.

Chapter 7
Stem Cell Therapy for Diabetic Foot Ulcers

Hallie J. Quiroz, Zhao-Jun Liu, and Omaida C. Velazquez

7.1 Introduction

Diabetes mellitus (DM) and its many complications involving the lower extremities are well characterized. Diabetic foot ulcers (DFU) are the most commonly recognized lower extremity complication of DM with a global prevalence of 6.4% (13% in North America) [1] and an estimated lifetime incidence up to 25%. [2] They develop due to a complex, multifactorial process consisting of peripheral neuropathy, external trauma or abnormal weight distribution, and concomitant peripheral vascular disease, which results in a chronic, nonhealing wound susceptible to infection. The peripheral neuropathy develops due to chronically elevated systemic blood glucose levels, which damages nerve conduction and progressively alters sensation in the foot. Patients with severe peripheral neuropathy are at higher risk of foot injury as they have diminished sensation to pain, which then results in wounds that develop over time with chronic trauma and poor blood flow. Preventative strategies involve primarily achieving glycemic control, periodic foot inspection, patient education, and other risk reduction strategies such as avoidance of smoking. If a DFU does develop, current treatment modalities involve early detection, continued glycemic control, off-loading pressure from the wound, debridement of necrotic tissue, infection control, revascularization procedures (if peripheral vascular disease is present), and aggressive wound care. These treatments often fail due to the aberrant wound healing found in the diabetic phenotype. Often these combined measures for wound closure fail, and patients require amputation, which occurs as high as 30 times more often in diabetic patients than in those of the general population. [3]. Due

H. J. Quiroz · Z.-J. Liu
University of Miami Leonard M. Miller School of Medicine, Miami, FL, USA

O. C. Velazquez (✉)
DeWitt Daughtry Department of Surgery, University of Miami Leonard M. Miller School of Medicine, Miami, FL, USA
e-mail: ovelazquez@med.miami.edu

© Springer Nature Switzerland AG 2021
T. P. Navarro et al. (eds.), *Stem Cell Therapy for Vascular Diseases*,
https://doi.org/10.1007/978-3-030-56954-9_7

to the high morbidity in this population and frequent failure rate of current medical and surgical options, novel therapies are warranted to assist in DFU wound healing.

7.1.1 Why Stem Cells?

The term "stem cell" is inherently a broad term, which describes the cell's ability to differentiate into other cellular phenotypes with the combined self-renewal capability. The two main types of stem cells are embryonic and somatic (adult) stem cells, which differ in their ability to differentiate into certain cell types. Embryonic stem cells have the ability to differentiate into any cell type (endodermal, mesodermal, ectodermal) and are considered totipotent as they can differentiate into all cell types, including embryonic structures. Somatic, or adult, stem cells are more limited in their abilities to differentiate and often are hindered by their lineage type. Currently, stem cells used therapeutically are exclusively adult stem cells, while ethical and scientific issues surround both embryonic and fetal stem cells and hinder their widespread implementation. In contrast, stem cells recovered postnatally from the umbilical cord, including the umbilical cord blood cells, amnion/placenta, umbilical cord vein, or umbilical cord matrix cells, are a readily available and inexpensive source of stem cells. Bone marrow-derived stem cells and adipose-derived stem cells are also popular sources of stem cells [4]. Moreover, with the discovery of induced pluripotent stem (iPS) cells, it is now possible to convert differentiated somatic cells into multipotent stem cells that have the capacity to generate all cell types of adult tissues. Thus, iPS cells have potential for regenerative medicine [5].

Stem cells utilized for DFU wound healing are a promising treatment modality as their therapeutic properties address many facets of the underlying pathophysiology of the impaired wound healing inherent in DFU. It has been shown that stem cells are able to mobilize and home to ischemic and wounded tissues, where they then embark on a cascade of pro-wound healing strategies. They are able to synthesize and secrete cytokines, which recruit other types of cells needed for the reconstruction of the wound bed, secrete growth factors, modulate the tissue immune response, assist in remodeling of the extracellular matrix, and promote angiogenesis and neuroregeneration. Taken together, stem cells utilize a vast array of tactics to promote wound healing. [6] In addition to their extrinsic pro-healing capabilities, stem cells are able to undergo differentiation into cells that may also assist and participate in wound healing such as myofibroblasts, keratinocytes, and endothelial cells. [7, 8] This chapter will discuss the aberrant wound healing inherent to those with long-standing DM, the types of stem cells utilized for DFU treatments, the delivery methods for stem cell therapy in DFU, and the future of stem cell therapies for DFU patients.

7.2 Wound Healing and Its Aberration in Diabetics

The cascade of physiologic wound healing is divided into these four overlapping phases: hemostasis, inflammatory, proliferative, and maturation/remodeling. Physiologic wound healing is a complex interplay between the immune system, signaling molecules, growth factors, and the vascular system that delivers cells and soluble factors to the newly injured tissue. After injury, the tissue releases cytokines, and the complement system activates which results in an increase of endothelial surface molecules that act as receptors for the capture of neutrophils, endothelial progenitor cells (EPC), and other cells necessary for tissue repair. The neutrophils then enter the injured tissue via diapedesis, which is enhanced due to the edema caused by the inflammatory cytokines, and begin killing tissue microbes with superoxide and reactive oxygen particles; however, this also results in increased tissue damage. Macrophages then arrive to begin clearing the wound of debris, which will allow for the remodeling phase of wound healing to begin. The wound remodeling and maturation phase consist of angiogenesis, fibroblasts, and T-lymphocytes. Angiogenesis, the development of new blood vessels, develops simultaneously to ensure proper blood flow to the tissue and that newly developed tissues will have the required nutrients for survival. The fibroblasts are essential for tissue repair and the development of granulation tissue by the placement of collage fibers. Once the wound has closed, the T-lymphocytes are heavily involved in the post-closure wound remodeling by assisting in collagenous fiber maturation and other tissue remodeling functions [9].

Chronic wounds are defined as wounds that fail to proceed through the normal phases of wound healing in an orderly and timely manner [10]. Often, chronic wounds stall in the inflammatory phase with an excessive neutrophilic response and non-progression to the macrophage/fibroblastic phase, which results in wounds that are prone to infection and difficult to heal. Poor wound healing in the diabetic phenotype occurs due to extrinsic as well as intrinsic wound characteristics. The extrinsic factors include peripheral neuropathy, which leads to continued wound trauma and mechanical stress and poor blood flow due to peripheral micro/macrovascular ischemic disease. Intrinsically, the wounds of diabetics also have impaired inflammation [11, 12], cellular proliferation and differentiation, and decreased ability to form collagen [13]. The diabetic phenotype is associated with an increased propensity for inflammatory cytokines over the wound healing cytokines and, due to chronic hypoxic conditions inherent in diabetic tissues, has decreased eNOS production, which is associated with bone marrow mobilization of cells necessary for wound healing and angiogenesis [14]. Diabetic neutrophils are less likely to arrive to the site of injury due to poor adherence and chemotaxis, and those that do arrive have an impairment in phagocytosis and bacterial killing. They also tend to linger in the wound tissue and create an excessive inflammatory response. Like the neutrophils, the macrophages also have impaired tissue recruitment and also maintain a pro-inflammatory response as opposed to a pro-wound healing phenotype. Overall this results in a tissue microenvironment with aberrant inflammatory responses that hinder both the development of granulation tissue by fibroblasts and eventual remodeling [9]. Stem cells may provide the diabetic wound environment with the necessary cells required for wound healing and ability to restore the microenvironment from inflammatory to healing and may also differentiate themselves into required cells for successful wound healing (Fig. 7.1).

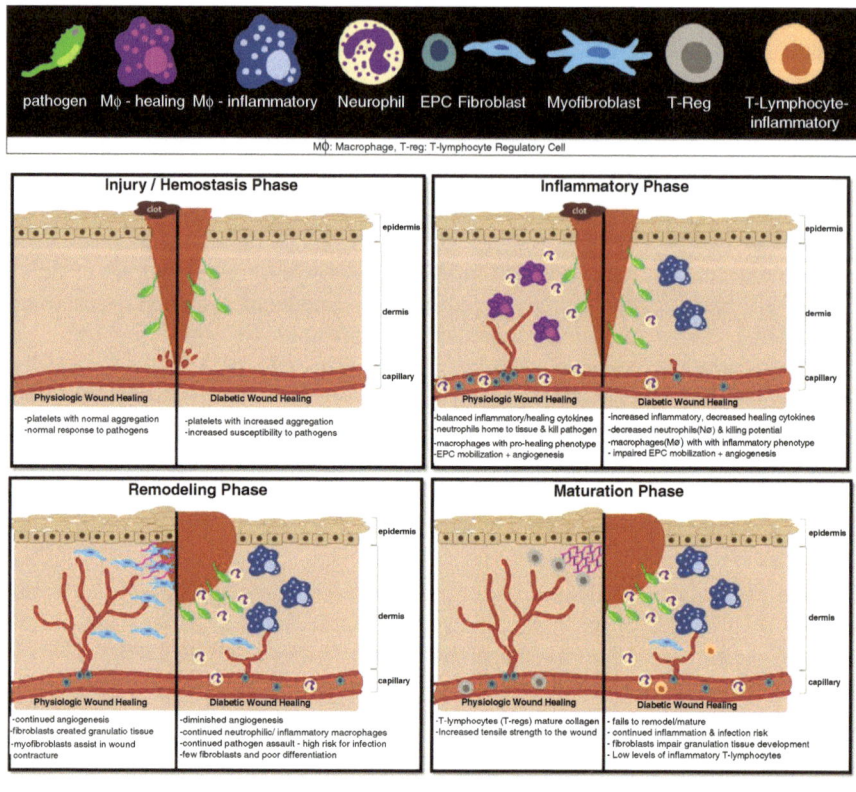

Fig. 7.1 Comparison between physiologic wound healing and diabetic wound healing

7.3 Stem Cells and Their Utilization in DFU Treatment

Stem cells are unspecialized and thus are able to differentiate into most cell types of the host organism and are also able to self-renew. They are found from embryonic to adult developmental stages; however with organismal growth and differentiation, the stem cells tend to lose their developmental potency. Due to this, stem cells range from totipotency to unipotency, with varying levels of differentiation potential depending upon the growth of the organism and other factors. Totipotent stem cells have the ability to self-renew and differentiate to form the entirety of the organism, including extraembryonic structures. The zygote, a sperm fertilized egg, is a bundle of totipotent stem cells that form the placental and all three germ layers. After further divisions, the zygote forms the blastocyst, which has an inner cell full of pluripotent stem cells. Pluripotent stem cells form all three germ layers, but not extraembryonic structures, an example of which would be embryonic stem cells (ESCs), which are harvested from the inner cell mass of embryos. Pluripotency describes a spectrum of development potency ranging from complete pluripotency to multipotent, oligopotent, and ending in unipotent cell lines. Multipotent stem cell lines have the ability to differentiate into specific cell lineages (within same germ layer), such as the hematopoietic stem cell (HSC), which can form many types of blood cells. HSC may then further differentiate into a myeloid cell, which is an oligopotent stem cell, which, depending upon host factors, will develop into different cell types within its own cell lineage, but cannot develop into, say, a red blood cell [5]. The stem cell classification with the least amount of differentiation capacity is the unipotent cell, which can only differentiate into one cell type, however, and has the ability to self-renew. This innate self-renewal capacity makes them important cell types for regenerative medicine. Utilizing stem cells for clinical applications ranges from neurodegenerative disorders to wound healing applications. The purpose of this text is to describe the applications of stem cell therapy for the treatment of DFUs. For this purpose, the stem cells utilized will be grossly categorized into two main categories, allogeneic and autologous stem cells, and are then subcategorized based upon whether they are embryonic or somatic and their tissues of origin.

7.3.1   Allogeneic Stem Cells

Allogeneic stem cells are donor cells from tissues foreign to the recipient but within the same species. Typically, allogeneic stem cells are totipotent or pluripotent such as ESCs or stem cells from extraembryonic structures such as the placenta or umbilical cord (UC). Because they are extracted from donors, the advantages are the ability to use younger/healthier donors, increased developmental potency, and ability to form donation banks or use cadaveric cells. However, their utilization may result in immunological incompatibility and contains some inherent ethical and legal issues with the utilization of donor tissues. The three main types of allogeneic stem cells that have been utilized for investigations into enhanced wound healing are placental, umbilical cord (UC), and embryonic stem cells. Human placental and UC are both sources of pluripotent mesenchymal stem cells (MSC) that have multi-lineage differentiation capabilities and are associated with noninvasive procurement procedures.

Human placental MSC is harvested from the expulsed placenta after the birth process has been completed and has the advantage of being a high-yield source of stem cells and comes from typically young and healthy donors. Placentas function as the immunoregulatory organ throughout pregnancy and regulate the fetal-maternal interphase. Likely due to this innate immunomodulatory function, the stem cells from placentas tend to express low immunogenicity when xenotransplanted in both *in vitro* and *in vivo* [15, 16]. For the purpose of this chapter, we will include MSCs from all placental tissue (amnion, chorion, chorionic villi, and decidua) and describe them as human placental MSC. These cells exhibit the typical MSC characteristics which include plastic adherence and expression of specific cell surface markers (+CD105, +CD73, +CD90, -CD34, -CD45, -CD14, -CD19,

-HLA-DR) and can differentiate into different mesodermal lineages [17]. These cells, while MSC, have advantages in their utilization over adult MSC due to their ease of extraction; a more homogenous, primitive population; and a higher proliferative rate when compared with bone marrow-derived MSC (BM-MSC). A higher proliferative rate allows for *ex vivo* expansion with a decreased risk for passage senescence, which leads to an older phenotype and less therapeutic potential [18]. Preclinical studies of human placental MSC have been utilized to increase angiogenesis in ischemia models [19, 20] and have also demonstrated accelerated wound healing and closure when compared to controls (human adipose-derived stem cells (ADSC) and human fibroblasts) [21, 22]. Despite promising results, there have yet to be any clinical studies of human placental MSC for the treatment of DFU, while currently a phase III trial for critical limb ischemia is underway [23].

Another type of MSC derived from extraembryonic structures are from the umbilical cord (UC), which includes both MSC extracted from Wharton's jelly, the connective tissue enveloping cord blood vessels, and the umbilical cord blood itself. These UC-MSCs also meet the minimum criteria for MSC designation and have similar advantages of utilization as the placental MSC, which include ease of procurement, homogenous/primitive population, and higher proliferation [24]. Preclinical studies of UC-MSC have demonstrated accelerated wound healing in a murine diabetic wound model [25] and in immunodeficient mice [26]. The only finalized randomized clinical trial utilizing UC-MSC was also designed to test the utilization of angioplasty with or without intra-arterial UC-MSC in diabetic patients with Fontaine II-IV diabetic feet and lower extremity peripheral arterial disease (PAD). The 3-month follow-up of these patients demonstrated that treatment with angioplasty plus intra-arterial and intramuscular UC-MSC resulted in better ulcer healing, skin temperature, and transcutaneous oxygen pressure($TcPO_2$) and decreased claudication [27]. Despite the success of the clinical trial utilizing UC-MSC, there remains a lack of an FDA-approved therapy. This is likely due to risks of immunocompatibility and future malignancy; however more robust studies and longer follow-up are required to answer these questions.

Embryonic stem cells (ESC), as opposed to the MSC of the placenta and umbilical cords, are an example of a totipotent stem cell. The advantage of ESC for regenerative medicine relies on their ability to form any type of cell, the donor source is primitive, and the cell source is typically banked for future use. However, due to their allogeneic nature, immune compatibility is a barrier to their usage. Furthermore, due to their procurement method (via the inner cell mass of in vitro fertilized embryos), their utilization remains ethically controversial and thus limits its capacity for human clinical trials. They have been used in preclinical studies of diabetic wound healing and have shown enhanced wound healing [28] along with increased levels of associated growth factors such as epidermal growth factor (EGF), vascular endothelial growth factor (VEGF), and fibronectin when compared to controls [28]. Despite the current ethical limitations of its use in human subjects, this cell type has an immense potential for regenerative medicine for DFUs and other diseases. Future investigations in the clinical realm need to be seriously considered to afford the best chance of a curative therapeutic for difficult disease processes such as DFU.

7.3.2   Autologous Stem Cells

Autologous stem cells are harvested from the same person for which they are intended to treat. These cells tend to have developmental potency ranging from pluripotent to unipotent, due to their procurement from fully developed tissues. The method of cell harvest is highly dependent upon the location of the stem cell niche, and thus procurement procedures vary from minimally invasive (peripheral blood) to invasive (bone marrow aspiration). Autologous cells have the advantage of being fully immunocompatible, have no risk of disease transmission, and have very few ethical limitations with their use. However, especially in the diabetic patient, the donors are typically older and have diminished stem cell niches as compared to younger (or embryonic) donors. It has been demonstrated that diabetic patients have stem cells with decreased developmental potency, decreased therapeutic efficacy, and increased risk of overall complications [29, 30]. Despite these concerns, autologous cells are the most commonly utilized cell type in both preclinical and clinical trials, underlining their importance and efficacy for the investigational treatment of DFU [4].

7.3.2.1   Bone Marrow-Derived Stem Cells (BMDSC)

The bone marrow houses a heterogenous population of adult stem cells and acts as a reservoir to repair damaged tissues and replace senescent cells. Normal skin is known to contain BM-derived cells, and the BM-derived stem cells have the ability to home to injured skin tissues and participate in the repair and regeneration [8]. The two main subpopulations of bone marrow-derived stem cells (BMDSC) are mesenchymal stromal/stem cells (MSC) and hematopoietic stem cells (HSC); however these also give rise to another important stem cell niche, the endothelial progenitor cells (EPC). These three types of stem cells, which primarily reside in the bone marrow, have all been shown to have regenerative effects, and thus this section will detail each BMDSC and discuss their utilization in the treatment of DFU.

7.3.2.2   Mesenchymal Stem Cells (MSC)

The term "mesenchyme" relates to the development of loose, connective tissues during embryogenesis and is a derivative of the mesoderm. Most mesenchymal tissues are comprised of terminally differentiated cells, which are derived from committed, lineage-directed mesenchymal precursor cells. However, mesenchymal stem cells, which are pluripotent, have the capability of multi-lineage differentiation, immunomodulation, and the ability to home to tissues where repair and regeneration are required, which make them ideal cell types for a multitude of chronic diseases. They are typically harvested from the bone marrow (BM-MSC) and peripheral blood (PB-MSC) but also have been found in the scalp, skeletal muscles, teeth, and adipose tissues [8]. To determine whether cells are in fact MSC, they must adhere to the International Society for Cellular Therapy standard criteria, which were mentioned earlier in this chapter. In brief, these include adherence to plastic, specific cell surface markers, and ability to differentiate into different mesodermal lineages [17].

MSC protocols for extraction and isolation are dependent upon the location of the stem cell niche. Whether from bone marrow aspiration (BM-MSC) or from a peripheral venous blood draw (PB-MSC), the cells are typically isolated using Ficoll density gradient methods and then seeding onto cell culture plates. MSCs have been shown to have high proliferative assays; however as mentioned earlier, not all MSCs are created equally. MSCs derived from placental and UC have been shown to have higher proliferation than those derived from adult tissues such as BM-MSCs. Due to the relative low concentration of MSC in both bone marrow and peripheral blood, most investigations require culture expansion in order to achieve the necessary cell count for adequate engraftment and therapeutic potential. Thus, cell passage is an important consideration for MSC due to the correlation of high passage number with decreased homing capabilities and therapeutic potential [30].

BM-MSCs have been shown efficacious in the treatment of chronic wounds [31], promotion of neovascularization in limb ischemia [32], and DFU wound healing [4]. Currently MSCs are the most commonly utilized stem cell in both preclinical and clinical trials of DFU wound healing. Falanga et al. demonstrated a direct correlation between the numbers of cells applied to the chronic wound with the percentage of wound size decreased. Therefore, it is likely that wound surface area directly correlates with the amount of MSC required to attain maximal therapeutic effect [31]. The BM-MSCs have been tested in multiple randomized controlled trials (RCT) and has repeatedly shown improved wound healing among other symptomatologies [4]. Unfortunately, there exists a heterogenic component to these trials and thus makes drawing discrete conclusions on MSC therapy for DFU difficult; however evidence highly suggests that MSCs are a safe and efficacious alternative therapy. Continued investigations into MSC therapy are required, as there is still a lack of any FDA-approved cell-based therapy for DFU.

7.3.2.3   Endothelial Progenitor Cells (EPC)

EPCs are housed in the bone marrow but can also be isolated from peripheral blood, umbilical cord blood, and adipose tissues [33]. Their progenitor population has been reported to be from multiple cell types such as hematopoietic stem cells, myeloid cells, or other EPCs. Unlike the MSCs, which have a clear specification for their characterizations, EPCs lack a consensus on the cell surface markers used for isolation; however this is thought to be due to their dynamic display of surface markers due to epigenetic cues from their microenvironment. However, despite this, the most commonly used criteria for EPC isolation from UC blood, peripheral blood, and bone marrow is a combination of CD34+/VEGFR-2+/CD133+/CD45-/CD14- followed by Fluorescent Activated Cell Sorting (FACS) analysis with EC surface markers such as platelet endothelial cell adhesion molecule-1 (PECAM-1) and von Willebrand factor (vWF), to name a few [33].

EPCs are released into the peripheral bloodstream in response to tissue damage and ischemia and, once engrafted, promote healing and angiogenesis in the affected tissues. They home to damaged tissues via stromal cell-derived factor-1-α (SDF-1α)-induced dual pairs of E-selectin cell adhesion molecule/ligand which increase capture of EPCs to the areas of critical ischemia [34]. Unfortunately, EPC mobilization in diabetics is impaired (due to low activated eNOS levels in the bone marrow and low SDF-1α levels in the wound tissue) which results in a sub-therapeutic level of circulating EPCs and decreased EPC capture in ischemic tissues [14]. EPCs of diabetic patients have also been shown to have diminished proliferative potential and are more likely to undergo apoptosis [35], all of which negatively affects wound healing. Due to derangement of normal EPC levels and functionality, cell-based approaches utilizing autologous EPCs require assistance via *ex vivo* enhancement of the extracted EPCs or additional therapies to enhance wound susceptibility to the EPCs.

Studies have shown that *ex vivo* expanded EPCs applied topically to a murine diabetic wound model promoted wound healing via increased local cytokine production and enhanced neovascularization [36] and have also increased wound healing with improved EPC functionality after systemic treatment of H_2S (depleted in DM patients/mice), when compared to controls [37]. Another study by Castilla et al. primed BMDSC with SDF-1α and reported that application of these cells to the diabetic murine wounds resulted in faster healing rates and enhanced neovascularization when compared with control cell therapy [38], indicating that cell-based therapies can be improved with *ex vivo* activation via cytokines, such as SDF-1α.

7.3.2.4 Hematopoietic Stem Cells (HSC)

Hematopoietic stem cells (HSC) are pluripotent stem cells contained in the myeloid tissue and peripheral blood and give rise to all blood cell lineages while maintaining a very high self-renewal capacity. These cells are able to regenerate all blood cell lines after transplantation (either autogenous or allogeneic) to the recipient. These cells are the most abundant cell type in the bone marrow but can also be extracted from the peripheral blood and have also been extracted from umbilical cord blood [39]. These cells are identified via the cell surface antigen CD34+ and CD45+ (which differentiates them from the stromal cells found in the bone marrow) and are isolated via density gradients. Typically, they are isolated after intravenous pretreatment with cytokines such as granulocyte colony-stimulating factor (G-CSF), which is utilized to mobilize the HSC from the myeloid tissue into the peripheral circulation, which are then extracted via venous blood draw.

It has been shown in physiologic wound healing models that HSCs have increased abundance after tissue injury, and methods to increase circulating HSCs (CXCR4 antagonists) result in improved wound angiogenesis, cellular proliferation, and wound closure [8, 40]. Preclinical studies of HSCs in DFU models have demonstrated enhanced DFU healing at both the inflammatory and proliferative phases of wound healing [41]. HSCs isolated from UC have also been utilized as topical treatment with a fibrin gel and accelerated wound closure in diabetic mice when compared to control treatments [39]. However, a study by Lu et al. demonstrated superior DFU healing with MSC [42], which may explain their relative low number of clinical trials. A clinical trial by Wettstein et al. utilized autologous HSC in a pressure sore model and reported decreased ulcer size in the treatment group; although the study was underpowered to adequately assess statistical significance, there were no safety concerns and no malignancy in the 2-year follow-up [43]. Although no current clinical trials are utilizing HSCs for wound healing, there is a trial utilizing a CXCR4 antagonist (Plerixafor™), known to increase circulating HSCs, currently underway at the writing of this text.

7.3.2.5 Adipose Stromal Cells (ASCs)

Stromal cells found in the adipose tissue are similar to mesenchymal stem cells and as such are named adipose stromal cells (ASCs). Adipose tissue is a more abundant tissue source in the body than bone marrow, with a more simplified extraction method (liposuction), which makes ASCs a promising resource for cell-based DFU treatments. ASCs have demonstrated differentiation into multiple cell lines including cardiomyocytes, endothelial cells, adipocytes, and myocytes, among others [44], and have similar in vitro characteristics to MSC such as plastic adherence, self-renewal, rapid proliferation, and lack of MHC-II. Interestingly, it has been demonstrated that ASCs have more immune privilege than BM-MSC and have demonstrated superior proliferative rates and genetic stability [45, 46].

Extraction of these cells is accomplished via liposuction, and the cells are then extracted via either mechanical or chemical means, which yields a heterogeneous population of cells called the stromal vascular fraction (SVF). The SVF contains preadipocytes, fibroblasts, vascular smooth muscle cells, endothelial cells, monocytes/macrophages, lymphocytes, and ASC [44, 47]. Characterization of these cells, like most stem cells, requires analysis of cell surface markers, albeit there are no international guidelines for their characterization. The ASC cell surface markers which have been uniformly reported as having a positive expression are CD13, CD29, CD34, CD44, CD73, CD90, and CD105, while CD14, CD31, CD45, and CD133 have all been reported as having little to no expression [48]. The therapeutic potential for ASC is inherent in the cells but also in the clinical applicability of their extraction and isolation process, which yields a much higher stem cell count than other methods (BM, PB), which often diminishes the need for in vitro expansion. The ideal isolation of ASC would include mechanical isolation methods (as enzymatic isolation in the USA is considered a drug [49]), with relative low risk for contamination and high cell yield count, and would be rapid enough for utilization in the same clinical setting. Raposio et al. have described a simplified, mechanical method for ASC isolation after liposuction that was complete within 15 minutes of the liposuction, with high cell count and viability [50]. The continued perfection of extraction and isolation protocols will make ASCs highly sought after for a wide range of clinical applications.

ASCs have been shown to aid in diabetic wound healing in mouse and rat models via increased granulation formation and epithelialization and have been shown to incorporate into the dermal/subdermal tissues and contribute to blood vessel formation [51–53]. They have also demonstrated capability of engrafting into the wound tissue and releasing growth factors to promote angiogenesis in a hind limb ischemia model [54]. Other studies have utilized platelet-rich plasma or 3D scaffolds (fibrin glue, collagen, etc.) in combination with ASC therapy as they are believed to work synergistically to repair tissues [55]. Although currently the utilization of ASCs for clinical studies is less frequent than BM-MSC, their usage is increasing in popularity. Currently there are multiple ongoing phase I-II trials in the utilization of ASCs for DFU.

7.3.3 Xenotransplantation

Xenotransplantation refers to the utilization of cell types transplanted from one species to another. The advantages of utilizing another species for stem cell therapy are the lack of ethical conflict and healthy stem cell source, lack of harvest risk for DFU patient, and the ability to create donor banking; however these advantages are dampened by the high risk of immunoincompatibility and the need to screen donors for disease that could pose a threat to the recipients. Xenotransplantation has been attempted in preclinical studies by utilizing human adult stem cells in diabetic wound models and had promising results without any adverse immunological reactions. However, there is currently still a lack of utilization of other species' cells utilized in human tissues for clinical trials. Methods to decrease species-specific cell markers involved in immunological graft rejections are still needed before these types of therapies will be able to be utilized in human tissues.

7.4 Delivery Systems

When determining cell-based therapeutic options for DFU, the determination of delivery method for the stem cells is also an important decision. Currently, no evidence suggests a superior delivery method for cell delivery to the wound bed, although both systemic and local injections have been proven effective. It is known that the therapeutic effect of stem cell therapies for tissue repair and regenerative purposes is highly dependent upon the number of viable cells that can reach the tissues. Thus, the ideal delivery method would provide an adequate number of intact and healthy cells available for tissue engraftment directly to the injured tissue with minimal procedural risk to the patient. Each delivery method has its advantages and disadvantages, and this section will discuss each delivery method and future endeavors to increase their efficiency.

7.4.1 Systemic Intra-Arterial/Intravenous Injections

Systemic injections involve either direct injection of cells into the arterial or venous system, which mimics the circulatory route of endogenous stem cells that eventually home to sites of ischemia or injury. Intra-arterial injections have the advantage of delivering cells directly to ischemic tissues, which is likely why this methodology is utilized for post-infarction regenerative purposes. However, for cutaneous wound healing, this approach is limited by the concomitant peripheral arterial disease inherent in DFU and the added risk of intra-arterial (IA) injections. IA has been associated with potential embolic formation and development of an arterial pseudoaneurysm at the injection site [56]. While the intravenous route decreases procedural and embolic formation risk, this methodology is widely criticized for its lack of targeted cell delivery and increased risk of cell filtration into the liver, lungs, and spleen, which results in a sub-therapeutic number of cells in the injured tissue. Recently, a targeted cell delivery system has been developed. A nanocarrier for targeted delivery of stem cells consisting of a dendrimer as the vehicle and adhesion molecules (E-selectin or E-selectin/VEGF) as the "GPS" to direct the "nanovehicle" carrying the "passenger cells" allows for the cells to park at the desired location. These adhesion molecules conjugated on nanocarriers can recognize their counterpart adhesion molecules, which are highly expressed on endothelial cells lining wound vasculature due to the stimulation of inflammatory cytokines/chemokines within wound tissues. They then attach to the surface of wound endothelial cells, deliver the stem cells to the desired tissues, and achieve therapeutic effects [57].

7.4.2 Local Injection/Topical Delivery

Direct injection or topical delivery of stem cells for cutaneous healing requires a highly concentrated population of cells that need to be placed either on top of the wound or injected adjacent to the wound tissue. Local injections involve the utilization of a small caliber needle with stem cells and delivery vehicle (usually saline) to inject aliquots either into the dermal/subcutaneous tissues around the wound or intramuscularly around the wound. This methodology increases the likelihood of the cells being available for tissue engraftment, however, is also met with both technical and environmental issues that can decrease stem cell survival. First, the mechanical shear forces exerted on the stem cells are increased in localized injections due to the smaller needle-gauge, which can significantly damage the cells and decrease their tissue viability. Secondly, the chronic wound tissue in DFU is a hostile environment that may also lead to decreased cell viability. For this reason, some investigators have attempted to prime the tissue environment or stem cells to increase cell engraftment and thus aid in wound healing [38]. Others have also speculated that a protective delivery vehicle may also aid cell engraftment and therapeutic effects. Topical delivery of stem cells is dependent upon the constant contact with the wound tissue and cell viability, which is often diminished in the hostile wound microenvironment. For this reason, topically delivered cells are prepared with either fibrin sealants, hydrogels, collagen gels, or extracellular membrane (ECM)-like materials and macromolecules which have all been shown to increase wound closure rates. Many of these are currently still under investigation but have shown promising results in accelerated wound closure rates.

7.5   Combination of Therapeutic Modalities to Enhance Stem Cell Effectiveness

As discussed previously, diabetic patients do not only have deficient wound healing abilities but also have a diminished bone marrow mobilization response and decreased lower extremity blood flow due to concomitant peripheral vascular disease. Thus, combined therapies that assist in both increased cell availability via increased bone marrow mobilization and increased peripheral blood flow are important adjuncts in the treatment of DFU. Many diabetic patients suffer concomitantly with peripheral arterial disease (PAD) and may require surgical interventions such as angioplasty to assist in the restoration of adequate blood flow to the lower extremities. Clinical studies investigated patients with critical limb ischemia (the most severe form of PAD) that contributed to their DFU to determine whether a combination approach is a superior option. Although the heterogeneity of clinical trials for this question makes it difficult to draw discrete conclusions, the overall results suggest that DFU patients with critical limb ischemia have improved wound healing and ankle-brachial index and decreased claudication distances [4]. Another study of patients deemed "high risk" for surgical revascularization received bone marrow cell therapy and demonstrated high rates of improved wound healing, improved rest pain, and decreased amputation rates [58]. Another adjunct to stem cell therapy in DFU is the utilization of G-CSF therapy, which stimulates the bone marrow to release stem and progenitor cells into the peripheral circulation. Clinical trials have found that the addition of G-CSF to stem cell therapy is safe and promotes wound healing and as such should be considered [4]. Other attempts at augmenting the regenerative potential of stem cells have utilized systemic hyperoxia with localized cytokine injections to increase the mobilization and homing of diabetic bone marrow cells [14].

7.6   Future of Stem Cell Therapy in DFUs

Currently the trend in stem cell therapy for DFU is autologous MSC injected locally to increase wound healing. However, there remain technologies and stem cell therapy adjacent treatments that are underutilized due to a fundamental lack of knowledge of stem cell biology and its interactions with the wound microenvironment. One avenue worth further investigation for utilization in diabetic patients is induced pluripotent stem cell (iPSC) therapies. In 2006, scientists discovered that adult stem cells were able to reverse pluripotency. They accomplished this by transducing mouse fibroblasts with four transcription factors (Oct3/4, Sox2, KLF4, and c-MYC) [5]. These transcription factors are mainly found in embryonic tissues and thus act to reprogram the cells into an embryonic-like pluripotent state. Since this discovery, human adult cell lines have been transformed to iPSC including the reprograming of DFU-derived fibroblast cell lines, which were able to then further differentiate into fibroblasts [59]. Utilization of these cell types in clinical trials requires the utilization of differentiation protocols using recombinant factors to allow these cells to differentiate into the desired cell types. Unfortunately, these recombinant factors are costly and thus diminish the feasibility of their use in large-scale clinical applications. Another risk is their higher malignancy risk and teratoma formation risk. Taken together, iPSCs are a promising cell technology for regenerative medicine, and no doubt their use in clinical medicine will increase with more knowledge and expertise in their use. Another promising therapeutic option in stem cell therapy is the utilization of stem cell extracellular vesicles (EVs). EVs carry cytokines and growth factors, signaling lipids, mRNAs, and regulatory miRNAs and are thought to be responsible for cell-cell communications and mediate stem cell's paracrine effects, via the formation of epigenetic modifications to recipient cells [5]. Studies utilizing EVs have been used to enhance cutaneous wounds and have also been shown to promote angiogenesis and ulcer healing in a murine DFU model [60]. The obvious advantage of this stem cell therapy approach is the decreased immunocompatibility and malignancy risk; however consistent procurement methodologies need to be developed before their utilization in clinical studies.

Genetic modifications of stem cells in preclinical studies of limb ischemia have also shown enhanced limb revascularization and improved leg functionality. Specifically, E-selectin supercharged MSC (overexpression of E-selectin on surface of MSC) has been developed via ex vivo transduction with an adeno-associated virus (data presented at the American College of Surgeons Clinical Congress 2019).

Overall the field of stem cell therapies for the treatment of DFU is promising and growing in popularity as the application of these therapies has been shown to be safe and efficacious. Continued investigations into the optimal stem cell type (whether modified or not), delivery method, and protocols need to occur before the widespread utilization of stem cell therapies for DFU treatment will occur.

References

1. International Diabetes Federation. IDF Diabetes Atlas, 8th ed. 2017.; http://www.diabetesatlas.org. Accessed October 1, 2019.
2. Singh N, Armstrong DG, Lipsky BA. Preventing foot ulcers in patients with diabetes. JAMA. 2005;293(2):217–28.

3. Trautner C, Haastert B, Giani G, Berger M. Incidence of lower limb amputations and diabetes. Diabetes Care. 1996;19(9):1006–9.
4. Lopes L, Setia O, Aurshina A, et al. Stem cell therapy for diabetic foot ulcers: a review of preclinical and clinical research. Stem Cell Res Ther. 2018;9(1):188.
5. Zakrzewski W, Dobrzynski M, Szymonowicz M, Rybak Z. Stem cells: past, present, and future. Stem Cell Res Ther. 2019;10(1):68.
6. Kanji S, Das H. Advances of stem cell therapeutics in cutaneous wound healing and regeneration. Mediat Inflamm. 2017;2017:–5217967.
7. Wu Y, Chen L, Scott PG, Tredget EE. Mesenchymal stem cells enhance wound healing through differentiation and angiogenesis. Stem Cells. 2007;25(10):2648–59.
8. Wu Y, Zhao RCH, Tredget EE. Concise review: bone marrow-derived stem/progenitor cells in cutaneous repair and regeneration. Stem Cells (Dayton, Ohio). 2010;28(5):905–15.
9. Ahmed AS, Antonsen EL. Immune and vascular dysfunction in diabetic wound healing. J Wound Care. 2016;25(Sup7):S35–s46.
10. Falanga V. Wound healing and its impairment in the diabetic foot. Lancet. 2005;366(9498):1736–43.
11. Fahey TJ, Sadaty A, Jones WG, Barber A, Smoller B, Shires GT. Diabetes impairs the late inflammatory response to wound healing. J Surg Res. 1991;50(4):308–13.
12. Marhoffer W, Stein M, Maeser E, Federlin K. Impairment of Polymorphonuclear leukocyte function and metabolic control of diabetes. Diabetes Care. 1992;15(2):256–60.
13. Hennessey PJ, Ford EG, Black CT, Andrassy RJ. Wound collagenase activity correlates directly with collagen glycosylation in diabetic rats. J Pediatr Surg. 1990;25(1):75–8.
14. Gallagher KA, Liu ZJ, Xiao M, et al. Diabetic impairments in NO-mediated endothelial progenitor cell mobilization and homing are reversed by hyperoxia and SDF-1 alpha. J Clin Invest. 2007;117(5):1249–59.
15. Bailo M, Soncini M, Vertua E, et al. Engraftment potential of human amnion and chorion cells derived from term placenta. Transplantation. 2004;78(10):1439–48.
16. Vegh I, Grau M, Gracia M, Grande J, de la Torre P, Flores AI. Decidua mesenchymal stem cells migrated toward mammary tumors in vitro and in vivo affecting tumor growth and tumor development. Cancer Gene Ther. 2013;20(1):8–16.
17. Parolini O, Alviano F, Bagnara GP, et al. Concise review: isolation and characterization of cells from human term placenta: outcome of the first international workshop on placenta derived stem cells. Stem Cells (Dayton, Ohio). 2008;26(2):300–11.
18. Barlow S, Brooke G, Chatterjee K, et al. Comparison of human placenta- and bone marrow-derived multipotent mesenchymal stem cells. Stem Cells Dev. 2008;17(6):1095–107.
19. Tran TC, Kimura K, Nagano M, et al. Identification of human placenta-derived mesenchymal stem cells involved in re-endothelialization. J Cell Physiol. 2011;226(1):224–35.
20. Prather WR, Toren A, Meiron M, Ofir R, Tschope C, Horwitz EM. The role of placental-derived adherent stromal cell (PLX-PAD) in the treatment of critical limb ischemia. Cytotherapy. 2009;11(4):427–34.
21. Kim SW, Zhang HZ, Guo L, Kim JM, Kim MH. Amniotic mesenchymal stem cells enhance wound healing in diabetic NOD/SCID mice through high angiogenic and engraftment capabilities. PLoS One. 2012;7(7):e41105.
22. Kong P, Xie X, Li F, Liu Y, Lu Y. Placenta mesenchymal stem cell accelerates wound healing by enhancing angiogenesis in diabetic Goto-Kakizaki (GK) rats. Biochem Biophys Res Commun. 2013;438(2):410–9.
23. Norgren L, Weiss N, Nikol S, et al. PLX-PAD cell treatment of critical limb Ischaemia: rationale and design of the PACE trial. Eur J Vasc Endovasc Surg. 2019;57(4):538–45.
24. Blumberg SN, Berger A, Hwang L, Pastar I, Warren SM, Chen W. The role of stem cells in the treatment of diabetic foot ulcers. Diabetes Res Clin Pract. 2012;96(1):1–9.
25. Tark KC, Hong JW, Kim YS, Hahn SB, Lee WJ, Lew DH. Effects of human cord blood mesenchymal stem cells on cutaneous wound healing in leprdb mice. Ann Plast Surg. 2010;65(6):565–72.

26. Luo G, Cheng W, He W, et al. Promotion of cutaneous wound healing by local application of mesenchymal stem cells derived from human umbilical cord blood. Wound Rep Regener. 2010;18(5):506–13.

27. Qin HL, Zhu XH, Zhang B, Zhou L, Wang WY. Clinical evaluation of human umbilical cord mesenchymal stem cell transplantation after angioplasty for diabetic foot. Exp Clin Endocrinol Diab. 2016;124(8):497–503.

28. Lee MJ, Kim J, Lee KI, Shin JM, Chae JI, Chung HM. Enhancement of wound healing by secretory factors of endothelial precursor cells derived from human embryonic stem cells. Cytotherapy. 2011;13(2):165–78.

29. Yan J, Tie G, Wang S, et al. Type 2 diabetes restricts multipotency of mesenchymal stem cells and impairs their capacity to augment postischemic neovascularization in db/db mice. J Am Heart Assoc. 2012;1(6):e002238.

30. Duscher D, Rennert RC, Januszyk M, et al. Aging disrupts cell subpopulation dynamics and diminishes the function of mesenchymal stem cells. Sci Rep. 2014;4:7144.

31. Falanga V, Iwamoto S, Chartier M, et al. Autologous bone marrow-derived cultured mesenchymal stem cells delivered in a fibrin spray accelerate healing in murine and human cutaneous wounds. Tissue Eng. 2007;13(6):1299–312.

32. Parikh PP, Liu ZJ, Velazquez OC. A molecular and clinical review of stem cell therapy in critical limb ischemia. Stem Cells Int. 2017;2017:3750829.

33. Kaushik K, Das A. Endothelial progenitor cell therapy for chronic wound tissue regeneration. Cytotherapy. 2019;21(11):1137–50.

34. Liu ZJ, Tian R, Li Y, et al. SDF-1alpha-induced dual pairs of E-selectin/ligand mediate endothelial progenitor cell homing to critical ischemia. Sci Rep. 2016;6:34416.

35. Albiero M, Menegazzo L, Boscaro E, Agostini C, Avogaro A, Fadini GP. Defective recruitment, survival and proliferation of bone marrow-derived progenitor cells at sites of delayed diabetic wound healing in mice. Diabetologia. 2011;54(4):945–53.

36. Asai J, Takenaka H, Ii M, et al. Topical application of ex vivo expanded endothelial progenitor cells promotes vascularisation and wound healing in diabetic mice. Int Wound J. 2013;10(5):527–33.

37. Liu F, Chen DD, Sun X, et al. Hydrogen sulfide improves wound healing via restoration of endothelial progenitor cell functions and activation of angiopoietin-1 in type 2 diabetes. Diabetes. 2014;63(5):1763–78.

38. Castilla DM, Liu ZJ, Tian R, Li Y, Livingstone AS, Velazquez OC. A novel autologous cell-based therapy to promote diabetic wound healing. Ann Surg. 2012;256(4):560–72.

39. Pedroso DC, Tellechea A, Moura L, et al. Improved survival, vascular differentiation and wound healing potential of stem cells co-cultured with endothelial cells. PLoS One. 2011;6(1):e16114.

40. Fathke C, Wilson L, Hutter J, et al. Contribution of bone marrow-derived cells to skin: collagen deposition and wound repair. Stem Cells (Dayton, Ohio). 2004;22(5):812–22.

41. Awad O, Dedkov EI, Jiao C, Bloomer S, Tomanek RJ, Schatteman GC. Differential healing activities of CD34+ and CD14+ endothelial cell progenitors. Arterioscler Thromb Vasc Biol. 2006;26(4):758–64.

42. Lu D, Chen B, Liang Z, et al. Comparison of bone marrow mesenchymal stem cells with bone marrow-derived mononuclear cells for treatment of diabetic critical limb ischemia and foot ulcer: a double-blind, randomized, controlled trial. Diabetes Res Clin Pract. 2011;92(1):26–36.

43. Wettstein R, Savic M, Pierer G, et al. Progenitor cell therapy for sacral pressure sore: a pilot study with a novel human chronic wound model. Stem Cell Res Ther. 2014;5(1):18.

44. Fraser JK, Wulur I, Alfonso Z, Hedrick MH. Fat tissue: an underappreciated source of stem cells for biotechnology. Trends Biotechnol. 2006;24(4):150–4.

45. Meza-Zepeda LA, Noer A, Dahl JA, Micci F, Myklebost O, Collas P. High-resolution analysis of genetic stability of human adipose tissue stem cells cultured to senescence. J Cell Mol Med. 2008;12(2):553–63.

46. Gonzalez-Rey E, Gonzalez MA, Varela N, et al. Human adipose-derived mesenchymal stem cells reduce inflammatory and T cell responses and induce regulatory T cells in vitro in rheumatoid arthritis. Ann Rheum Dis. 2010;69(01):241–8.
47. Kokai LE, Marra K, Rubin JP. Adipose stem cells: biology and clinical applications for tissue repair and regeneration. Transl Res. 2014;163(4):399–408.
48. Yoshimura K, Shigeura T, Matsumoto D, et al. Characterization of freshly isolated and cultured cells derived from the fatty and fluid portions of liposuction aspirates. J Cell Physiol. 2006;208(1):64–76.
49. U.S. Food and Drug Administration. CFR- Code of Federal Regulations Title Wq. Part 1271: Human Cells, Tissues and Cellular and Tissue-based Products. 2013.
50. Raposio E, Caruana G, Bonomini S, Libondi G. A novel and effective strategy for the isolation of adipose-derived stem cells: minimally manipulated adipose-derived stem cells for more rapid and safe stem cell therapy. Plast Reconstr Surg. 2014;133(6):1406–9.
51. Nambu M, Kishimoto S, Nakamura S, et al. Accelerated wound healing in healing-impaired db/db mice by autologous adipose tissue-derived stromal cells combined with atelocollagen matrix. Ann Plast Surg. 2009;62(3):317–21.
52. Maharlooei MK, Bagheri M, Solhjou Z, et al. Adipose tissue derived mesenchymal stem cell (AD-MSC) promotes skin wound healing in diabetic rats. Diabetes Res Clin Pract. 2011;93(2):228–34.
53. Di Rocco G, Gentile A, Antonini A, et al. Enhanced healing of diabetic wounds by topical administration of adipose tissue-derived stromal cells overexpressing stromal-derived factor-1: biodistribution and engraftment analysis by bioluminescent imaging. Stem Cells Int. 2010;2011:304562.
54. Nie C, Yang D, Morris SF. Local delivery of adipose-derived stem cells via acellular dermal matrix as a scaffold: a new promising strategy to accelerate wound healing. Med Hypotheses. 2009;72(6):679–82.
55. Bertozzi N, Simonacci F, Grieco MP, Grignaffini E, Raposio E. The biological and clinical basis for the use of adipose-derived stem cells in the field of wound healing. Ann Med Surg (2012). 2017;20:41–8.
56. Walczak P, Zhang J, Gilad AA, et al. Dual-modality monitoring of targeted intraarterial delivery of mesenchymal stem cells after transient ischemia. Stroke. 2008;39(5):1569–74.
57. Liu ZJ, Daftarian P, Kovalski L, et al. Directing and potentiating stem cell-mediated angiogenesis and tissue repair by cell surface E-selectin coating. PLoS One. 2016;11(4):e0154053.
58. Giles KA, Rzucidlo EM, Goodney PP, Walsh DB, Powell RJ. Bone marrow aspirate injection for treatment of critical limb ischemia with comparison to patients undergoing high-risk bypass grafts. J Vasc Surg. 2015;61(1):134–7.
59. Gerami-Naini B, Smith A, Maione AG, et al. Generation of induced pluripotent stem cells from diabetic foot ulcer fibroblasts using a nonintegrative Sendai virus. Cell Reprogram. 2016;18(4):214–23.
60. Li X, Xie X, Lian W, et al. Exosomes from adipose-derived stem cells overexpressing Nrf2 accelerate cutaneous wound healing by promoting vascularization in a diabetic foot ulcer rat model. Exp Mol Med. 2018;50(4):29.

Chapter 8
Venous Foot and Leg Ulcers

Edith Tzeng and Kathy Gonzalez

8.1 Introduction

Normal wound healing is a complex process comprised of well-orchestrated inter-actions between a variety of cell types, cytokines, and growth factors [1]. Chronic, nonhealing wounds result from conditions such as diabetes, pressure, arterial insuf-ficiency, and venous disease that lead to the disruption of the cellular and molecular events found in normal wound healing [2]. These wounds represent a major eco-nomic burden to the health-care system, affecting 1–2% of the general population and costing Medicare more than $20 billion annually [3].

Venous leg ulcerations (VLUs) are estimated to affect 500,000 to 600,000 people annually in the United States alone, contributing to health-care costs approaching $1.5 billion to $3 billion each year. The mean total cost of treating a venous ulcer over a 6-month follow-up period is $15,732 [4]. These estimates only take into account the direct treatment costs and fail to consider the additional financial burden incurred by the patient's loss of work and disability. Additionally, chronic wounds have a significant impact on quality of life, causing patients substantial pain, limit-ing their mobility and thus restricting their ability to work and perform activities of daily living, resulting in feelings of depression and social isolation [5].

Despite a wide array of therapies available for the management of chronic wounds, up to 50% of wounds that have been present for over a year remain resis-tant to treatment [6]. Thus, efforts have been concentrated on developing more inno-vative therapies to improve wound healing. In particular, the rapidly advancing field

E. Tzeng (✉)
VA Pittsburgh Healthcare System and University of Pittsburgh, Pittsburgh, PA, USA

Division of Vascular Surgery, University of Pittsburgh Medical Center, Pittsburgh, PA, USA
e-mail: tzenge@upmc.edu

K. Gonzalez
Division of Vascular Surgery, University of Pittsburgh Medical Center, Pittsburgh, PA, USA

© Springer Nature Switzerland AG 2021
T. P. Navarro et al. (eds.), *Stem Cell Therapy for Vascular Diseases*,
https://doi.org/10.1007/978-3-030-56954-9_8

of regenerative medicine has emerged as a promising alternative to improve wound repair. Regenerative therapy focuses on utilizing stem cells to restore the conditions for physiologic tissue renewal. A number of preclinical and clinical trials have demonstrated positive outcomes and safety profiles for stem cell therapy in this application. However, questions remain regarding the ideal stem cell population to utilize and how to optimally deliver the cells to the site of injury [7, 8].

8.2   Epidemiology of Venous Ulceration

Venous leg ulcers represent a substantial clinical challenge and health care burden. The overall prevalence of this condition in westernized countries is estimated to be 1%, increasing to greater than 3% in those over 65 years of age [9]. VLUs are estimated to affect 500,000 to 600,000 people annually in the United States. They account for 80–90% of all lower extremity ulcers and are estimated to cost the US health-care system between $1.5 billion and $3 billion annually [4]. These costs do not take into account the financial loss incurred by the patient's inability to work and disability. Additionally, these wounds negatively impact quality of life because of pain and restricted mobility that present daily challenges to patients, leading to feelings of depression and social isolation [10].

Contributing significantly to the socioeconomic cost of these wounds is the fact that VLUs are prone to chronicity and recurrence. Approximately 30% of venous ulcers remain unhealed after a 6-month period, and recurrence rates are as high as 60 to 70% [11]. Ma et al. concluded that the mean total cost of treating VLU during a 6-month follow-up period in a cohort of 84 patients was $15,732. Those that healed without recurrence cost $10,563, but those who failed to heal had a total cost that was three times higher at $33,907 [4]. While the costs of treating these wounds are already high, the global prevalence of VLUs is predicted to increase exponentially as people are living longer with multiple comorbidities [12]. The projected costs of these wounds are staggering and support the need for wound care strategies that accelerate venous wound healing and prevent recurrence.

8.3   Normal Wound Healing

The normal wound healing process is traditionally divided into three overlapping but distinct phases – inflammation, proliferation, and maturation.

8.3.1   Inflammation

The inflammatory phase is characterized by a cellular and vascular response to injury that functions to eliminate devitalized tissue in the wound, prevent infection, and set the stage for tissue regeneration [1]. The initial vascular response to injury is vasoconstriction to prevent hemorrhage. Platelets adhere to the exposed collagen in the subendothelial layers of the blood vessel wall and form the initial hemostatic plug. This is followed by activation of the coagulation and complement cascades. Prothrombin is converted to thrombin, which then converts fibrinogen to fibrin. The thrombus formed from cross-linked fibrin, platelets, and plasma fibronectin is the first line of defense against microbial invasion and serves as a scaffold for infiltrating cells [13]. Platelets in the clot release chemotactic factors that are essential to the recruitment of inflammatory cells to the wound. They also release many growth factors, including transforming growth factor (TGF)-α, TGF-β, and platelet-derived growth factor (PDGF) [14]. Fibrin binds to integrin CD11b/CD18 on infiltrating monocytes and neutrophils. It also binds to $\alpha_v\beta_3$ integrin on endothelial and fibroblast cells, as well as fibroblast growth factor-2 (FGF-2) and vascular endothelial growth factor (VEGF), thus aiding in angiogenesis [7, 13].

Polymorphonuclear cells (PMNs) are the first inflammatory cells to arrive at the wound and do so between 24 and 48 hours post-wounding. They protect the wound from infection by killing bacteria and phagocytizing devitalized tissue and cellular debris [1]. In addition, they serve as a major source of pro-inflammatory cytokines, including IL-1α, IL-1β, IL-6, and tumor necrosis factor-α (TNF-α) [7]. After 2–3 days, monocytes are recruited into the wound bed where they differentiate into macrophages, which play a pivotal role in the transition from inflammation toward repair. Macrophages also phagocytize and kill bacteria, scavenge tissue debris, and remove apoptotic neutrophils. They secrete cytokines and growth factors that are essential for the later stages of wound repair. These include chemotactic factors that attract fibroblasts to the wound area and growth factors such as PDGF, FGF, VEGF, TGF-β, and TGF-α, all of which play a role in cell migration, proliferation, and matrix production [14, 15].

8.3.2 Proliferation

The proliferative phase of wound repair occurs 2–10 days after injury and is characterized by cellular proliferation and migration of different cell types, resulting in extracellular matrix (ECM) deposition, angiogenesis, and reepithelialization [16]. Fibroblasts attracted to the wound become the predominant cell type in the wound by 3–5 days post-injury. The fibroblasts proliferate and produce fibronectin, hyaluronic acid, collagen, and proteoglycans, leading to the construction of new ECM and a platform for keratinocyte migration [13]. About 4 days after injury, the provisional fibrin matrix begins to be replaced by granulation tissue, which is composed of fibroblasts, collagen, blood vessels, and macrophages [7].

Angiogenesis accompanies granulation tissue formation to provide the oxygen and nutrients necessary to support cell metabolism. In the form of developing capillary sprouts, endothelial cells (ECs) digest and penetrate the underlying vascular basement membrane, invade the ECM, and form tube-like structures that extend, branch, and create capillary networks. EC migration is stimulated by FGF, VEGF, and other angiogenesis factors. To facilitate migration through the basement membrane into the fibrin clot, endothelial capillary sprouts express $\alpha_v\beta_3$ integrin, which is able to recognize all provisional matrix proteins [17].

Stimulated by PDGF, TGF-β, epidermal growth factor (EGF), and a number of other growth factors, fibroblasts secrete collagen and enhance collagen cross-linking, resulting in increased mechanical strength in the healing wound. The provisional fibrin matrix is gradually replaced by type III collagen followed by type I collagen during the remodeling phase. Fibroblasts also differentiate into myofibroblasts, which exert contractile forces via focal adhesion contacts that link the intracellular cytoskeleton to the ECM, leading to wound contraction and reduction in wound area [7, 13].

Reepithelialization is the process of restoring an intact epidermis after cutaneous injury. It involves the migration of adjacent epithelial cells into the wound, proliferation of keratinocytes behind the advancing epithelial tongue, restoration of the basement membrane, and differentiation of keratinocytes into a stratified epidermis [14]. Keratinocyte migration and proliferation are modulated by multiple factors, including the ECM, integrin receptors, matrix metalloproteinases (MMPs), and growth factors, including EGF, TGF-α, and keratinocyte growth factor (KGF) [14, 18]. The ECM provides a scaffold for keratinocytes to migrate across. The direction of keratinocyte migration is coordinated by their surface integrin interaction with newly formed collagen in the wound bed. MMPs release keratinocytes from their substratum and facilitate migration through the matrix by degrading type IV collagen and laminin in the basement membrane and disrupting attachment to fibrillar collagen. Once migration is completed, likely secondary to contact inhibition, keratinocytes and fibroblasts secrete type IV collagen to restore the basement membrane, and keratinocytes terminally differentiate to form a stratified epidermis [13, 14].

8.3.3   Maturation

The maturation phase begins 2–3 weeks after injury and lasts for a year or more. It involves ECM turnover and a significant decrease in cellularity, as most of the cells in the healing wound exit the wound or undergo apoptosis. The ECM is transformed from mainly type III collagen to type I collagen through the actions of MMPs secreted by local fibroblasts, macrophages, and endothelial cells. MMPs are inhibited by tissue inhibitors of metalloproteinases (TIMPs), and the balance between MMP and TIMP activity is essential for appropriate wound repair and remodeling. During the maturation phase, the healing wound continues strengthen but never achieves the properties of uninjured skin [14, 16].

8.4   Pathophysiology of Venous Ulceration

Acute cutaneous wounds undergo the linear and overlapping events of the three wound healing phases and result in benign scar formation [14]. Chronic wounds fail to progress through the orderly series of these events. While the pathogenesis of venous ulceration is multifactorial, the underlying causative factor is ambulatory venous hypertension which results in microcirculatory dysfunction, chronic inflammation, fibroblast senescence, and altered protease activity (Fig. 8.1) [19].

Both venous reflux and obstruction can contribute to the development of venous hypertension [20]. Suprainguinal venous obstructive lesions from thrombotic and nonthrombotic lesions (e.g., May-Thurner syndrome) can occur alone or in combination with infrainguinal venous incompetence [21]. Approximately 50% of patients with venous ulcers have superficial and perforating vein valvular incompetence [19]. Varicose vein formation may occur as a result of venous valvular incompetence and further contribute to ambulatory venous hypertension [22]. The vein wall in varicose veins is characterized by the loss of smooth muscle cell contractile shape and an increased collagen-elastin ratio; these changes result in vein wall fibrosis and abnormal venous contractility [21].

Changes in the vein wall and valve are considered primary events leading to venous disease, although it is unclear which one precedes the other [20]. Increased venous pressure transmitted from the macrocirculation to the microcirculation alters the shear and mechanical stress experienced by the ECs, causing them to express selectins and release vasoactive agents, inflammatory molecules, chemokines, and prothrombotic precursors [23]. Patients with venous disease have increased expression of intercellular adhesion molecule-1 (ICAM-1), and likely vascular cell adhesion molecule-1 (VCAM-1) and endothelial leukocyte adhesion molecule-1 (E-selectin), which sense the altered mechanical forces and shear stress and

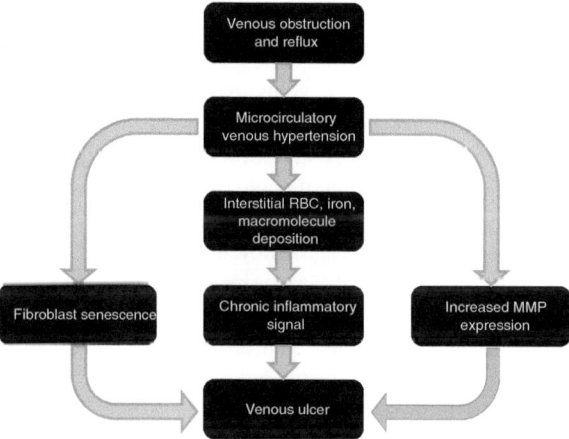

Fig. 8.1 Pathophysiology of venous ulceration. Abbreviations: MMP, matrix metalloproteinase; RBC, red blood cell

subsequently activate the recruitment and diapedesis of leukocytes. This results in leukocyte transmigration into the vein wall and valve, stimulating an inflammatory cascade, production of multiple pro-inflammatory cytokines (TGF-β1, TNF-α, IL-1), and increased expression of MMPs. These lead to pathologic changes in the vein wall, valve, endothelium, and surrounding tissues, ultimately causing dermal destruction with skin changes and ulcer formation [20, 23].

Microcirculatory venous hypertension also leads to the extravasation of macromolecules and red blood cells (RBCs) into the dermal interstitium [24, 25]. The extravasated RBCs cause excessive interstitial iron deposition. RBC degradation products, iron, and extravasated interstitial proteins create a continuous inflammatory signal leading to a chronic cycle of leukocyte recruitment and activation, secretion of inflammatory mediators, and tissue destruction [26–28].

The predominant leukocytes present in the dermis of chronic venous insufficiency patients are macrophages and mast cells [27]. Two phenotypes of macrophages have been described: a pro-inflammatory M1 phenotype associated with microbicidal capacity and the secretion of high levels of pro-inflammatory cytokines (TNF-α, IL-1, IL-6, and IL-23), and an anti-inflammatory M2 phenotype, which decreases pro-inflammatory cytokine levels, secretes components of the ECM, and is essential for the later phases of tissue repair [29]. It has been demonstrated that dermal iron deposition results in persistence of the pro-inflammatory M1 phenotype with continued tissue destruction and impaired wound healing, likely secondary to excessive TNF-α production.

Cytokines play an important role in the pathophysiology of venous ulcers, coordinating inflammation, leukocyte activation, expression of cytokines in the interstitial space, and MMP activation [20]. Healing venous ulcers are associated with increased levels of TGF-β1, likely reflecting the important role TGF-β1 plays in fibrogenesis, matrix deposition, and proliferation [30]. Chronic, nonhealing venous ulcers are characterized by elevated levels of inflammatory cytokines including IL-1β, IL-6, IFN-γ, and TNF-α. Four weeks of compression therapy, an important component of treatment for chronic venous wounds, reduces these cytokines while increasing TGF-β1 levels [31].

MMP overexpression in varicose veins and venous ulcers contributes significantly to the pathogenesis of venous insufficiency and ulceration. Increased venous pressure leads to altered mechanical stretch, induction of hypoxia inducible factor (HIF) and other MMP inducers, leukocyte infiltration, and expression of pro-inflammatory cytokines, all of which contribute to increased MMP expression [32]. In the vein wall, MMPs degrade ECM proteins such as collagen and elastin and inhibit vascular smooth muscle contraction, resulting in impaired venous contractility, venous dilation, and varicose vein formation. In venous wounds, MMP overexpression leads to excessive matrix degradation, preventing normal matrix formation and remodeling. Fluid from chronic venous wounds contains markedly elevated levels of several metalloproteinases, including MMP-1, MMP-2, MMP-8, and MMP-9, compared to fluid from healthy acute wounds [33–37]. Four weeks of compression therapy have also been demonstrated to reduce MMP levels in venous wounds [38].

Venous wounds are also associated with aberrant fibroblast activity. Fibroblasts isolated from these wounds produce less collagen than normal fibroblasts [39]. They also proliferate at a slower rate and are morphologically distinct with characteristics of senescent cells [40, 41]. This senescent state is induced by venous hypertension [42]. It has been demonstrated that fibroblasts from venous ulcers fail to proliferate or produce collagen in response to TGF-β1 due to decreased expression of TGF-β Type II receptors [43, 44]. Venous ulcer fibroblasts also have diminished proliferation to growth factors such as PDGF, bFGF, and EGF [45]. Venous hypertension induces fibroblast differentiation into myofibroblasts that increase the tension in the dermis and make the skin vulnerable to injury. When injury occurs, the increased tension in the dermis increases wound separation and venous ulcer formation [21].

8.5 Current Therapies for Venous Ulceration

The management of chronic wounds requires a systematic approach to properly identify and target the underlying precipitating and perpetuating factors [7]. The basic tenets of wound care involve appropriate medical management of comorbid conditions (diabetes, renal insufficiency, and poor nutrition), the use of antibiotics in the setting of acute infection, revascularization of ischemic limbs, and sharp debridement of nonviable tissue [46].

In venous ulcers, where venous hypertension acts as the main etiological and exacerbating factor, external compression therapy is the cornerstone of management. Compression applied to the calf increases local interstitial pressure, decreases superficial and deep venous hydrostatic pressure, and improves venous return, decreasing venous hypertension and reducing the leakage of solutes and fluid into the interstitial space (Fig. 8.2) [47]. Four weeks of compression therapy have been shown to decrease many of the inflammatory cytokines and MMPs present in venous ulcers [31, 38]. Multiple forms of external compression exist, including the Unna's boot, three- or four-layer compression bandages, and short stretch compression bandages [46]. A Cochrane review concluded that multilayer compression bandages containing an elastic component are more effective at increasing ulcer healing rates compared to single-layer systems or those composed of only inelastic components [48]. Regular use of high-grade compression hosiery after completion of ulcer healing is essential for preventing ulcer recurrence [49]. In one study examining the 15-year results of compression therapy for venous ulcers, patients who were compliant with compression had ulcer healing rates of greater than 90% with a recurrence rate of less than 20% [50]. Those who were noncompliant showed lower ulcer healing rates of 55% and 100% recurrence by 36 months.

In addition to compression therapy, local wound care is essential for the management of venous wounds. As with other wound types, regular debridement must be performed to remove necrotic tissue, wound exudates, and bacteria in order to expose healthy granulation tissue [20]. Multiple types of wound dressings are

Mechanism of Action	Therapy
Decrease venous hypertension	• Compression therapy • Endovenous ablation of incompetent superficial and perforator veins • Endovascular or open surgery for deep venous obstruction
Maintain moist, granulating wound	• Regular debridement • Dressings (e.g., hydrocolloid, alginate)
Reduce microbial burden and infection	• Regular debridement • Antibiotics for active infection
Provide scaffold for cell migration and secrete growth factors	• Bioengineered skin substitutes (e.g., Apligraf ®, Dermagraft®, OASIS®)

Fig. 8.2 Mechanism of action of the current therapies for venous ulcers

available and classified into nonocclusive (simple nonadhering), semiocclusive/occlusive, and advanced (either growth factor or human dermal equivalent) [51]. A moist wound environment is preferable to provide the optimal conditions for cells involved in the healing process and to allow for autolytic debridement, ultimately resulting in accelerated revascularization and development of granulation tissue [52]. However, excess moisture can lead to maceration of the surrounding skin and may predispose wounds to infection. Therefore, the type of wound dressing applied should depend on the characteristics of the wound. Currently, hydrocolloid is recommended for wounds with granulating bases while alginate-based dressings are preferred in highly exudative wounds [51]. However, there is insufficient evidence to support the use of any particular type of dressing to improve healing in venous ulcers [52].

Venous ulcers that persist or fail to reduce in size after 4 weeks of standard treatment may be considered for advanced adjunctive therapies. These include bioengineered skin replacement therapies, such as Apligraf®, Dermagraft®, and OASIS® [20]. These agents provide a biological scaffold for cell attachment, migration, and secretion of multiple growth factors that induce wound healing. In small randomized clinical trials, these biologic therapies combined with compression therapy have been found to be more effective at achieving complete venous wound healing compared to compression therapy alone [53–55].

Other biological therapies that have been investigated for use in chronic wounds include autologous platelet-rich plasma (PRP) and recombinant human (rh) growth factors [46]. The initial interest in growth factor therapies evolved from early studies on autologous PRP, and the cascade of growth factors released from activated platelets when whole blood is centrifuged [46, 56]. Becaplermin (rhPDGF-BB) is the only FDA-approved growth factor therapy and has been demonstrated to be effective, in combination with standard wound care, for the treatment of neuropathic diabetic foot wounds but not those of venous or pressure etiology [57]. This growth factor therapy has also been associated with the concern about the development of distant malignancies, limiting the application of this treatment widely [58]. Other growth factors that have been studied in other countries but are not available in the United States include rhEGF and FGF [46, 59].

In addition to compression therapy and local wound management with the modalities described above, the Society for Vascular Surgery and the American Venous Forum clinical practice guidelines recommend venous surgery for the treatment of superficial venous incompetence or deep venous reflux or obstruction to aid in venous wound healing and to prevent recurrence through the reduction of venous pressures and tissue congestion. Endovenous ablation is the therapy of choice for superficial venous reflux and pathologic perforating veins near a wound, while endovascular angioplasty and stenting or open surgical bypasses are utilized for deep venous obstruction [60]. The ESCHAR trial compared surgical correction of superficial venous reflux and compression therapy to compression therapy alone and found that the addition of surgery significantly reduced ulcer recurrence, although it did not affect ulcer healing time [61, 62]. Harlander-Locke et al. demonstrated that endovenous ablation of incompetent superficial and perforator veins accelerated wound healing in patients who had failed compression therapy [63]. Moreover, patients with healed wounds following endovenous ablation of incompetent superficial and perforator veins had reduced ulcer recurrence rates [64].

Biophysical modalities such as ultrasound, negative pressure therapy, and hyperbaric oxygen therapy have been studied but are not currently recommended for adjunctive use in the management or prevention of venous ulcers by the SVS-AVF guidelines [20, 60].

8.6 Exogenous Stem Cell Therapy for Venous Ulceration

Despite the wide array of therapeutic modalities available for the treatment of venous wounds, none have really improved healing better than good compression. While approximately 70% of venous wounds heal in a 6-month period, recurrence rates are as high as 60–70% [11]. Stem cell-based therapies have generated significant interest as a promising approach to enhance healing of all types of wounds. Stem cells are defined by their capacity to both self-renew and differentiate into multiple cell lines [65]. They can also secrete growth factors and cytokines involved in tissue regeneration, which may modulate the chronic wound environment to improve wound healing. Stem cells from numerous sources are being studied for their capacity to accelerate wound repair with both preclinical and clinical trials supporting potential efficacy (Fig. 8.3) [66].

Stem Cell Type	Advantages	Disadvantages
Embryonic stem cells (ESCs)	• Pluripotent • Unlimited proliferation	• Ethical and legal restrictions • Immunogenicity • Teratogenicity • No clinical evidence
Induced pluripotent stem cells (iPSCs)	• Pluripotent • Unlimited proliferation • No ethical or legal restrictions • Non-immunogenic	• Teratogenicity • No clinical evidence
Bone marrow-derived stem cells (BM-MSCs)	• No ethical or legalrestrictions • Non-immunogenic • Non-teratogenic	• Invasive harvest procedure • Low yield • Limited proliferative capacity in vitro • Decline innumber and proliferative and differentiation potential with age and disease • Limited clinical evidence
Adipose-derived stem cells (ADSCs)	• Abundance of tissue • Minimally invasive harvest procedure • High yield • No ethical or legal restrictions • Non-immunogenic • Non-teratogenic	• Limited proliferativecapacity in vitro • Limited clinical evidence
Umbilical cord blood and Extra-fetal tissue-derived stem cells	• Abundance of tissue • Non-invasive harvest procedure • No ethical or legal restrictions • Non-immunogenic • Non-teratogenic	• Limited clinical evidence

Fig. 8.3 Advantages and disadvantages of the different stem cell types being investigated for venous wound healing

8.6.1   Embryonic Stem Cells

Embryonic stem cells (ESCs) are pluripotent cells isolated from the inner cell mass of blastocyst-stage embryos. They are able to differentiate into any of the three primary germ layers – endoderm, mesoderm, and ectoderm [67]. ESCs have been successfully differentiated into functional keratinocytes that are able to form a stratified epidermis in vitro, offering the possibility of bioengineering skin substitutes for patients needing skin grafts or other wound coverage [68]. However, ethical and legal concerns have limited the use of ESCs for research and clinical purposes [69]. Additionally, the potential for immune rejection and teratoma formation further hinder the clinical application of these cells [70].

8.6.2   Induced Pluripotent Stem Cells

Induced pluripotent stem cells (iPSCs) are adult somatic cells reprogrammed into pluripotent cells [71]. Because iPSCs are derived from differentiated adult tissues, the ethical concerns associated with human ESCs are eliminated [69]. Unlike ESCs, autologous iPSCs are nonimmunogenic [72, 73]. They are also easily harvested from cutaneous sources such as skin fibroblasts [74]. iPSCs have been successfully differentiated into dermal stem cells, fibroblasts, melanocytes, keratinocytes, and mesenchymal cells capable of forming dermal papilla [75–79]. iPSC-derived keratinocytes have been utilized to generate 3D skin equivalents in vitro that exhibit a multilayered epidermis and cornified layer at the surface of the epidermis [80].

In a murine excisional wound healing model, topical application of human-induced pluripotent stem cell-derived ECs (hiPSC-EC) accelerated wound healing with increased wound perfusion and capillary density as well as increased collagen deposition and macrophage infiltration. Angiogenic gene expression, including platelet endothelial cell adhesion molecule (PECAM) and VEGF, was also significantly upregulated [81]. Similarly, in another murine model, co-application of hiPSC-ECs and hiPSC-smooth muscle cells (SMCs) accelerated wound closure with enhanced SMC migration and neovascularization. In vitro, hiPSC-ECs secreted high levels of VEGF, EGF, and FGF-4 compared to primary cells [82]. However, despite their great potential for accelerating wound repair, the use of iPSCs is also limited by their potential for teratoma formation [83].

8.6.3 Mesenchymal Stem Cells

Mesenchymal stem cells (MSCs) are multipotent cells that can be isolated from various tissue sources, including bone marrow, adipose tissue, umbilical cord blood, nerve tissue, and dermis [66]. Similar to iPSCs, the use of MSCs avoids the ethical controversies of ESC use, and allogeneic transplantation is associated with minimal immunoreactivity [7]. Bone marrow-derived MSCs (BM-MSCs) have been extensively studied with regard to their potential for wound healing and tissue regeneration [66].

While it was originally hypothesized that stem cell regenerative therapies were effective due to the stem cells' ability to differentiate into repair cells, it is now recognized that they function predominantly as a source of biomolecules that recruit native cells to the wound. Stem cells secrete cytokines, growth factors, and extracellular matrix (ECM) that act in an autocrine or paracrine manner to influence the local wound environment. Growth factors produced by stem cells induce cell proliferation, cytoprotection, and migration. Stem cells are able to protect other cells from oxygen-free radicals by producing antioxidants and anti-apoptotic molecules. They also secrete angiogenic factors, antifibrotic factors, anti-inflammatory or immunomodulatory factors, and factors essential for ECM maintenance, including collagen, MMPs, and TIMPs [84]. Therefore, stem cells offer not only the ability to replenish deficient progenitor cells via differentiation, but they can also correct the dysregulated chronic wound environment by restoring autocrine and paracrine signaling.

MSCs have been reported to play an important role in all three phases of wound healing (Fig. 8.4). Current evidence suggests that the contribution of MSC differentiation to wound healing is limited due to poor engraftment and survival of these cells in the wound bed. Their therapeutic benefit is more likely attributable to paracrine signaling with the release of trophic factors that reduce inflammation, promote angiogenesis, and induce cell migration and proliferation [85, 86].

Exogenous BM-MSCs have been shown to home to sites of tissue injury. In vitro, BM-MSCs migrate in response to multiple chemotactic factors, including

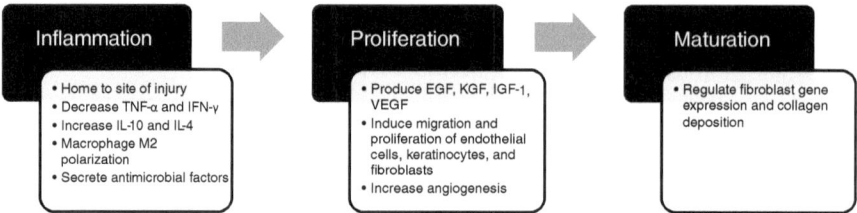

Fig. 8.4 Role of mesenchymal stem cells in each phase of wound healing. Abbreviations: EGF, epidermal growth factor; IFN, interferon; IGF, insulin-like growth factor; IL, interleukin; KGF, keratinocyte growth factor; TNF, tumor necrosis factor; VEGF, vascular endothelial growth factor

insulin-like growth factor (IGF-1), PDGF, IL-1β, IFN-γ, and TNF-α. They express multiple chemokine receptors whose expression can be upregulated by inflammatory cytokines such as TNF-α [87]. In vivo, fluorescently labeled BM-MSCs have been found to preferentially migrate to sites of cutaneous injury in a murine model [88].

At sites of injury, MSCs exert anti-inflammatory actions that make them particularly attractive for the treatment of venous wounds, which are characterized by a protracted inflammatory state. When co-cultured with immune cells in vitro, MSCs decreased the secretion of pro-inflammatory cytokines TNF-α and IFN-γ and increased anti-inflammatory cytokines IL-10 and IL-4 [89] by the immune cells. MSCs have other immunomodulatory effects including suppression of T-cell proliferation and NK cell activation, inhibition or promotion of B cell proliferation, and modulation of the cytokine secretory profile of dendritic cells and macrophages [90]. MSCs are able to induce the anti-inflammatory M2 phenotype of macrophages in vitro. In vivo, systemically infused MSCs are able to home to the wound site and promote macrophage M2 polarization to modulate the local inflammatory response via decreased infiltration of inflammatory cells, decreased production of TNF-α and IL-6, and increased production of IL-10 [91]. MSCs also exhibit antimicrobial activity by secreting antimicrobial factors such as LL-37 and upregulating bacterial killing and phagocytosis by immune cells [92, 93].

MSCs secrete many known mediators of tissue repair, including EGF, KGF, IGF-1, and VEGF, that support cell migration, proliferation, and angiogenesis. BM-MSC-conditioned medium significantly enhances migration of macrophages, keratinocytes, and ECs, as well as proliferation of keratinocytes and ECs in vitro. In vivo, murine wounds treated with BM-MSC-conditioned medium demonstrate increased recruitment of macrophages and endothelial progenitor cells [94]. When co-cultured with MSCs, dermal fibroblasts undergo increased proliferation and migration, as well as altered expression of genes involved in ECM homeostasis and cell adhesion [95]. MSC-treated wounds also express higher levels of VEGF with increased angiogenesis and capillary density. Additionally, though MSCs exhibit relatively low levels of engraftment, they have been shown to contribute to cells in the epidermis and skin appendages via differentiation, thus contributing to dermal regeneration [96]. Multiple studies have reported that application of MSCs to acute or diabetic rodent wounds accelerates wound closure with histology demonstrating improved epithelialization, increased granulation tissue formation, and increased angiogenesis [86].

Clinical trials utilizing BM-MSCs to accelerate wound healing have also yielded positive results. Badiavas and Falanga demonstrated that topically applied and locally injected autologous bone marrow aspirate stimulated healing of chronic wounds with evidence of dermal rebuilding [97]. In a series of 20 patients, Yoshikawa et al. treated a variety of nonhealing wounds with topical autologous BM-MSCs using an artificial dermis made of collagen sponge. Eighteen of the 20 wounds completely healed, and histology revealed regeneration of fibrous, fat, and vascular tissues [98]. Falanga et al. developed a unique fibrin polymer spray delivery system to topically apply cultured autologous bone marrow-derived MSCs to treat both acute and chronic wounds. The acute wounds consisted of surgical defects created during Mohs surgery. These wounds healed within 8 weeks postop, faster than acute wounds treated with a control fibrin spray, suggesting that the spray application of MSCs accelerated resurfacing. The chronic wounds consisted of lower extremity diabetic or venous ulcerations present for greater than 1 year. These wounds significantly decreased in size or healed completely within 20 weeks, with a correlation noted between the number of MSCs applied to the wounds and the percent reduction in ulcer area [99]. No adverse events were reported suggesting a good safety profile for BM-MSC use.

The clinical use of BM-MSCs still faces several challenges. The invasiveness of the bone marrow harvest is painful and can be complicated by infection and hemorrhage [100]. The procedure itself yields a limited number of MSCs because only a fraction (0.001–0.01%) of the harvested bone marrow cells are MSCs [101]. As a result, time and resources are required to expand the cells in culture to achieve therapeutic concentrations [66]. Diabetic and elderly patients also have fewer bone marrow-derived MSCs, and these cells may be dysfunctional, raising concerns about the function of MSCs harvested from these disadvantaged populations [59, 102].

8.6.4 Adipose-Derived Mesenchymal Stem Cells

Unlike BM-MSCs, adipose-derived MSCs (ADSCs) can be harvested from excess adipose tissue using minimally invasive techniques (i.e., liposuction) [103]. Additionally, these lipoaspirates contain much higher stem cell numbers (3.5×10^5 to 1×10^6 ADSCs per gram of lipoaspirate) as compared to bone marrow aspirate (500 to 5×10^4 MSCs per gram of bone marrow aspirate) [104]. Therefore, ADSCs can be isolated in high numbers immediately after harvest, avoiding the need for culture and ex vivo expansion [105]. ADSCs are non-immunogenic and more genetically stable in long-term culture with higher proliferation rates than BM-MSCs [106]. For all of these reasons, adipose tissue has surpassed bone marrow as the preferred source of MSCs for wound repair and other applications [106, 107].

ADSCs have also demonstrated efficacy in cutaneous wound healing in both preclinical and clinical trials. In a murine excisional wound healing model, application of ADSC-seeded hydrogels accelerated wound closure and increased vascularity [108]. Locally applied autologous ADSCs improved skin graft survival, enhanced angiogenesis, and increased epithelialization in a diabetic rat model [109].

In a non-randomized, prospective, single-center pilot study, Konstantinow et al. investigated the efficacy of autologous adipose tissue-derived stromal vascular fraction (SVF), the cellular extract from adipose tissue that contains the regenerative mesenchymal progenitor and stem cell populations, for the treatment of chronic lower extremity ulcers. Sixteen patients with chronic leg ulcers of at least 6-month duration (45% venous, 55% mixed arterial-venous), who had refused skin grafting and vascular surgery and had failed conservative management with compression and negative pressure therapy, received a single topical application of SVF cells. Four microliters of autologous SVF-suspension was injected into the ulcer and bordering area, and an additional 2.5 mL of cell suspension was topically applied via a wound-sized collagen sponge. All the venous patients and 4 of the 9 arterial-venous patients experienced complete wound healing within 9–26 weeks. The 5 arterial-venous patients who did not heal had larger ulcers and ABI scores below 0.8. All of the patients experienced a significant reduction in wound pain [110].

Kavala and Turkyilmaz applied autologous ADSCs to venous leg ulcerations in conjunction with treatment of underlying venous hypertension. Thirty-one patients with primary venous insufficiency, normal deep venous systems, and first-time ulceration were included in the study. All patients underwent greater saphenous vein radiofrequency ablation, and those with perforator incompetence underwent perforator ligation. Despite surgical management of the venous hypertension, all the wounds persisted after 6 months. These wounds were subsequently treated with a single local injection of autologous ADSCs. Eighteen of these wounds completely healed by 12 months, and 13 ulcers exhibited significant contraction and epithelialization with ulcer size reduced by 96%. Patients were followed for a year after healing, and only 3 of the 31 patients developed recurrent ulceration. No adverse events were observed [111].

A systematic review conducted by Holm et al. summarizing the clinical trials studying the use of ADSCs for chronic lower extremity ulcers concluded that ADSCs consistently proved to be safe, improved healing of chronic ulcers, and reduced pain despite differences in study design, ADSC isolation and application methods, and overall poor study quality. While these studies are promising, improved clinical evidence is necessary to define the long-term safety and efficacy of ADSCs for venous wound repair [107].

8.6.5   Umbilical Cord Blood and Extra-Fetal Tissue

Multipotent MSCs have been isolated from human umbilical cord blood and extra-fetal tissues, including amniotic fluid, Wharton's jelly, and placental tissue. In most cases, these tissues are discarded at birth; thus, cells can be harvested without risk to the baby or the mother. Therefore, perinatal tissues potentially represent an unlimited source of MSCs with easy access and minimal ethical or legal considerations [102]. In addition to serving as a reservoir for MSCs, placental tissues also express multiple growth factors critical for wound healing, including EGF, KGF, bFGF, and the family of TGFs [112].

The use of placental tissue for wound healing dates back more than a century. The first reported clinical use of amniotic membrane was in 1910 when it was used in skin transplantation [113]. It was also utilized as a skin substitute for the treatment of burned and ulcerated skin [114, 115]. In 1957, Denkewalter treated 22 lower extremity venous wounds with fresh placental dressings and compression therapy. Sixteen of the wounds healed completely over a 7-week period [116]. In this application, placental membrane serves as a biological scaffold containing multiple growth factors as well as viable cells, including MSCs, neonatal fibroblasts, and epithelial cells, all of which promote wound healing [117].

More recently, there have been multiple studies on the efficacy of placental tissue on the healing of venous wounds. Mermet et al. conducted a prospective pilot study to evaluate the safety and efficacy of amniotic membrane grafting for wound healing in 15 patients with chronic venous wounds refractory to standard therapy for at least 3 months. During the 3-month follow-up period, 12 patients exhibited at least a 50% reduction in ulcer size with three patients who completely healed. All patients reported a significant reduction in pain [118]. Similarly, Francis et al. applied amniotic membrane to 40 chronic venous ulcers resistant to conventional therapies for at least 3 months. By day 90, 80% of the patients demonstrated greater than 50% reduction in ulcer area with increased granulation tissue formation and epithelialization with decreased bacterial colonization of the wound [119].

Commercially available placental tissue allografts include Grafix®, EpiFix®, and AmnioExcel®. A prospective, single-arm cohort study found that application of Grafix®, which consists of cryopreserved placental membrane, to 30 venous wounds that failed to heal using standard local wound care and multilayered compression bandaging resulted in complete wound healing in 53% of the patients. Eighty percent experienced a reduction in wound size by half as compared with only 25% of the patients treated with standard therapy [120]. A randomized controlled trial was conducted with 109 subjects to evaluate the efficacy of Epifix®, a dehydrated human amnion/chorion membrane allograft, as an adjunct to multilayer compression therapy for the treatment of venous wounds [121]. The study found that patients treated with EpiFix® and compression were more likely to experience complete wound healing as compared to those who received standard wound care and compression alone. At 16 weeks, 71% of the intervention group experienced complete ulcer healing compared to only 44% in the control group [121].

8.7 Optimizing Stem Cell Therapy for Wound Healing

While stem cell therapy offers a promising therapeutic modality for venous wound healing, further study is required to maximize its potential efficacy. Specific considerations that must be addressed before this therapy can be clinically applied include optimal donor selection, tissue source, cell isolation method, and mechanism of cell delivery [59].

8.7.1 Donor and Tissue Selection

There is evidence that aging and disease negatively impact stem cell function and therapeutic potential, which will limit the effectiveness of autologous stem cell therapy in elderly and diabetic patients. Aged MSCs have decreased proliferative and differentiation capacity as well as alterations in the profile of therapeutic gene expression and cytokine production [122–125]. Recent studies suggest that these age-related changes are secondary to a shift in MSC subpopulation composition with the loss of certain functional cell populations. Duscher et al. showed that aged MSCs have reduced angiogenic potential and do not improve wound healing in aged mice. Using single-cell transcriptional analysis, aged MSCs were found to be depleted of a subpopulation that exhibits a provascular transcriptional profile [125]. Khong et al. demonstrated that murine wounds treated with BM-MSCs harvested from elderly patients healed more slowly than those treated with young BM-MSCs. The young BM-MSCs contained a higher proportion of cells expressing genes involved in angiogenesis, immunomodulation, and migration [126].

Stem cells derived from diabetic patients are similarly impaired with decreased angiogenic potential, increased pro-inflammatory cytokine secretion, and decreased proliferation and differentiation [127]. In a rat model of hindlimb ischemia, administration of normal BM-MSCs significantly increased limb perfusion and capillary density, while administration of diabetic BM-MSCs had no therapeutic effect. This correlated with transcriptional analysis of the BM-MSCs derived from the diabetic rats, which showed decreased expression of angiogenic genes, including VEGF-A, VEGF-C, angiopoietin-1, and angiopoietin-2, as compared with BM-MSCs from healthy rats [128]. Rennert et al. reported that ADSCs harvested from diabetic mice had decreased angiogenic gene expression and angiogenic potential in vivo compared to those derived from control mice. Single-cell transcriptional analysis revealed that a subpopulation of ADSCs characterized by high expression of angiogenic genes was depleted in diabetic mice as compared to the normal mice [129]. Madhira et al. found that BM-MSCs isolated from obese, type 2 diabetic mice express higher levels of IL-6 and TNF-α compared to BM-MSCs from control mice, suggesting that diabetic MSCs may contribute to the chronic inflammation present in diabetic wounds [130]. Multiple studies have suggested that diabetes impairs the proliferative and differentiation capacity of both BM-MSCs and ADSCs, increasing their tendency to differentiate into adipocytes [128, 129].

The therapeutic efficacy of stem cells can vary according to tissue of origin. BM-MSCs, ADSCs, and UCB-MSCs have differences in gene expression and protein production [131, 132]. UCB-MSCs exhibit increased expression of genes related to matrix remodeling via metalloproteinases and angiogenesis compared to BM-MSCs [132]. In vitro, more ECs migrate toward Wharton's jelly-derived MSCs (WJ-MSCs) than toward BM-MSCs. Additionally, these cells form longer vessels when incubated with WJ-MSC conditioned medium than with BM-MSC conditioned medium [133]. In one study, amniotic mesenchymal stem cells (AMSCs) accelerated murine diabetic wound closure compared to ADSCs and dermal fibroblasts. When compared to ADSCs, AMSCs showed higher expression of angiogenic genes and proteins as well as higher engraftment and keratinocyte differentiation in the wounds [134]. On the other hand, a different study comparing the effect of ADSCs, AMSCs, and BM-MSCs on murine wound healing concluded that ADSCs produced the most pronounced effect on wound closure. Wound bed histology showed enhanced reepithelialization and healthier granulation tissue in the ADSC-treated wounds compared to the AMSC- and BM-MSC-treated wounds. In vitro, ADSCs were better than AMSCs and BM-MSCs at promoting dermal fibroblast migration and type I collagen production. Additionally, fibroblasts cultured with AMSCs expressed higher levels of VEGF, bFGF, KGF, and TGF-β [135]. These findings indicate that further studies are necessary to better understand the impact of aging, disease, and tissue source on stem cell applications in wound healing.

8.7.2 Delivery Methods

MSCs have been delivered to wound beds by several different methods. Local injection of the cells is the most common and preferred approach but is limited by poor cell retention, survival, and engraftment. Potential contributors to these consequences include mechanical shear resulting in membrane disruption during the injection process and the harsh microenvironment of the wound bed [136]. MSCs have also been delivered topically through the use of phosphate-buffered saline, matrigel, fibrin polymer, or hydrogel seeding [100]. Novel cell delivery systems are currently being developed that will optimize MSC survival. Rustad et al. seeded BM-MSCs into hydrogels and demonstrated enhanced viability, engraftment, secretion of angiogenic cytokines, and expression of transcription factors associated with stemness. Wounds treated with MSC-seeded hydrogels exhibited accelerated healing and enhanced angiogenesis as compared to wounds treated with MSC injection alone [137]. Lee et al. developed a porous biodegradable polymeric microsphere scaffold for MSC delivery which increased in vivo engraftment and maintenance of stemness when administered to myocardium [138]. Guo et al. encapsulated BM-MSCs in cytoprotective alginate beads before embedding them in an injectable hydrophobic scaffold. Injecting BM-MSCs embedded in this scaffold into excisional murine wounds increased BM-MSC survival and improved new tissue formation [139].

Genetic engineering is also being harnessed to enhance stem cell survival, migration, and therapeutic potential. Herberg et al. genetically engineered BM-MSCs to overexpress stromal cell-derived factor-1 (SDF-1) under tight doxycycline control. SDF-1β overexpression improved BM-MSC survival under oxidative stress by increasing autophagy and decreasing caspase-3-dependent apoptosis [140]. Ho Wang Yin et al. silenced PHD2, a regulator of hydroxia-inducible transcription factor-1α (HIF-1α), in BM-MSCs, which activated HIF-1α and increased the expression of its target gene VEGF-A. This increased MSC survival and therapeutic angiogenesis in a murine model of critical limb ischemia [141].

The interaction between SDF-1/CXCL12 and its receptor CXCR4 mediates MSC migration to sites of injury [142]. Hu et al. demonstrated that BM-MSC migration to murine burn wounds was associated with significantly increased levels of CXCL12 and CXCR4 at the wound margins. Pre-treating the BM-MSCs with a CXCR4 antagonist inhibited their mobilization in vitro and in vivo and impaired wound healing [143]. Human MSC CXCR4 surface expression decreases significantly during ex vivo expansion, so researchers are working to improve CXCR4 expression with genetic engineering techniques. Overexpression of CXCR4 in UCB-MSCs improved cell migration toward an SDF-1 gradient [142].

MSCs can also be genetically modified to function as a source of paracrine factors. Transfection of v-myc into ADSCs increased VEGF secretion and augmented angiogenesis in vitro. Further modification of the v-myc ADSCs with Akt1 led to even greater VEGF secretion and vasculogenesis. Application of these cells to murine wounds accelerated wound closure, decreased inflammation, and improved collagen regeneration [144]. Kosaric et al. engineered BM-MSCs to overexpress and secrete PDGF-B. Local injection of these genetically modified BM-MSCs into diabetic murine wounds led to accelerated wound healing compared to treatment with normal BM-MSCs [145].

8.8 Conclusion

Chronic venous leg wounds continue to pose a significant clinical challenge despite the availability of numerous modalities for their treatment. These wounds represent a significant economic and social burden, costing the health-care system billions annually and negatively impacting patients' quality of life. Stem cell therapy has emerged as a promising adjunctive therapy for the management of these wounds, offering the potential to restore the conditions of physiologic wound healing by modulating inflammation, enhancing angiogenesis, and stimulating cell migration and proliferation. Mesenchymal stem cells, which can be derived from multiple tissue sources, including bone marrow, fat, and extra-fetal tissues, have been preferentially studied compared to embryonic stem cells and induced pluripotent stem cells due to the lack of ethical or legal considerations, immunogenicity, and teratogenicity associated with their use. Multiple preclinical and small clinical trials have demonstrated the efficacy of mesenchymal stem cells for the treatment of venous ulcers, but more studies are necessary to elucidate the ideal source of stem cells and method of cell delivery. Furthermore, larger, more standardized clinical trials are needed to confirm that stem cell therapy is efficacious and safe for this class of chronic wounds.

References

1. Stadelmann WK, Digenis AG, Tobin GR. Physiology and healing dynamics of chronic cutaneous wounds. Am J Surg. 1998;176:26S–38S.

2. Martin P, Nunan R. Cellular and molecular mechanisms of repair in acute and chronic wound healing. BrJ Dermatol. 2015;173:370–8.
3. Nussbaum SR, Carter MJ, Fife CE, DaVanzo J, Haught R, Nusgart M, et al. An economic evaluation of the impact, cost, and Medicare policy implications of chronic nonhealing wounds. Value Health. 2018;21:27–32.
4. Ma H, O'Donnell TF, Rosen NA, Iafrati MD. The real cost of treating venous ulcers in a contemporary vascular practice. J Vasc Surg Venous Lymphat Disord. 2014;2:355–61.
5. Herber OR, Schnepp W, Rieger MA. A systematic review on the impact of leg ulceration on patients' quality of life. Health Qual Life Outcomes. 2007;5:44.
6. Cha J, Falanga V. Stem cells in cutaneous wound healing. Clin Dermatol. 2007;25:73–8.
7. Kanji S, Das H. Advances of stem cell therapeutics in cutaneous wound healing and regeneration. Mediators Inflamm [Internet]. 2017 [cited 2019 Sep 17];2017. Available from: https://www.ncbi.nlm.nih.gov/pmc/articles/PMC5682068/.
8. Sorice S, Rustad KC, Li AY, Gurtner GC. The role of stem cell therapeutics in wound healing: current understanding and future directions. Plast Reconstr Surg. 2016;138:31S.
9. Xie T, Ye J, Rerkasem K, Mani R. The venous ulcer continues to be a clinical challenge: an update. Burns Trauma. [Internet]. 2018. [cited 2019 Nov 21];6. Available from: https://www.ncbi.nlm.nih.gov/pmc/articles/PMC6003071/.
10. Green J, Jester R, McKinley R, Pooler A. The impact of chronic venous leg ulcers: a systematic review. J Wound Care. 2014;23:601–12.
11. Parker CN, Finlayson KJ, Edwards HE. Predicting the likelihood of delayed venous leg ulcer healing and recurrence: development and reliability testing of risk assessment tools. Ostomy Wound Manage. 2017;63:16–33.
12. Franks PJ, Barker J, Collier M, Gethin G, Haesler E, Jawien A, et al. Management of patients with venous leg ulcers: challenges and current best practice. J Wound Care. 2016;25:S1–67.
13. MT F, Mohapatra D, Kumar D, Chittoria R, Nandhagopal V. Current concepts in the physiology of adult wound healing. Plas Aesthet Res. 2015;2:250–6.
14. Li J, Chen J, Kirsner R. Pathophysiology of acute wound healing. Clin Dermatol. 2007;25:9–18.
15. Martins-Green M, Petreaca M, Wang L. Chemokines and their receptors are key players in the orchestra that regulates wound healing. Adv Wound Care. 2013;2:327–47.
16. Gurtner GC, Werner S, Barrandon Y, Longaker MT. Wound repair and regeneration. Nature. 2008;453:314–21.
17. Tonnesen MG, Feng X, Clark RAF. Angiogenesis in wound healing. J Investig Dermatol Symp Proc. 2000;5:40–6.
18. Pastar I, Stojadinovic O, Yin NC, Ramirez H, Nusbaum AG, Sawaya A, et al. Epithelialization in wound healing: a comprehensive review. Adv Wound Care. 2014;3:445–64.
19. Agren MS, Eaglstein WH, Ferguson MW, Harding KG, Moore K, Saarialho-Kere UK, et al. Causes and effects of the chronic inflammation in venous leg ulcers. Acta Derm Venereol Suppl (Stockh). 2000;210:3–17.
20. Chi Y-W, Raffetto JD. Venous leg ulceration pathophysiology and evidence based treatment. Vasc Med Lond Engl. 2015;20:168–81.
21. Crawford JM, Lal BK, Durán WN, Pappas PJ. Pathophysiology of venous ulceration. J Vasc Surg Venous Lymphat Disord. 2017;5:596–605.
22. Bradbury AW. Pathophysiology and Principles of Management of Varicose Veins. In: Fitridge R, Thompson M, editors. Mech Vasc Dis Ref Book Vasc Spec [Internet]. Adelaide (AU): University of Adelaide Press; 2011 [cited 2019 Nov 22]. Available from: http://www.ncbi.nlm.nih.gov/books/NBK534256/.
23. Raffetto JD. Pathophysiology of chronic venous disease and venous ulcers. Surg Clin North Am. 2018;98:337–47.
24. Burnand KG, Clemenson G, Whimster I, Gaunt J, Browse NL. The effect of sustained venous hypertension on the skin capillaries of the canine hind limb. BJS. 1982;69:41–4.
25. Burnand KG, Whimster I, Naidoo A, Browse NL. Pericapillary fibrin in the ulcer-bearing skin of the leg: the cause of lipodermatosclerosis and venous ulceration. BMJ. 1982;285:1071–2.

26. Pappas PJ, Fallek SR, Garcia A, Araki CT, Back TL, Durán WN, et al. Role of leukocyte activation in patients with venous stasis ulcers. J Surg Res. 1995;59:553–9.
27. Pappas PJ, DeFouw DO, Venezio LM, Gorti R, Padberg FT, Silva MB, et al. Morphometric assessment of the dermal microcirculation in patients with chronic venous insufficiency. J Vasc Surg. 1997;26:784–95.
28. Pappas PJ, Teehan EP, Fallek SR, Garcia A, Araki CT, Back TL, et al. Diminished mononuclear cell function is associated with chronic venous insufficiency. J Vasc Surg. 1995;22:580–6.
29. Sindrilaru A, Peters T, Wieschalka S, Baican C, Baican A, Peter H, et al. An unrestrained pro-inflammatory M1 macrophage population induced by iron impairs wound healing in humans and mice. J Clin Invest. 2011;121:985–97.
30. Gohel MS, Windhaber RAJ, Tarlton JF, Whyman MR, Poskitt KR. The relationship between cytokine concentrations and wound healing in chronic venous ulceration. J Vasc Surg. 2008;48:1272–7.
31. Beidler SK, Douillet CD, Berndt DF, Keagy BA, Rich PB, Marston WA. Inflammatory cytokine levels in chronic venous insufficiency ulcer tissue before and after compression therapy. J Vasc Surg. 2009;49:1013–20.
32. MacColl E, Khalil RA. Matrix metalloproteinases as regulators of vein structure and function: implications in chronic venous disease. J Pharmacol Exp Ther. 2015;355:410–28.
33. Wysocki AB, Staiano-Coico L, Grinnell F. Wound fluid from chronic leg ulcers contains elevated levels of metalloproteinases MMP-2 and MMP-9. J Invest Dermatol. 1993;101:64–8.
34. Weckroth M, Vaheri A, Lauharanta J, Sorsa T, Konttinen YT. Matrix metalloproteinases, gelatinase and collagenase, in chronic leg ulcers. J Invest Dermatol. 1996;106:1119–24.
35. Herouy Y, May AE, Pornschlegel G, Stetter C, Grenz H, Preissner KT, et al. Lipodermatosclerosis is characterized by elevated expression and activation of matrix metalloproteinases: implications for venous ulcer formation. J Invest Dermatol. 1998;111:822–7.
36. Saito S, Trovato MJ, You R, Lal BK, Fasehun F, Padberg FT, et al. Role of matrix metalloproteinases 1, 2, and 9 and tissue inhibitor of matrix metalloproteinase-1 in chronic venous insufficiency. J Vasc Surg. 2001;34:930–8.
37. Amato B, Coretti G, Compagna R, Amato M, Buffone G, Gigliotti D, et al. Role of matrix metalloproteinases in non-healing venous ulcers. Int Wound J. 2015;12:641–5.
38. Beidler SK, Douillet CD, Berndt DF, Keagy BA, Rich PB, Marston WA. Multiplexed analysis of matrix metalloproteinases in leg ulcer tissue of patients with chronic venous insufficiency before and after compression therapy. Wound Repair Regen Off Publ Wound Heal Soc Eur Tissue Repair Soc. 2008;16:642–8.
39. Herrick SE, Ireland GW, Simon D, McCollum CN, Ferguson MW. Venous ulcer fibroblasts compared with normal fibroblasts show differences in collagen but not fibronectin production under both normal and hypoxic conditions. J Invest Dermatol. 1996;106:187–93.
40. Stanley AC, Park HY, Phillips TJ, Russakovsky V, Menzoian JO. Reduced growth of dermal fibroblasts from chronic venous ulcers can be stimulated with growth factors. J Vasc Surg. 1997;26:994–9; discussion 999–1001
41. Mendez MV, Stanley A, Park H-Y, Shon K, Phillips T, Menzoian JO. Fibroblasts cultured from venous ulcers display cellular characteristics of senescence. J Vasc Surg. 1998;28:876–83.
42. Stanley AC, Fernandez NN, Lounsbury KM, Corrow K, Osler T, Healey C, et al. Pressure-induced cellular senescence: a mechanism linking venous hypertension to venous ulcers. J Surg Res. 2005;124:112–7.
43. Hasan A, Murata H, Falabella A, Ochoa S, Zhou L, Badiavas E, et al. Dermal fibroblasts from venous ulcers are unresponsive to the action of transforming growth factor-β 11. J Dermatol Sci. 1997;16:59–66.
44. Kim B-C, Kim HT, Park SH, Cha J-S, Yufit T, Kim S-J, et al. Fibroblasts from chronic wounds show altered TGF-beta-signaling and decreased TGF-beta type II receptor expression. J Cell Physiol. 2003;195:331–6.
45. Agren MS, Steenfos HH, Dabelsteen S, Hansen JB, Dabelsteen E. Proliferation and mitogenic response to PDGF-BB of fibroblasts isolated from chronic venous leg ulcers is ulcer-age dependent. J Invest Dermatol. 1999;112:463–9.

46. Frykberg RG, Banks J. Challenges in the treatment of chronic wounds. Adv Wound Care. 2015;4:560–82.
47. Burnand KG, Layer GT. Graduated elastic stockings. Br Med J Clin Res Ed. 1986;293:224–5.
48. O'Meara S, Cullum N, Nelson EA, Dumville JC. Compression for venous leg ulcers. Cochrane Database Syst Rev [Internet]. 2012 [cited 2019 Nov 24]; Available from: https://www.cochranelibrary.com/cdsr/doi/10.1002/14651858.CD000265.pub3/full.
49. Shenoy MM. Prevention of venous leg ulcer recurrence. Indian Dermatol Online J. 2014;5:386–9.
50. Mayberry JC, Moneta GL, Taylor LM, Porter JM. Fifteen-year results of ambulatory compression therapy for chronic venous ulcers. Surgery. 1991;109:575–81.
51. O'Donnell TF, Balk EM. The need for an intersociety consensus guideline for venous ulcer. J Vasc Surg. 2011;54:83S–90S.
52. Norman G, Westby MJ, Rithalia AD, Stubbs N, Soares MO, Dumville JC. Dressings and topical agents for treating venous leg ulcers. Cochrane Database Syst Rev [Internet]. 2018 [cited 2019 Nov 24]; Available from: https://www.cochranelibrary.com/cdsr/doi/10.1002/14651858.CD012583.pub2/full.
53. Falanga V, Margolis D, Alvarez O, Auletta M, Maggiacomo F, Altman M, et al. Rapid healing of venous ulcers and lack of clinical rejection with an allogeneic cultured human skin equivalent. Human Skin Equivalent Investigators Group. Arch Dermatol. 1998;134:293–300.
54. Harding K, Sumner M, Cardinal M. A prospective, multicentre, randomised controlled study of human fibroblast-derived dermal substitute (Dermagraft) in patients with venous leg ulcers. Int Wound J. 2013;10:132–7.
55. Mostow EN, Haraway GD, Dalsing M, Hodde JP, King D, OASIS Venus Ulcer Study Group. Effectiveness of an extracellular matrix graft (OASIS wound matrix) in the treatment of chronic leg ulcers: a randomized clinical trial. J Vasc Surg. 2005;41:837–43.
56. Knighton DR, Ciresi K, Fiegel VD, Schumerth S, Butler E, Cerra F. Stimulation of repair in chronic, nonhealing, cutaneous ulcers using platelet-derived wound healing formula. Surg Gynecol Obstet. 1990;170:56–60.
57. Smiell JM, Wieman TJ, Steed DL, Perry BH, Sampson AR, Schwab BH. Efficacy and safety of becaplermin (recombinant human platelet-derived growth factor-BB) in patients with non-healing, lower extremity diabetic ulcers: a combined analysis of four randomized studies. Wound Repair Regen Off Publ Wound Heal Soc Eur Tissue Repair Soc. 1999;7:335–46.
58. Papanas N, Maltezos E. Benefit-risk assessment of becaplermin in the treatment of diabetic foot ulcers. Drug Saf. 2010;33:455–61.
59. Kosaric N, Kiwanuka H, Gurtner GC. Stem cell therapies for wound healing. Expert Opin Biol Ther. 2019;19:575–85.
60. O'Donnell TF, Passman MA, Marston WA, Ennis WJ, Dalsing M, Kistner RL, et al. Management of venous leg ulcers: clinical practice guidelines of the Society for Vascular Surgery® and the American venous forum. J Vasc Surg. 2014;60:3S–59S.
61. Barwell JR, Davies CE, Deacon J, Harvey K, Minor J, Sassano A, et al. Comparison of surgery and compression with compression alone in chronic venous ulceration (ESCHAR study): randomised controlled trial. Lancet Lond Engl. 2004;363:1854–9.
62. Gohel MS, Barwell JR, Taylor M, Chant T, Foy C, Earnshaw JJ, et al. Long term results of compression therapy alone versus compression plus surgery in chronic venous ulceration (ESCHAR): randomised controlled trial. BMJ. 2007;335:83.
63. Harlander-Locke M, Lawrence PF, Alktaifi A, Jimenez JC, Rigberg D, DeRubertis B. The impact of ablation of incompetent superficial and perforator veins on ulcer healing rates. J Vasc Surg. 2012;55:458–64.
64. Harlander-Locke M, Lawrence P, Jimenez JC, Rigberg D, DeRubertis B, Gelabert H. Combined treatment with compression therapy and ablation of incompetent superficial and perforating veins reduces ulcer recurrence in patients with CEAP 5 venous disease. J Vasc Surg. 2012;55:446–50.
65. Behr B, Ko SH, Wong VW, Gurtner GC, Longaker MT. Stem cells. Plast Reconstr Surg. 2010;126:1163–71.

66. Duscher D, Barrera J, Wong VW, Maan ZN, Whittam AJ, Januszyk M, et al. Stem cells in wound healing: the future of regenerative medicine? A mini-review. Gerontology. 2016;62:216–25.
67. Odorico JS, Kaufman DS, Thomson JA. Multilineage differentiation from human embryonic stem cell lines. Stem Cells Dayt Ohio. 2001;19:193–204.
68. Guenou H, Nissan X, Larcher F, Feteira J, Lemaitre G, Saidani M, et al. Human embryonic stem-cell derivatives for full reconstruction of the pluristratified epidermis: a preclinical study. Lancet Lond Engl. 2009;374:1745–53.
69. Lo B, Parham L. Ethical issues in stem cell research. Endocr Rev. 2009;30:204–13.
70. Wu DC, Boyd AS, Wood KJ. Embryonic stem cell transplantation: potential applicability in cell replacement therapy and regenerative medicine. Front Biosci J Virtual Libr. 2007;12:4525–35.
71. Takahashi K, Yamanaka S. Induction of pluripotent stem cells from mouse embryonic and adult fibroblast cultures by defined factors. Cell. 2006;126:663–76.
72. Guha P, Morgan JW, Mostoslavsky G, Rodrigues NP, Boyd AS. Lack of immune response to differentiated cells derived from syngeneic induced pluripotent stem cells. Cell Stem Cell. 2013;12:407–12.
73. Lu Q, Yu M, Shen C, Chen X, Feng T, Yao Y, et al. Negligible Immunogenicity of Induced Pluripotent Stem Cells Derived from Human Skin Fibroblasts. PLoS ONE [Internet]. 2014 [cited 2019 Oct 22];9. Available from: https://www.ncbi.nlm.nih.gov/pmc/articles/PMC4263724/.
74. Gorecka J, Kostiuk V, Fereydooni A, Gonzalez L, Luo J, Dash B, et al. The potential and limitations of induced pluripotent stem cells to achieve wound healing. Stem Cell Res Ther [Internet]. 2019 [cited 2019 Oct 22];10. Available from: https://www.ncbi.nlm.nih.gov/pmc/articles/PMC6416973/.
75. Sugiyama-Nakagiri Y, Fujimura T, Moriwaki S. Induction of skin-derived precursor cells from human induced pluripotent stem cells. PLoS One. 2016;11:e0168451.
76. Hewitt KJ, Shamis Y, Hayman RB, Margvelashvili M, Dong S, Carlson MW, et al. Epigenetic and phenotypic profile of fibroblasts derived from induced pluripotent stem cells. PLoS One. 2011;6:e17128.
77. Ohta S, Imaizumi Y, Okada Y, Akamatsu W, Kuwahara R, Ohyama M, et al. Generation of human melanocytes from induced pluripotent stem cells. PLoS One. 2011;6:e16182.
78. Bilousova G, Chen J, Roop DR. Differentiation of mouse induced pluripotent stem cells into a multipotent keratinocyte lineage. J Invest Dermatol. 2011;131:857–64.
79. Veraitch O, Mabuchi Y, Matsuzaki Y, Sasaki T, Okuno H, Tsukashima A, et al. Induction of hair follicle dermal papilla cell properties in human induced pluripotent stem cell-derived multipotent LNGFR(+)THY-1(+) mesenchymal cells. Sci Rep. 2017;7:42777.
80. Itoh M, Kiuru M, Cairo MS, Christiano AM. Generation of keratinocytes from normal and recessive dystrophic epidermolysis bullosa-induced pluripotent stem cells. Proc Natl Acad Sci U S A. 2011;108:8797–802.
81. Clayton ZE, Tan RP, Miravet MM, Lennartsson K, Cooke JP, Bursill CA, et al. Induced pluripotent stem cell-derived endothelial cells promote angiogenesis and accelerate wound closure in a murine excisional wound healing model. Biosci Rep. 2018;38
82. Kim KL, Song S-H, Choi K-S, Suh W. Cooperation of endothelial and smooth muscle cells derived from human induced pluripotent stem cells enhances neovascularization in dermal wounds. Tissue Eng Part A. 2013;19:2478–85.
83. Gutierrez-Aranda I, Ramos-Mejia V, Bueno C, Munoz-Lopez M, Real PJ, Mácia A, et al. Human induced pluripotent stem cells develop teratoma more efficiently and faster than human embryonic stem cells regardless the site of injection. Stem Cells Dayt Ohio. 2010;28:1568–70.
84. Baraniak PR, McDevitt TC. Stem cell paracrine actions and tissue regeneration. Regen Med. 2010;5:121–43.

85. Maxson S, Lopez EA, Yoo D, Danilkovitch-Miagkova A, Leroux MA. Concise review: role of mesenchymal stem cells in wound repair. Stem Cells Transl Med. 2012;1:142–9.
86. Hocking AM, Gibran NS. Mesenchymal stem cells: paracrine signaling and differentiation during cutaneous wound repair. Exp Cell Res. 2010;316:2213–9.
87. Ponte AL, Marais E, Gallay N, Langonné A, Delorme B, Hérault O, et al. The in vitro migration capacity of human bone marrow mesenchymal stem cells: comparison of chemokine and growth factor chemotactic activities. Stem Cells Dayt Ohio. 2007;25:1737–45.
88. Ishii G, Sangai T, Sugiyama K, Ito T, Hasebe T, Endoh Y, et al. In vivo characterization of bone marrow-derived fibroblasts recruited into fibrotic lesions. Stem Cells Dayt Ohio. 2005;23:699–706.
89. Aggarwal S, Pittenger MF. Human mesenchymal stem cells modulate allogeneic immune cell responses. Blood. 2005;105:1815–22.
90. Meirelles L d S, Fontes AM, Covas DT, Caplan AI. Mechanisms involved in the therapeutic properties of mesenchymal stem cells. Cytokine Growth Factor Rev. 2009;20:419–27.
91. Zhang Q-Z, Su W-R, Shi S-H, Wilder-Smith P, Xiang AP, Wong A, et al. Human gingiva-derived mesenchymal stem cells elicit polarization of m2 macrophages and enhance cutaneous wound healing. Stem Cells Dayt Ohio. 2010;28:1856–68.
92. Krasnodembskaya A, Song Y, Fang X, Gupta N, Serikov V, Lee J-W, et al. Antibacterial effect of human mesenchymal stem cells is mediated in part from secretion of the antimicrobial peptide LL-37. Stem Cells Dayt Ohio. 2010;28:2229–38.
93. Mei SHJ, Haitsma JJ, Dos Santos CC, Deng Y, Lai PFH, Slutsky AS, et al. Mesenchymal stem cells reduce inflammation while enhancing bacterial clearance and improving survival in sepsis. Am J Respir Crit Care Med. 2010;182:1047–57.
94. Chen L, Tredget EE, Wu PYG, Wu Y. Paracrine factors of mesenchymal stem cells recruit macrophages and endothelial lineage cells and enhance wound healing. PLoS One. [Internet]. 2008. [cited 2019 Oct 27];3. Available from: https://www.ncbi.nlm.nih.gov/pmc/articles/PMC2270908/.
95. Smith AN, Willis E, Chan VT, Muffley LA, Isik FF, Gibran NS, et al. Mesenchymal stem cells induce dermal fibroblast responses to injury. Exp Cell Res. 2010;316:48–54.
96. Wu Y, Chen L, Scott PG, Tredget EE. Mesenchymal stem cells enhance wound healing through differentiation and angiogenesis. Stem Cells Dayt Ohio. 2007;25:2648–59.
97. Badiavas EV, Falanga V. Treatment of chronic wounds with bone marrow-derived cells. Arch Dermatol. 2003;139:510–6.
98. Yoshikawa T, Mitsuno H, Nonaka I, Sen Y, Kawanishi K, Inada Y, et al. Wound therapy by marrow mesenchymal cell transplantation. Plast Reconstr Surg. 2008;121:860–77.
99. Falanga V, Iwamoto S, Chartier M, Yufit T, Butmarc J, Kouttab N, et al. Autologous bone marrow-derived cultured mesenchymal stem cells delivered in a fibrin spray accelerate healing in murine and human cutaneous wounds. Tissue Eng. 2007;13:1299–312.
100. Hu MS, Borrelli MR, Lorenz HP, Longaker MT, Wan DC. Mesenchymal stromal cells and cutaneous wound healing: a comprehensive review of the background, role, and therapeutic potential [internet]. Stem Cells Int. 2018; [cited 2019 Nov 1]. Available from: https://www.hindawi.com/journals/sci/2018/6901983/.
101. Mohamed-Ahmed S, Fristad I, Lie SA, Suliman S, Mustafa K, Vindenes H, et al. Adipose-derived and bone marrow mesenchymal stem cells: a donor-matched comparison. Stem Cell Res Ther. 2018;9:168.
102. Bieback K, Brinkmann I. Mesenchymal stromal cells from human perinatal tissues: from biology to cell therapy. World J Stem Cells. 2010;2:81–92.
103. Tsuji W, Rubin JP, Marra KG. Adipose-derived stem cells: implications in tissue regeneration. World J Stem Cells. 2014;6:312–21.
104. De Ugarte DA, Morizono K, Elbarbary A, Alfonso Z, Zuk PA, Zhu M, et al. Comparison of multi-lineage cells from human adipose tissue and bone marrow. Cells Tissues Organs. 2003;174:101–9.

105. Hassanshahi A, Hassanshahi M, Khabbazi S, Hosseini-Khah Z, Peymanfar Y, Ghalamkari S, et al. Adipose-derived stem cells for wound healing. J Cell Physiol. 2019;234:7903–14.
106. Bertozzi N, Simonacci F, Grieco MP, Grignaffini E, Raposio E. The biological and clinical basis for the use of adipose-derived stem cells in the field of wound healing. Ann Med Surg. 2017;20:41–8.
107. Holm JS, Toyserkani NM, Sorensen JA. Adipose-derived stem cells for treatment of chronic ulcers: current status. Stem Cell Res Ther. 2018;9:142.
108. Garg RK, Rennert RC, Duscher D, Sorkin M, Kosaraju R, Auerbach LJ, et al. Capillary force seeding of hydrogels for adipose-derived stem cell delivery in wounds. Stem Cells Transl Med. 2014;3:1079–89.
109. Zografou A, Papadopoulos O, Tsigris C, Kavantzas N, Michalopoulos E, Chatzistamatiou T, et al. Autologous transplantation of adipose-derived stem cells enhances skin graft survival and wound healing in diabetic rats. Ann Plast Surg. 2013;71:225–32.
110. Konstantinow A, Arnold A, Djabali K, Kempf W, Gutermuth J, Fischer T, et al. Therapy of ulcus cruris of venous and mixed venous arterial origin with autologous, adult, native progenitor cells from subcutaneous adipose tissue: a prospective clinical pilot study. J Eur Acad Dermatol Venereol JEADV. 2017;31:2104–18.
111. Kavala AA, Turkyilmaz S. Autogenously derived regenerative cell therapy for venous leg ulcers. Arch Med Sci Atheroscler Dis. 2018;3:e156–63.
112. Koizumi NJ, Inatomi TJ, Sotozono CJ, Fullwood NJ, Quantock AJ, Kinoshita S. Growth factor mRNA and protein in preserved human amniotic membrane. Curr Eye Res. 2000;20:173–7.
113. Davis JS II. Skin grafting at the Johns Hopkins Hospital. Ann Surg. 1909;50:542–9.
114. Stern M. The grafting of preserved amniotic membrane to burned and ulcerated surfaces, substituting skin grafts: a preliminary report. J Am Med Assoc. 1913;60:973–4.
115. Sabella N. Use of the fetal membranes in skin grafting. Med Rec 1866-1922. 1913;83:478–80.
116. Denkewalter FR. Ambulatory treatment of varicose leg ulcers with fresh placental dressings. AMA Arch Surg. 1957;74:316–21.
117. Pourmoussa A, Gardner DJ, Johnson MB, Wong AK. An update and review of cell-based wound dressings and their integration into clinical practice. Ann Transl Med. [Internet]. 2016. [cited 2019 Nov 25];4. Available from: http://atm.amegroups.com/article/view/12913
118. Mermet I, Pottier N, Sainthillier JM, Malugani C, Cairey-Remonnay S, Maddens S, et al. Use of amniotic membrane transplantation in the treatment of venous leg ulcers. Wound Repair Regen Off Publ Wound Heal Soc Eur Tissue Repair Soc. 2007;15:459–64.
119. Francis J, Shajimon CR, Bhat AK, Kanakambaran B. Use of amnion transfer in resistant nonhealing venous leg ulcers. Indian J Surg. 2015;77:457–62.
120. Farivar BS, Toursavadkohi S, Monahan TS, Sharma J, Ucuzian AA, Kundi R, et al. Prospective study of cryopreserved placental tissue wound matrix in the management of chronic venous leg ulcers. J Vasc Surg Venous Lymphat Disord. 2019;7:228–33.
121. Bianchi C, Cazzell S, Vayser D, Reyzelman AM, Dosluoglu H, Tovmassian G, et al. A multicentre randomised controlled trial evaluating the efficacy of dehydrated human amnion/ chorion membrane (EpiFix®) allograft for the treatment of venous leg ulcers. Int Wound J. 2018;15:114–22.
122. Marędziak M, Marycz K, Tomaszewski KA, Kornicka K, Henry BM. The influence of aging on the regenerative potential of human adipose derived mesenchymal stem cells [internet]. Stem Cells Int. 2016; [cited 2019 Nov 5]. Available from: https://www.hindawi.com/journals/sci/2016/2152435/abs/.
123. Zaim M, Karaman S, Cetin G, Isik S. Donor age and long-term culture affect differentiation and proliferation of human bone marrow mesenchymal stem cells. Ann Hematol. 2012;91:1175–86.
124. De Barros S, Dehez S, Arnaud E, Barreau C, Cazavet A, Perez G, et al. Aging-related decrease of human ASC angiogenic potential is reversed by hypoxia preconditioning through ROS production. Mol Ther J Am Soc Gene Ther. 2013;21:399–408.
125. Duscher D, Rennert RC, Januszyk M, Anghel E, Maan ZN, Whittam AJ, et al. Aging disrupts cell subpopulation dynamics and diminishes the function of mesenchymal stem cells. Sci

Rep. [Internet]. 2014. [cited 2019 Nov 5];4. Available from: https://www.ncbi.nlm.nih.gov/pmc/articles/PMC4239576/.

126. Khong SML, Lee M, Kosaric N, Khong DM, Dong Y, Hopfner U, et al. Single-cell transcriptomics of human mesenchymal stem cells reveal age-related cellular subpopulation depletion and impaired regenerative function. Stem Cells. 2019;37:240–6.

127. Fijany A, Sayadi LR, Khoshab N, Banyard DA, Shaterian A, Alexander M, et al. Mesenchymal stem cell dysfunction in diabetes. Mol Biol Rep. 2019;46:1459–75.

128. Kim H, Han JW, Lee JY, Choi YJ, Sohn Y-D, Song M, et al. Diabetic mesenchymal stem cells are ineffective for improving limb ischemia due to their impaired Angiogenic capability. Cell Transplant. 2015;24:1571–84.

129. Rennert RC, Sorkin M, Januszyk M, Duscher D, Kosaraju R, Chung MT, et al. Diabetes impairs the angiogenic potential of adipose-derived stem cells by selectively depleting cellular subpopulations. Stem Cell Res Ther. 2014;5:79.

130. Madhira SL, Challa SS, Chalasani M, Nappanveethl G, Bhonde RR, Ajumeera R, et al. Promise(s) of mesenchymal stem cells as an in vitro model system to depict pre-diabetic/diabetic milieu in WNIN/GR-Ob mutant rats. PLoS One. [Internet]. 2012. [cited 2019 Nov 6];7. Available from: https://www.ncbi.nlm.nih.gov/pmc/articles/PMC3483309/

131. Noël D, Caton D, Roche S, Bony C, Lehmann S, Casteilla L, et al. Cell specific differences between human adipose-derived and mesenchymal-stromal cells despite similar differentiation potentials. Exp Cell Res. 2008;314:1575–84.

132. Panepucci RA, Siufi JLC, Silva WA, Proto-Siqueira R, Neder L, Orellana M, et al. Comparison of gene expression of umbilical cord vein and bone marrow-derived mesenchymal stem cells. Stem Cells Dayt Ohio. 2004;22:1263–78.

133. Hsieh J-Y, Wang H-W, Chang S-J, Liao K-H, Lee I-H, Lin W-S, et al. Mesenchymal stem cells from human umbilical cord express preferentially secreted factors related to neuroprotection, neurogenesis, and angiogenesis. PLoS One. [Internet]. 2013. [cited 2019 Nov 6];8. Available from: https://www.ncbi.nlm.nih.gov/pmc/articles/PMC3749979/.

134. Kim S-W, Zhang H-Z, Guo L, Kim J-M, Kim MH. Amniotic Mesenchymal stem cells enhance wound healing in diabetic NOD/SCID mice through high angiogenic and engraftment capabilities. PLoS ONE [Internet]. 2012 [cited 2019 Nov 6];7. Available from: https://www.ncbi.nlm.nih.gov/pmc/articles/PMC3398889/.

135. Liu X, Liu X, Wang Z, Wang Z, Wang R, Wang R, et al. Direct comparison of the potency of human mesenchymal stem cells derived from amnion tissue, bone marrow and adipose tissue at inducing dermal fibroblast responses to cutaneous wounds. Int J Mol Med. 2013;31:407–15.

136. Aguado BA, Mulyasasmita W, Su J, Lampe KJ, Heilshorn SC. Improving viability of stem cells during syringe needle flow through the design of hydrogel cell carriers. Tissue Eng Part A. 2012;18:806–15.

137. Rustad KC, Wong VW, Sorkin M, Glotzbach JP, Major MR, Rajadas J, et al. Enhancement of mesenchymal stem cell angiogenic capacity and stemness by a biomimetic hydrogel scaffold. Biomaterials. 2012;33:80–90.

138. Lee YS, Lim KS, Oh J-E, Yun A, Joo WS, Kim HS, et al. Development of porous PLGA/PEI1.8k biodegradable microspheres for the delivery of Mesenchymal Stem Cells (MSCs). J Control Release Off J Control Release Soc. 2015;205:128–33.

139. Guo R, Ward CL, Davidson JM, Duvall CL, Wenke JC, Guelcher SA. A transient cell shielding method for viable MSC delivery within hydrophobic scaffolds polymerized in situ. Biomaterials. 2015;54:21–33.

140. Herberg S, Shi X, Johnson MH, Hamrick MW, Isales CM, Hill WD. Stromal cell-derived factor-1β mediates cell survival through enhancing autophagy in bone marrow-derived mesenchymal stem cells. PLoS One. [Internet]. 2013. [cited 2019 Nov 7];8. Available from: https://www.ncbi.nlm.nih.gov/pmc/articles/PMC3589360/

141. HoWangYin K-Y, Loinard C, Bakker W, Guérin CL, Vilar J, D'Audigier C, et al. HIF-prolyl hydroxylase 2 inhibition enhances the efficiency of mesenchymal stem cell-based therapies for the treatment of critical limb ischemia. Stem Cells. 2014;32:231–43.

142. Marquez-Curtis LA, Gul-Uludag H, Xu P, Chen J, Janowska-Wieczorek A. CXCR4 transfection of cord blood mesenchymal stromal cells with the use of cationic liposome enhances their migration toward stromal cell-derived factor-1. Cytotherapy. 2013;15:840–9.
143. Hu C, Yong X, Li C, Lü M, Liu D, Chen L, et al. CXCL12/CXCR4 axis promotes mesenchymal stem cell mobilization to burn wounds and contributes to wound repair. J Surg Res. 2013;183:427–34.
144. Song S-H, Lee M-O, Lee J-S, Jeong H-C, Kim H-G, Kim W-S, et al. Genetic modification of human adipose-derived stem cells for promoting wound healing. J Dermatol Sci. 2012;66:98–107.
145. Kosaric N, Srifa W, Gurtner GC, Porteus MH. Abstract 100: human mesenchymal stromal cells engineered to overexpress PDGF-B using CRISPR/Cas9/rAAV6-based tools improve wound healing. Plast Reconstr Surg Glob Open. [Internet]. 2017. [cited 2019 Nov 7];5. Available from: https://www.ncbi.nlm.nih.gov/pmc/articles/PMC5417952/.

Chapter 9
Induced Pluripotent Stem Cell-Derived Vascular Smooth Muscle Cells for Vascular Regeneration

Biraja C. Dash

9.1 Introduction

Cardiovascular disease (CVD) such as atherosclerosis and critical limb ischemia remains the leading cause of mortality and morbidity across the world [1]. This led to the emergence of vascular tissue engineering research thrust with an interest in developing tissue-engineered vascular grafts (TEVGs) and microvasculature [2]. Synthetic grafts are often the first choice, as vascular conduits, to reconstruct or bypass vascular occlusion in the absence of autologous and allogenic grafts [3, 4]. However, these synthetic grafts exhibit several shortcomings such as low patency rates, higher infection, and lack of growth potential [5, 6]. Thus, there has always been a need for biological TEVGs. Since its conception in 1986, the vascular regeneration strategy is evolving from finding a choice of biomaterials and cell source to building a vascular bed [6–8]. Engineering of this microvasculature is critical for tissue regeneration, wound healing, and organ transplantation. Numerous strategies to engineer vascular bed have been accomplished and are an emerging area in the field of vascular tissue engineering [2, 9, 10].

Vascular regeneration strategies often comprise of cells and scaffolds for them to grow [11]. Recent advances in vascular regeneration have considered blood vessel components for rational scaffold design and selecting appropriate cell sources [2]. The extracellular matrix (ECM) components in large blood vessels such as arteries and veins are mainly collagen, elastin, and proteoglycans. The predominant cells found in larger blood vessels are endothelial (ECs) lining the inner layer and vascular smooth muscle cells (VSMCs) on the periphery. Microvasculatures such as small capillaries are composed of ECs and pericytes as support cells [12–14]. The vascular tissue engineering field has made many achievements including the development

B. C. Dash (✉)
Department of Surgery (Plastic Surgery), Yale School of Medicine, Yale University, New Haven, CT, USA
e-mail: biraja.dash@yale.edu

© Springer Nature Switzerland AG 2021
T. P. Navarro et al. (eds.), *Stem Cell Therapy for Vascular Diseases*,
https://doi.org/10.1007/978-3-030-56954-9_9

of novel scaffold and bioreactor systems [10, 15] and autologous adult and induced pluripotent stem cells (iPSCs) as a renewable cell source for ECs and VSMCs [16].

The VSMCs are a major component of blood vessels and support the vasculature and maintain the barrier function in the blood vessels. VSMCs have widely been used in vascular regeneration with limitations such as lack of a renewable source and an abundant number of cells [16, 17]. Current pluripotent stem cell (PSC) technology such as embryonic stem cell (ESC) and induced PSCs (iPSCs) alleviates this concern with their ability to produce any cell type of the body especially functional VSMCs in abundance [18, 19]. Furthermore, these iPSC-derived VSMCs mimic the disease phenotype by carrying disease-causing mutations. Eventually, human iPSC-derived VSMCs can be used for developing TEVGs, vascular bed, and disease models to develop personalized therapy [20–22]. This book chapter will cover briefly the technical advances in vascular regeneration and iPSC reprogramming and differentiation strategies. We will then discuss how these advances have opened the door for the application of hiPSC-VSMCs in regenerative therapy, disease modeling, and drug screening.

9.2   Vascular Regeneration Strategies

Functional blood vessels categorized as arteries, arterioles, capillaries, venules, and veins perform the essential job of delivering oxygen and nutrients to various parts of the body. A typical blood vessel consists of an inner lining of ECs supported by pericytes and VSMCs. These cells in the blood vessels play an important role not only in maintaining a barrier for pathogens but also in many other physiological processes [23]. Numerous studies on vascular development and vascular disease pathophysiology form a blueprint for vessel engineering [11]. Vascular regeneration is critical for the success of organ and tissue transplantation efforts and first consolidated as a field around the goal of developing vascular graft replacements for individual vessels [2]. With the discovery of first TEVG by Weinberg and Bell in 1986, the field is evolving (Fig. 9.1) toward the creation of complex vascular networks [15, 24].

9.2.1   Tissue-Engineered Vascular Grafts

Since the discovery of the first TEVG [24], substantial effort has been made to improve mechanical and biological properties comparable to artery and vein. The desirable characteristics of a TEVG are i) higher mechanical strength to support the hemodynamics of arterial flow and withstand long-term implantation, ii) improved potency without inflammatory and/or immunogenic response, and iii) ability to remodel, repair, and integrate into the host. Most importantly, the holy grail is to

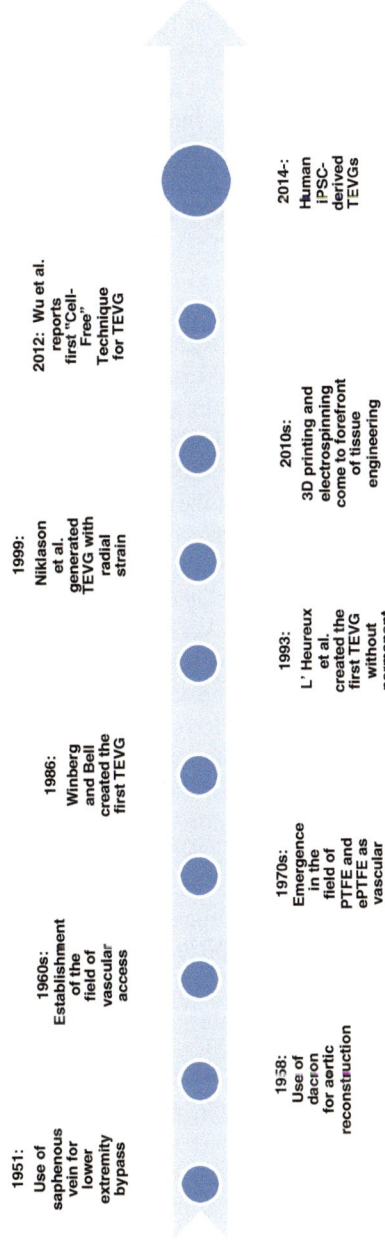

Fig. 9.1 A schematic showing evolution of tissue-engineered vascular grafts

develop technology that can generate a readily available, large scale of patient-specific TEVGs [15, 25–29].

TEVGs, based on their fabrication method, can be divided into two categories i) scaffold-based and ii) scaffold-free [15]. The scaffold-based method involves the use of a biodegradable biomaterial in a tubular form to support cell growth. These scaffolds are generally produced either using synthetic polymers such as polyglycolic acid (PGA) or natural biopolymers fibrin and collagen. Niklason and Langer used tubular PGA and bovine VSMCs in a bioreactor for 8 weeks to develop a robust TEVG. PGA being biodegradable degrades by the end of 8 weeks and leaves the cellular TEVGs with dense collagen matrix [25]. Similarly, collagen and fibrin are widely utilized for the fabrication of TEVGs [26, 28–30]. On the other hand, the cell-free method has been used to develop TEBVs without the use of a biomaterial. L'Heureux et al. first reported a cell sheet-based TEVG [27]. In this method, VSMCs and fibroblasts were cultured for a month to form the cell sheets. The cell sheets were then peeled off and wrapped around a mandrel, followed by their culture in a bioreactor for 8 weeks to produce the TEVGs. The TEVGs were mechanically robust with ECM content such as collagen. In addition to this strategy, a vascular ring method was used to form TEVGs [31]. VSMCs-based rings were fabricated using an agarose mold. The VSMCs self-assemble around the agarose pillar to form a ring structure and secrete collagen to form the ECM of the rings in static culture. Several rings were joined together to form a TEVG but with poor mechanical strength [31].

In addition to finding the right biomaterial, the choice of a renewable cell source is crucial for the fabrication of TEVGs [16]. VSMCs, fibroblast, and ECs are major cell types that have been explored for the last few decades [25, 26, 32]. These cells remain in culture for 8–24 weeks and undergo 45–60 population doublings to form the TEBV [33]. The cells generated from elderly patients will either dedifferentiate or undergo apoptosis within 10–15 PDs resulting in poor ECM secretion and eventually resulting in weak TEVGs [33]. It is difficult to generate robust TEVGs with adequate mechanical strength using older cells. Thus, success is dependent on the source and age of the donors [34–36]. Mesenchymal stem cells (MSCs) are the other cell type that is explored. Andreadis and colleagues successfully derived VSMCs using MSCs and used in fibrin hydrogel to form TEVGs [37]. In another study, Niklason and colleagues used human bone marrow-derived MSCs to form the TEVGs [38]. Adipose-derived stem cells (ASCs) have also been pursued as an attractive cell source for vascular regeneration. Wang et al. successfully engineered small-diameter vessels utilizing human ASCs-derived VSMCs [39]. In another instance, Andreadis and colleagues generated VSMCs from hair follicle stem cells to develop TEVGs [40–42]. Although MSCs, ASCs, and hair follicle stem cells show their potential to generate VSMCs and TEVGs, none of these studies resulted in robust TEVGs comparable to human arteries or veins. ESCs and iPSCs are emerging as an alternative source of VSMCs and discussed in detail in this book chapter.

9.2.2 Engineered Microvasculature

Fabrication strategy for engineering a network of vessels is different than that of fabricating a single vessel. The technique is heavily dependent on a biomaterial with cell-specific regenerative cues. In addition to promoting microvasculature, these cues often provide support and maintain the network both in vitro and in vivo [9, 10]. Natural polymers such as fibrin, a proangiogenic biomaterial, have been widely used to engineer vasculature [43]. Other naturally derived materials such as collagen, hyaluronic acid, dextran, agarose, gelatin, and silk protein [44–47] were seen to support a vascular bed formation. Synthetic materials are not the best choice of material as they need additional ligands to support vessel formation. In one of the reports, Cuchiara et al. engineered a modified polyethylene glycol (PEG)-based hydrogel system to support prevascularization [48].

The approaches to generate this microvasculature can be divided into two categories, (i) top-down and (ii) bottom-up [2]. In the top-down approach, the geometry and architecture of the vascular bed are predesigned and pre-fabricated before the vascular cells are seeded. However, in the bottom-up setting, the vascular cells are encouraged to mimic physiological mechanisms for the new vessel formation via angiogenesis or vasculogenesis. The top-down approach use 3D printing [49], laser degradation [50], and layer-by-layer fabrication [51] methods to incorporate the desired architecture. The bottom-up approach works through providing a chemical gradient such as proangiogenic factors chemoattractant protein-1 (MCP-1), vascular endothelial cell growth factor (VEGF), basic fibroblast growth factor (bFGF), stromal cell-derived growth factor (SDF)-1α, phorbol 12-myristate 13-acetate (PMA), and sphingosine-1-phosphate (S1P) and fluid shear stress [52–55]. In addition to chemical and mechanical stimuli, low oxygen tension also aids to the vascularization through the regulation of hypoxia-inducible factor (HIF) in vascular cells [55–57].

Engineering a realistic microvasculature requires cellular components such as ECs, pericytes, and VSMCs. EC is the major cell type that is used for forming a microvasculature, while fibroblasts, pericytes, or MSCs are co-cultured as support cells to accelerate vascularization and to prolong the stability of this resulting microvasculature [52, 58–61]. Perivascular cells like VSMCs or pericytes when co-cultured with ECs regulate vascular barrier function, integrity, and stability through paracrine and adhesive interactions [62]. An array of stem cell technologies such as ESC, iPSC, MSC, ASC, umbilical cord-derived stem cells, and hemangioblasts have evolved as potential sources for these ECs and perivascular cells [2, 11]. Although these new stem cell sources for perivascular cells have made it possible to move beyond primary cell culture, their success is dependent upon further investigation.

9.3   Induced Pluripotent Stem Cells: A Renewable Source of VSMCs

9.3.1   Methods for Reprogramming

Takahashi and Yamanaka reprogrammed fibroblast cells with the induction of pluripotency-related genes Oct4, Klf4, Sox2, and c-Myc [63]. This study published in 2006 formed a firm ground for today's iPSC technology. The iPSCs have the potential to differentiate into any cell type of interest similar to ESCs without any ethical concern. Since its initial discovery, there is a lot of progress made in reprogramming and differentiation methods, and regenerative therapy [64], disease modeling, and drug screening [65, 66].

The iPSCs were initially reprogrammed using retroviruses as a method of inducing the pluripotent genes [63, 67, 68]. This use of retroviruses comes with the risk of tumor formation and transgene activation [69]. Since its initial discovery, the technology has advanced toward achieving a better reprogramming efficiency and safety [65, 68]. Many of these reprogramming methods involve the use of episomal plasmids, minicircle vectors, and transient adenoviral expression to achieve integration-free iPSCs [70–74]. These iPSCs are safer than the earlier retroviral ones but with low reprogramming efficiency. Several other reprogramming methods use safer and more efficient Cre/LoxP system [75] or PiggyBac transposons [76], Sendai viruses, direct delivery of RNA [77], miRNA [78], small molecules [79], and cell-permeable proteins to achieve integration-free iPSCs [18, 80]. As of now, protein- and RNA-based methods are considered safer and efficient means for reprogramming [79].

9.3.2   VSMC Differentiation Method

Differentiation protocols to generate VSMCs have been designed using both ESCs and iPSCs. The differentiation protocol can be broadly classified into the embryoid body (EB) and monolayer methods irrespective of the stem cell source (ESC or iPSC) [18]. The protocols are further altered using a combination of growth factors and small molecules to achieve VSMCs of specific lineages such as mesoderm and neural crest and have huge implications on their differentiation efficiency and application [20]. Once differentiated the VSMCs are characterized for purity and functionality by evaluating their morphology, cellular markers, contractility, and calcium transients (Fig. 9.2).

9.3.3   Embryoid Body Method

The EB method mimics early embryonic development and generates VSMCs from all three different lineages including mesoderm [19]. Initial EB differentiation protocol generated cells from cardiovascular progenitor fate followed by enrichment of

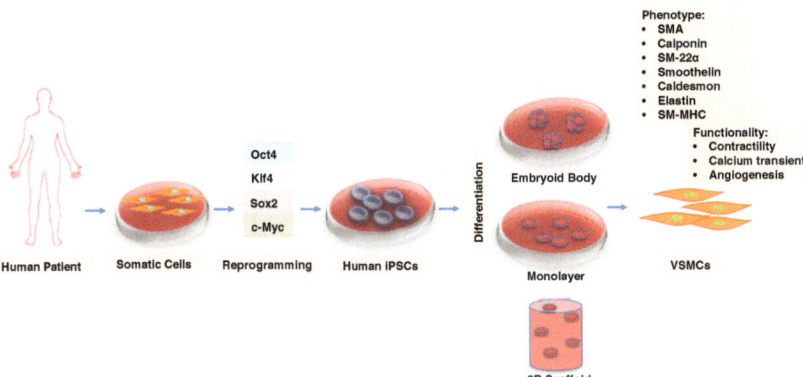

Fig. 9.2 A schematic illustrating existing VSMC differentiation methods

hiPSC-derived VSMCs using FACS sorting [19, 21]. In one of the reports, iPSCs were generated using human aortic vascular smooth muscle cells (HASMCs). The iPSCs were then differentiated back to VSMCs using an EB method. The differentiated cell population expressed VSMC genes and exhibited contractility similar to HASMCs [81]. However, the method resulted in VSMCs with a residual expression of lentiviral transgenes and low differentiation efficiency suggesting an incomplete commitment to the VSMC phenotype [21, 81].

In another protocol, Ge et al. cultured EBs in suspension followed by culturing them on gelatin-coated plates in an EB differentiation medium (10% FBS, 1% non-essential amino acids, 0.1 mmol/L β-mercaptoethanol, and 1% L-glutamine). Finally, the cells were cultured in a smooth muscle-specific SmGM-2 medium on Matrigel-coated plates. The cells were found positive for smooth muscle α-actin (SMA) and calponin [82]. A modification to this method was reported to scale up the production. In this method, Dash et al. used iPSC from feeder-free culture. EBs were initially cultured in mTeSR medium and various ratios of mTeSR and EB differentiation medium. The protocol followed similar steps afterward and generated as many as 40 million cells in 15 days [83]. The VSMCs were of synthetic phenotype and were positive for early VSMC markers including SMA, calponin, and SM-22α. The cells under low serum and high TGF-β1 culture conditions developed into mature phenotype as shown by their staining with mature markers smooth muscle myosin heavy chain (SM-MHC) and elastin. The resulting VSMCs were contractile in response to agonists carbachol and KCl. This most important output of this method was its scalability without the need for any enrichment step. Furthermore, the cells mimic the properties of VSMCs from the lateral plate mesoderm lineage [83]. To produce clinically relevant VSMCs, a serum-free, the chemically defined medium (CDM) was used to grow the EBs and differentiated VSMCs. The method yielded VSMCs within 28 days of EB formation and maintenance of the VSMC phenotype needed VEGF and bFGF [84]. While this method could be used to generate GMP-grade VSMCs, the scalability of this method should further be investigated.

9.3.4   Monolayer Method

The monolayer method of differentiation circumvents major limitations of the EB-based methods such as (i) heterogeneous cell population, (ii) serum-dependent differentiation, and (iii) lengthy differentiation time [18]. The monolayer method uses feeder-free hiPSC and generates VSMCs from mesoderm or neural crest lineage [18, 21]. Briefly, the hiPSCs are grown under the feeder-free condition as single cells. This step is followed by the use of growth factors and small molecules or combinations to differentiate the naïve hiPSCs toward mesodermal or neural crest fate. These intermediate cells are then cultured under pro-VSMC growth factors PDGF-BB and TGF-β1 to achieve final differentiation into VSMCs [20].

In one such study, Cao et al. used CDM with bone morphogenetic protein 4 (BMP4), glycogen synthase kinase 3 (GSK3) inhibitor CHIR99021, and ascorbic acid to generate mesodermal cardiovascular progenitor cells (CVPCs) from hESCs and hiPSCs [85]. The CVPCs were then cultured under PDGF-BB and TGF-β1 to differentiate into VSMCs with phenotype and functionality similar to HASMCs [85]. CD34+ progenitor cells were another source of progenitor cells that were used to produce VSMCs. In this study, hiPSCs were differentiated into CD34+ progenitor cells by combined modulation of two signaling pathways mitogen-activated protein kinase (MAPK) extracellular signal-regulated protein kinase (MEK)/extracellular signal-regulated kinase (ERK) signaling and bone morphogenetic protein 4 (BMP4) signaling [86]. These progenitor cells were then cultured under PDGF-BB and bFGF until their final differentiation to functional VSMCs [86]. Gerecht and colleagues seeded hiPSCs on collagen IV-coated plates and supplemented with PDGF-BB and TGF-β1 for final VSMC differentiation. 98% of the cells were positive for SMA, calponin, and SM22 and 50% positive for SM-MHC. The method could generate both synthetic and contractile VSMCs [87].

The method by Sinha and colleagues took the leap from the existing methods and differentiated hiPSCs into developmental origin-specific VSMC subtypes. Briefly, they grew hiPSCs on a feeder-free condition in CDM and differentiated them toward intermediate cell populations with combinations of small molecules and growth factors such as neuroectoderm (SB431542/FGF2), lateral plate mesoderm (FGF2/BMP4), and paraxial mesoderm (FGF2/LY294002) lineages. These intermediate cell populations were then spiked with PDGF-BB and TGF-β1 to produce a pure population of functional VSMCs. This method generates a range of VSMC subtypes that have potentials in disease modeling and vascular tissue engineering [88]. Patsch et al. developed a two-step protocol to efficiently differentiate VSMCs from hiPSC within a short duration of time. In the first step, vascular progenitor cells were produced from hiPSC using a cocktail of key growth factors BMP4/FGF2/VEGF followed by culturing these cells on collagen IV-coated dishes on the second step [89]. This was a rapid and efficient protocol with an ability to generate 99% of pure VSMCs within 6 days.

Transient cell populations like neural crest cells and MSCs have been explored in differentiating VSMCs from hiPSCs. Menendez et al. manipulated the Wnt signaling and SMAD pathway using small molecules to get multipotent NCSCs. The method generated a pure population of NCSCs and was used to derive VSMCs [90]. Similarly, MSCs generated from hiPSCs were used to derive VSMCs. This multi-step method generates synthetic VSMCs with a high proliferation rate. The first stage of the differentiation protocol yields multipotent MSCs, and these MSCs were then treated with a combination of TGF-β1 and heparin to differentiate into VSMCs expressing SMA, SM-MHC, calponin, and caldesmon [91].

Alternative methods of generating VSMCs include direct differentiation of somatic cells to VSMCs. Karamariti et al. used human embryonic lung fibroblast cells and performed direct differentiation using Yamanaka factors to generate partially induced pluripotent stem cells (PiPS). These PiPS were cultured on a collagen IV plate and VSMC differentiation medium, generated functional PiPS-SMCs with 42.5% calponin$^+$ and 38% SM22α^+ [92]. This method has the potential to reduce the risks of the tumorigenic effects of iPSCs.

9.3.5   3D Scaffold Method

Recently a 3D method has been reported to generate a large scale of hiPSC-VSMCs. The method used alginate hydrogel microtubes to provide the cells with a suitable environment for differentiation. The VSMCs were generated in 10 days and exhibited contractility and the ability to form vasculature along with ECs. The method used differentiation protocol developed by Patsch et al. and an alginate hydrogel tubes to generate VSMCs with high purity and abundance. Furthermore, transcriptome analysis of these VSMCs showed an enhancement in proangiogenic gene expression [93].

9.4   iPSC-VSMC and Vascular Regeneration

iPSC technology brings a renewable cell source, scalability, and efficiency to regenerative therapies [18, 20, 83, 94]. iPSC-derived TEVGs and microvasculature thus are promising strategies for CVD [15]. However, the success of these iPSC-derived vessels is dependent upon their ability to maintain robust mechanical properties with reduced thrombogenic and immunogenic risks and anastomosis with the host vessel in addition to maintaining their survival and phenotype [15, 16].

9.4.1   Tissue-Engineered Vascular Grafts

Toward this goal, several attempts were made to engineer TEVGs using iPSC-VSMCs. Hibino et al. were the first one to report the use of iPSC-VSMCs in generating an implantable TEVGs [95]. They made a cell sheet using mouse iPSC-derived

ECs and VSMCs. The sheet was then placed on the top of a biodegradable scaffold composed of polyglycolic acid (PGA)-poly-l-lactide and poly(L-lactide-co-ε-caprolactone). This TEVG with an internal diameter of 0.8 mm was then implanted as an interposition graft in the inferior vena cava in an immunodeficient mice model. The TEVGs remained patent, and all the animals survived 10 weeks post-implantation with no thrombosis, aneurysm formation, graft rupture, or calcification. Histological evaluation of the graft suggested neotissue formation with ECs and VSMCs migration. However, the survival of implanted iPSC-vascular cells was negatively affected [95]. In another study, Xie et al. seeded iPSC-VSMCs on a nanofibrous, poly(L-lactide) scaffolds and implanted the grafts subcutaneously in nude mice [96]. The implanted cells maintained VSMC phenotypes and were positive for myocardin and SM22α but were negative for smoothelin and SM-MHC showing incomplete iPSC differentiation [96]. Similarly, Wang et al. used iPSC-derived VSMCs and poly(L-lactide) nanofibrous scaffolds to fabricate the TEVG. The TEVGs were then implanted into nude mice for 2 weeks. The implanted TEVGs maintained the phenotype and deposited collagen on the matrix [97]. A significant improvement was made when Karamiriti et al. [92] used PiPS to derive ECs and VSMCs. These cells were seeded on decellularized vascular grafts. This method resulted in a functional TEVG similar to the mouse artery. The TEVGs, when transplanted into nude mice, showed effective grafting and successful anastomosis in the host [92].

Few reports suggested the use of intermediate cells CVPCs and MSCs in generating vascular grafts. Hu et al. generated integration-free iPSC-VSMCs from human peripheral blood mononuclear cells and differentiated them into CVPCs via a mesodermal intermediate [98]. The CVPCs were then seeded onto fibronectin-coated nanofibrous poly(L-lactide) scaffolds and subcutaneously implanted into nude mice. Histological analysis after 14 days post-implantation revealed uniform cell growth in the scaffold, collagen deposition, and no tumor formation [98]. Similarly, Sundaram et al. derived MSCs from hiPSC using CDM. The MSCs were then seeded onto tubular PGA scaffolds and grown under pulsatile culture conditions in a bioreactor for 8 weeks [99]. The grafts showed calponin-positive cells and matrix with an abundant amount of type I collagen and burst pressure of 700 mmHg. The suture retention was found to be 30 g and dry collagen % was 14%, which is approximately half that of native veins. The key finding was how karyotype plays a key role in the development of these vascular grafts. They reported normal karyotype is essential to form functional TEVGs as chromosomal abnormalities may result in calcified vessel constructs. However, the hiPSC-MSC-derived TEVGs were not mechanically robust and could not be tested in animals [99].

Gui et al. used a similar bioreactor method [25, 100] and fully differentiated hiPSC-VSMCs to develop a mechanically stronger and functional TEVG [100]. In this study, the hiPSC-VSMCs were generated from an integration-free hiPSCs and using the EB-based differentiation method [83]. The terminally differentiated synthetic VSMCs with high proliferation rates were seeded on gelatin-coated PGA scaffold for 8 weeks under a static condition and medium containing TGF-β1 and PDGF-BB [100]. The hiPSC-based TEVGs contained abundant collagenous matrix and cells maintained the phenotype. The TEVGs with collagen as the major ECM composition had burst pressure and suture retention of 500 mmHg and 30–70 g, respectively. The TEVGs, when implanted into a rat aorta model for 14 days, showed no sign of rupture and calcification. The animals survived for 2 weeks. TEVGs were patent and displayed active vascular remodeling without teratoma formation. The TEVGs maintained the phenotype and survival of hiPSC-VSMCs in vivo. Although the TEVGs were not robust or had mature elastin fibers as native vascular grafts [15, 25], this report provided initial blueprints for the use of fully differentiated hiPSC-VSMCs in engineering hiPSC-derived TEVGs [100].

Most recently, Luo et al. improvised the existing EB differentiation method of hiPSC-VSMC, bioreactor culture condition, and pulsatile stretching to engineer a TEVG with mechanical strength comparable to native vessels [94]. Incremental addition of pulsatile radial stress at 110–120 beats per minute (bpm) along with medium containing TGF-β1 significantly improved the collagen deposition (43.1% ± 4.4%) and mechanical strength indicated by rupture pressure (1419.0 ± 174.4 mmHg) and suture retention strength (157.5 ± 16.5 g). The TEVG, when implanted into a rat aortic model, maintained patency and was able to withstand aortic blood pressure with no sign of rupture or aberrant deformation. Furthermore, ultrasonography did not reveal any radial dilation or longitudinal elongation. No teratoma formation was seen during this 1-month implantation. The explants showed robust mechanical strength and contractile function post-implantation in addition to increased viability and maintaining the phenotype of hiPSC-VSMCs. Contrary to native blood vessels, mature elastin fibers were not detected in these improved hiPSC-TEVGs. This study has established an improved method to develop mechanically robust TEVGs on large scale and provides a foundation for future production of non-immunogenic, cellular hiPSC-derived TEVGs composed of allogeneic vascular cells [94].

In another effort to better mimic blood vessels, Nakayama et al. developed a bilayer nanofibrous collagen scaffold [101]. The inner layer with longitudinally aligned nanofibers was seeded with hiPSC-ECs, and the outer layer was seeded with hiPSC-VSMCs on circumferentially aligned nanofibers. The iPSC-derived VSMCs and ECs oriented themselves on the aligned collagen nanofibers mimicking the behavior of primary VSMCs and ECs. The iPSC-derived VSMCs and ECs maintained their phenotype with reduced inflammation. However, the mechanical strength, collagen production, and in vivo performance of these hiPSC-based TEVGs were not evaluated [101].

9.4.2 Engineered Microvasculature

iPSC-VSMCs have widely been used to engineer larger blood vessels, but their use as support cells in engineering microvasculature needs more attention. Gerecht and colleagues developed a self-organized vascular network using hiPSC-derived early vascular cells. These early vascular cells were composed of VE-cadherin+ early ECs and PDGFRβ⁺ early pericytes with VSMC-like phenotype [102]. These prevascular cells, when embedded in a synthetic hyaluronic acid-based hydrogel, formed complex vascular networks by day 3. The microvascular structures contained ECs in the lumen and the early perivascular cells encircling them. An in vivo subcutaneous study in a murine model showed the integration of this microvasculature into the host vessels [102]. In another report, Ren et al. used iPSC-ECs and VSMCs to generate functional vasculature in decellularized rat and human lung scaffolds [103]. This was achieved by the co-seeding of ECs and VSMCs in a two-stage culture protocol in the vascular compartments of rat and human lungs. They achieved around 75% endothelial coverage in rat lung compared to the native rat lungs with reduced vascular resistance and improved barrier function. The endothelium was found to be patent for 3 days in an orthotopic implantation model in rats [103].

Sinha and colleagues revealed the key role of lineage-specific VSMCs in maintaining a robust vasculature [104]. In this study, hiPSC-VSMCs were generated using a monolayer method from lateral plate mesoderm, neuroectoderm, and paraxial mesoderm [88]. These VSMCs were then used along with HUVECs on Matrigel to form vasculature. The lateral plate mesoderm compared to other VSMC subtypes were found to be more proangiogenic in supporting the vasculature. In-depth transcriptome analysis pointed toward the role of Midkine, also known as neurite growth-promoting factor 2, as one of the important mediators for the enhanced vasculogenic potential. This study highlights the essential role of paracrine secretion in lineage-dependent therapeutic revascularization [104]. In a few recent studies, Gorecka et al. and Dash et al. (unpublished) have independently shown the proangiogenic and anti-inflammatory potential of hiPSC-VSMCs. The hiPSC-VSMCs generated using an already established EB-based method [83] were shown to promote wound healing in both acute and diabetic wound models via paracrine factor secretion. The hiPSC-VSMCs, when embedded in a biomimetic collagen scaffold, experienced a hypoxic environment and secreted proangiogenic growth factors VEGF, bFGF, and angiopoietin-1 and anti-inflammatory cytokines SDF-1α and IL-10. The hiPSC-VSMCs embedded in this collagen scaffolds promoted healing via enhanced angiogenesis and reduced inflammation in acute and diabetic wound models in nude mice.

9.5   iPSC-VSMCs and Vascular Disease Modeling

iPSC-VSMCs have been used effectively in investigating disease mechanisms of Marfan syndrome, SVAS, WBS, and Hutchinson-Gilford progeria syndrome. Marfan syndrome is a connective tissue disorder and results in thoracic aortic aneurysms in the patients. The disease phenotype of VSMCs includes defects in fibrillin-1 accumulation, ECM degradation, TGF-β1 signaling, contraction, and apoptosis [105]. Granata et al. generated iPSC-VSMCs from Marfan syndrome patients. They followed Cheung et al. [88] monolayer protocol to generate the VSMCs. The generated iPSC-VSMCs recapitulated the disease phenotype and identified several important downstream targets, including KLF4 and p38. Also, they showed the use of the CRISPR-Cas9 system as a therapeutic tool. The gene editing of fibrillin-1 mutation by CRISPR-Cas9 restored the abnormal fibrillin-1, TGF-β1, and abnormal matrix metalloproteinase levels [105].

Similarly, Ge et al. established iPSC lines from patients with supravalvular aortic stenosis (SVAS) and Williams-Beuren syndrome (WBS) [82]. These vascular diseases are characterized by narrowing or complete blockage of the ascending aorta because of aberrant VSMC proliferation. The iPSC-VSMCs from these diseased cell lines were generated using EB-based methods of differentiation. The SVAS-VSMCs exhibited disease phenotype with higher proliferation and reduced contractility compared to healthy iPSC-VSMCs. The disease phenotype was found to be due to an abnormality in elastin gene expression accompanied by GTPase RhoA signaling and extracellular signal-regulated kinase (ERK)1/2 activity. Similar findings were observed in the case of WBS-VSMCs [82]. Furthermore, Dash et al. created a 3D disease model of SVAS. They seeded SVAS hiPSC-VSMCs onto ring-shaped agarose gel to form a 3D rings [83]. The SVAS patient-derived rings exhibited higher cellular proliferation, decreased actin bundle filament formation, and reduced contractility [83] mimicking the SVAS disease phenotype. Kinnear et al. treated the WBS phenotype with an mTOR (mechanistic target of rapamycin) inhibitor, rapamycin [106]. The rapamycin was able to restore the contractile response and tubular formation of WBS hiPSC-VSMCs. This study provides a candidate drug for patients with WBS and SVAS [106]. Another therapeutic target in SVAS hiPSC-VSMC is integrin-β3. The study showed an upregulation of integrin-β3 and enhanced integrin-β3 signaling in SVAS hiPSC-VSMCs, and thus a β3-blockade is a promising and much needed noninvasive therapeutic approach for SVAS [107].

iPSC-VSMCs were also used to understand the underlying mechanism of early aging in children with Hutchinson-Gilford progeria syndrome (HGPS). The disease pathophysiology shows early atherosclerosis due to aberrant VSMC loss [108]. The HGPS-derived iPSC-VSMCs recapitulate the disease phenotype with less proliferation and accumulation of progerin in the nucleus [109]. Truskey and colleagues developed a disease model of HGPS. They developed a TEVG using HGPS-derived hiPSC-VSMCs [110]. They seeded hiPSC-VSMCs on a collagen hydrogel to construct the TEVGs. The resulting HGPS hiPSC-VSMCs-based TEVGs exhibited atherosclerotic conditions such as reduced vasocontractility, thickened vessel walls, and increased rates of calcification and apoptosis. Furthermore, these TEVGs were used to study the therapeutic effect of everolimus, a rapamycin analog. The treatment enhanced the vasoactivity of the VSMCs [110].

Patients with congenital cardiovascular malformation such as bicuspid aortic valves (BAV) suffer from aortopathy in their ascending aorta [111]. Jiao et al. created a disease model of BAV aortopathy by generating BAV-derived hiPSC-VSMCs from the neural crest and paraxial mesoderm. The differentiated VSMCs from neural crest and paraxial mesoderm resemble in vivo counterparts from ascending and descending aorta, respectively [112]. The BAV-derived hiPSC-VSMCs from neural crest lineage exhibited disease phenotype with reduced contractility and aberrant proliferation. However, paraxial mesoderm-derived VSMCs, which populate the descending aorta, generated from the same patients did not demonstrate disease pathophysiology. Furthermore, a mechanistic study revealed mTOR pathways as the therapeutic target. These findings suggest the role of altered hemodynamics in addition to the immature neural crest-derived VSMCs behind aortopathy in the ascending aorta of BAV patients [112].

Hypertension is a disease involving vascular cells especially VSMCs, and therefore hiPSC-VSMCs might help identify new targets and develop novel therapies for this condition. Beil et al. established patient-derived iPSCs from multiple patients with hypertension and differentiated them to functional VSMCs using an EB method [113]. The study shows the contractility response of these differentiated VSMCs in response to phorbol 12-myristate 13-acetate and endothelin-1 and inflammatory stimuli such as TNFα [113]. These hiPSC-VSMCs from hypertension patients have the potential to be used for screening of antihypertensive drugs. In future, this will help in finding optimal antihypertensive treatments for individual patients.

9.6   Concluding Remarks

The progress in iPSC technology is transforming vascular tissue engineering and disease modeling strategies. The hiPSC-VSMCs have huge potential in regenerative therapy, disease modeling, drug screening, and precision medicine (summarized in Fig. 9.3). Efficient and integration-free reprogramming approaches are increasing the possibility of hiPSC-derived VSMCs in translating to the clinic, while a generation of the lineage-specific and large scale of VSMCs is growing our understanding of various disease pathologies and their regenerative potential. As of now, hiPSC-VSMCs provide a reliable model system to develop patient-specific disease models for drug screening. However, regenerative application of hiPSC-VSMC-derived tissue-engineered products needs further investigation.

Safety is of primary concern as iPSCs are known for their tumorigenic potential. In a recent study, scientists from Japan used a hiPSC-derived retinal pigment epithelium cell sheet to treat macular degeneration in a patient [64]. Although the long-term safety and efficacy is not yet known, caution should be taken, and efforts should be made toward the production of GMP-grade iPSCs. The initial strategy should involve developing a well-defined differentiation protocol by making sure the cells are 100% differentiated with no transgene. The second strategy should consider long-term in vivo efficacy and safety study in large animals.

Recently, hiPSC-VSMCs have been used in bioreactors to engineer robust hiPSC-derived TEVGs. The collagen deposition by hiPSC-VSMCs provides the strength to these constructs. However, none of these TEVGs show mature elastic fibers in them. A recent study attempted to engineer vascular constructs with elastic fibers [114]. In this study, Eoh et al. used contractile hiPSC-VSMCs and seeded them on PEGdma-PLA [poly(ethylene glycol) dimethacrylate/poly(L-lactide)] scaffolds followed by culturing them in a pulsatile flow bioreactor. A quiescent culture medium was containing TGF-β1 and 0.5% fetal calf serum was used. The

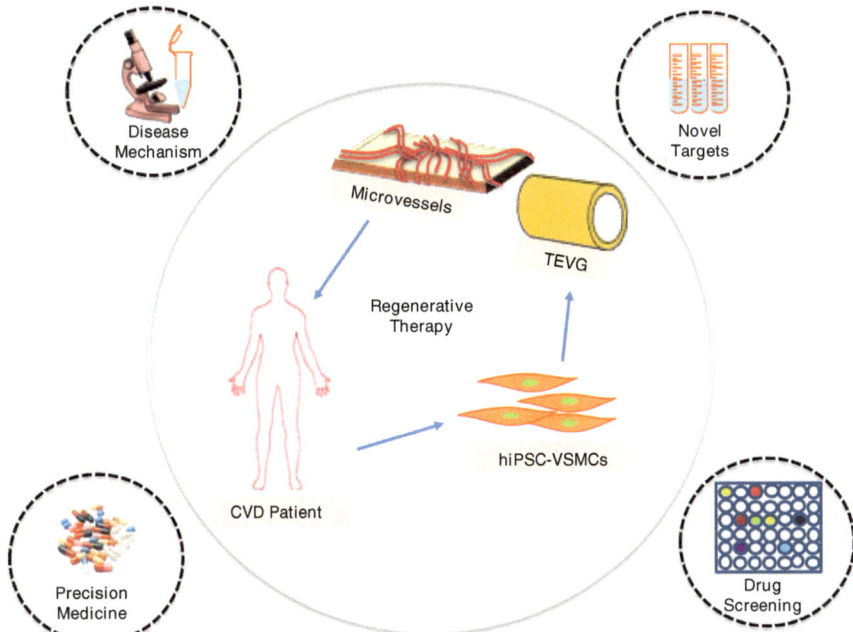

Fig. 9.3 A schematic showing hiPSC-VSMCs and their application in regenerative therapy, disease modeling, identifying novel targets, drug screening, and precision medicine

hiPSC-VSMCs in peristaltic flow in a bioreactor system resulted in the formation of robust elastic fibers [114]. This work is the first and the only one so far, which presented an effective approach to produce mature elastin fibers from hiPSC-VSMCs [114]. Further efforts should be made to use these conditions to engineer TEVG with elastic fibers.

hiPSC-VSMCs and their use in neovascularization strategy are still in its infancy. A very few studies have reported their ability to support angiogenesis via paracrine secretion. Although our recent studies have explored their paracrine secretion and ability to promote wound healing, further efforts should be carried out to investigate their full regenerative potential to broaden their therapeutic application.

Conflicts of Interest The author declares no conflict of interest.

References

1. Mortality GBD, Causes of Death C. Global, regional, and national life expectancy, all-cause mortality, and cause-specific mortality for 249 causes of death, 1980–2015: a systematic analysis for the Global Burden of Disease Study 2015. Lancet. 2016;388:1459–544.

2. Greco Song HH, Rumma RT, Ozaki CK, Edelman ER, Chen CS. Vascular tissue engineering: progress, challenges, and clinical promise. Cell Stem Cell. 2018;22:608.
3. DeBakey ME, Crawford ES, Garrett HE, Beall AC Jr, Howell JF. Surgical considerations in the treatment of aneurysms of the thoraco-abdominal aorta. Ann Surg. 1965;162:650–62.
4. Sciarretta JD, Macedo FI, Otero CA, Figueroa JN, Pizano LR, Namias N. Management of traumatic popliteal vascular injuries in a level I trauma center: a 6-year experience. Int J Surg. 2015;18:136–41.
5. Schild AF, Perez E, Gillaspie E, Seaver C, Livingstone J, Thibonnier A. Arteriovenous fistulae vs. arteriovenous grafts: a retrospective review of 1,700 consecutive vascular access cases. J Vasc Access. 2008;9:231–5.
6. Chard RB, Johnson DC, Nunn GR, Cartmill TB. Aorta-coronary bypass grafting with polytetrafluoroethylene conduits. Early and late outcome in eight patients. J Thorac Cardiovasc Surg. 1987;94:132–4.
7. Shum-Tim D, Stock U, Hrkach J, Shinoka T, Lien J, Moses MA, et al. Tissue engineering of autologous aorta using a new biodegradable polymer. Ann Thorac Surg. 1999;68:2298–304. discussion 305
8. Canver CC. Conduit options in coronary artery bypass surgery. Chest. 1995;108:1150–5.
9. Sun G, Gerecht S. Vascular regeneration: engineering the stem cell microenvironment. Regen Med. 2009;4:435–47.
10. Park KM, Gerecht S. Harnessing developmental processes for vascular engineering and regeneration. Development. 2014;141:2760–9.
11. Lowenthal J, Gerecht S. Stem cell-derived vasculature: a potent and multidimensional technology for basic research, disease modeling, and tissue engineering. Biochem Biophys Res Commun. 2016;473:733–42.
12. Zhang WJ, Liu W, Cui L, Cao Y. Tissue engineering of blood vessel. J Cell Mol Med. 2007;11:945–57.
13. Vaz CM, van Tuijl S, Bouten CV, Baaijens FP. Design of scaffolds for blood vessel tissue engineering using a multi-layering electrospinning technique. Acta Biomater. 2005;1:575–82.
14. Ziegler T, Nerem RM. Tissue engineering a blood vessel: regulation of vascular biology by mechanical stresses. J Cell Biochem. 1994;56:204–9.
15. Cong X, Zhang SM, Batty L, Luo J. Application of human induced pluripotent stem cells in generating tissue-engineered blood vessels as vascular grafts. Stem Cells Dev. 2019;28:1581–94.
16. Sundaram S, Niklason LE. Smooth muscle and other cell sources for human blood vessel engineering. Cells Tissues Organs. 2012;195:15–25.
17. Lawson JH, Glickman MH, Ilzecki M, Jakimowicz T, Jaroszynski A, Peden EK, et al. Bioengineered human acellular vessels for dialysis access in patients with end-stage renal disease: two phase 2 single-arm trials. Lancet. 2016;387:2026–34.
18. Dash BC, Jiang Z, Suh C, Qyang Y. Induced pluripotent stem cell-derived vascular smooth muscle cells: methods and application. Biochem J. 2015;465:185–94.
19. Ayoubi S, Sheikh SP, Eskildsen TV. Human induced pluripotent stem cell-derived vascular smooth muscle cells: differentiation and therapeutic potential. Cardiovasc Res. 2017;113:1282–93.
20. Klein D. iPSCs-based generation of vascular cells: reprogramming approaches and applications. Cell Mol Life Sci. 2018;75:1411–33.
21. Maguire EM, Xiao Q, Xu Q. Differentiation and application of induced pluripotent stem cell-derived vascular smooth muscle cells. Arterioscler Thromb Vasc Biol. 2017;37:2026–37.
22. Ji H, Kim HS, Kim HW, Leong KW. Application of induced pluripotent stem cells to model smooth muscle cell function in vascular diseases. Curr Opin Biomed Eng. 2017;1:38–44.
23. Smith Q, Gerecht S. Going with the flow: microfluidic platforms in vascular tissue engineering. Curr Opin Chem Eng. 2014;3:42–50.
24. Weinberg CB, Bell E. A blood vessel model constructed from collagen and cultured vascular cells. Science. 1986;231:397–400.

25. Niklason LE, Gao J, Abbott WM, Hirschi KK, Houser S, Marini R, et al. Functional arteries grown in vitro. Science. 1999;284:489–93.
26. Syedain ZH, Meier LA, Bjork JW, Lee A, Tranquillo RT. Implantable arterial grafts from human fibroblasts and fibrin using a multi-graft pulsed flow-stretch bioreactor with noninvasive strength monitoring. Biomaterials. 2011;32:714–22.
27. L'Heureux N, Dusserre N, Konig G, Victor B, Keire P, Wight TN, et al. Human tissue-engineered blood vessels for adult arterial revascularization. Nat Med. 2006;12:361–5.
28. Syedain Z, Reimer J, Lahti M, Berry J, Johnson S, Bianco R, et al. Corrigendum: tissue engineering of acellular vascular grafts capable of somatic growth in young lambs. Nat Commun. 2017;8:14297.
29. Syedain ZH, Graham ML, Dunn TB, O'Brien T, Johnson SL, Schumacher RJ, et al. A completely biological "off-the-shelf" arteriovenous graft that recellularizes in baboons. Sci Transl Med. 2017;9
30. Fernandez CE, Yen RW, Perez SM, Bedell HW, Povsic TJ, Reichert WM, et al. Human vascular microphysiological system for in vitro drug screening. Sci Rep. 2016;6:21579.
31. Strobel HA, Hookway TA, Piola M, Fiore GB, Soncini M, Alsberg E, et al. Assembly of tissue-engineered blood vessels with spatially controlled heterogeneities. Tissue Eng Part A. 2018;24:1492–503.
32. Konig G, McAllister TN, Dusserre N, Garrido SA, Iyican C, Marini A, et al. Mechanical properties of completely autologous human tissue engineered blood vessels compared to human saphenous vein and mammary artery. Biomaterials. 2009;30:1542–50.
33. L'Heureux N, Paquet S, Labbe R, Germain L, Auger FA. A completely biological tissue-engineered human blood vessel. FASEB J. 1998;12:47–56.
34. Niklason LE, Abbott W, Gao J, Klagges B, Hirschi KK, Ulubayram K, et al. Morphologic and mechanical characteristics of engineered bovine arteries. J Vasc Surg. 2001;33:628–38.
35. Solan A, Niklason L. Age effects on vascular smooth muscle: an engineered tissue approach. Cell Transplant. 2005;14:481–8.
36. Han J, Liu JY, Swartz DD, Andreadis ST. Molecular and functional effects of organismal aging on smooth muscle cells derived from bone marrow mesenchymal stem cells. Cardiovasc Res. 2010;87:147–55.
37. Liu JY, Swartz DD, Peng HF, Gugino SF, Russell JA, Andreadis ST. Functional tissue-engineered blood vessels from bone marrow progenitor cells. Cardiovasc Res. 2007;75:618–28.
38. Gong Z, Calkins G, Cheng EC, Krause D, Niklason LE. Influence of culture medium on smooth muscle cell differentiation from human bone marrow-derived mesenchymal stem cells. Tissue Eng Part A. 2009;15:319–30.
39. Wang C, Cen L, Yin S, Liu Q, Liu W, Cao Y, et al. A small diameter elastic blood vessel wall prepared under pulsatile conditions from polyglycolic acid mesh and smooth muscle cells differentiated from adipose-derived stem cells. Biomaterials. 2010;31:621–30.
40. Peng HF, Liu JY, Andreadis ST, Swartz DD. Hair follicle-derived smooth muscle cells and small intestinal submucosa for engineering mechanically robust and vasoreactive vascular media. Tissue Eng Part A. 2011;17:981–90.
41. Liu JY, Peng HF, Andreadis ST. Contractile smooth muscle cells derived from hair-follicle stem cells. Cardiovasc Res. 2008;79:24–33.
42. Liu JY, Peng HF, Gopinath S, Tian J, Andreadis ST. Derivation of functional smooth muscle cells from multipotent human hair follicle mesenchymal stem cells. Tissue Eng Part A. 2010;16:2553–64.
43. Ceccarelli J, Putnam AJ. Sculpting the blank slate: how fibrin's support of vascularization can inspire biomaterial design. Acta Biomater. 2014;10:1515–23.
44. Burdick JA, Prestwich GD. Hyaluronic acid hydrogels for biomedical applications. Adv Mater. 2011;23:H41–56.
45. Park KM, Gerecht S. Hypoxia-inducible hydrogels. Nat Commun. 2014;5:4075.

46. Trappmann B, Baker BM, Polacheck WJ, Choi CK, Burdick JA, Chen CS. Matrix degradability controls multicellularity of 3D cell migration. Nat Commun. 2017;8:371.
47. Han H, Ning H, Liu S, Lu QP, Fan Z, Lu H, et al. Silk biomaterials with vascularization capacity. Adv Funct Mater. 2016;26:421–36.
48. Cuchiara MP, Gould DJ, McHale MK, Dickinson ME, West JL. Integration of self-assembled microvascular networks with microfabricated PEG-based hydrogels. Adv Funct Mater. 2012;22:4511–8.
49. Miller JS, Stevens KR, Yang MT, Baker BM, Nguyen DH, Cohen DM, et al. Rapid casting of patterned vascular networks for perfusable engineered three-dimensional tissues. Nat Mater. 2012;11:768–74.
50. Heintz KA, Bregenzer ME, Mantle JL, Lee KH, West JL, Slater JH. Fabrication of 3D biomimetic microfluidic networks in hydrogels. Adv Healthc Mater. 2016;5:2153–60.
51. Zhang B, Montgomery M, Chamberlain MD, Ogawa S, Korolj A, Pahnke A, et al. Biodegradable scaffold with built-in vasculature for organ-on-a-chip engineering and direct surgical anastomosis. Nat Mater. 2016;15:669–78.
52. Kim S, Lee H, Chung M, Jeon NL. Engineering of functional, perfusable 3D microvascular networks on a chip. Lab Chip. 2013;13:1489–500.
53. Nguyen DH, Stapleton SC, Yang MT, Cha SS, Choi CK, Galie PA, et al. Biomimetic model to reconstitute angiogenic sprouting morphogenesis in vitro. Proc Natl Acad Sci U S A. 2013;110:6712–7.
54. Galie PA, Nguyen DH, Choi CK, Cohen DM, Janmey PA, Chen CS. Fluid shear stress threshold regulates angiogenic sprouting. Proc Natl Acad Sci U S A. 2014;111:7968–73.
55. Bekhite MM, Finkensieper A, Rebhan J, Huse S, Schultze-Mosgau S, Figulla HR, et al. Hypoxia, leptin, and vascular endothelial growth factor stimulate vascular endothelial cell differentiation of human adipose tissue-derived stem cells. Stem Cells Dev. 2014;23:333–51.
56. Semenza GL. Hypoxia-inducible factors in physiology and medicine. Cell. 2012;148:399–408.
57. Kusuma S, Peijnenburg E, Patel P, Gerecht S. Low oxygen tension enhances endothelial fate of human pluripotent stem cells. Arterioscler Thromb Vasc Biol. 2014;34:913–20.
58. Moya ML, Hsu YH, Lee AP, Hughes CC, George SC. In vitro perfused human capillary networks. Tissue Eng Part C Methods. 2013;19:730–7.
59. Whisler JA, Chen MB, Kamm RD. Control of perfusable microvascular network morphology using a multiculture microfluidic system. Tissue Eng Part C Methods. 2014;20:543–52.
60. Lin SL, Kisseleva T, Brenner DA, Duffield JS. Pericytes and perivascular fibroblasts are the primary source of collagen-producing cells in obstructive fibrosis of the kidney. Am J Pathol. 2008;173:1617–27.
61. Jeon JS, Bersini S, Whisler JA, Chen MB, Dubini G, Charest JL, et al. Generation of 3D functional microvascular networks with human mesenchymal stem cells in microfluidic systems. Integr Biol (Camb). 2014;6:555–63.
62. Jamieson J, Macklin B, Gerecht S. Pericytes derived from human pluripotent stem cells. Adv Exp Med Biol. 2018;1109:111–24.
63. Takahashi K, Yamanaka S. Induction of pluripotent stem cells from mouse embryonic and adult fibroblast cultures by defined factors. Cell. 2006;126:663–76.
64. Takagi S, Mandai M, Gocho K, Hirami Y, Yamamoto M, Fujihara M, et al. Evaluation of transplanted autologous induced pluripotent stem cell-derived retinal pigment epithelium in exudative age-related macular degeneration. Ophthalmol Retina. 2019;3:850–9.
65. Shi Y, Inoue H, Wu JC, Yamanaka S. Induced pluripotent stem cell technology: a decade of progress. Nat Rev Drug Discov. 2017;16:115–30.
66. Soldner F, Jaenisch R. Medicine. iPSC disease modeling. Science. 2012;338:1155–6.
67. Park IH, Zhao R, West JA, Yabuuchi A, Huo H, Ince TA, et al. Reprogramming of human somatic cells to pluripotency with defined factors. Nature. 2008;451:141–6.
68. Chen IY, Matsa E, Wu JC. Induced pluripotent stem cells: at the heart of cardiovascular precision medicine. Nat Rev Cardiol. 2016;13:333–49.
69. Lee AS, Tang C, Rao MS, Weissman IL, Wu JC. Tumorigenicity as a clinical hurdle for pluripotent stem cell therapies. Nat Med. 2013;19:998–1004.

70. Ban H, Nishishita N, Fusaki N, Tabata T, Saeki K, Shikamura M, et al. Efficient generation of transgene-free human induced pluripotent stem cells (iPSCs) by temperature-sensitive Sendai virus vectors. Proc Natl Acad Sci U S A. 2011;108:14234–9.
71. Stadtfeld M, Nagaya M, Utikal J, Weir G, Hochedlinger K. Induced pluripotent stem cells generated without viral integration. Science. 2008;322:945–9.
72. Yu J, Vodyanik MA, Smuga-Otto K, Antosiewicz-Bourget J, Frane JL, Tian S, et al. Induced pluripotent stem cell lines derived from human somatic cells. Science. 2007;318:1917–20.
73. Okita K, Matsumura Y, Sato Y, Okada A, Morizane A, Okamoto S, et al. A more efficient method to generate integration-free human iPS cells. Nat Methods. 2011;8:409–12.
74. Jia F, Wilson KD, Sun N, Gupta DM, Huang M, Li Z, et al. A nonviral minicircle vector for deriving human iPS cells. Nat Methods. 2010;7:197–9.
75. Soldner F, Hockemeyer D, Beard C, Gao Q, Bell GW, Cook EG, et al. Parkinson's disease patient-derived induced pluripotent stem cells free of viral reprogramming factors. Cell. 2009;136:964–77.
76. Woltjen K, Michael IP, Mohseni P, Desai R, Mileikovsky M, Hamalainen R, et al. piggyBac transposition reprograms fibroblasts to induced pluripotent stem cells. Nature. 2009;458:766–70.
77. Warren L, Manos PD, Ahfeldt T, Loh YH, Li H, Lau F, et al. Highly efficient reprogramming to pluripotency and directed differentiation of human cells with synthetic modified mRNA. Cell Stem Cell. 2010;7:618–30.
78. Sandmaier SE, Telugu BP. MicroRNA-mediated reprogramming of somatic cells into induced pluripotent stem cells. Methods Mol Biol. 2015;1330:29–36.
79. Qin H, Zhao A, Fu X. Small molecules for reprogramming and transdifferentiation. Cell Mol Life Sci. 2017;74:3553–75.
80. Kim D, Kim CH, Moon JI, Chung YG, Chang MY, Han BS, et al. Generation of human induced pluripotent stem cells by direct delivery of reprogramming proteins. Cell Stem Cell. 2009;4:472–6.
81. Lee TH, Song SH, Kim KL, Yi JY, Shin GH, Kim JY, et al. Functional recapitulation of smooth muscle cells via induced pluripotent stem cells from human aortic smooth muscle cells. Circ Res. 2010;106:120–8.
82. Ge X, Ren Y, Bartulos O, Lee MY, Yue Z, Kim KY, et al. Modeling supravalvular aortic stenosis syndrome with human induced pluripotent stem cells. Circulation. 2012;126:1695–704.
83. Dash BC, Levi K, Schwan J, Luo J, Bartulos O, Wu H, et al. Tissue-engineered vascular rings from human iPSC-derived smooth muscle cells. Stem Cell Rep. 2016;7:19–28.
84. El-Mounayri O, Mihic A, Shikatani EA, Gagliardi M, Steinbach SK, Dubois N, et al. Serum-free differentiation of functional human coronary-like vascular smooth muscle cells from embryonic stem cells. Cardiovasc Res. 2013;98:125–35.
85. Cao N, Liang H, Huang J, Wang J, Chen Y, Chen Z, et al. Highly efficient induction and long-term maintenance of multipotent cardiovascular progenitors from human pluripotent stem cells under defined conditions. Cell Res. 2013;23:1119–32.
86. Park SW, Jun Koh Y, Jeon J, Cho YH, Jang MJ, Kang Y, et al. Efficient differentiation of human pluripotent stem cells into functional CD34+ progenitor cells by combined modulation of the MEK/ERK and BMP4 signaling pathways. Blood. 2010;116:5762–72.
87. Wanjare M, Kuo F, Gerecht S. Derivation and maturation of synthetic and contractile vascular smooth muscle cells from human pluripotent stem cells. Cardiovasc Res. 2013;97:321–30.
88. Cheung C, Bernardo AS, Trotter MW, Pedersen RA, Sinha S. Generation of human vascular smooth muscle subtypes provides insight into embryological origin-dependent disease susceptibility. Nat Biotechnol. 2012;30:165–73.
89. Patsch C, Challet-Meylan L, Thoma EC, Urich E, Heckel T, O'Sullivan JF, et al. Generation of vascular endothelial and smooth muscle cells from human pluripotent stem cells. Nat Cell Biol. 2015;17:994–1003.
90. Menendez L, Kulik MJ, Page AT, Park SS, Lauderdale JD, Cunningham ML, et al. Directed differentiation of human pluripotent cells to neural crest stem cells. Nat Protoc. 2013;8:203–12.

91. Menendez L, Yatskievych TA, Antin PB, Dalton S. Wnt signaling and a Smad pathway block-ade direct the differentiation of human pluripotent stem cells to multipotent neural crest cells. Proc Natl Acad Sci U S A. 2011;108:19240–5.

92. Karamariti E, Margariti A, Winkler B, Wang X, Hong X, Baban D, et al. Smooth muscle cells differentiated from reprogrammed embryonic lung fibroblasts through DKK3 signaling are potent for tissue engineering of vascular grafts. Circ Res. 2013;112:1433–43.

93. Lin H, Qiu X, Du Q, Li Q, Wang O, Akert L, et al. Engineered microenvironment for manu-facturing human pluripotent stem cell-derived vascular smooth muscle cells. Stem Cell Rep. 2019;12:84–97.

94. Luo J, Qin L, Zhao L, Gui L, Ellis MW, Huang Y, et al. Tissue-engineered vascular grafts with advanced mechanical strength from human iPSCs. Cell Stem Cell. 2020;26:251–61 e8.

95. Hibino N, Duncan DR, Nalbandian A, Yi T, Qyang Y, Shinoka T, et al. Evaluation of the use of an induced puripotent stem cell sheet for the construction of tissue-engineered vascular grafts. J Thorac Cardiovasc Surg. 2012;143:696–703.

96. Xie C, Hu J, Ma H, Zhang J, Chang LJ, Chen YE, et al. Three-dimensional growth of iPS cell-derived smooth muscle cells on nanofibrous scaffolds. Biomaterials. 2011;32:4369–75.

97. Wang Y, Hu J, Jiao J, Liu Z, Zhou Z, Zhao C, et al. Engineering vascular tissue with functional smooth muscle cells derived from human iPS cells and nanofibrous scaffolds. Biomaterials. 2014;35:8960–9.

98. Hu J, Wang Y, Jiao J, Liu Z, Zhao C, Zhou Z, et al. Patient-specific cardiovascular progenitor cells derived from integration-free induced pluripotent stem cells for vascular tissue regen-eration. Biomaterials. 2015;73:51–9.

99. Sundaram S, One J, Siewert J, Teodosescu S, Zhao L, Dimitrievska S, et al. Tissue-engineered vascular grafts created from human induced pluripotent stem cells. Stem Cells Transl Med. 2014;3:1535–43.

100. Gui L, Dash BC, Luo J, Qin L, Zhao L, Yamamoto K, et al. Implantable tissue-engineered blood vessels from human induced pluripotent stem cells. Biomaterials. 2016;102:120–9.

101. Nakayama KH, Joshi PA, Lai ES, Gujar P, Joubert LM, Chen B, et al. Bilayered vascular graft derived from human induced pluripotent stem cells with biomimetic structure and function. Regen Med. 2015;10:745–55.

102. Kusuma S, Shen YI, Hanjaya-Putra D, Mali P, Cheng L, Gerecht S. Self-organized vascular networks from human pluripotent stem cells in a synthetic matrix. Proc Natl Acad Sci U S A. 2013;110:12601–6.

103. Ren X, Moser PT, Gilpin SE, Okamoto T, Wu T, Tapias LF, et al. Engineering pulmonary vasculature in decellularized rat and human lungs. Nat Biotechnol. 2015;33:1097–102.

104. Bargehr J, Low L, Cheung C, Bernard WG, Iyer D, Bennett MR, et al. Embryological origin of human smooth muscle cells influences their ability to support endothelial network forma-tion. Stem Cells Transl Med. 2016;5:946–59.

105. Granata A, Serrano F, Bernard WG, McNamara M, Low L, Sastry P, et al. An iPSC-derived vascular model of Marfan syndrome identifies key mediators of smooth muscle cell death. Nat Genet. 2017;49:97–109.

106. Kinnear C, Chang WY, Khattak S, Hinek A, Thompson T, de Carvalho Rodrigues D, et al. Modeling and rescue of the vascular phenotype of Williams-Beuren syndrome in patient induced pluripotent stem cells. Stem Cells Transl Med. 2013;2:2–15.

107. Misra A, Sheikh AQ, Kumar A, Luo J, Zhang J, Hinton RB, et al. Integrin beta3 inhibition is a therapeutic strategy for supravalvular aortic stenosis. J Exp Med. 2016;213:451–63.

108. Olive M, Harten I, Mitchell R, Beers JK, Djabali K, Cao K, et al. Cardiovascular pathology in Hutchinson-Gilford progeria: correlation with the vascular pathology of aging. Arterioscler Thromb Vasc Biol. 2010;30:2301–9.

109. Liu GH, Barkho BZ, Ruiz S, Diep D, Qu J, Yang SL, et al. Recapitulation of premature age-ing with iPSCs from Hutchinson-Gilford progeria syndrome. Nature. 2011;472:221–5.

110. Atchison L, Zhang H, Cao K, Truskey GA. A tissue engineered blood vessel model of Hutchinson-Gilford progeria syndrome using human iPSC-derived smooth muscle cells. Sci Rep. 2017;7:8168.
111. Losenno KL, Goodman RL, Chu MW. Bicuspid aortic valve disease and ascending aortic aneurysms: gaps in knowledge. Cardiol Res Pract. 2012;2012:145202.
112. Jiao J, Xiong W, Wang L, Yang J, Qiu P, Hirai H, et al. Differentiation defect in neural crest-derived smooth muscle cells in patients with aortopathy associated with bicuspid aortic valves. EBioMedicine. 2016;10:282–90.
113. Biel NM, Santostefano KE, DiVita BB, El Rouby N, Carrasquilla SD, Simmons C, et al. Vascular smooth muscle cells from hypertensive patient-derived induced pluripotent stem cells to advance hypertension pharmacogenomics. Stem Cells Transl Med. 2015;4:1380–90.
114. Eoh JH, Shen N, Burke JA, Hinderer S, Xia Z, Schenke-Layland K, et al. Enhanced elastin synthesis and maturation in human vascular smooth muscle tissue derived from induced-pluripotent stem cells. Acta Biomater. 2017;52:49–59.

Chapter 10
Mesenchymal Stem Cell and Hematopoietic Stem Cell Transplantation for Vasculitis

Lianming Liao and Yongquan Gu

Vasculitis is a heterogeneous group of pathologies characterized by inflammation and necrosis of vessel walls. More than 30 kinds of vasculitis have been reported according to an international consensus [1]. It may present as a primary process or as a complication of some other pathologic conditions. Primary vasculitis is relatively rare but is associated with significant morbidity and mortality, particularly if diagnosis is delayed. Pathologic conditions, such as collagen-vascular, rheumatic, infectious, or malignant diseases, may sometimes be accompanied by vasculitis.

The cause of vasculitis is still mostly unknown. Risk factors of vasculitis include geography, age, ethnicity, gender, and genetic and environmental factors. For example, Behcet disease is more common in countries along the ancient Silk Route [2]. Takayasu disease is more prevalent in South Asian countries and in children less than 5 years of age, with a female to male ratio of 9 to 1 [3]. Giant cell arteritis (GCA) and granulomatosis with polyangiitis (GPA) occur predominantly in the White population [4]. Studies have found the association of hepatitis B with polyarteritis nodosa (PAN), hepatitis C with mixed cryoglobulinemia, and silica dust with pauci-immune vasculitis [5].

Selection of treatment regimens depends on the type and the severity of vasculitis. Treatment generally includes three components: remission induction, remission maintenance, and monitoring. Glucocorticoids are the first-line treatment for vasculitis and may be used with or without immunosuppressive agents.

A variety of immunosuppressive medications, newer biologic agents, and new treatment regimens have been introduced in the recent years to address this unmet

L. Liao
Department of Laboratory Medicine, Fujian Medical University Union Hospital, Fuzhou, China

Y. Gu (✉)
Department of Vascular Surgery, Xuan Wu Hospital of Capital Medical University, Beijing, China

© Springer Nature Switzerland AG 2021 221
T. P. Navarro et al. (eds.), *Stem Cell Therapy for Vascular Diseases*,
https://doi.org/10.1007/978-3-030-56954-9_10

medical need, which include methotrexate, azathioprine, mycophenolate, cyclophosphamide, rituximab, intravenous immunoglobulin, and plasma exchange.

10.1 Mesenchymal Stem Cell Characteristics

Mesenchymal stem cells (MSCs), also known as mesenchymal stromal cells, are adult fibroblast-like cells that are adherent to the surface of culture plastic and capable of differentiation into adipocytes, chondroblasts, and osteoblasts. MSCs were originally isolated from bone marrow and later from a variety of tissues, such as adipose tissue, tooth pulps, periodontal tissue, umbilical cord, and placenta. In 2006, the International Society for Cellular Therapy recommended a set of minimal criteria to uniformize MSC characteristics [6].

The immunoregulatory properties of different types of MSCs have been well studied. MSCs exhibit capabilities such as prompting T-cell expansion to a regulatory phenotype, shifting macrophages to anti-inflammatory and immunosuppressive M2 phenotypes, and inhibiting dendritic cells maturation. The functions of NK cells, B cells, and memory T cells are suppressed as well [7–10]. The immunoregulatory properties of MSCs have been harnessed to treat autoimmune diseases.

Importantly MSCs may migrate to the damaged tissue and secrete a number of cytokines and chemokines through paracrine, endocrine, and exosome mechanisms [11]. The secreted cytokines and chemokines include vascular endothelial growth factor, stromal cell-derived factor-1, fibroblast growth factor, insulin-like growth factor, keratinocyte growth factor, hepatocyte growth factor, and vascular endothelial growth factors. In addition MSCs can transfer mitochondria, functional proteins, mRNAs and microRNAs into the damaged cells via microvesicle-dependent cell-to-cell communication. These all help correct the course of injury and regulate the local immune response.

After numerous in vitro and in vivo preclinical studies, autologous and allogeneic MSCs have been applied in a range of immune-mediated conditions, including graft versus host disease, Crohn's disease, multiple sclerosis, refractory systemic lupus erythematosus, and systemic sclerosis. Hypothetically MSCs transplantation may be beneficial for vasculitis by reducing inflammation, inducing prosurvival genes, and downregulating pro-apoptotic genes.

10.2 Hematopoietic Stem Cell Characteristics

Vasculitis may develop into a chronic inflammatory disorder and presents as a relapsing-remitting illness. Therefore, an ideal therapeutic goal is to switch off the inflammation and halt disease progression. Immunoablation and reconstitution of the immune system via hematopoietic stem cell transplantation (HSCT) is a more intensive approach than immunosuppressants. This approach can switch off the autoreactive, inflammatory process and restoring self-tolerance.

Immunoablation and HSCT have been practiced as a therapy for various autoimmune diseases, including systemic sclerosis, systemic lupus erythematosus and Crohn's disease, for several decades [12]. The purpose of HSCT in the treatment of autoimmune diseases is to allow delivery of intensive chemotherapy or chemoradiotherapy in order to cause severe immunosuppression or even total immunoablation. Infused stem cells then repopulate the patient and give rise to new hematopoiesis and a complete immune system. In allogeneic HSCT, the immune system is provided by the donor cells.

10.3   HSP IgA vasculitis (Henoch–Schönlein purpura)

IgA vasculitis is the new term for Henoch-Schönlein purpura (HSP) and is the commonest systemic vasculitis in childhood [13]. It is defined in the latest Chapel Hill nomenclature (2012) as vasculitis with IgA1-dominant immune deposits affecting small vessels (predominantly capillaries, venules, or arterioles). HSP is associated with glomerulonephritis which is indistinguishable from IgA nephropathy [13]. The most important prognostic factor for poor outcome is renal involvement. Children with microscopic hematuria without renal dysfunction or proteinuria and those with non-persistent mild-moderate proteinuria usually do not require any specific therapeutic intervention other than a "watchful waiting approach" since the prognosis is excellent. HSP-associated arthritis responds well to non-steroidal anti-inflammatory drugs [14]. Severe skin lesions and gastrointestinal involvement could require a short course of an oral corticosteroid. However controlled studies have shown that corticosteroids do not prevent renal disease [15]. Immunosuppressants including azathioprine, MMF, or intravenous cyclophosphamide may be considered as second-line agents.

Mu et al. reported a 12-year-old boy treated with cord-derived mesenchymal stem cells for liver cirrhosis and refractory HSP [16]. The patient presented with purpura in the skin of the bilateral lower limbs and thrombocytopenia. He had chronic itching skin rash for the past 2 years and received prednisone treatment. At admission, ultrasonography of the abdomen showed diffuse lesions and multiple solid nodules in the liver. Abdominal computed tomography showed hepatomegaly with small nodules under the right lobe of the liver and enlarged splenic sinuses. The patient received MSC transplantation for eight times in 2 months. Then methylprednisolone was tapered off after 1 month with disappearance of skin rash and normalization of platelet count and liver transaminase level. Abdominal ultrasound showed fewer round nodules in the liver and decreased spleen size. Follow-up at 6 months revealed there was no skin rash, and no nodules in the liver and the platelet count remained normal. This is a rare case of HSP with thrombocytopenia and liver cirrhosis that responded to MSC treatment.

10.4   ANCA-Associated Vasculitis (AAV)

Antineutrophil cytoplasmic autoantibody (ANCA)-associated vasculitis (AAV) comprises granulomatosis with polyangiitis (GPA, previously referred to as Wegener's granulomatosis), microscopic polyangiitis (MPA), eosinophilic granulomatous polyangiitis (EGPA), and renal-limited vasculitis. GPA may present sequentially as a predominantly granulomatous form or as an acute small vessel vasculitic form. These two presentations may also co-exist.

There is a rapid expansion in the therapeutic agents for AAV, including purine, pyrimidine, mycophenolate mofetil, leflunomide, 15-deoxyspergualin, immunoglobulin, TNF-alpha antagonism infliximab, IL-5 antagonism mepolizumab, rituximab (for induction of B-lymphocyte depletion), alemtuzumab (for induction for T-lymphocyte depletion), and antithymocyte globulin (for induction for T-lymphocyte depletion). Due to the fact that AAV is associated with abnormal immune function, immunoablation, and HSCT to switch off the autoreactive, inflammatory process of the patients is reasonable.

In a phase I–II trial of autologous peripheral blood stem cell transplantation for refractory autoimmune disease, one patient with GPA was enrolled [17]. The patient was male and 21 years old. He has been treated with corticosteroids, cyclophosphamide, and cyclosporin A before. Peripheral blood stem cells were mobilized with granulocyte colony-stimulating factor after administration of cyclophosphamide (2 g/m^2) for 2 days. 5×10^6 CD34$^+$ cells/kg were collected by apheresis and infused. After hematopoietic reconstitution, the size of the left orbital granuloma decreased substantially and the exophthalmos was reduced. Monthly steroid pulse therapy was discontinued. At 3 months after transplantation serum proteinase 3 (PR3)-anti neutrophil cytoplasmic antibodies (ANCA) level decreased to 39 IU/ml, which was 72 IU/ml before transplantation. However, it increased again to 157 IU/ml at 12 months. Thus high dose cyclophosphamide with autologous peripheral blood stem cell transplantation is promising. However why GPA relapses in the long-term remains unclear.

Additionally, in an international meeting taking place in 2000, four patients with GPA receiving autologous peripheral stem cell transplantation were reported. All patients had an initially complete response, but two patients relapsed at 2.3 and 3 years, respectively, which was easier to control [18]. However the detailed treatment protocol was not described.

Secondary autoimmune diseases are a known complication after autologous stem cell transplantations [19]. Indeed, p-ANCA-associated vasculitis was induced in a 43-year-old man who had received autologous stem cell transplantation for systemic sclerosis. The patient received a conditioning regimen with cyclophosphamide and antithymocyte globulin before receiving cyclophosphamide and granulocyte colony-stimulating factor mobilized stem cell transplantation. He responded well to HSCT. One year and 4 months after transplantation mild erythrocyturia without acanthocytes and proteinuria were seen on routine urinalysis. During the following year, erythrocyturia increased to 131 erythrocytes/μl and protein excretion to 628 mg/g creatinine. Renal biopsy revealed mild global and focal-segmental sclerosing and focal-segmental proliferative glomerulonephritis that supported the diagnosis of p-ANCA-positive glomerulonephritis. The patient responded well to Rituximab treatment.

10.5 Kawasaki Disease (KD)

Kawasaki disease (KD) is a systemic inflammatory disease that predominantly affects medium and small-sized arteries. The principal clinical features of KD include polymorphous exanthema and acute non-purulent cervical lymphadenopathy, which are manifestation of abnormal immune function [20].

Early recognition and treatment of KD with aspirin and intravenous immunoglobulin (IVIG) are crucial. However, IVIG resistance has been reported in up to 20% of cases [21]. Other treatments include corticosteroids and corticosteroids plus IVIG. In some case report, anti-TNF-α, anakinra, plasmapheresis, and immunoglobulin plus ciclosporin were shown to be effective [22].

Most recently Uchimura et al. evaluated if adipose-derived MSCs could suppress KD-associated vasculitis in a *Candida albicans* water-soluble fraction (CAWS)-induced severe coronary arteritis. *Candida albicans*-derived substances, such as *C. albicans* water-soluble fraction (CAWS), induce coronary arteritis similar to KD in mice [23]. Mice were treated with intravenous MSCs or phosphate-buffered saline. On day 29, the mice were sacrificed. MSC infusion significantly inhibited coronary arteritis and decreased the levels of pro-inflammatory cytokines IL-1β, IL-12, IL-17, RANTES, INF-γ, and TNF-α. Most importantly MSC infusion improved animal survival. These findings highlight that MSC transplantation is potentially a novel therapeutic strategy for severe KD due to their anti-inflammatory and immunoregulatory functions.

10.6 Polyarteritis Nodosa (PAN)

Polyarteritis nodosa (PAN) is characterized by necrotizing vasculitis in medium- or small-sized arteries or angiographic abnormalities. Patients may also have other symptoms of the skin, muscle, kidneys, gastrointestinal tract, and heart. Treatment of severe PAN includes corticosteroids, cyclophosphamide, and mycophenolate mofetil. Despite therapy, mortality remains high. Biologic agents including rituximab were also described for children with systemic PAN.

Similar to other autoimmune disorders, intense immunosuppression followed by reconstitution of immune system with a stem cell transplant has been proposed as a last-ditch treatment. A 22-year-old Caucasian female with an 8-year history of juvenile-onset PAN was treated with autologous peripheral blood stem cell transplantation [24]. Over the following 8 years, she had multiple flares of disease which could not be controlled by oral and i.v. corticosteroids, cyclophosphamide (to a total dose of 51 g), oral colchicine, IVIG, and plasmapheresis. In the 18 months before autologous HSCT, she suffered increasingly frequent flares and repeat angiography showed new aneurysms in the hepatic arteries. She was therefore offered autologous HSCT. After administration of cyclophosphamide ($1.5 \, g/m^2$), stem cells were harvested by leucopheresis after stem cell mobilization with granulocyte-colony stimulating factor from the bone marrow. $CD34^+$ cells were purified by magnetic bead selection. Immunosuppressive conditioning regimen was compromised of 20 mg CAMPATH-1H (days −9 to −5), fludarabine 30 mg/m2 (days −8 to −4), and cyclophosphamide $1 \, g/m^2$ on days −3 and − 2. After HSCT she remained well and discontinued immunosuppressive medication other than low-dose prednisolone (<10 mg/day) for the next 5 months. Unfortunately she developed a new vasculitic rash on the lower extremities that were not present before HSCT over the ensuing year. Fourteen months after HSCT, she developed autoimmune hyperthyroidism. In addition she was positive for thyroglobulin antibodies and p-ANCA. At 18 months, the patient developed autoimmune thrombocytopenia. The platelet count recovered with IVIG and oral steroids. By sequence-specific T-cell receptor (TCR) heteroduplex (HD) analysis of purified T-cell subsets, the researchers showed that clonal T-cell expansions, present within 2 months of HSCT when the majority of the T cells express $CD45RO^+$, were subsequently within the $CD45RA^+$ T-cell subset at 1 year after HSCT. These data suggested that T cells underwent reversion from $CD45RO^+$ to RA^+. Thus in patients who may have a genetic background which predisposes them to autoimmunity, immune reconstitution after HSCT can be associated with new autoimmune phenomena [19].

10.7   Takayasu Arteritis

Takayasu arteritis (TA) is the large vessel vasculitis (LVV). The clinical diagnosis of TA is usually challenging. Due to the non-specific symptoms and the absence of specific laboratory parameters, TA is often unrecognized in the acute early phase. There have been few evidence-based therapies for TA. The general therapeutic approach is induction of remission (high dose corticosteroid combined with another immunosuppressant), followed by maintenance therapy (lower dose corticosteroid combined with a maintenance immunosuppressive agent, usually methotrexate). About half of patients respond to steroids and the non-responders may benefit from other forms of immunosuppression [25]. In addition, methotrexate, azathioprine, mycophenolate mofetil, leflunomide, chlorambucil, antimalarials, and cyclophosphamide have been used in children as first- or second-line agents. Biologic therapies, including anti-TNFα mAb and tocilizumab (a monoclonal antibody against interleukin 6 receptor), were reported to be effective [26, 27].

Autologous HSCT for TA was reported in a Brazilian woman [28]. She was diagnosed in June 1990 when she was 41 years old. The arteriography showed irregularities and stenosis of the abdominal aorta. The patient was treated with various immunosuppressive   agents,   such   as   steroids,   oral   cyclophosphamide, mycophenolate mofetil, methotrexate, and chlorambucil, but all of those therapies failed. In October 2002, a magnetic resonance angiogram showed narrowing and irregularities in both carotid and subclavian arteries and in the brachiocephalic artery. The worsening of clinical symptoms prompted the patient and her physician to choose experimental autologous HSCT in April 2003. Hematopoietic stem cells were mobilized with cyclophosphamide ($2\,g/m^2$) and granulocyte colony-stimulating factor. Conditioning regimen included cyclophosphamide ($50\,mg/kg/day \times 4$) plus rabbit anti-thymocyte globulin. After transplantation the clinical condition improved rapidly; there was complete resolution of headache, dizziness, and malaise, while limb claudication was significantly reduced. Sixty days after HSCT, magnetic resonance angiography showed correction of the stenosis of the brachiocephalic artery and reduction in the irregularities of the left carotid artery and of the left subclavian artery. On day 320, arterial pulses of the left lower limbs and of the carotid arteries showed normal shape and speed by Doppler US, and the wave speed of abdominal aorta increased to 73 cm/s. In this case the surprisingly fast improvement in artery structure and function is unexpected and deserve further studies.

10.8   DADA2

Deficiency of adenosine deaminase type 2 (DADA2) is an autosomal recessive disease resembling polyarteritis nodosa and is caused by mutations in the *CECR1* gene [29, 30]. The principal clinical features include livedo racemosa, vasculitic peripheral neuropathy, digital ischemia, and cutaneous ulceration. Anti-TNF-alpha mAb is particularly efficacious for this form of monogenic vasculitis [31].

Allogeneic HSCT has been reported to be successful in a DADA2 patient [32]. Two brothers with ADA2 deficiency had a homozygous mutation in *CECR1* (p.R169Q). One brother presented in 1999, at 6 months of age. He underwent HSCT in 2003 from a matched unrelated donor after myeloablative conditioning. The patient showed rapid immune reconstitution, with resolution of cytopenias, skin lesions, hepatosplenomegaly and hypercoagulability, and recovery of serum ADA2 levels to the normal range for his age. MRI revealed the brain was negative for vasculopathic changes. The absence of vasculopathy and the resolution of hypercoagulability after HSCT suggests that the correction of ADA2 blood levels reduces macrophage activation and endothelial disruption, both of which probably contribute to vasculitis. This patient's younger brother presented in 2009 at 6 years of age. Treatment with an anti-TNF alpha mAb (etanercept) stabilized his clinical condition, although he has persisting profound lymphopenia and low-grade inflammation.

Patients with DADA2 demonstrate skewed macrophage development toward the M1 pro-inflammatory phenotype as opposed to the M2 anti-inflammatory phenotype. M1 macrophages are known to produce TNF alpha, which could explain why anti-TNF alpha mAb seems particularly effective in DADA2. Due to the fact that MSC may skew macrophage from M1 to M2 phenotype, we hypothesize that MSC may be beneficial for DADA2 patients. Future clinical trials are needed to support our hypothesis.

10.9   CANDLE and SAVI

CANDLE (chronic atypical neutrophilic dermatosis with lipodystrophy and elevated temperature) syndrome is a recessive disease caused by gene mutations in the proteasome pathway and is classified as a proteasome-associated autoinflammatory syndrome (PRAAS). Mutations in *PSMB8*, *PSMB4*, *PSMB9*, *PSMA3*, and *POMP* are proposed to be responsible for CANDLE syndrome. Effective treatments for CANDLE syndrome are still elusive. Oral corticosteroids, methotrexate, cyclosporine, azathioprine, or intravenous immunoglobulins have achieved some improvements. CANDLE is associated with dysregulated type I interferon production; therefore targeting this pathway with selective JAK1/2 kinase inhibitor baricitinib has been proposed and a treatment protocol has been started.

Stimulator of interferon genes (STING)-associated vasculitis of infancy (SAVI) arises from sporadic/dominant mutation in the *TMEM173* gene and presents early in life with a vasculitic rash affecting the cheeks, nose, and peripheries. Standard vasculitis therapies are ineffective. Cutaneous vasculitis and deteriorating lung function usually continue relentlessly throughout childhood, with development of pulmonary hypertension and lung fibrosis, often with fatal outcome. Reports again suggest that early treatment targeting the interferon pathway (e.g., with JAK inhibitors) may offers some benefits to the patients.

Although no clinical trials have been reported for CANDLE and SAVI with either MSCs or HSCT, we consider that both strategies may be helpful in alleviating the patients' symptoms and improve their quality of life.

10.10   Conclusion

Considerable therapeutic advances for the treatment of vasculitis have been made in the past 10 years, including application of MSCs and HSCT. As new treatments that facilitate corticosteroid sparing are emergently needed, robust randomized controlled trials are expected to confirm the preliminary results of MSCs and HSCT. However it is a great challenge to enroll enough patients for randomized controlled trials aiming the rare diseases. Thus international cooperation is necessary in the future.

References

1. Jennette JC, Falk RJ, Bacon PA, et al. 2012 revised international Chapel Hill consensus conference nomenclature of Vasculitides. Arthritis Rheum. 2013;65(1):1–11.
2. Sakane T, Takeno M, Suzuki N, Inaba G. Behçet's disease. N Engl J Med. 1999;341(17):1284–91.
3. Barron KS, Shulman ST, Rowley A, et al. Report of the National Institutes of Health workshop on Kawasaki disease. J Rheumatol. 1999;26(1):170–90.

4. Hoffman GS, Kerr GS, Leavitt RY, et al. Wegener granulomatosis: an analysis of 158 patients. Ann Intern Med. 1992;116(6):488–98.
5. Scott DG, Watts RA. Systemic vasculitis: epidemiology, classification and environmental factors. Ann Rheum Dis. 2000;59(3):161–3.
6. Dominici M, Le Blanc K, Mueller I, et al. Minimal criteria for defining multipotent mesenchymal stromal cells. The International Society for Cellular Therapy position statement. Cytotherapy. 2006;8(2):315–7.
7. Figueroa FE, Carrión F, Villanueva S, Khoury M. Mesenchymal stem cell treatment for autoimmune diseases: a critical review. Biol Res. 2012;45(3):269–77.
8. Zhao RC, Liao L, Han Q. Mechanisms of and perspectives on the mesenchymal stem cell in immunotherapy. J Lab Clin Med. 2004;143(5):284–91.
9. Klinker MW, Wei CH. Mesenchymal stem cells in the treatment of inflammatory and autoimmune diseases in experimental animal models. World J Stem Cells. 2015;7(3):556–67.
10. Lee HK, Lim SH, Chung IS, et al. Preclinical efficacy and mechanisms of mesenchymal stem cells in animal models of autoimmune diseases. Immune Netw. 2014;14(2):81–8.
11. Rad F, Ghorbani M, Mohammadi Roushandeh A, Habibi Roudkenar M. Mesenchymal stem cell-based therapy for autoimmune diseases: emerging roles of extracellular vesicles. Mol Biol Rep. 2019;46(1):1533–49.
12. Jantunen E, Myllykangas-Luosujärvi R. Stem cell transplantation for treatment of severe autoimmune diseases: current status and future perspectives. Bone Marrow Transplant. 2000;25(4):351–6.
13. Gardner-Medwin JM, Dolezalova P, Cummins C, Southwood TR. Incidence of Henoch-Schonlein purpura, Kawasaki disease, and rare vasculitides in children of different ethnic origins. Lancet. 2002;360(9341):1197–202.
14. Ozen S. The spectrum of vasculitis in children. Best Pract Res Clin Rheumatol. 2002;16(3):411–25.
15. Chartapisak W, Opastiraku S, Willis NS, Craig JC, Hodson EM. Prevention and treatment of renal disease in Henoch-Schonlein purpura: a systematic review. Arch Dis Child. 2009;94(1):132–7.
16. Mu K, Zhang J, Gu Y, et al. Cord-derived mesenchymal stem cells therapy for liver cirrhosis in children with refractory Henoch-Schonlein purpura: a case report. Medicine (Baltimore). 2018;97(47):e13287.
17. Tsukamoto H, Nagafuji K, Horiuchi T, et al. A phase I-II trial of autologous peripheral blood stem cell transplantation in the treatment of refractory autoimmune disease. Ann Rheum Dis. 2006;65(4):508–14.
18. Tyndall A, Passweg J, Gratwohl A. Haemopoietic stem cell transplantation in the treatment of severe autoimmune diseases 2000. Ann Rheum Dis. 2001;60(7):702–7.
19. Ashihara E, Shimazaki C, Hirata T, et al. Autoimmune thrombocytopenia following peripheral blood stem cell autografting. Bone Marrow Transplant. 1993;12(3):297–9.
20. Mccrindle BW, Rowley AH, Newburger JW, et al. Diagnosis, treatment, and long-term management of Kawasaki disease: a scientific statement for health professionals from the American Heart Association[J]. Circulation. 2017;135(17):e927–99.
21. Eleftheriou D, Levin M, Shingadia D, Tulloh R, Klein NJ, Brogan PA. Management of Kawasaki disease. Arch Dis Child. 2014;99(1):74–83.
22. Noguchi S, Saito J, Kudo T, et al. Safety and efficacy of plasma exchange therapy for Kawasaki disease in children in intensive care unit: case series. JA Clin Rep. 2018;4(1):25.
23. Uchimura R, Ueda T, Fukazawa R, et al. Adipose tissue-derived stem cells suppress coronary arteritis of Kawasaki disease in vivo. Pediatr Int. 2019; https://doi.org/10.1111/ped.14062.
24. Wedderburn LR, Jeffery R, White H, et al. Autologous stem cell transplantation for paediatric-onset polyarteritis nodosa: changes in autoimmune phenotype in the context of reduced diversity of the T- and B-cell repertoires, and evidence for reversion from the CD45RO(+) to RA(+) phenotype. Rheumatology (Oxford). 2001;40(11):1299–307.
25. Maffei S, Renzo MD, Bova G, et al. Takayasu's arteritis: a review of the literature. Intern Emerg Med. 2006;1(2):105–12.

26. Tanaka F, Kawakami A, Iwanaga N, et al. Infliximab is effective for Takayasu arteritis refractory to glucocorticoid and methotrexate. Intern Med. 2006;45(2):313–6.
27. Nakaoka Y, Higuchi K, Arita Y, et al. Tocilizumab for the treatment of patients with refractory takayasu arteritis. Int Heart J. 2013;54(2):405–11.
28. Voltarelli JC, Oliveira MC, Stracieri AB, et al. Haematopoietic stem cell transplantation for refractory Takayasu's arteritis. Rheumatology (Oxford). 2004;43(10):1308–9.
29. Zhou Q, Yang D, Ombrello AK, et al. Early-onset stroke and vasculopathy associated with mutations in ADA2. N Engl J Med. 2014;370:911–20.
30. Navon Elkan P, Pierce SB, Segel R, et al. Mutant adenosine deaminase 2 in a polyarteritis nodosa vasculopathy. N Engl J Med. 2014;370(9):921–31.
31. Nanthapisal S, Murphy C, Omoyinmi E, et al. Deficiency of adenosine deaminase type 2 (DADA2): a description of phenotype and genotype in 15 cases. Arthritis Rheumatol. 2016;68(9):2314–2.
32. Van Montfrans J, Zavialov A, Zhou Q. Mutant ADA2 in vasculopathies. N Engl J Med. 2014;371(5):478–9.

Chapter 11
Mesenchymal Stem Cell and Endothelial Progenitor Cell Transplantation for Buerger's Disease

Lianming Liao and Yongquan Gu

Thromboangiitis obliterans (TAO), also known as Buerger's disease, was first described by von Winiwarter in a person in 1879 [1]. In 1908, Leo Buerger published a detailed description of the pathological findings on 11 amputated limbs and named the disease [2]. It is a nonatherosclerotic inflammatory disorder of unknown etiology that affects small- and medium-sized vessels of the extremities. TAO may also affect gastrointestinal, cerebrovascular, coronary, and renal arteries in some cases [3, 4].

Although smoking is the strongest risk factor in the development and progression of TAO, the specific mechanism of tobacco in the etiopathogenesis of TAO is not fully understood. It is not known which exact components of tobacco are involved in the pathogenesis of TAO. Hereditary factors (related to specific human leukocyte antigen haplotypes) may also contribute to the development of TAO. Endothelial dysfunction is associated with inflammation and thereby impaired endothelium-dependent vasorelaxation [4]. Most importantly a body of literature has addressed TAO as an autoimmune disease [5]. However, the exact etiology of TAO is still elusive.

A staging system for clinical symptoms was proposed by Rutherford (Table 11.1).

There is no standard treatment for TAO. The most effective intervention for TAO is smoking cessation as smoking is the strongest risk factor for TAO. Platelet inhibitors, such as aspirin and clopidogrel, may reduce secondary events in TAO patients with atherosclerotic disease. Vasodilators, such as amlodipine, nifedipine, and verapamil, can alleviate symptoms by dilating vessels proximal to the stenotic or occlusive lesion. Other drugs that have been proven beneficial include pentoxifylline,

L. Liao
Department of Laboratory Medicine, Fujian Medical University Union Hospital, Fuzhou, China

Y. Gu (✉)
Department of Vascular Surgery, Xuan Wu Hospital of Capital Medical University, Beijing, China

© Springer Nature Switzerland AG 2021
T. P. Navarro et al. (eds.), *Stem Cell Therapy for Vascular Diseases*, https://doi.org/10.1007/978-3-030-56954-9_11

Table 11.1 Rutherford classification

Grade	Category	Clinical
0	0	Asymptomatic
I	1	Mild claudication
I	2	Moderate claudication
I	3	Severe claudication
II	4	Rest pain
III	5	Ischemic ulcer not exceeding digits
IV	6	Severe ischemic ulcer or gangrene

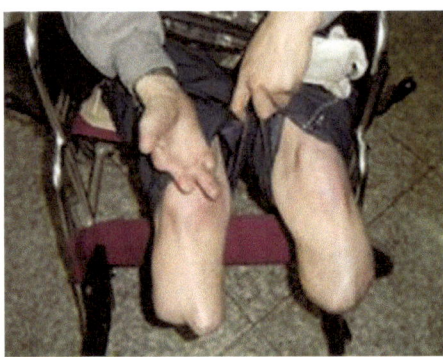 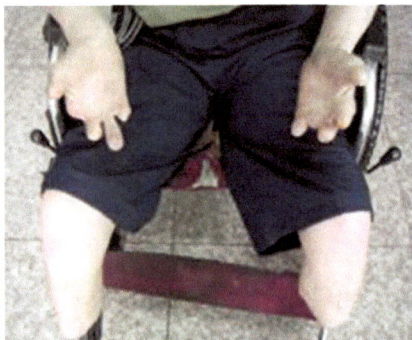

Fig. 11.1 Photographs showing healed amputation stumps

cilostazol naftidrofuryl, levocarnitine, arginine, buflomedil, ketanserin, niacin, lovastatin, bosentan, treprostinil, and prostacyclin derivatives. Overall, the long-term outcomes of the pharmacological inventions are unfavorable. Administration of growth factors and gene vectors for vascular endothelial growth factor (VEGF) gene to improve endothelial cell proliferation, migration, and blood vessel formation in the ischemic limb has also been reported with encouraging results. Spinal cord stimulators may modulate painful stimuli and alleviate pain in severe TAO. Surgical revascularization is rarely possible for TAO patients due to the diffused vascular damage of the distal vessels. Endovascular therapy may be technically challenging because of the prevalent location of lesions in distal vessels. Thus other innovative therapies are crucial to decrease amputation rate or even avoid amputation (Fig. 11.1).

A promising treatment for critical limb ischemia is stem cell therapy, in which stem cells are injected into the affected area to solicit the so-called therapeutic angiogenesis. Stem cells are undifferentiated cells that theoretically have the ability to differentiate into a specialized adult cell type in a specific tissue in the human body. Multipotent adult stem cells are found in differentiated tissues. The first reported trial of therapeutic angiogenesis using stem cells was the therapeutic angiogenesis by cell transplantation (TACT) trial published in 2002 [6]. Since then many clinical trials have been performed using various types of cells that are capable of promoting ulcer healing and neovascularization in animal models.

11.1 Endothelial Progenitor Cells

The formation of new blood vessels in response to tissue injury or ischemia is a complex physiological process. Postnatal angiogenesis was once thought to be exclusively mediated by sprouting of endothelial cells from pre-existing blood vessels. Now endothelial progenitor cells (EPCs) are well recognized to participate in new vessel formation [7]. EPCs belong to an immature cell population that is capable of differentiating into mature endothelial cells. EPCs can be isolated as CD34+ or AC133+ mononuclear cells (MNCs) from bone marrow or peripheral blood. Tissue ischemia or systemic administration of G-CSF, GM-CSF, vascular endothelial growth factor, or estrogen mobilizes EPCs from bone marrow into peripheral blood and the mobilized EPCs specifically home to sites of nascent neovascularization, thereby contributing to vascular repair.

The number and function of EPCs are crucial for endothelial function, especially in chronic ischemic diseases, including TAO [8–10]. Katsuki et al. found that the numbers of circulating EPCs were similar between the healthy controls and TAO patients, although the number of early outgrowth EPCs was significantly decreased in TAO patients [8]. On the contrary, Park et al. showed the number of EPCs and EPC colonies in TAO patients was significantly lower compared to the healthy control [9]. Although both teams used the same isolation and culture methods for EPCs, there was discrepancy in terms of circulating EPCs and colony-forming units in TAO patients in their reports. This discrepancy may be due to the fact that they used different definition for EPCs. Katsuki defined EPCs as CD34+/KDR+ or CD133+/KDR+ MNCs. Park et al. counted all of the cultured cells as EPCs, which were positive for vWF and VE cadherin (51% and 47%, respectively) and negative for CD34 and CD133. Idel et al. used a somewhat different method for the culture of EPCs [10]. They cultured MNCs in wells coated with human fibronectin and gelatin and maintained in endothelial cell basal medium-2 (EBM-2) supplemented with EGM-2 microvascular single aliquots and 5% fetal bovine serum. They defined ECPs as cells double-positive for lectin and Di-AcLDL. They showed the numbers of circulating EPCs were similar in the TAO group and the control group. Nevertheless, migration capacity of EPCs was not impaired in TAO patients in all of the three studies.

Yamamoto et al. quantitated mRNA expression of EPC-specific molecules (e.g., Flk-1, Flt-1, CD133, VE-cadherin, etc.) in bone marrow-derived or peripheral blood-derived MNCs obtained from four patients with ischemic limbs (two with TAO). They reported mRNA expression of EPC-specific molecules decreased in the circulating and bone marrow EPCs (CD45^{low}CD34+CD133+) [11].

In respect of the involvement of endothelial cells in the pathology of TAO, it is reasonable to propose that EPC transplantation may benefit TAO patients. As CD133+ is a marker of early EPCs, Burt et al. injected CD133+ stem cells collected from the peripheral blood of one TAO patient and eight other patients with critical limb ischemia to induce therapeutic angiogenesis [12]. All patients were not candidates for surgical revascularization and faced risk of amputation of the affected leg.

Stem cells were mobilized by administering G-CSF at 10 mcg/kg/day for 4–5 days. MNCs were collected by leukapheresis. CD133$^+$ stem cells were selected and injected into the patient's affected limb. Each injection delivered 2.5–5 million cells. At 12 months, two patients, both with lower extremity ulcers before treatment, underwent amputation of the treated leg. For the other seven patients, rest pain resolved within days of injection. Some functional parameters, such as treadmill pain-free walking time and treadmill exercise capacity, tended to improve but did not reach statistical significance. The authors did not describe the detailed response of the TAO patient after EPC injection.

11.2 Mononuclear Cells from Bone Marrow, Peripheral Blood, and Umbilical Cord Blood

Local injection of both bone marrow mononuclear cells (BMMNCs) and peripheral blood mononuclear cells (PBMNCs) into the ischemic limb has been proposed to initiate therapeutic angiogenesis. The strategy exploits the concept that MNCs contain EPCs that incorporate into new capillaries and other cells that will secrete factors and cytokines that may promote vessel formation.

Many studies have shown efficiency of autologous bone marrow cell injections for limb ischemia. Yamamoto et al. aspirated 400–500 mL of bone marrow from the posterior iliac crest of two TAO patients and isolated MNCs by centrifugation. Concentrated MNCs were intramuscularly injected into 40 sites of the ischemic limb. The two TAO patients were a 38-year-old woman with a painful ulcer in her left foot and a 51-year-old man with an ischemic lesion in his right foot, respectively. Ischemic status (e.g., rest pain, transcutaneous oxygen pressure, regional blood flow evaluated by thermography, and ulcer size) was dramatically improved after cell transplantation [11]. Soon Gu' team at Xuanwu Hospital reported a large clinical trial with 43 ischemic limbs in 35 patients, including 3 TAO patients. Bone marrow of each patient was stimulated by an injection of the recombinant human G-CSF (300 µg/d) for 2–3 days. In addition, heparin (12,500 units/day) was administered to avoid thrombosis. Then approximately 200 ml bone marrow (130–200 ml) was drawn from the iliac spine for MNCs. After depletion of red blood cells, concentrated BMMNCs were delivered by intramuscular injection and/or arterial intraluminal injection. Overall pain relief was remarked [13]. It is worthy to know that they administered G-CSF for 2–3 days, which may reduce cardiovascular adverse events caused by remarked increase in PBMNCs when G-CSF was administered for 5 days.

Koshikawa et al. used BMMNCs to improve symptoms of the ischemic hands in patients with peripheral arterial diseases. They enrolled six patients with TAO and one with collagen disease. Mean digital/brachial pressure index in those patients was 0.15 before transplantation and significantly increased to 0.67 at 6 months after transplantation. All patients showed improvement of pain scale and ischemic ulcers [14].

In a relatively large clinical trial, 28 homogenous TAO patients were enrolled. They were nonresponders to iloprost infusion and smoking cessation and were not candidates for nonsurgical or surgical revascularization. They all had unilateral critical limb ischemia. The patients received multiple injections of BMMNC [15]. The mean follow-up time was 16.6 months (range, 7.6–33.8 months). Only one patient required toe amputation during follow-up. A change in the ankle-brachial pressure index >0.15 was achieved in 8 patients at 3 months and in 14 patients at 6 months compared with baseline values. Patients demonstrated a significant improvement in rest pain scores, peak walking time, and quality of life. Total healing of the most important lesion was achieved in 15 patients (83%) with ischemic ulcers. Most importantly, digital subtraction angiography studies showed vascular collateral networks had formed across the affected arteries in 22 patients (78.5%).

There was another clinical trial with a large sample size that evaluated autologous BMMNC transplantation in 36 nonreconstructible TAO patients [16]. All of the patients were deemed having limb-threatening ischemia. Bone marrow was aspirated from the posterior iliac crests. The marrow was depleted of red blood cells and injected into the calf muscles of the affected limbs. At 6 months, three patients (12%) underwent major amputation. Significant improvement in skin ulcers, mean ankle-brachial index, and mean transcutaneous oximetry was observed.

The long-term effect of BMMNCs for TAO was also excellent in a study with eight TAO patients [17]. Eleven limbs (3 with rest pain and 8 with an ischemic ulcer) of 8 TAO patients were followed up for clinical events for a mean of 684 ± 549 days (range 103–1466 days) after BMMNC transplantation. At 4 weeks, improvement in pain was observed in all 11 limbs, with complete relief in 4 (36%). VAS pain score decreased from 5.1 ± 0.7 to 1.5 ± 1.3. An improvement in skin ulcers was observed in all eight limbs with an ischemic ulcer, with complete healing in seven (88%).

In the 3-year-follow-up study of TACT trial [6], which included 115 patients (74 with peripheral arterial disease and 41 with TAO), 3-year mortality and leg amputation-free interval were accessed as primary end points [18]. The median follow-up time for surviving patients was 25.3 months. In the TAO subgroup, the 3-year overall survival rate was 100% (no death), and the 3-year amputation-free rate was 91%. The significant improvement in the leg pain scale, ulcer size, and pain-free walking distance was maintained for at least 2 years after the therapy. They concluded that the safety and efficacy of BMMNC transplantation were not inferior to the conventional revascularization therapies.

Most recently, Gu's team reported their 10-year follow-up of TAO patients after BMMNC transplantation [19]. This is so far the longest follow-up report of the similar studies, and the results confirmed the safety and efficacy of BMMNCs for TAO. During January 2005 and July 2006, 59 patients with TAO were treated with either aspirin alone ($n = 19$) or aspirin plus BMMNC injection ($n = 40$). Concentrated ABMMNCs were injected at 5 cm proximal to the obstructive lesion (Fig. 11.2). The 10-year amputation-free survival was 85.3% (29/34) in patients treated with BMMNCs compared to 40% (6/15) in patients treated with aspirin alone. Ulcer

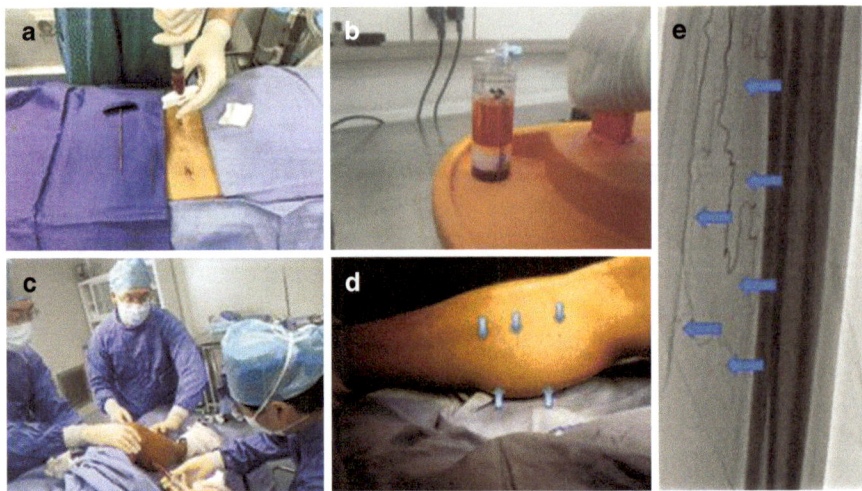

Fig. 11.2 Representative photos of BMMNC treatment. (**a**) Bone marrow was harvested from the posterior superior iliac spine. (**b**) Separation of red cells and BMMNCs. (**c**) BMMNC injection. (**d**) Injection sites. (**e**) Representative angiogram. Arrows indicate injection sites along the tibial arteries

area, toe-brachial index, transcutaneous oxygen pressure, and pain score were also significantly improved with BMMNC treatment (Fig. 11.3).

Another long-term follow-up study by Baran et al. also supported the benefit of autologous BMMNC transplantation in TAO patients, even though this study had a smaller sample size [20]. Twenty-eight patients (25 males and 3 females) were enrolled between April 2003 and August 2005. BMMNCs were injected into the gastrocnemius muscle, the intermetatarsal region, and the dorsum of the foot ($n = 26$) or forearm ($n = 2$), and saline was injected into the contralateral limbs. The mean follow-up time was 139.6 ± 10.5 months. The ankle-brachial pressure index evaluated at 6 months and 120 months was improved compared to the baseline scores. The angiographic improvement was 78.5% and 57.1% at 6 and 120 months, respectively. The 10-year amputation-free rate was 96% in BMMNC-implanted limbs and 93% in saline-injected limbs. The high amputation-free rate in the saline-injected limbs was interesting. We think this is because BMMNCs secrete many proangiogenic factors into the peripheral circulation and exert proangiogenic effect in the distal saline-injected limbs.

Kim et al. achieved autologous whole bone marrow stem cell transplantation via fenestration of the tibia bone [21]. Twenty-seven TAO patients (34 lower limbs) who were not candidates for surgical revascularization or radiologic intervention were enrolled. Fenestration through the tibia bone was performed under general or spinal anesthesia. Six tibial sites were fenestrated with a 2.5-mm-diameter screw under fluoroscopic guidance. This procedure allowed bone marrow stem cells to be released into ischemic calf muscle through fenestrated posterior tibia holes. The mean follow-up time was 19.1 months. Before treatment all of the 34 limbs had symptoms

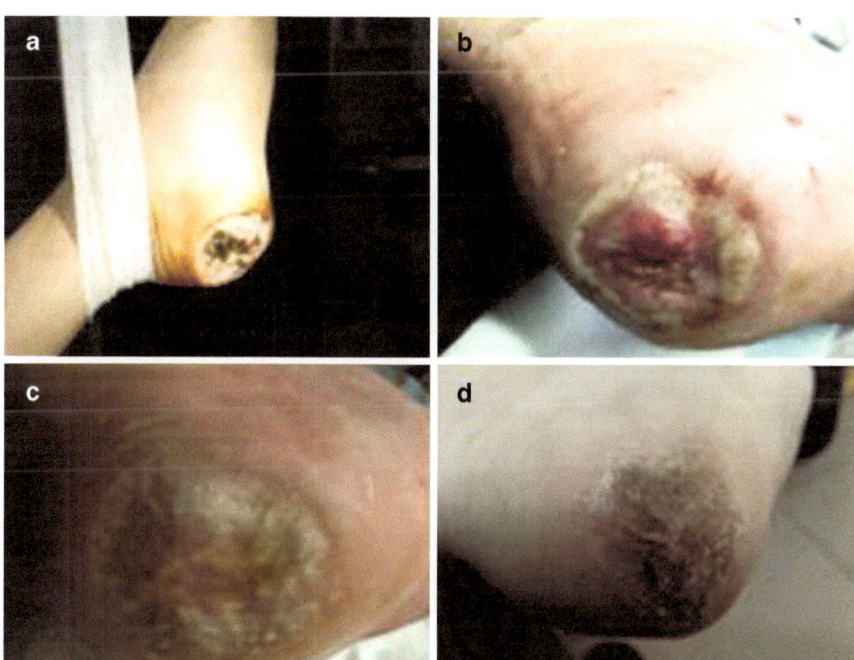

Fig. 11.3 Representative photographs showing the gradual healing of an ulcer during the follow-up period. (**a**) Before BMMNC transplantation. (**b**) Three months after BMMNC transplantation. (**c**) Six months after BMMNC transplantation. (**d**) Ten years after BMMNC transplantation

that were more than category 3 (severe claudication). During the follow-up period, 23 limbs (67.6%) had symptoms of category 2 (moderate claudication). One limb achieved a +3 (markedly improved) outcome, 26 (76.5%) achieved a +2 (moderately improved) outcome, and 7 (20.6%) limbs were unchanged. Thirteen of 17 limbs with nonhealing ulcer healed during follow-up. Although the authors concluded this method was effective in inducing therapeutic angiogenesis in TAO patients, we think it is more invasive compared to intramuscular injection of BMMNCs.

Although MNC transplantation for ischemic limb disease was first performed with BMMNCs, PBMNCs are also widely used. PBMNCs can be harvested in an easier and less invasive approach. The mononuclear cell fraction is usually enriched by Ficoll density gradient system centrifugation and by use of blood centrifugation and plasmapheresis systems after G-CSF or GM-CSF mobilization. Moriya et al. retrospectively evaluated 14 TAO patients who were treated between July 2002 and December 2005 and analyzed the data in December 2007. Improvement of ischemic symptoms was remarked. Only one TAO patient underwent major amputation during the observation period [22]. Horie et al. reported excellent long-term clinical outcomes for patients with lower limb ischemia implanted with G-CSF-mobilized autologous PBMNCs [23]. Among 11 patients with TAO, the 2-year survival rate was 100%; the 1-year amputation-free rates were 79%. Ishida et al. enrolled five patients with TAO and one patient with arteriosclerosis obliterans. PBMNCs were harvested and injected intramuscularly (five legs and one arm) for 2 days. Improvement in the ankle-brachial pressure index was seen in four patients at 4 weeks, and ischemic ulcer improved in three patients at 3 weeks. The mean maximum walking distance significantly increased from 203 m to 559 m at 4 weeks and was sustained for 24 weeks [24].

Furthermore, Kim AK et al. used human umbilical cord blood-derived mononuclear cells (UCBMNCs) for TAO [25] after they had tried BMMSCs [21]. UCBMNCs should be associated with less graft-versus-host disease, and the human leucocyte antigen (HLA) matching should be less stringent because of the immunological naiveté of UCBMNCs. In their study, seven TAO patients (seven lower limbs) who had intermittent claudication, rest pain, and foot ulcer for a minimum of 3 months without evidence of improvement with medical treatment were enrolled. The patients continued their medications during the study period. A total of 4×10^8 ABO type-matched HCBMNCs were injected into 20 sites of the ischemic calf muscles along the tibial and peroneal arteries. After the procedures, the patients were followed up at 1, 3, 6, and 9 months. The patients did not receive any immunosuppressive drugs and did not experience any graft-versus-host disease during the follow-up period. However, the authors did not report specifically the efficacy of HCBMNC transplantation in the TAO patients [25].

We notice that most of the studies using MNCs for TAO did not observe any serious adverse events. Surprisingly, one patient suffered sudden death at 20 months after transplantation of BMMNCs, and the authors thought it was associated with injection of BMMNCs [14]. The sudden death happened when the patient was 30 years old. He had no risk factors for atherosclerosis and stopped smoking before BMMNC injection. Furthermore, [201]thallium scintigraphy performed before injection revealed no sign of myocardial ischemia. Considering the patient's background and the natural course of TAO, the authors thought that his death was related to BMMNC transplantation. Indeed, several studies have suggested the possible role of BMMNCs in atherogenesis. Silvestre et al., for example, demonstrated that transplantation of BMMNCs into ischemic limbs of apolipoprotein E-knockout mice led to a significant increase in atherosclerotic plaque size in the aortic sinus despite the fact that the total cholesterol levels were within normal range and there was no significant change in plaque stability [26]. Therefore they suggested transplantation of BMMNCs may contribute to "silent" progression of atherosclerosis, which could be harmful in the long term. More recently, George et al. have also shown that an intravenous injection of bone marrow cells into apolipoprotein E-knockout mice resulted in an increase in atherosclerotic lesion size, whereas an injection of EPCs influenced plaque stability [27]. We should note that in the experiments with apolipoprotein E-knockout mice, BMMNCs were intravenously injected, whereas in the human clinical trials, BMMNCs were injected locally in the affected legs. In fact, three long-term follow-ups did not observe similar adverse events [18–20]. Nevertheless, more patients are needed to establish a definite relationship between BMMNC transplantation and atherosclerosis.

11.3   Hematopoietic Stem Cell

Hematopoietic stem cells (HSCs) play important roles in angiogenesis. In a study by Kinoshita et al., 15 TAO patients received intramuscular injection of G-CSF mobilized CD34$^+$ cells from peripheral blood [28]. PBMNCs were harvested after bone marrow mobilization with G-CSF (10 mg/kg per day) for 5 days. Leukapheresis was performed to harvest PBMNCs, and magnetic separation was used for CD34$^+$ cells. Purified CD34$^+$ cells were intramuscularly injected into 40 sites (30 sites in the calf, 6 sites in the sole, and 4 sites in the intertoe muscle) of the leg. Dose of CD34$^+$ cells was 10^5 cells/kg, 5×10^5 cells/kg, or 10^6 cells/kg. Favorable results were observed. Rutherford scale significantly improved by week 8, and the improvement sustained until week 208. CLI-free ratio increased and peaked (100%) at week 156. Due to the high cost of magnetic separation for purification of CD34$^+$ cells, we think HSCs are not preferred cells for the treatment of TAO unless HSCs are proved to be superior to other types of cells in terms of efficacy and safety.

11.4   Mesenchymal Stem Cells

As we have mentioned in the other chapter, mesenchymal stem cells (MSCs) were originally isolated from bone marrow and later from a variety of tissues, such as adipose tissue, tooth pulps, periodontal tissue, umbilical cord, and placenta. MSCs from umbilical cord, adipose tissue, and bone marrow have been used for TAO. The invasive procedure for harvesting autologous MSCs from bone marrow or adipose tissue is a disadvantage.

MSCs are well studied for their ability to promote angiogenesis and arteriogenesis through stromal and paracrine activity. Theoretically, UCBMSCs have many advantages because of abundant resource and the putative stronger stemness of newborn cells compared with adult stem cells. Cell therapy using UCBMSCs also have the merit of being less invasive and less expensive because it is easy to mass-produce UCBMSCs as a commercial product.

Interestingly, in vitro experiment evaluating the promoting effects of MSCs on human umbilical vein endothelial cell proliferation, migration, and tube formation and in vivo experiment evaluating the effects of MSCs in animal models of hindlimb ischemia showed that UCMSCs were superior to BMMSCs and adipose tissue-derived MSCs (ATMSCs) were superior to UCMSCs [29, 30].

Dash et al. first conducted a randomized controlled trial using BMMSCs for chronic nonhealing ulcers of the lower extremities. A total of 24 patients, 6 with diabetic foot ulcers and 18 with TAO, were enrolled and randomized into implant and control groups. In the implant group, the patients received autologous cultured BMMSCs along with standard wound dressing; the control group received only the standard wound dressing regimen. They assessed ulcer size at the beginning of the study and 12 weeks after treatment. A larger decrease in ulcer area in the BMMSC group was observed: mean ulcer area decreased from 5.04 cm² to 1.48 cm². In the control group, the mean ulcer area decreases from 4.68 cm² to 3.59 cm². Pain-free walking distance increased from 38.33 meters to 284.44 meters in the BMMSC group. On the contrary, mean pain-free walking distance increased from 35.66 meters to 78.22 meters in the control group [31].

A prospective, double-blind randomized placebo-controlled multicenter study was conducted by Gupta et al. that used allogeneic BMMSCs to patients with established arterial occlusive disease (Rutherford II-4, III-5, or III-6) and was not suitable for or had failed revascularization treatment. Twenty patients (BMMSC: placebo = 1:1) were administered with at a dose of 2 million cells/kg or placebo (PlasmaLyte A) at the gastrocnemius muscle of the ischemic limbs. Significant increase in ankle-brachial pressure index and ankle pressure was seen in the BMMSC group compared to the placebo group. However, the authors did not reported how many TAO were included in their cohort [32]. They further conducted a prospective, dose-finding phase II study assessing the efficacy and safety of intramuscular administration of allogeneic BMMSCs in TAO patients. Cells were injected intramuscularly in the gastrocnemius muscle and locally around the nonhealing ulcer. Significant reduction of rest pain and healing of ulcers in an accelerated fashion were observed [33].

Kim reported for the first time a clinical trial on TAO patients using UCBMSCs [34]. They first proved that transplantation of UCBMSCs augmented arteriogenesis in the ischemic limb of immunodeficient nude mice. Then four TAO patients were enrolled for UCBMSC transplantation. All patients had already received medical treatment, surgical interventions, and even amputations, but they had to take painkillers to sleep at night. The human leukocyte antigen (HLA) typings were done to get a proper match between the patients and preserved umbilical cord blood. UCBMSCs (1×10^6) were injected into the adjacent area of the lesions with a 23-gauge needle syringe. Strikingly, the pain of the patients was alleviated more rapidly than the formation of the new capillaries, which happened between 5 hours and 14 days in all patients. The unhealed skin lesions of the two patients showed skin regeneration within 120 days. Allograft rejection was not observed, and even no immunosuppressants were administered during the follow-up periods of up to 25 months in the first enrolled patient.

In another phase I study with 8 patients (5 with TAO), Yang et al. injected a total of 1×10^7 UCBMSCs into 20 sites on each limb using 23-gauge needle. Injection sites were selected below the knee at 20 different sites of ischemic calf muscle along the tibial and peroneal arteries [35]. During the 6-month follow-up period, no death or serious adverse events were observed, and there were no amputations. Angiography revealed increasing scores compared with those at baseline in three of eight patients. Improvement in ulcer healing and an increase in pain-free walking distance were also observed.

Several groups used ATMSCs for proangiogenic therapy. In a phase I trial the safety and efficacy of autologous cultured ATMSCs to treat patients with non-revascularizable critical limb ischemia were evaluated. There was one male TAO patient with Rutherford grade III-6. Adipose tissues were obtained by simple liposuction from the abdominal subcutaneous fats and digested with collagenase I. Patients were treated with ATMSCs by intramuscular injection into the ischemic leg. Rest pain and TcPO2 all improved during the 6-month follow-up [36].

In the study by Lee et al., 12 TAO patients and 3 patients with diabetic foot were treated with intramuscular injections of ATMSCs [37]. A total of 3×10^8 ATMSCs (each syringe had 5×10^6 ATMSCs) were injected at 60 points into the lower extremities of 12 patients. Clinical improvement occurred in 10 patients (66.7%), including 7 of 12 TAO patients (58.3%). Four TAO patients required minor amputation during follow-up, and all amputation sites healed completely. Digital subtraction angiography before and 6 months after ATMSC implantation showed formation of numerous vascular collateral networks across affected arteries. Improvement of more than one grade in collateral vessel formation was observed in two of the three patients with diabetic foot (66.7%) and in eight of the ten patients with TAO (80%). A two-year long studies with ATMSCs in 17 TAO patients also showed the onetime ATMSC therapy can provide long-term benefit to patients as indicated by decreased rest pain, increased pain-free walking distance, increased toe-brachial pressure index, increased transcutaneous oxygen pressure, and increased arterial brachial pressure index and freedom from amputations during the follow-up [38].

11.5 Conclusions

TAO represents a most severe disease that profoundly influences patient quality of life. Prompt recognition, medication, and revascularization are the current standards of care. Nevertheless, this care strategy is not completely effective. Researches for new pharmacological and angiogenic therapies are underway to meet this unmet medical need. Current literature supports that intramuscular administration of BMMNCs, PBMNCs, and ATMSCs is a relatively safe and effective therapy for TAO patients not suitable to conventional revascularization. Adverse events are mostly mild and are related to local implantation/injection. Although encouraging results from multiple studies have been reported, unfortunately such studies involved small numbers of patients. There is a need for larger, placebo-controlled, randomized multicenter trials to confirm safety and efficacy of these cell therapies.

Animal studies indicate that paracrine, anti-apoptotic growth factor, or other factors produced by stem cells may mediate the response independent of direct differentiation into endothelial cells. However, the precise molecular mechanisms of stem cell therapy are still unknown. The specific mechanisms for the improvement in the patients' pain remain to be fully explained because the quick reduction of rest pain was noticed before vessel formation. In addition, many questions remain unanswered with regard to stem cell therapy, including identification of the ideal cell types, autologous versus allogeneic cells, optimal cell number, and route and frequency of administration. Effective protocols regarding in vitro cell methods for augmentation of cell potency, which may include stimulation of the stem cells with small molecule, cytokines, and various growth factors and use of bioactive microspheres, are also needed to be explored and evaluated in clinical trials.

References

1. Winiwarter F. A peculiar form of endarteritis and endophlebitis with gangrene of the foot [Ueber eine eigenthümliche Form von Endarteriitis und Endophlebitis mit Gangrän des Fusses]. Archiv für Klinische Chirurgie. 1879;23:202-26.
2. Buerger L. Thromboangiitis obliterans: a study of the vascular lesions leading to presenile spontaneous gangrene. Am J Med. 1908;136:567-80.
3. Kröger K. Buerger's disease: what has the last decade taught us? Eur J Intern Med. 2006;17(4):227-34.
4. Azizi M, Boutouyrie P, Bura-Rivière A, et al. Thromboangiitis obliterans and endothelial function. Eur J Clin Investig. 2010;40(6):518-26.
5. Moghaddam AS, Modaghegh MHS, Rahimi H, et al. Molecular mechanisms regulating immune responses in thromboangiitis obliterans: a comprehensive review. Iran J Basic Med Sci. 2019;22(3):215-24.
6. Tateishi-Yuyama E, Matsubara H, Murohara T, et al. Therapeutic angiogenesis for patients with limb ischaemia by autologous transplantation of bone-marrow cells: a pilot study and a randomised controlled trial. Lancet. 2002;360(9331):427-35.
7. Asahara T, Murohara T, Sullivan A, et al. Isolation of putative progenitor endothelial cells for angiogenesis. Science. 1997;275(5302):964-7.
8. Katsuki Y, Sasaki K, Toyama Y, et al. Early outgrowth EPCs generation is reduced in patients with Buerger's disease. Clin Res Cardiol. 2011;100(1):21-7.
9. Park HS, Cho KH, Kim KL, et al. Reduced circulating endothelial progenitor cells in thromboangiitis obliterans (Buerger's disease). Vasc Med. 2013;18(6):331-9.
10. Idei N, Nishioka K, Soga J, et al. Vascular function and circulating progenitor cells in thromboangiitis obliterans (Buerger's disease) and atherosclerosis obliterans. Hypertension. 2011;57(1):70-8.
11. Yamamoto K, Kondo T, Suzuki S, et al. Molecular evaluation of endothelial progenitor cells in patients with ischemic limbs. Therapeutic effect by stem cell transplantation. Arterioscler Thromb Vasc Biol. 2004;24(12):e192-6.
12. Burt RK, Testori A, Oyama Y, et al. Autologous peripheral blood CD133+ cell implantation for limb salvage in patients with critical limb ischemia. Bone Marrow Transplant. 2010;45(1):111-6.
13. Gu Y, Zhang J, Qi L. A clinical study on implantation of autologous bone marrow mononuclear cells after bone marrow stimulation for treatment of lower limb ischemia. Zhongguo Xiu Fu Chong Jian Wai Ke Za Zhi. 2006;20(10):1017-20. [Article in Chinese]
14. Koshikawa M, Shimodaira S, Yoshioka T, et al. Therapeutic angiogenesis by bone marrow implantation for critical hand ischemia in patients with peripheral arterial disease: a pilot study. Curr Med Res Opin. 2006;22(4):793-8.
15. Durdu S, Akar AR, Arat M, et al. Autologous bone-marrow mononuclear cell implantation for patients with Rutherford grade II-III thromboangiitis obliterans. J Vasc Surg. 2006;44(4):732-9.
16. Motukuru V, Suresh KR, Vivekanand V, et al. Therapeutic angiogenesis in Buerger's disease (thromboangiitis obliterans) patients with critical limb ischemia by autologous transplantation of bone marrow mononuclear cells. J Vasc Surg. 2008;48(6 Suppl):53S-60S.
17. Miyamoto K, Nishigami K, Nagaya N, et al. Unblinded pilot study of autologous transplantation of bone marrow mononuclear cells in patients with thromboangiitis obliterans. Circulation. 2006;114(24):2679-84.
18. Matoba S, Tatsumi T, Murohara T, et al. Long-term clinical outcome after intramuscular implantation of bone marrow mononuclear cells (Therapeutic Angiogenesis by Cell Transplantation [TACT] trial) in patients with chronic limb ischemia. Am Heart J. 2008;156(5):1010-8.
19. Guo J, Guo L, Cui, et al. Autologous bone marrow-derived mononuclear cell therapy in Chinese patients with critical limb ischemia due to thromboangiitis obliterans: 10-year results. Stem Cell Res Ther. 2018;9(1):43.
20. Baran Ç, Durdu S, Özçınar E, et al. Long-term follow-up of patients with Buerger's disease after autologous stem cell therapy. Anatol J Cardiol. 2019;21(3):155-62.

21. Kim DI, Kim MJ, Joh JH, et al. Angiogenesis facilitated by autologous whole bone marrow stem cell transplantation for Buerger's disease. Stem Cells. 2006;24(5):1194–200.
22. Moriya J, Minamino T, Tateno K, et al. Long-term outcome of therapeutic neovascularization using peripheral blood mononuclear cells for limb ischemia. Circ Cardiovasc Intervent. 2009;2(3):245–54.
23. Horie T, Onodera R, Akamastu M, et al. Long-term clinical outcomes for patients with lower limb ischemia implanted with G-CSF-mobilized autologous peripheral blood mononuclear cells. Atherosclerosis. 2010;208(2):461–6.
24. Ishida A, Ohya Y, Sakuda H, Ohshiro K, et al. Autologous peripheral blood mononuclear cell implantation for patients with peripheral arterial disease improves limb ischemia. Circ J. 2005;69(10):1260–5.
25. Kim AK, Kim MH, Kim S, et al. Stem-cell therapy for peripheral arterial occlusive disease. Eur J Vasc Endovasc Surg. 2011;42(5):667–75.
26. Silvestre J-S, Gojova A, Brun V, Potteaux S, et al. Transplantation of bone marrow-derived mononuclear cells in ischemic apolipoprotein E-knockout mice accelerates atherosclerosis without altering plaque composition. Circulation. 2003;108(23):2839–42.
27. George J, Afek A, Abashidze A, et al. Transfer of endothelial progenitor and bone marrow cells influences atherosclerotic plaque size and composition in Apolipoprotein E knockout mice. Thromb Vasc Biol. 2005;25(12):2636–41.
28. Kinoshita M, Fujita Y, Katayama M, et al. Long-term clinical outcome after intramuscular transplantation of granulocyte colony stimulating factor-mobilized CD34 positive cells in patients with critical limb ischemia. Atherosclerosis. 2012;224(2):440–5.
29. Yin C, Liang Y, Zhang J, et al. Umbilical cord-derived mesenchymal stem cells relieve hindlimb ischemia through enhancing angiogenesis in tree shrews. Stem Cells Int. 2016;2016:9742034.
30. Lu H, Wang F, Mei H, et al. Human adipose mesenchymal stem cells show more efficient angiogenesis promotion on endothelial colony-forming cells than umbilical cord and endometrium. Stem Cells Int. 2018;2018:7537589.
31. Dash NR, Dash SN, Routray P, et al. Targeting nonhealing ulcers of lower extremity in human through autologous bone marrow-derived mesenchymal stem cells. Rejuvenation Res. 2009;12(5):359–66.
32. Gupta PK, Chullikana A, Parakh R, et al. A double blind randomized placebo controlled phase I/II study assessing the safety and efficacy of allogeneic bone marrow derived mesenchymal stem cell in critical limb ischemia. J Transl Med. 2013;11:143.
33. Gupta PK, Krishna M, Chullikana A, et al. Administration of adult human bone marrow-derived, cultured, pooled, allogeneic mesenchymal stromal cells in critical limb ischemia due to Buerger's disease: phase II study report suggests clinical efficacy. Stem Cells Transl Med. 2017;6(3):689–99.
34. Kim SW, Han H, Chae GT, et al. Successful stem cell therapy using umbilical cord blood-derived multipotent stem cells for Buerger's disease and ischemic limb disease animal model. Stem Cells. 2006;24(6):1620–6.
35. Yang SS, Kim NR, Park KB, et al. A phase 1 study of human cord blood-derived mesenchymal stem cell therapy in patients with peripheral arterial occlusive disease. Int J Stem Cells. 2013;6(1):37–44.
36. Bura A, Planat-Benard V, Bourin P, et al. Phase I trial: the use of autologous cultured adipose-derived stroma/stem cells to treat patients with non-revascularizable critical limb ischemia. Cytotherapy. 2014;16(2):245–57.
37. Lee HC, An SG, Lee HW, et al. Safety and effect of adipose tissue-derived stem cell implantation in patients with critical limb ischemia: a pilot study. Circ J. 2012;76(7):1750–60.
38. Ra JC, Jeong EC, Kang SK, et al. A prospective, nonrandomized, no placebo-controlled, phase I/II clinical trial assessing the safety and efficacy of intramuscular injection of autologous adipose tissue-derived mesenchymal stem cells in patients with severe Buerger's disease. Cell Med. 2016;9(3):87–102.

Chapter 12
Changing the Course of Peripheral Arterial Disease Using Adult Stem Progenitor Cells

Mark Niven, Galit Sivak, Shlomo Baytner, Roman Liberson, Shlomo Bulvik, Yael Porat, Michael Frogel, Louis Shenkman, Martin Grajower, Frank Veith, and Michael Belkin

Abbreviations

ABI	Ankle-brachial Index
ACE	Angiotensin-converting enzyme
AcLDL	Acetylated low-density lipoprotein
ACP	Angiogenic cell precursor
AE	Adverse events
AFS	Amputation-free survival
ATMP	Advanced therapy medicinal products

M. Niven · S. Baytner · R. Liberson · S. Bulvik
Sanz Medical Center, Laniado Hospital, Netanya, Israel

G. Sivak
Rabin Medical center, Tel Aviv University, Tel Aviv, Israel

Y. Porat (✉)
BioGenCell, Ltd., Laniado Hospital, Netanya, Israel
e-mail: Yael.Porat@biogencell.net

M. Frogel
Cohen's Children's Medical Center, New Hyde Park, NY, USA

L. Shenkman
Tel Aviv University, Tel Aviv, Israel

M. Grajower
Albert Einstein College of Medicine, Bronx, NY, USA

F. Veith
NYU-Langone Medical Center, New York, NY, USA

The Cleveland Clinic, Cleveland, OH, USA

M. Belkin
Sanz Medical Center, Laniado Hospital, Netanya, Israel

Tel Aviv University, Tel Aviv, Israel

© Springer Nature Switzerland AG 2021
T. P. Navarro et al. (eds.), *Stem Cell Therapy for Vascular Diseases*,
https://doi.org/10.1007/978-3-030-56954-9_12

AP	Ankle pressure
BM	Bone marrow
CFA	Common femoral artery
CLI	Critical Limb Ischemia
CLTI	chronic limb-threatening ischemia
CTCAE	Common Terminology Criteria for Adverse Events
CPK	Creatine phosphokinase
CV	Cardiovascular
DC	Dendritic cell
Del-1 and DELTA 1	Developmentally regulated endothelial locus
DSMB	Data and Safety Monitoring Board
EC	Endothelial cells
EnEPC	Enriched endothelial progenitor cells
EPC	Endothelial progenitor cells
ESC	European Society for Cardiology
EVT	Endovascular therapy
FGF	Fibroblast growth factor
FIH	First in human
GVHD	Graft-versus-host disease
GSV	Great saphenous vein
G-CSF	Granulocyte colony-stimulating factor
GCP	Good clinical practice
GMP	Good manufacturing practice
GTP	Good tissue practice
Hg	Hemoglobin
HGF	Hepatocyte growth factor
HIF	Hypoxia inducible factor
HSPC	Hematopoietic stem/progenitor cells
IA	Intra-arterial
IC	Intermittent claudication
ICH	International Conference on Harmonization of Technical Requirements for Registration of Pharmaceuticals for Human Use
IL-10	Interleukin-10
IM	Intramuscular
IV	Intravenous
LEAD	Lower extremity arterial disease
LOCF	Last observation carried forward
MedDRA	Medical Dictionary for Regulatory Activities
MI	Myocardial infarction
MNC	Mononuclear cells
MSC	Mesenchymal stem cells
NIH	National Institutes of Health
NO	Nitric oxide
PAD	Peripheral artery disease

PBMC	Peripheral blood mononuclear cell
PB-MNC	Peripheral blood-derived mononuclear cells
PI	Principal investigator
PTA	Percutaneous transluminal angioplasty
PVR	Pulse volume recording
QoL	Quality of life
RCT	Randomized controlled trial
RNA	Ribonucleic acids
SAE	Severe adverse effect
SOC	System organ class
SPC	Stem/progenitor cells
TASC	Trans-Atlantic Inter-Society Consensus
TBI	Toe-brachial index
TcPO2	Transcutaneous oxygen pressure
TGF-β	Transforming growth factor beta
TP	Toe pressure
TTF	Treatment failure
Ulex	Plant *Ulex europaeus*
VAS	Visual Analogue Scale
VascuQol	Vascular Quality of Life
VEGF	Vascular endothelial growth factor
WBC	White blood cells
WIfI	Wound, Ischemia, and foot Infection

12.1 Introduction

Peripheral artery disease (PAD) is caused by atherosclerotic occlusion of the arteries of the body. PAD can affect the brain, internal organs, and limbs. Most commonly this vascular disease causes partial or total occlusion of the blood supply to the legs and is sometimes referred to as lower extremity arterial disease (LEAD). LEAD affects more than 200 million people worldwide with about 12 million people in the USA and 17 million in the EU (https://www.nhlbi.nih.gov/health/educational/pad/materials/pad_extfctsht_general.html, [45, 62]). Clinically, it is characterized by intermittent claudication (IC), pain in the muscles of the lower limb brought on physical activity and rapidly relieved by rest. When PAD worsens, it reaches the stage of Critical Limb Ischemia (CLI), a life-threatening disease with comorbidities and an extremely low quality of life (QoL). CLI, also referred to as chronic limb-threatening ischemia (CLTI), is the major cause of ischemic amputation [1, 21, 61]. CLI presents clinically as rest pain, ischemic ulceration, or gangrene of the foot or the leg (Fig. 12.1) and requires immediate treatment [48].

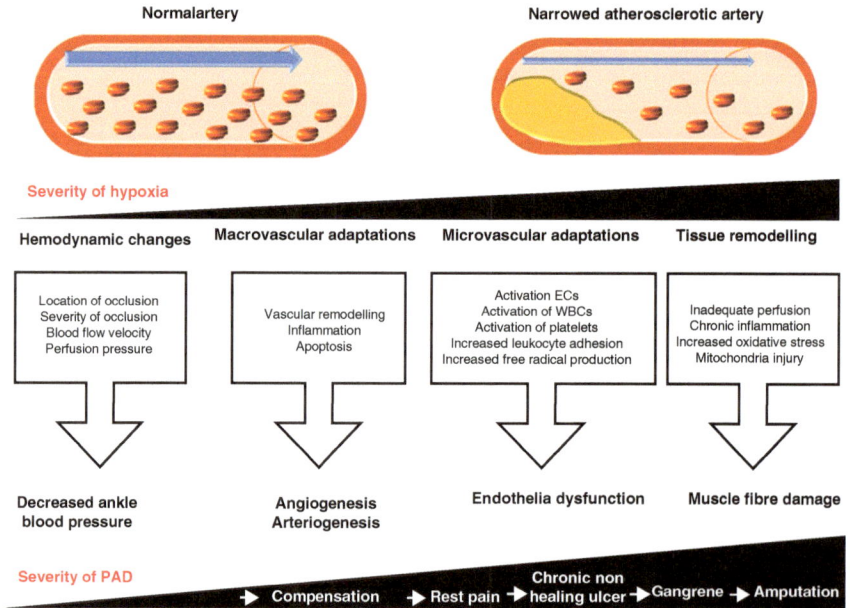

Fig. 12.1 Schematic representation of the response to ischemia in peripheral artery disease [48] Initially the ischemic limb compensates for the hypoxia by altering the hemodynamics and promoting microvascular adaptations by induction of angiogenesis and/or arteriogenesis. As the severity of the hypoxia increases, the microvascular adaptations are not sufficient. These changes lead to mitochondrial injury, free radical generation and subsequent muscle fiber damage, myofiber degeneration, and fibrosis. Additional decreases in oxygen supply and increased metabolic demands lead to rest pain, chronic non-healing wounds and gangrene, threatening limb function, and viability. In this figure, the blue arrows show the direction of blood flow in the artery, and the white arrows show the increase in severity of disease. Abbreviations: ECs endothelial cells, HIF-1α hypoxia inducible factor-1α, NO Nitric oxide, PAD peripheral artery disease, VEGF vascular endothelial growth factor, WBCs white blood cells

12.1.1   CLI Diagnostics and Current Best Practice

The assessment of the severity of PAD is traditionally based on the Fontaine or Rutherford classifications [31, 37, 72]. Rutherford suggested classification for grading the severity of chronic arterial occlusive disease for the purposes of standardized reporting practices is outlined in Table 12.1, where symptomatic disease is stratified into six categories.

Pressure indexes such as the ankle-brachial index (ABI) may be better for comparing groups of patients, as well as for monitoring a given patient over time after intervention (e.g., after bypass surgery). In addition, to claim cause and effect and attribute the improvement to a treatment, some objective evidence of hemodynamic change needs to be included, and a change in the ABI of more than 0.10 was recommended. This was later adopted by the Trans-Atlantic Inter-Society Consensus (TASC) [25].

Table 12.1 Rutherford classification of PAD and CLI

Category	Symptoms	Objective criteria
0	Asymptomatic	Normal treadmill Reactive hyperemia test
1	Mild claudication	Completes treadmill exerciser AP after exercise >50 mm Hg
2	Moderate claudication	Exercise between categories 1 and 3
3	Severe claudication	Cannot complete standard treadmill exercise AP after exercise <50 mm Hg
4	Ischemic rest pain	Resting AP < 40 mm Hg, fiat or barely pulsatile ankle or metatarsal PVR; TP < 30 mm Hg
5	Minor tissue loss non-healing ulcer, focal gangrene with diffuse pedal ischemia	Resting AP < 60 mm Hg, ankle or metatarsal PVR fiat or barely pulsatile; TP < 40 mm Hg
6	Major tissue loss Extending above transmetatarsal level, functional foot no longer salvageable	Same as category 5

AP Ankle pressure, *PVR* pulse volume recording, *TP* toe pressure, Rutherford's Categories 4, 5, and 6 are embraced by the term chronic CLI.; Normal treadmill = Five minutes at 2 mph (2 Miles per hour = 3.6 Km per hour 60 meter per minute) on a 12% incline

Rest pain scores on rating scales ranging from 0 for the best (completely resolved) to 4 points for the worst condition (severe pain unresolved with paracetamol or non-steroidal anti-inflammatory drugs) were suggested by Tateishi-Yuyama [83].

The 6-minute walking test is considered informative and a predictor of further deterioration for CLI patients. Typically, annual decline in 6-minute walk performance (−73.0 ft (~22 meter) is observed in CLI patients with ABI <0.50. Smith et al. defined "mild claudication" as the ability to walk 2 to 3 blocks (900 ft) (~270 meter) before stopping; "moderate claudication," 1 or 2 blocks (600 ft) (~180 meter); and "severe claudication," less than 1 block (300 ft) (~90 meter) [77]. Perera defined a small meaningful change in 6-minute walk as a change of 20 meters and a large meaningful change of 50 meters or more [55, 64].

A more recent classification system (WIfI classification) has been proposed by the Society of Vascular Surgery. This classification evaluates the prognosis of the affected lower limb by considering the following three factors which are graded into four categories (0 = none, 1 = mild, 2 = moderate, 3 = severe): wound (W), ischemia (I), and foot infection (fI) (Table 12.2) [56]. In the last revision of the European Society of Cardiology guidelines, the definition of CLI was replaced by the new concept of CLTI. While the term CLI mainly defined the degree of severe ischemia as the underlying cause of the disease, the CLTI definition also takes into account the degree of infections and wounds, which are perceived as crucial in estimating the prognosis of the lower limb [1, 21]. Unlike Rutherford's classification, the WIfI does not include pain and walking ability that might also affect CLI prognosis.

Table 12.2 Wound, Ischemia, and foot Infection (WIfI) [37, 56]

Wound		
Grade	Ulcer	Gangrene
0	No ulcer	No gangrene
1	Small, shallow ulcer on distal leg or foot; no exposed bone, unless limited to distal phalanx	No gangrene
2	Deeper ulcer with exposed bone, joint, or tendon; generally not involving the heel; shallow heel ulcer, without calcaneal involvement	Gangrenous changes limited to digits
3	Extensive, deep ulcer involving forefoot and/or midfoot; deep, full-thickness heel ulcer ± calcaneal involvement	Extensive gangrene involving the forefoot/ midfoot; full-thickness heel necrosis ± calcaneal involvement

Ischemia			
Grade	ABI	Ankle systolic pressure	TP, TcPO$_2$
0	≥0.80	>100 mm Hg	≥60 mm Hg
1	0.6–0.79	70–100 mm Hg	40–59 mm Hg
2	0.4–0.59	50–70 mm Hg	30–39 mm Hg
3	ʿ0.39	<50 mm Hg	<30 mm Hg

Infection	
Grade	Clinical manifestation of infection
0	No symptoms or signs of infection Infection present, as defined by the presence of at least two of the following items: Local swelling or induration Erythema 0.5–2 cm around the ulcer Local tenderness or pain Local warmth Purulent discharge (thick, opaque to white, or sanguineous secretion)
1	Local infection involving only the skin and the subcutaneous tissue Exclude other causes of an inflammatory response of the skin (trauma, gout, acute Charcot, fracture, thrombosis, venous stasis)
2	Local infection with erythema >2 cm, or involving structures deeper than skin and subcutaneous tissues, and no systemic inflammatory response signs
3	No systemic inflammatory response signs Local infection with the signs of SIRS, as manifested by two or more of the following: Temperature > 38 or <36 °C Heart rate > 90 beats/min Respiratory rate > 20 breaths/min or PaCO$_2$ < 32 mm Hg White blood cell count > 12,000 or <4000 cu/mm or 10% immature bands

ABI ankle brachial index, *PaCO2* partial pressure of carbon dioxide, *SIRS* systemic inflammatory response syndrome, *TcPO2* transcutaneous oximetry, *TP* toe pressure

Notes: Patient's symptoms are graded by three categories: foot wound severity, tissue perfusion by ABI or transcutaneous oximetry, and the presence of infection

CLI is associated with high risks for cardiovascular events, including myocardial infarction, stroke, and death. All current CLI guidelines support the use of statins and medications aimed at improving blood flow (e.g., phosphodiesterase inhibitor cilostazol), reducing blood viscosity (aspirin and anticoagulants), antiplatelet therapy (Plavix), and angiotensin-converting enzyme (ACE) inhibitors to reduce cardiovascular events and mortality [85]. In addition, pain is controlled with several levels of analgesics and narcotic medications. Secondary prevention by lifestyle changes (smoking cessation, healthy diet, weight loss, and regular physical exercise) are also useful [1, 85]. In patients with diabetes, glycemic control is particularly important for improved outcome [1]. While there is no drug specifically approved for the treatment of CLI, promising interventional methods are constantly improving. Veith et al. showed that frequent follow-up of CLI patients and aggressive intervention can dramatically decrease major amputation rates, reporting a decrease from 41% to 5% in primary amputations between the years 1974 and 1989. This approach is now accepted as the standard of care, with further establishment of multidisciplinary wound healing centers in most middle-sized and large hospitals around the world [34, 38, 89]. The therapeutic approach to patients with PAD includes two aspects. The first is to address the risk related to a specific lesion's symptoms, length, level of occlusion, and localization, while the second is the management of the patients' increased risk of any cardiovascular (CV) event [1, 21]. A flowchart summarizing the proposed therapeutic strategies is presented in Fig. 12.2. Revascularization should be attempted as much as possible; bypass surgery or angioplasty should be considered depending on the anatomical region and lesion complexity [21]. For some CLI patients, these interventional procedures are not suitable for several of reasons, such as the distribution of the occlusive disease in medium and small vessels, lesions too numerous and too small to revascularize, and comorbidities [48]. Yet, starting from the 1980s, it was shown that with a more aggressive limb salvage approach, less than 6% of CLI patients were not candidates for interventional treatment [88]. According to Aboyans et al. and Conte et al., the majority of CLTI patients are anatomically suitable for revascularization and establishing direct in-line flow to the foot is the primary technical goal [1, 21]. Recently, Abualhin et al. reported that distal anastomosis performed on 73 patients with Rutherford' categories 5–6 resulted in technical success in 98.6%, with 1-month bypass patency in 87.8% of the patients, bypass assisted patency in 91.9%, and secondary patency in 93.2%. The 1-year results of these parameters were 54.4%, 71.4%, and 75.1%, respectively. Limb salvage and amputation-free survival (AFS) at 1-year were 84.3% and 79.1%, respectively, with most of the failures occurring within the 6-month follow-up (6-month limb salvage 85.8% and AFS 82.1%) [2]. Thus, it seems that despite good technical revascularization, clinical success is considerably less than 100%. Furthermore, due to the ulcers and subsequent gangrene and recurrent infections, these patients are frequently infected and require treatment with antibiotics, often

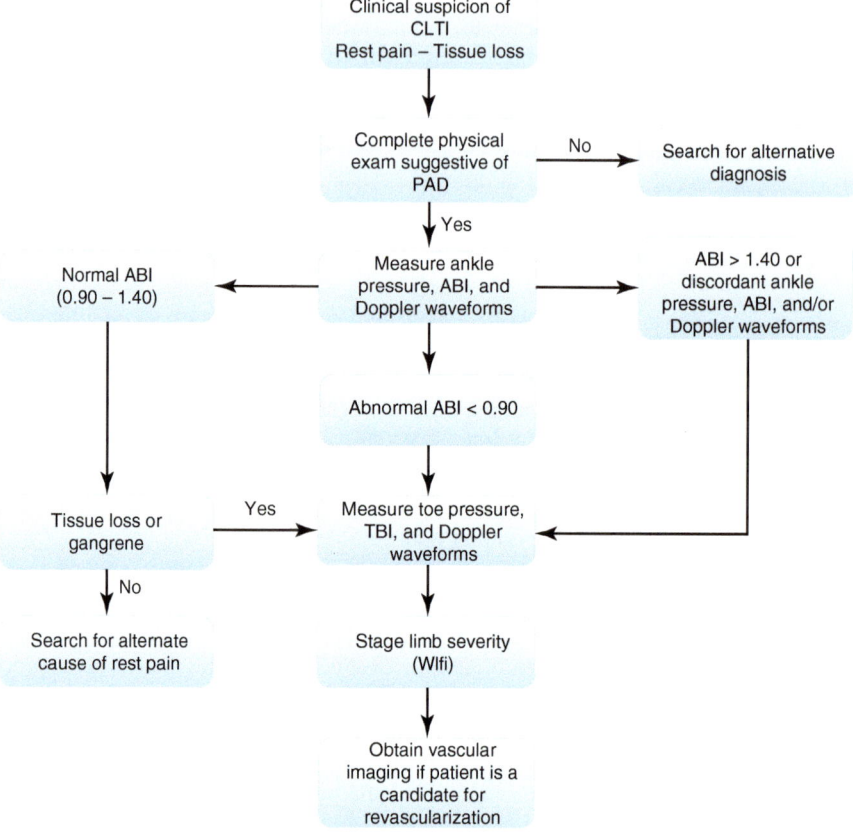

Fig. 12.2 Flow diagram for the investigation of patients presenting with suspected chronic limb-threatening ischemia (CLTI) [21]. ABI Ankle-brachial index, PAD peripheral artery disease, TBI toe-brachial index, WIfI Wound, Ischemia, and foot Infection

leading to the development of antibiotic resistance. When revascularization attempts fail and for nonrevascularizable patients, new therapies, such as gene or SPC therapy, are required since the current available therapy only includes symptomatic treatments.

12.1.2 Demographic Data

From January 2007 to December 2008, the prevalence and incidence of CLI in the USA was 0.23% and 0.20%, respectively. Overall, the success rates of the current therapies and prevention measures are limited, and once PAD progresses to CLI, the risks of limb loss and mortality increase. It is estimated that 220,000–240,000 amputations are carried out in the USA and Europe annually due to failure of revascularization [4]. The risk of amputations because of vascular diseases is dramatically increased in diabetes, which affects more than 230 million people worldwide [10, 94].

It is estimated that CLI will affect more than 3 million patients in the western world with an annual 2% US growth rate [53]. Based on historical data, within 6–12 months after the diagnosis of CLI, approximately 30% of patients will undergo amputation and 20% will die [23, 61, 76]. The 2-year and 5-year mortality rates are approximately 35% and 70%, respectively [66]. Despite advances in medical and interventional therapies, the amputation rate has increased from 19 per 100,000 person/year to 30–50 per 100,000 person/year over the past decades, mainly driven by an increase in the number of diabetics and older patients [3, 62]. Successful rehabilitation is achieved in less than two-thirds and one-half of patients after below-knee and above-knee amputations, respectively. Fewer than 50% of amputees achieve full mobility [4], and in patients who survive the first major amputation, a second amputation is required in 30% of the cases. Amputations cause devastating psychological effects and diminished QoL and also have a negative impact on survival. Even with the current best practice, the 5-year mortality rate for CLI is >60%, exceeding that of prostate cancer (<1%), breast cancer (11%), acute MI (20%), colorectal cancer (36%), and stroke (41%) [9].

12.1.3 Cost of CLI

The estimated total costs of treating CLI in the USA alone are $10 to $20 billion per year [4, 10, 42]. The cost of follow-up, long-term care, and treatment for an amputee who remains at home is $49,000 per year versus only $600 to $800 per year after limb salvage. Amputations are associated with substantial costs (e.g., hospitalization, surgery, fitting and building of prosthesis, rehabilitation process, home health aides, adaptations at the patients' homes, influence on family and economic productivity, long-term healthcare costs, etc.) [5]. The CLI economic burden is very high. Thus a 25% reduction in amputations could save $2.9 to $3.0 billion yearly in US healthcare costs.

From what has been described above, CLI is a progressive devastating illness with significant disability, poor quality of life, and morbidity and mortality that exceed cancer. The economic toll is enormous, and the number of cases is increasing dramatically. There is an unmet, immediate need for the development of new therapies to stabilize or reverse the disease course, especially in "no option" patients.

This chapter describes new innovative approaches to treat CLI patients who failed or are not eligible for revascularization procedures and/or those suffering from occlusive disease in medium and small vessels, too numerous and small to revascularize, and suffering from multiple comorbidities. It will review several gene and cell therapy approaches and present preliminary first-in-human (FIH) results of a novel treatment that combines immune cell therapy and a stepwise activation and differentiation of stem/progenitor cells (SPC). Utilizing this innovative technology, peripheral blood cells from a standard blood draw (with no pretreatment or mobilization) can be transformed, within a day, into a cellular therapeutic product code-named BGC101, composed of early endothelial progenitor cells (EPCs), SPCs, alternatively activated pro-tolerogenic and pro-angiogenic dendritic cells (DCs), and T helper cells. [67]. As will be described in detail below, this treatment has shown promising therapeutic effects in patients with otherwise untreatable CLI after a single treatment. The first cohort results have met the expected safety and efficacy primary endpoints. BGC101 has been found to be safe with 6-month amputation-free survival (AFS) in all patients. Additional beneficial effects were observed on increased leg blood flow, wound healing, walking ability, reduction of pain, decreased usage of narcotic medications, and improved quality of life (QoL).

12.2   Review of Gene and Cell Therapy Investigations

12.2.1   Gene Therapy

Gene therapies using naked/plasmid-encoding angiogenic factors such as vascular endothelial growth factor (VEGF), hepatocyte growth factor (HGF), fibroblast growth factor (FGF), hypoxia inducible factor (HIF), and developmentally regulated endothelial locus (Del-1 and DELTA 1) aimed at promoting neovascularization were highly promising in animal models, but were not effective in inducing functionally significant angiogenesis in clinical trials. Evidence accumulated from 22 phase 1 and phase 2 studies in 2008 supports the safety of these approaches in humans and also provides indications of bioactivity in patients with these dreaded conditions. Even so, true breakthroughs have been elusive [21, 46, 86]. An important example is the report by Powell et al. who tested the safety and bioactivity of HGF plasmid injection for CLI. In this randomized double-blind, placebo-controlled, dose-escalating, multi-center HGF-STAT trial, 104 patients with rest pain or tissue loss due to severe lower extremity ischemia were assigned to receive injections of placebo or 1 of 3 dosing regimens of HGF plasmid into the ischemic leg muscle. A unique, prespecified analysis plan allowed the investigators to identify an increase in TcPO2 in the high-dose group that was not present in other treatment groups, thus providing objective evidence for bioactivity. However, other end points, such as amputation rate, wound healing, and ankle/brachial or toe/brachial index, did not reveal differences between treatment groups [69]. Despite advances in the understanding of the diseases and the gene delivery tools, growth factor therapy results have been inconclusive. New modalities using gene therapy with biomaterials and cell-mediated delivery are very promising, but at this stage they are still in the pre-clinical research stage [92]

12.2.2 Stem/Progenitor Cells (SPC) Therapy for PAD and CLI

Adult bone marrow-derived cells (BM) that contains hematopoietic SPC (HSPC) and mesenchymal stem cells (MSC) has been widely used for numerous clinical applications. For more than 50 years HSPCs, the oldest form of therapeutic adult stem cells, have been administered in over 50,000 implantations, providing physicians with a thorough understanding of their utility, mainly for replacing blood and immune cells. More than 29,000 autologous transplants performed thus far have proven that they significantly lower the risk of infection due to the rapid recovery of immune function and the avoidance of rejection and graft-versus-host disease (GVHD). These advantages have established autologous HSPC transplants as a standard second-line treatment for various malignant conditions, enabling the use of more intense chemotherapy [17, 35]. In addition, autologous HSPC infusion was also found to be safe and has been used to treat approximately 900 patients with autoimmune diseases, leading to sustained remissions in about 30% [63]. SPCs are capable of self-renewal and differentiation into organ-specific cell types as well as having paracrine effects via the release of pro-angiogenic growth factors/cytokines. A combination of cellular activities that contribute to the effects of SPCs transplantation include: the cells' vasculogenic properties; paracrine effect resulting from secretion of multiple growth factors; and secretion of exosomes containing proteins, ribonucleic acids (RNAs), and microRNAs which stimulate both receptor-mediated and genetic mechanisms [32]. Cellular therapies also provide a treatment solution that addresses multiple aspects of CLI, including reduction of inflammation, tissue remodeling, and increased perfusion [9]. Since regenerative medicine treatment began in 1997, the feasibility and safety of BM-derived SPC has been established in over 3000 patients with refractory angina, ischemic cardiomyopathy, and chronic end-stage heart failure [33, 11]. In these studies, HSPCs and MSCs from BM aspirates and mobilized BM, both with and without ex vivo culturing steps, all showed high safety profiles, regardless of the administration method (intramuscular injections (IM), intravenous infusion (IV), or via angiography).

Progress has also been achieved in establishing therapeutic protocols for treating a variety of conditions, such as critical limb ischemia, acute myocardial ischemia, and infarction by using SPC. A variety of allogeneic and autologous tissues have been suggested as SPC sources, such as BM, peripheral blood mobilized cells, and mesenchymal organs. Overall, studies applying cells produced in compliance to good manufacturing practice (GMP) and good tissue practice (GTP) show that cell implantation was well tolerated and improved clinical status and survival, while most of the reported adverse effects stemmed from pre-procedural treatments connected to acquiring cells for the treatment [28, 33, 35].

12.2.3 Results of Stem/Progenitor Cell (SPC)-Based Therapy in PAD and CLI

Results of non-controlled as well as randomized controlled trials (RCT) applying SPC-based therapy in PAD and CLI are summarized in Table 12.3. One of the most promising and innovative treatments for PAD and CLI is the use of SPC that promotes small-to-medium sized blood vessel neovascularization and supports tissue reperfusion in a more physiological way with potentially high effectiveness. More than 70 studies have demonstrated the safety and clinical benefits of autologous BM mononuclear cells (BM-MNC), BM-MSC, G-CSF-mobilized peripheral blood-derived mononuclear cells (PB-MNC), or EPCs for patients with CLI. BM aspiration necessitates systemic/epidural or local anesthesia and aspiration of large amounts of marrow (300–500 mL) that many CLI patients cannot tolerate [52]. For those who undergo the procedure, the most frequent adverse reaction was local pain, responsive to non-steroidal anti-inflammatory drugs [28].

12.2.3.1 BM Mononuclear Cells (BM-MNC)

In the first published study, patients with chronic CLI conditions that were not amenable to revascularization received BM concentrate or peripheral blood mononuclear cells (PBMC) implantation. Cell implantation induced no local inflammatory reaction or edema of the gastrocnemius up to 72 hours after injection. Concentrations of serum creatine phosphokinase (CRP) increased after implantation (maximum after 1 day) and reverted to baseline within 7 days. 25 patients were treated with BM-MNC ($1.6 \pm 0.6 \times 10e9$ cells) and injected at 40 points into the gastrocnemius of the more ischemic limb (ankle-brachial index; ABI <0.6). 20 patients were in the control treatment, 4 obtained saline solution, and 16 patients were treated with PBMC ($1.5 \pm 0.6 \times 10e9$ cells) injected into the contralateral leg. The cell injection procedure was safe. 2 patients out of 47 died from myocardial infarction judged as unrelated to treatment, and no other treatment-related adverse events (AE) were reported. These results reflect a mortality rate of 4.3% compared to the 20% mortality expected based on historical data with the existing best practice methods [21, 23, 76]. PBMC control group showed moderate effects on stabilizing and improving blood flow and pain. A significant improvement in the BM-MNC group compared with the PBMC or saline was observed in ABI, transcutaneous oxygen pressure (TcPO2), rest pain, and the pain-free walking distance at 4 and 24 weeks [83].

Miyamoto et al. administered autologous BM-MNC and investigated their safety and efficacy in recovering refractory chronic PAD of limbs and hands. No serious adverse events were reported, and the treatment was effective in relieving severe pain of PAD, especially for Buerger's disease. The maximum pain level before implantation was 66.5 ± 5.0 (VAS 0–100), and it decreased to 12.1 ± 2.2 after implantation ($p < 0.001$). Rest pain in legs and fingers was resolved in 11 of 12 cases

Table 12.3 Summary of results from published clinical studies treating CLI with SPC product therapies

Cell source	Admin. route	No. of patients	Study level	Safety outcome	Efficacy outcome	Ref
BM-MNC – Purified only Autologous	IM 40 sites	25	RCT	Short-term 72 h No inflammatory reaction or edema of gastrocnemius Long-term 2Y Reduced mortality rate – 4.3% (2/47) No AE	↑ABI, TcPO2 ↓Pain ↓Amputation ↓Mortality	Tateishi-Yuyama et al. [83]
Non-mobilized PBMC Purified only Autologous	IM 40 sites	16	RCT	Short-term 72 h No inflammatory reaction or edema of gastrocnemius Long-term 2Y Reduced mortality rate – 4.3% (2/47) No AE	↑ AB⁻, TcPO2 ↓Pain ↓Amputation	Tateishi-Yuyama et al. [83]
Mobilized BM-MNC Purified only Autologous	IM 65 sites	30	Un-controlled	Long-term No transplantation-related AE	↑ ABI, TcPO2 ↓Pain ↓Amputation	Kawamura et al. [43]
Mobilized BM-MNC Purified only Autologous	IM 40 sites	28	RCT	Long-term 3 M No transplantation-related AE	↑ABI, TcPO2 ↓Ulcers ↓Amputation	Huang et al. [40]
Mobilized BM-MNC Purified only Autologous	IM 50–70 sites	92	Un-controlled	Short-term 24 h No transplantation-related AE	↑ABI, TcPO2 ↓Pain ↓Amputation	Kawamura et al. [44]
BM-MNC Purified only Autologous	IM 40 sites	74	Controlled	Long-term No transplantation-related AE	↑ABI, TcPO2 ↓Pain	Huang et al. [41]
Mobilized BM-MNC Purified only Autologous	IM 40 sites	76	Controlled	Long-term No transplantation-related AE	↑ABI, TcPO2 ↓Pain	Huang et al. [41]

(continued)

Table 12.3 (continued)

Cell source	Admin. route	No. of patients	Study level	Safety outcome	Efficacy outcome	Ref
Non-mobilized blood Tissue-directed Autologous	IM 30 sites	6	Un-controlled	Short-term 48 h – No AE Long-term 6 M No transplantation-related AE No mortality (100% survival)	↑ABI, ↓Ulcers, ↓Amputation	Mutirangura et al. (2009)
BM-MNC Purified only Autologous	IM 45 sites	51	Un-controlled	Short-term 72 h No swelling, pain, infectious complications or discomfort at the injected leg Long-term 6 M and post study 2Y No AE	↑ABI, TcPO2 ↑Walking distance ↓Rutherford ↓Ulcers ↓Pain ↓Amputation	Amann et al. [6]
BM-MSC Ex-vivo expanded Autologous	IM 20 sites	20	Double-blind RCT	Short-term Transplantation was well tolerated with no or mild discomfort Long-term 6 M No treatment elated AE	↑ABI, TcPO2 ↑pain-free Walking distance ↓Ulcers ↓Pain ↓Amputation	Lu et al. [52]
BM-MNC Purified only Autologous	IM 20 sites	21	Double-blind RCT	Short-term Transplantation was well tolerated with no or mild discomfort Long-term 6 M No treatment elated AE	↑ABI, TcPO2 ↑pain1-free Walking distance ↓Ulcers ↓Pain ↓Amputation	Lu et al. [52]
BM-contrate Autologous	IA Catheter at 800 ml/h IM not specified	41	RCT	Long-term 3, 6 M AE and SAEs characteristic of the disease	↓Ulcers[a] ↓Pain Amputation[a] ABI[a] ↓Death[a] ↓Rutherford ↑QoL	Klepanec et al. [47]

Cell source	Admin. route	No. of patients	Study level	Safety outcome	Efficacy outcome	Ref
BM-MSC and Macrophages Ex-vivo expanded and activated Ixmyelocel-T Autologous	IM >20 sites	86	Double-blind RCT	Short-term 2 h Long-term 1 W, 3, 6, 9, 12 M AE and SAEs characteristic of the disease	↓Ulcers[a] ↓Pain ↓Amputation[a]	Powell et al. (2012)
Mobilized BM-CD34 Purified only Autologous	IM 8 sites	28	Double-blind RCT	During Mobilization Long-term 2 W–12 M No transplantation-related AE	↑ABI[a] ↓Walking distance ↑QoL[a] ↓Rutherford[a] ↓Ulcers[a] ↓Pain[a] ↓Amputation[a]	Losordo et al. [51]
BM-MNC Autologous	IA 3 repeated every 3 weeks by slow hand injection in the CFA	81	Double-blind RCT	Long-term 2, 6 M	↓Ulcers[a] ↓Pain Amputation[a] ↑ABI[a] ↓Death[a] ↑QoL	Teraa et al. [84]

(continued)

Table 12.3 (continued)

Cell source	Admin. route	No. of patients	Study level	Safety outcome	Efficacy outcome	Ref
Mobilized BM-CD34 Purified only Autologous	IM	25	Open labelled 3 Doses	Long-term 3 M 6 M	↑ABI, TcPO2 ↑Walking distance ↓Ulcers, ↓Amputation	Dong et al. [24]
Mobilized BM- MNC Purified only Autologous	IM	28	RCT	Long-term 6 M and post study 3 Y No AE	↑TcPO2 ↓Amputation	Dubsky et al. [27]
Non-mobilized Blood Ex vivo tissue- directed angiogenic cells Autologous	IM 30 sites	20	RCT	Short-term 48 h – No AE Long-term 6 M No transplantation-related AE No mortality (100% survival)	↑ABI, TcPO2, ↑Walking distance ↓Ulcers, ↓Amputation	Szabo et al. [81]
BM-MSC Ex vivo expanded Allogeneic	IM 40–60 sites	10	Double-blind RCT	Short-term Transplantation was well tolerated Long-term 6 M 13 AEs and 6 SAEs No transplantation-related AE	↑ABI, TcPO2, Ulcers, Amputation Death	Gupta et al. [36]
Placenta MSC Allogeneic	IM 3 treatments once every 4 weeks	4	Open labelled	One short-term mild AE (fever)	↑ABI ↑Pain-free walking distance ↓Ulcers ↓Pain Amputation	Wang et al., ([91]
Mobilized BM-MNC Autologous	IM and intra-arterial	700	Meta-analysis	Long-term 2 M-3 Y Reduced mortality rate – 2.8% (21/761) – No AE	↑ ABI, TcPO2, ↑Walking distance ↓Pain	Fadini et al. [28]
Variety of Autologous cells	IM and Intra-arterial	2332	Meta-analysis	Long-term 2 M-3 Y Reduced risk of amputation by 37% No effect on mortality rate Low rate of AEs	↑ABI, TcPO2, ↑Walking distance ↓Pain	Rigato et al. [74]

Abbreviations used in this table: *BM-MNC* Bone marrow-mononuclear cells, *MSC* mesenchymal stem cells, *PBMC* peripheral blood mononuclear cell, *IM* intramuscular, *CFA* common femoral artery, *RCT* randomized controlled trial, *AE* adverse events, *SAE* severe adverse effect, *H* hour, *W* week, *M* month, *Y* Year,

(92%). Pain-free walking time on a treadmill improved significantly (140 ± 53 seconds before implantation to 451 ± 74 seconds after implantation, $p = 0.034$). Resting ABI in legs implanted with BM mononuclear cells also improved (0.65 ± 0.08 before implantation vs. 0.73 ± 0.07 after implantation, $p = 0.055$). Significant perfusion improvement was demonstrated by 99mTc-tetrofosmin perfusion scintigraphy [57].

12.2.3.2 Mobilized BM (PB-MNC) Versus BM Mononuclear Cells (BM-MNC)

Several studies with growth factor mobilization of BM (also referred to as PB-MNC) were performed with safety and efficacy results similar to those of the BM-MNC trials. Overall, reported AE stemmed from pre-procedural treatments with G-CSF. AE included flu-like symptoms, myalgia, fever, and bone pain. A smaller number of AE included three patients who had to discontinue G-CSF due to chest pain, muscle pain, and anaphylaxis, respectively, one patient with ventricular fibrillation who recovered after cardioversion, and one patient who had minor retinal bleeding [27, 28, 43, 44, 49]. The long-term mortality rate in these studies was 2.8%, with 21 deaths reported between 2 months and 3 years after therapy, as compared to the 20% expected based on historical data. Thus, based on data from 761 patients, the authors concluded that no safety concerns exist with this type of cell therapy [28]. Among these, Huang et al. studied the effect of G-CSF mobilized PB-MNC ($3.0 \times 10e9$ cells) in a RCT design on 28 diabetic patients with CLI. The control group received conventional wound care, and both groups were supplemented with an intravenous injection of prostaglandin E1. The study patients received G-CSF for a total of 5 days before PB-MNC collection. Huang reported improvements in pain-free walking distance, healing of diabetic foot ulcers, and significant increase in ABI (from 0.50 ± 0.21 to 0.63 ± 0.25 ($p < 0.001$)) and in angiographic scores [40]. Despite the limitations of the lack of compatibility between the studies, the outcome of BM-derived cell therapy (as well as that of Mobilized PB-MNC) on perfusion parameters (ABI, TcPO2) and the clinical course (wound healing, walking distance) remains consistent and positive throughout the different reports. Pooled results show that autologous cell therapy can induce an increase in ABI values between 0.1 and 0.2 points, which is considered a significant clinical outcome [72], and an increase in TcPO2 between 10 and 20 mmHg O2. Depending on baseline values, walking distance can improve about 100 to 200 meters. No serious side effects were reported [28, 41].

Dubsky et al. conducted a comparative study of patients with diabetic foot disease, 28 in the treatment arm and 22 control patients (standard care). 17 were treated by BM-MNC cells and 11 by PBMNC. At 6 months, 10 major amputations occurred in the control group, 2 in the BM-MNC group, and 1 in the PB-MNC group. A beneficial effect of cell therapy was observed with no difference between the two cell treatment groups [27].

12.2.3.3 Intramuscular (IM) Versus Intra-arterial (IA) Administration of BM Cells

Rigato and Fadini reported 4 studies utilizing IA administration including one RCT on 41 advanced CLI patients (Rutherford category 5 and 6) comparing IM (21 patients) and IA (20 patients) and one double-blind RCT on 160 CLI patients (Rutherford category 3–6) comparing 3 repeated treatments (once every 3 weeks) of IA administration of BM-MNC or placebo red blood cells. In both studies there was no difference in outcome between the groups. At 6-month follow-up, Klepanec reported 4 deaths (9.7%) and 10 major amputations (24%) without clearly detailing the group-associated events. Teraa reported 4 deaths (4.9%) and 10 major amputations (18.5%) in the IA BM-MNC group and 5 deaths (6.3%) and 10 major amputations (12.3%) in the IA placebo group. Indeed, in Rigato's analysis of delivery route, only IM but not IA administration was associated with a significant improvement in amputation rate, amputation-free survival, complete wound healing, ABI, and TcO2, while both IM an IA significantly improved rest pain score [47, 74, 84].

12.2.3.4 BM Mononuclear Cells (BM-MNC) Versus BM Mesenchymal Stem Cells (BM-MSC)

As of 2017 Rigato et al. reported 4 studies utilizing BM-MSC obtained either by BM aspiration or by mobilization. Lu et al. conducted a double-blind RCT study in 41 diabetic patients comparing BM-MNC (20 patients) and BM-MSC (21 patients). Selected BM-MNC were injected immediately, while BM-MSC were first expanded ex vivo for 12–15 days. Saline was used as a control and was injected into the second leg. Lu reported that a BM aspiration volume of 30 ml was sufficient for generation of BM-MSC, while 300–500 ml was needed for preparation of BM-MNC. Cells were administrated intramuscularly (20 injections, 3 cm intervals, 1–1.5 cm in depth, (0.5–1 mL BM-MSCs or BM-MNCs per site). There were no serious adverse events. BM-MSC were superior over BM-MNC in limb perfusion, wound healing, and pain-free walking time, but there was no significant difference between the groups in amputations or pain relief [52].

12.2.3.5 Dose Dependency

Losordo et al. assessed dose dependency in a RCT utilizing two doses of mobilized BM purified CD34 SPC. 28 CLI patients were treated with $1 \times 10e5$ autologous CD34+ cells/kg (low-dose; 7 patients), $1 \times 10e6$ (high-dose; 9 patients), or placebo (control; 12 patients). 8 IM injections were administered to the ischemic leg. No adverse safety signal was associated with cell administration. 60 SAEs occurred in 22 subjects during the study. 1 occurred during mobilization before treatment (moderate hypotension which required prolonged hospitalization) and 59 after treatment. The majority of SAEs were considered unrelated to the study with 1 judged as possibly related (severe worsening of CLI in the target leg after injection which required prolonged hospitalization). There were 2 deaths during the study (group was not reported) and 11 major amputations. Major amputation incidence and AFS were significantly lower in the combined cell-treated groups compared with the control group with no significant dose related effect. Most amputations occurred within 6-month post injection, 4 in the control group (33%), 3 in the low-dose group (42%), and 2 in the high-dose group (22%) with 2 amputations between 6 and 12 months in the control group (a total of 50%). No treatment-related differences were found in wound healing, rest pain and QoL, whereas 6-min walking test improved in the cell treated groups. Lack of dose dependency in this preliminary study might be due to the small size of the groups [51].

12.2.3.6 Allogeneic Ex Vivo Expanded Cells

Gupta et al. described a double-blind RCT using allogeneic BM-MSC. Patients graded as Rutherford 4 (5 patients), Rutherford 5 (10 Patients), and Rutherford 6 (5 Patients) received a single treatment of 180–220 × 10e6 BM-MSC (10 patients) or placebo suspension (10 patients) via 40–60 IM injections in the gastrocnemius. Incidence of AEs in the BM-MSC arm was 13 vs. 45 in the placebo arm, and serious SAE including death, infected gangrene, and amputations were similar in both arms (5 in BM-MSC and 4 in the placebo group). Two deaths in the BM-MSC were not attributed by the study DSMB to the cell therapy. Two amputations occurred in each group. Nonetheless, a significant increase in ABI and ankle pressure was seen in BM-MSC arm compared to the placebo group. These results may reflect the inclusion of unsalvageable Rutherford 6 patients as suggested by Benoit et al. in their 2011 report [13, 52]. In a preliminary study, applying allogeneic ex vivo expanded placenta-derived MSC, 4 patients obtained 3 sets of IM once every 4 weeks. Safety results were promising with only one mild transient AE of fever. Ulcer healing, pain, pain-free walking test, and ABI improvement were reported, but no ABI or patient grading were provided. One patient had a major amputation [91].

12.2.3.7 Ex Vivo Activated/Differentiated Cell Products

In a double-blind RCT, Powell et al. tested the safety and efficacy of Ixmyelocel-T, a mixture of ex vivo expanded BM-MSC and alternately activated macrophages, in 86 patients (46 Ixmyelocel-T and 24 placebo). Patients received 20 IM injections and were followed for 12 months. Ixmyelocel-T treatment was well tolerated. The occurrence of adverse events and serious adverse events was similar between the two groups. There were four deaths (8%) in the Ixmyelocel-T group. This represented a decreased death rate compared to the 20% mortality expected based on historical data. However, the placebo group had the same mortality rate of 8%. There were ten major amputations (21%) in the Ixmyelocel-T group and six (25%) in the placebo. In both groups, most of the amputations occurred within 6 months. These results indicate that the therapy did not improve the one-year amputation or mortality rates. Improvement was observed in AFS and time to treatment failure (TTF based on one or more of: major amputation of the injected leg; mortality; doubling of total wound surface; and de novo gangrene) in ixmyelocel-T-treated patients compared with controls. In addition, the treatment effect for both TTF and AFS was even more pronounced in patients who entered the trial with baseline wounds (Powell et al. 2012).

While administration of fresh PBMC was inferior to BM-MNC [83], angiogenic cell precursors (ACP), a product resulted from non-mobilized peripheral blood after 5 days of pro-angiogenic ex vivo activation, showed a high safety profile and an improvement in circulation, ulcer healing, and reduced amputation rate. In the immediate follow-up after the intramuscular injection, patients were hemodynamically stable. There were no abnormalities in hematology, kidney and liver function tests, including serum myoglobin. One patient developed dyspnea that was caused by fluid overload, with immediate response to diuretic therapy. Elevated cardiac enzymes were detected in one patient, even though the patient had no symptoms of angina [60]. Similar results were obtained by Szabó et al. from applying ACP in a larger, controlled study of 20 patients (10 patients treated with ACP and 10 with standard care). The treatment was well-tolerated. At the 3-month follow-up, there were no major amputations and only two minor amputations in the treated group versus six major amputations in the controls and one death due to sepsis. Objective (ABI, TcO2) and subjective quality of life (QoL) improvement were seen in the treated group at 3 months. Post-study evaluation showed that the two-year major amputation free rate was 70% in the treated group versus 30% in the controls. The improvement in other objective and subjective parameters was sustained [81].

12.2.3.8 Summary of Cell-Based Therapies

Typical for early development stages of innovative therapeutic modalities, most studies were conducted on small patient groups ranging from 5 to 25 patients, and only part were RCTs or double-blind RCT trials. By 2015, more than 1000 CLI patients were treated with SPCs. The SPCs were directly obtained from organs, such as the BM or fat tissue or, alternatively, using mobilizing agents to induce massive proliferation of BM cells, followed by cell collection using an aphaeresis unit. Most of the studies were performed with autologous BM-derived cells, administrated locally to CLI patients in one treatment session of intramuscular injections. Overall, these studies showed that the cell implantation was well tolerated, not associated with severe adverse events and that they improved the clinical status of the patients. Safety analysis included the evaluation of death, cancer, unregulated angiogenesis, and procedural adverse events (AEs). The overall AE rate was low (4.2%) [12]. Most of the reported AEs were related to the pre-procedural activities for acquiring cells. Post cell therapy AEs were mainly injection site reactions and musculoskeletal disorders [28, 74].

Moreover, the data are supported by systematic reviews and meta-analyses of open labelled and RCTs. For example, Benoit et al. summarized 45 clinical trials, including 7 RCTs, with 1272 patients who received cell therapy. Efficacy analysis included the clinical endpoints of amputation and death as well as functional and surrogate endpoints. Cell therapy patients had a significantly lower amputation rate than controls (odds ratio 0.36, $p = 0.0004$). Cell therapy also improved a variety of functional and surrogate outcomes, such ABI, TcPO2, and quality of life (QoL) [12]. More recently, Rigato et al. reported a large meta-analysis on 2332 CLI patients, including 19 RCTs, 7 non-randomized, and 41 non-controlled studies [74]. The primary analysis (all randomized controlled trials) showed that cell therapy reduced the risk of amputation by 37% and improved amputation-free survival by 18% and wound healing by 59%, without affecting mortality. Taken together, the data indicate that cell therapy significantly increased ABI, TcPO2, reduced rest pain, and improved QoL. Cell therapy patients did not have a higher mortality rate than controls and demonstrated no increase in cancer incidence. Many of these studies show decreased mortality in comparison to the natural history of 20% mortality and 30% amputations that are expected within 6–12 months from CLI diagnosis [21, 23, 76]. As discussed above, Rigato and Fadini in 2017 showed that cell therapy reduced the risk of amputation and improved amputation-free survival but did not affect mortality. This may reflect the fact that the control group is also receiving better care. Indeed, in a summary of placebo-controlled groups of 11 cell therapy studies reported between 2001 and 2015, the average mortality was 9% (range 0–33%) at 6 months. The rate of major amputations was much closer to the expected value with an average of 28% (range 10–67%) at 6 months. The limitation in death rate comparison may stem from the fact that many studies have a 6-month follow-up, while mortality sometimes occurs at a later time after the end of the study. This is not an issue when amputation is measured, since at least 85% of the major amputations occur with the first 6 months after treatment [13, 27, 36, 51, 65, 66, 81, 84, 50, 70, 90].

12.3 Future Application

The promising results of the studies summarized above encouraged us to develop a new combination of cells for effective neovascularization, reduction of inflammation, and recruitment of additional SPC from endogenous resources. CLI is currently an incurable, life-threatening, and seriously debilitating disease. We therefore developed a patient-friendly method, based on a standard blood draw that is safe, accessible to patients in every clinic, and scalable. The goal beyond limb salvage is to extend lifespan and improve functionality and QoL.

Since the number of EPCs and HSPCs in the blood is relatively low in healthy individuals and even lower in diabetic patients [14, 29], an ex vivo method for the enrichment and augmentation of these specific cells was developed. DCs, originally identified by Steinman et al. in 1973 [78], regulate both innate and adaptive immunological responses by the triggering of antigen-specific T-cell responses [7, 18–20, 26, 58, 78, 87]. However, in the presence of anti-inflammatory molecules such as transforming growth factor beta (TGF-β), basic fibroblast growth factor (bFGF) and interleukin (IL)-10, DCs are alternatively activated in an antigen-independent manner and induce secretion of potent pro-angiogenic factors like vascular endothelial growth factor (VEGF) and nitric oxide, resulting in pro-angiogenic effects [8, 15, 54, 73, 79, 82]. In the presence of pro-angiogenic factors such as ischemia and the presence of VEGF, DCs were shown to contribute to neovascularization [16, 30, 75, 80, 93].

Autologous-enriched endothelial progenitor cells (EnEPC) is a defined cell population generated from a standard blood draw using a novel one-day technology employing alternatively activated DCs to specifically direct potentially therapeutic cell activity in vitro (Fig. 12.3). Previous in vitro and animal studies in the hind limb ischemia model have shown promising results in reversing induced limb ischemia

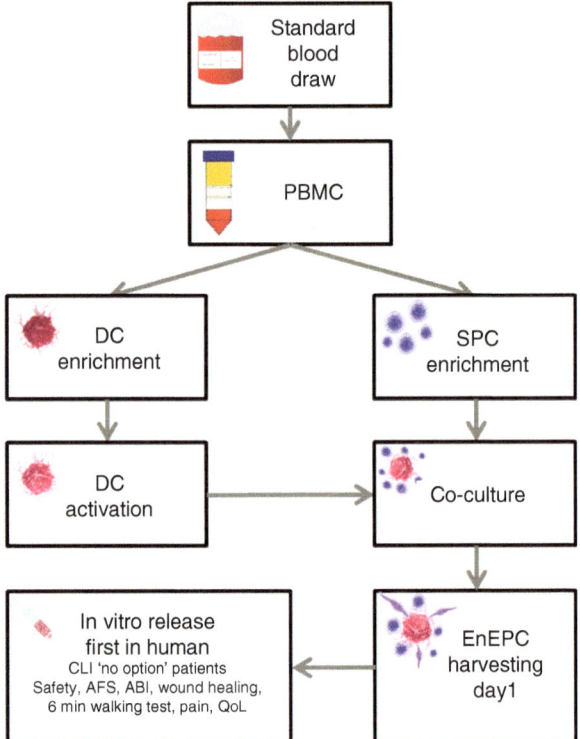

Fig. 12.3 Blood-derived SPC specifically activated by DCs
Flow chart depicting the generation of enriched EnEPC. BGC101 is a serum-free medium advanced therapy medicinal product (ATMP) designed to treat ischemic legs. It is produced in adherence to good tissue practice (GTP) and good manufacturing practice (GMP). Non-mobilized blood-derived plasmacytoid and myeloid DCs activated with pro-tolerogenic and pro-angiogenic cytokines (such as IL-10, VEGF) are used to specifically direct the in vitro activation of SPCs which were enriched from the same blood sample and co-cultured for 12–18 hours. Harvested EnEPCs were tested for safety (Gram stain, sterility, endotoxin and mycoplasma), identity (EPCs, SPC, DC and T helper cells), and potency (Ac-LDL and Ulex Lectin)

[67, 68]. BGC101 is the first EnEPC-derived advanced therapy medicinal product (ATMP) designed to treat ischemic legs. It is produced in adherence to GMP and GTP.

We report here a first-in-human (FIH), pilot clinical study assessing the safety and efficacy of BGC101 in the treatment of PAD with CLI.

12.3.1 Methods and Results

This FIH, non-controlled open-label pilot study assessing the safety and efficacy of BGC101 in the treatment of PAD with CLI was conducted in compliance with good clinical practice (GCP) and was closely reviewed by an independent Data and Safety Monitoring Board (DSMB) and sponsored by BioGenCell Ltd (NIH clinicaltrials.gov Identifier: NCT02805023).

Study Population Patients with severe disease and with no other treatment option ("no option") were selected. Patients had characteristics including very low to no blood flow in the legs as measured by ABI (<0.5), toe brachial pressure index (TBI), and ultrasound duplex test and had non-healing ulcers and infections. Between September 2006 and January 2017, six eligible patients underwent blood collection, and five patients were treated with BGC101. One patient withdrew before treatment due to gastrointestinal bleeding unrelated to the study. The five eligible patients, one Rutherford 4 and four Rutherford 5, were treated with a single session of 30 IM injections of BGC101 into the gastrocnemius muscle of the diseased leg, under local anesthesia with lidocaine cream (see Table 12.4 for baseline data; Fig. 12.4a for cell injection, 4b for injected leg 30 minutes after injection). Patients were followed for safety 48 hours and 1 week after cell administration. Further follow-up for safety and efficacy assessment was performed at 1, 3, and 6 months. 4 patients completed the 6-month follow-up period, and one patient withdrew from the study immediately prior to the 3-month follow-up visit. This patient had a computed tomography angiogram (CT angiogram) after therapy that showed improved run-off in the calf vessels. He was advised that he was now eligible again for an interventional procedure and underwent transluminal angioplasty (PTA). The patient was amputation-free several days before the 3-months follow-up (2.9 months). For this patient, documented data from the 1-month follow-up visit was used based on last observation carried forward (LOCF).

Study Investigational Product and Dose Starting with 250–350 ml of peripheral blood, co-culture of activated DCs for 12–18 hours with SPCs from the same patient sample generated a treatment dose of $91.0 \pm 23.4 \times 10e6$ (range $51.1–178.9 \times 10e6$) of BGC101 cells with $98.1 \pm 0.4\%$ viability. BGC101 comprises $58.1 \pm 7.0\%$ EPCs (expressing Ulex-lectin, acetylated low-density lipoprotein (AcLDL) uptake, Tie2, vascular endothelial growth factor receptor 1 and 2, and CD31) and $17.3 \pm 4.7\%$ SPCs (expressing CD34 and CD184 as well as plas-

Table 12.4 Patients data on screening

Parameter	Pt01-001	Pt01-002	Pt01-004	Pt01-005	Pt01-006
Gender	Male	Male	Female	Male	Male
Age (years)	71	67	67	56	68
Diabetes	Diabetic	Non-diabetic	Diabetic	Non-diabetic	Diabetic
Smoking habits	Non-smoker	Past heavy smoker >35Yrs	Non-smoker	Past heavy smoker >35Yrs	Heavy smoker >35Yrs
Rutherford	5 Minor tissue loss	4 Ischemic rest pain	5 Minor tissue loss	5 Minor tissue loss	5 Minor tissue loss
Intervention (surgery/ catheterization)	Peripheral arterial bypass surgery Catheterization	Peripheral arterial bypass surgery Catheterization	Amputation of contralateral Catheterization	Thrombectomy	Bypass for occluded artery
AFS	CTLI	CTLI	CTLI	CTLI	CTLI
ABI / TBI	ABI 0.48	ABI 0.29	ABI 0.36	ABI 0.4	ABI 0.33 TBI 0.13
Ulcers/ gangrene	4 Ulcers	NA	2 Blueness of toes	1 Gangrene	2 Ulcers 1 Gangrene
Walking	Could not perform treadmill Walking test was not done Can walk a few meters	Could not perform treadmill Walking test was not done Patient is dependent on a wheel chair	Amputated Walking test was not done Patient is dependent on a wheel chair	Could not perform treadmill Walking test was not done Can walk a few meters	Could not perform treadmill Walking test done: 0 minutes Patient is dependent on a wheel chair
Pain relief (narcotic medications)	NA	Percocet	NA	Oxycodone; fentanyl	Percocet
Pain (VAS)	VAS 6	VAS 8	VAS 0	VAS 5	VAS 9
Quality of life	83/203	94/203	71/203	134/203	76/203

ABI Ankle-brachial index, *TBI* toe-brachial index, *NA* not applicable, *AFS* amputation-free survival, *VAS* visual analogue scale

macytoid and myeloid DCs (expressing CD304 and CD141) and T helper cells (expressing CD3 and CD4).

Safety The primary outcome of the study was safety. AEs and SAEs were classified in accordance to International Conference on Harmonization of Technical Requirements for Registration of Pharmaceuticals for Human Use (ICH) Medical Dictionary for Regulatory Activities (MedDRA), System Organ Class Preferred Term (SOC) based on Common Terminology Criteria for Adverse Events (CTCAE) [22]. A total of 44 AEs were reported, including 4 SAEs that were all typical of CLI or its underlying disease (i.e., happened or could have happened

Fig. 12.4 BGC101 cell injection. (**a**) During cell injections. (**b**) About 30 minutes after transplantation

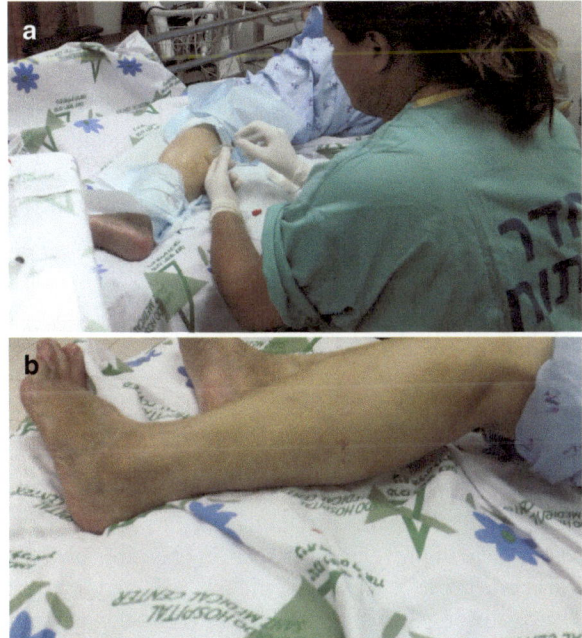

regardless of the therapy). 10 of the 44 AEs occurred during the screening period of 2 weeks prior to BGC101 administration (an average of 4AEs/patient/month), whereas 34 post-treatment AEs were reported during the 6-months follow-up (an average of 1.1AEs/patient/month). The 10 pretreatment AEs included one SAE of gastrointestinal bleeding after blood collection which was judged by the principal investigator (PI) and DSMB as an unrelated SAE. Of the 34 post-treatment AEs, 25 were defined as unrelated or unlikely related including the 3 SAEs (hospitalization due to foot infection and hypokalemia (same patient) and retroperitoneal hematoma due to angiography). Nine AEs were defined as a) possibly related (6 AEs; 4 recovered spontaneously; 1 recovered with medical treatment; 1 was ongoing with medical treatment at study termination), b) probably related (1 AE, recovered spontaneously), and c) related (2 AEs, recovered spontaneously). Based on review of the AEs and SAEs, the DSMB determined that the treatment protocol including blood collection as well as BGC101 IM administration was well tolerated and the BGC101 therapy was safe. The DSMB thus recommended continuing and expanding the study to a larger patient population with one amendment – shortening the post treatment in-patient follow-up time from 48 to 24 hours and thereby reducing the exposure to hospital risks such as nosocomial infections.

Efficacy   In this study, population prevention of deterioration (i.e., stabilizing the disease) or improvement were considered successful outcomes.

Amputation and Mortality Primary efficacy endpoints were major amputation rate (below or above the knee) and AFS at 6 months. All four patients completed the study with 6 months AFS (amputation and mortality rate = 0). The one patient who withdrew from the study immediately prior to the 3-month follow-up visit was amputation-free at that time. Secondary objectives endpoints included blood flow, assessed by ankle brachial pressure index (ABI), toe-brachial pressure index (TBI), ulcers number and severity score, walking capability, local pain, pain-control medications, and QoL.

Blood Flow Based on the Inter-Society Consensus for the Management of Peripheral Arterial Disease (TASC II) report, a changing ABI is possibly the best individual predictor, because if a patient's ABI deteriorates, it is most likely to continue to do so in the absence of successful treatment [61]. In addition, to claim cause and effect and attribute the improvement to the treatment, an objective evidence of the ABI or TBI of more than 0.10 is recommended [72]. Three out of the four patients who completed 6-month follow-up had >0.1 (ABI increase ranging from 0.13–0.54). On average ABI increased by from 0.37 ± 0.03 to 0.57 ± 0.13 (Delta of 0.19, 53% improvement). According to [56], patients with ABI <0.4 have severe ischemia grade 3, with ischemic rest pain and increased amputation risk. However, especially in patients with diabetes and wounds complicated by infection, correction of perfusion to 0.4 < ABI <0.8 may speed healing of wounds and leg salvage [56]. In this study, starting from 1 month after treatment the patients' average blood flow exceeded the level of 0.4, corresponding to moderate-severe arterial disease with possible limb salvage (Fig. 12.5). In one patient, only TBI could be measured and showed an increase from 0.13 to 0.32, which can support wound healing.

Wound Healing Four out of five patients had one or more wounds in the treated leg as detected in the screening visits. Each ulcer was defined based on its location and specifically traced and ranked by severity damage score (0 = no wound; 1 = limited to skin; 2 = penetrates the subcutaneous layer; 3 = involvement of tendons/fascia/muscle; 4 = bone exposure). A total and average damage score for each time point was calculated by summing the scores for all ulcers per patient and dividing by the number of tested patients. In all patients with wounds, ulcer worsening occurred during the screening period before treatment. In two patients, both the number of ulcers and the damage score increased and in one patient, who entered the study 2 years after amputation of the contralateral leg, the damage score increased dramatically, and a severe infection occurred before treatment. In two patients, deterioration continued after treatment, and in two others both the number and damage score were reduced, some of the wounds healed completely and some improved but were still present at 6 months.

Walking Capability Four out of five patients had two legs and were potentially capable of walking. At the study initiation, the test chosen to measure walking ability was a 6-minute walking test on a treadmill. However, the patients could not walk unaided on the treadmill or barely walked with a walker. Thus, after amending the

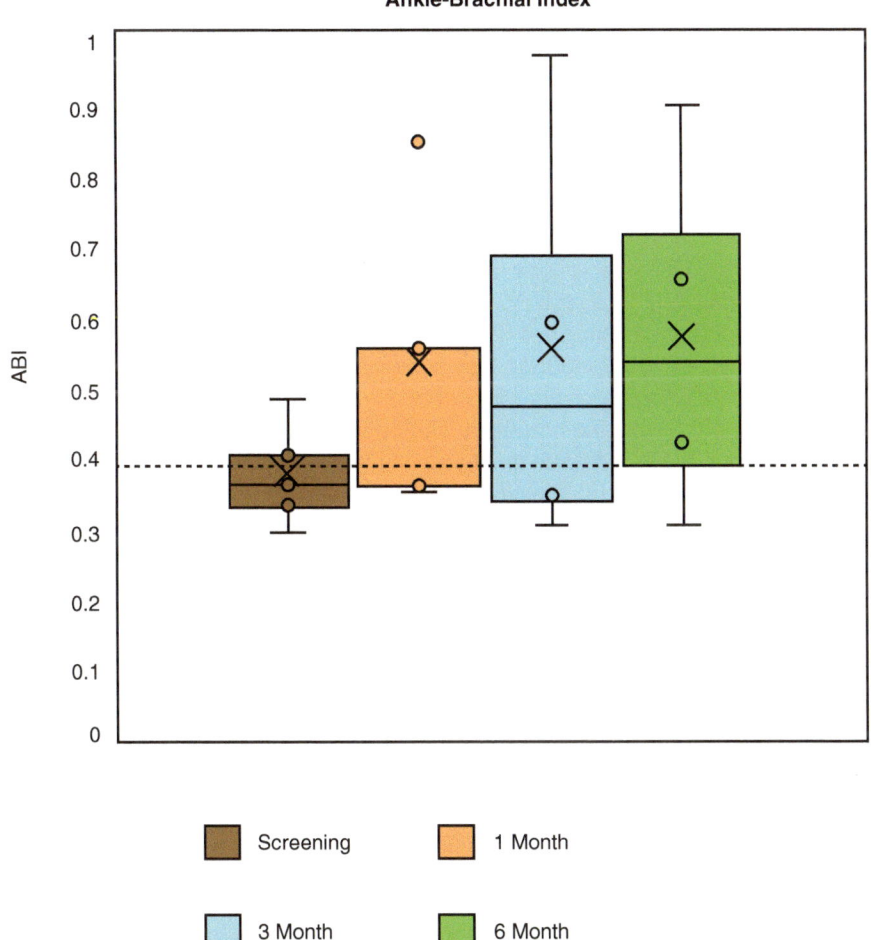

Fig. 12.5 Pilot study ABI results
ABI improvement trend is seen at all time points. Starting from 1 month after treatment the patients' average blood flow exceeded the level of 0.4 which corresponds to ischemic rest pain and risk of limb loss and reached the level of 0.40–0.80, corresponding to moderate-severe arterial disease

protocol, for patients who could not perform the treadmill test, a 6-minute walking test was performed on a flat surface. Distance and time were measured until the patient reported discomfort, for a maximum of 6 minutes.

One patient was not capable of walking at any stage from screening visits until the 1-month follow-up. Since this patient withdrew prior to the 3-month follow-up, this result was included in the study analysis as LOCF. By 6 months, all other patients showed improvement in walking time, distance, and stability that enabled them to go from using a wheelchair or a walker to using a walking stick and take daily walks or to walk more than 6 minutes on the treadmill. Large meaningful improvements from 36 to 115 meters, from 120 to 240 meters, and from 280 to 337.5 meters were observed in the walking distance at baseline and at 6 months in 3 patients. Furthermore, based on the improvement in blood flow and decrease in paresthesia, the amputated patient was allowed to re-use her leg prosthesis.

Pain Assessment

Visual Analogue Scale (VAS) of 1 (no pain) to 10 (worst possible pain) was used to assess the pain level. VAS scores showed moderate pain during the screening period (even though no physical tests or invasive tests were involved in the screening process). No increase in VAS scale was observed during blood collection (average VAS 5.4 and 3.2 during screening and blood collection, respectively). The acute effect of the cell transplantation by 30 IM injections into the gastrocnemius utilizing local anesthesia with lidocaine cream was assessed using the pain score before and 6, 24, and 48 hours following the injections. The mean VAS score prior to the procedure was 3.9, and 2.2, 2.7, and 3.0 at 6, 24, and 48 hours, respectively, indicating that the blood collection and the IM injection procedures were well tolerated. VAS scale continued at a level of 3.0–3.5 until the end of the follow-up visits at 6 months. A hallmark of CLI is severe rest pain caused by vascular insufficiency. CLI is dominated by pedal pain except in diabetic patients, where superficial pain sensation may be altered and they may experience only deep ischemic pain, such as calf claudication and ischemic rest pain. In most cases, the pedal pain is intolerably severe; it may respond to foot dependency, but otherwise responds only to opiates. This pain not only prevents physical activity, but it also alters the patient's QoL. In this study, a record of concomitant medications taken by patients was used in addition to other signs to assess the treatment effect on patients' pain relief and QoL. Medications were scored based on their relative strength as P1 = analgesics (e.g., ibuprofen); P2 = narcotic-like (e.g., Tramadex and Zaldiar), and P3 = narcotics (e.g., percocet, oxycodone, and fentanyl). Medications prescribed specifically for back pain and neuropathy were marked as NP1 and were not included in the assessment of pain severity.

Two patients reported pain or paresthesia relief starting as early as 1 week after treatment. In three patients, a reduction to zero use of P1, P2, and P3 medications between screening and 6 months after treatment was observed.

Quality of Life Assessment

QoL is as an important outcome measure for interventions designed to improve health, well-being, or both. The King's College Hospital's Vascular Quality of Life (VascuQol) is a disease-specific QoL Questionnaire for use in lower limb ischemia. It was designed to be an evaluative measure and sensitive to within-patient change [59]. A Hebrew translation of the questionnaire was utilized prior to treatment and 1, 3, and 6 months after the treatment. The questionnaire evaluated physical score, leg disease-related pain, pain not related to the leg, mental score, and patients' easement of their current condition vs. the last year. A gradual increase in QoL Total score from a base line average of 91.6 ± 11.3 to 135.5 ± 21.2 at 6-month was observed (Fig. 12.6). Improvement in walking capability correlated with a pain relief in these patients that can be seen by their concomitant medication

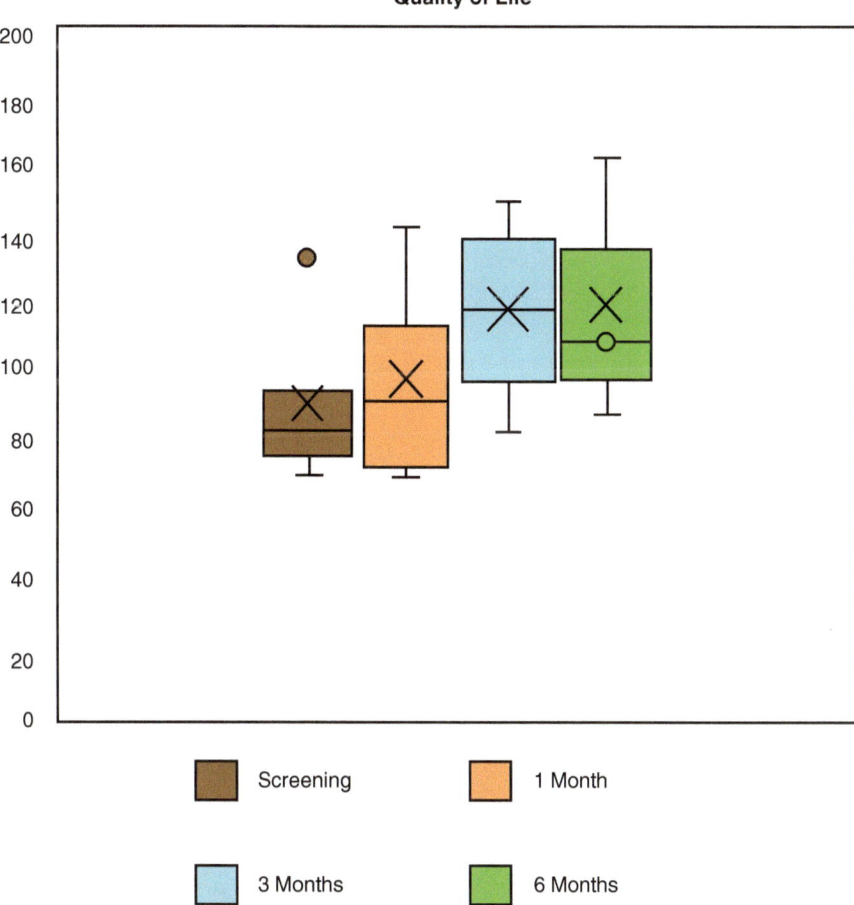

Fig. 12.6 Improvement trends in symptoms as assessed by QoL questionnaire during the study. Throughout the study VascuQol, QoL gradually rose with most of the effect obtained by 3 months after the treatment

consumption. These trends in reduction of pain should be further assessed as a possible potential early efficacy biomarker.

Summary of this Pilot Study Five severe CLI "no option" patients were treated in this pilot study. The main aim of the study was to evaluate the safety of the treatment. The study therapy procedures (blood collection and cell transplantation) were well-tolerated and safe. Since all the patients were severe "no option" CLI patients, efficacy endpoints including primary efficacy endpoint of AFS and secondary endpoints of blood flow (assessed by ABI/TBI), ulcers severity, walking capability, local pain, pain-control medications, and QoL were also measured. The primary endpoint of AFS was achieved in all patients that completed the 6-month follow-up period and in one patient who completed 2.9 months before becoming eligible for an interventional treatment option. As of Jun 2020, 3.5–3.8 years after the study, one post study amputation occurred due to sepsis of the foot. The number of tested parameters was different between patients. For example, one patient had no wound and another patient had only one leg, so wound healing and walking capability were not tested in them, respectively. For each patient, at least six of the tested parameters were stabilized or improved and at least three improved. Among the patients who completed the 6-months follow-up, there was a total of 27 improved results out of 31 tested parameters, representing a 77% improvement. Stabilizing the disease status and preventing the disease progression accounted for an additional 12% of the measured parameters. Taken together, in 89% of the tested parameters, BGC101 treatment delayed disease progression and improved the clinical status.

12.4   Conclusions

Despite positive clinical outcomes resulting from better classification of PAD and CLI characteristics (Fontaine, Rutherford, Wifi), more unified treatment protocols and the opening of multidisciplinary centers for treatment of ischemic low extremities and wounds, amputation rate has increased from 19 per 100,000 person/year to 30–50 per 100,000 person/year over the past decades, mainly driven by an increase in the number of diabetics and older patients [1, 3, 21, 34, 39, 61, 62, 89].

In addition to low survival rates, prognosis with respect to limb preservation in CLI patients is poor, particularly in nonrevascularizable, considered as "no-option" CLI patients, where 6-month major amputation rates range from 20% to 30%. Additionally, CLI is associated with a poor quality of life and high treatment costs, especially when amputation is inevitable. New treatment modalities using gene and SPC therapies have been slowly emerging during the last 15 years, but no gene or cell therapy for CLI has yet received a marketing authorization and CLI currently remains a major public health issue [46, 74, 85]. A few meta-analysis reports, with the largest by Rigato et al., in 2017 with data from 2332 patients from 19 RCTs, 7 nonrandomized trials, and 41 non-controlled studies, showed that cell therapy is safe, reduced the risk of amputation by 37%, improved amputation-free survival by 18%, and improved wound healing by 59% without affecting mortality. The latter fact is probably due to the relatively low mortality rate obtained in the placebo groups of the analyzed studies. In addition, cell therapy significantly increased ABI and TCPO2 and reduced rest pain. Thus, they concluded that cell therapy has the potential to modify the natural history of intractable CLI. Considering the severity of a disease burdened by high morbidity and mortality rates, they urged the scientific community to advance cell therapies to market [74]. Based on the summary presented here, ex vivo cultured, differentiated cells are the more promising SPC product. However, the safety issues of source cells collection (allogenic or autologous BM-derived) as well as the complicated and long culture periods required during which patients can further deteriorate make most of these methods unsuitable for mass treatments.

We report here a novel treatment based on a methodology that combines immune DCs specific activation of SPC that leads to differentiated EnEPCs, code-named BGC101, with a short time culture of 12–18 hours. The EnEPC based treatment addresses several biological features of the disease, including long-lasting effect on neovascularization and on chronic inflammation. This new approach is designed to enable mass production of patient friendly, safe personalized products that can be supplied within a day in every clinic and thus open the widespread availability of cell therapies for CLI. Furthermore, in order to address the entire CLI market and the full spectrum of PAD, we aim at developing a fully automated device for production of the EnEPC line of products that can be placed at regional hospitals and laboratories. BGC101 cells were found safe and effective in the FIH pilot study reported here, and further RCT studies on a larger population are planned to evaluate the potential of this new concept. If proven to be safe and effective in future clinical trials, this approach will disrupt current treatment strategies by developing accessible, safe, effective, and user-friendly cell-based treatment platform with the potential to reverse the disease process, save billions to payors, and offer patients the ability to return to their baseline quality of life. Furthermore, we believe that in the future, combining classical improved revascularization with cell therapies that stimulate regeneration and function of the microvasculature will enable a better long-term leg salvage and function. Such an approach may prove fruitful, improve the prognosis, and change the course of severe PAD worldwide.

References

1. Aboyans V, Ricco J, Bartelink M, Björck M, Brodmann M, Cohnert T, Collet J, Czerny M, De Carlo M, Debus S, Espinola-Klein C, Kahan T, Kownator S, Mazzolai L, Ross Naylor A, Roffi M, Röther J, Sprynger M, Tendera M, Tepe G, Venermo M, Vlachopoulos C, Desormais I. 2017 ESC guidelines on the diagnosis and treatment of peripheral arterial diseases, in collaboration with the European Society for Vascular Surgery (ESVS): document covering atherosclerotic disease of extracranial carotid and vertebral, mesenteric, renal, upper and lower extremity arteries "The Task Force for the Diagnosis and Treatment of Peripheral Arterial Diseases of the European Society of Cardiology (ESC) and of the European Society for Vascular Surgery (ESVS)". Eur Heart J. 2018;39(9):793–816.
2. Abualhin M, Sonetto A, Faggioli G, Mirelli M, Freyrie A, Gallitto E, Spath P, Stella A, Gargiulo M. Outcomes of duplex-guided paramalleolar and inframalleolar bypass in patients with critical limb ischemia. Ann Vasc Surg. 2018;53:154–64.
3. Allie D, Hebert C, Lirtzman M, Wyatt C, Keller V, Khan M, Khan M, Fail P, Vivekananthan K, Mitran E, Allie S, Chaisson G, Stagg S, Allie A, McElderry M, Walker C. Critical limb ischemia: a global epidemic. A critical analysis of current treatment unmasks the clinical and economic costs of CLI. EuroIntervention. 2005;1(1):75–84.
4. Allie D, Hebert C, Ingraldi A, Patlola R, Walker C. 24-carat gold, 14-carat gold, or platinum standards in the treatment of critical limb ischemia: bypass surgery or endovascular intervention? J Endovasc Ther. 2009;16(1):134–46.
5. Alonso A, Garcia L. The costs of critical limb ischemia. Endovascular Today. 2011:32–6.
6. Amann B, Luedemann C, Ratei R, Schmidt-Lucke JA. Autologous bone marrow cell transplantation increases leg perfusion and reduces amputations in patients with advanced critical limb ischemia due to peripheral artery disease. Cell Transplant. 2009;18(3):371–80.

7. Banchereau J, Steinman RM. Dendritic cells and the control of immunity. Nature. 1998;392:245–52.
8. Banchereau J, Briere F, Caux C, Davoust J, Lebecque S, Liu YJ, Pulendran B, Palucka K. Immunobiology of dendritic cells. Annu Rev Immunol. 2000;18:767–811.
9. Bartel R, Booth E, Cramer C, Ledford K, Watling S, Zeigler F. From bench to bedside: review of gene and cell-based therapies and the slow advancement into phase 3 clinical trials, with a focus on Aastrom's Ixmyelocel-T. Stem Cell Rev Rep. 2013;9:373–83.
10. Baser O, Verpillat P, Gabriel S, Wang L. Prevalence, incidence, and outcomes of critical limb ischemia in the US Medicare population. Vasc Dis Manag. 2013;10(2):E26–36.
11. Behfar A, Crespo-Diaz R, Nelson TJ, Terzic A, Gersh BJ. Stem cells: clinical trials results the end of the beginning or the beginning of the end? Cardiovasc Hematol Disord Drug Targets. 2010;10(3):186–201.
12. Benoit E, O'Donnell TF, Patel AN. Safety and efficacy of autologous cell therapy in critical limb ischemia: a systematic review. Cell Transplant. 2013;22(3):545–62.
13. Benoit E, O'Donnell TF, Iafrati E, Asher DF, Bandyk J, Hallett W, Lumsden AB, Pearl GJ, Roddy SP, Vijayaraghavan K, Patel AN. The role of amputation as an outcome measure in cellular therapy for critical limb ischemia: implications for clinical trial design. J Transl Med. 2011;9:165.
14. Berezin AE, Kremzer AA, Martovitskaya YV, Berezina TA, Gromenko EA. Pattern of endothelial progenitor cells and apoptotic endothelial cell-derived microparticles in chronic heart failure patients with preserved and reduced left ventricular ejection fraction. EBioMedicine. 2016;4:86–94. https://doi.org/10.1016/j.ebiom.2016.01.018
15. Bonifaz L, Bonnyay D, Mahnke K, Rivera M, Nussenzweig MC, Steinman RM. Efficient targeting of protein antigen to the dendritic cell receptor dec-205 in the steady state leads to antigen presentation on major histocompatibility complex class i products and peripheral cd8+ t cell tolerance. J Exp Med. 2002;196:1627–38.
16. Brassard DL, Grace MJ, Bordens RW. Interferon-alpha as an immunotherapeutic protein. J Leukoc Biol. 2002;71:565–81.
17. Canellos GP. CHOP may have been part of the beginning but certainly not the end: issues in risk-related therapy of large-cell lymphoma. J Clin Oncol. 1997;15(5):1713–6.
18. Caux C, Burdin N, Galibert L, Hermann P, Renard N, Servet-Delprat C, Banchereau J. Functional cd40 on b lymphocytes and dendritic cells. Res Immunol. 1994;145:235–9.
19. Cella M, Scheidegger D, Palmer-Lehmann K, Lane P, Lanzavecchia A, Alber G. Ligation of cd40 on dendritic cells triggers production of high levels of interleukin-12 and enhances t cell stimulatory capacity: T-t help via apc activation. J Exp Med. 1996;184:747–52.
20. Cheng P, Nefedova Y, Corzo CA, Gabrilovich DI. Regulation of dendritic-cell differentiation by bone marrow stroma via different notch ligands. Blood. 2007;109:507–15.
21. Conte MS, Bradbury AW, Kolh P, White JV, Dick F, Fitridge R, Mills JL, Ricco JB, Suresh KR, Murad MH, GVG Writing Group, Aboyans V, Aksoy M, Alexandrescu VA, Armstrong D, Azuma N, Belch J, Bergoeing M, Bjorck M, Chakfé N, Cheng S, Dawson J, Debus ES, Dueck A, Duval S, Eckstein HH, Ferraresi R, Gambhir R, Gargiulo M, Geraghty P, Goode S, Gray B, Guo W, Gupta PC, Hinchliffe R, Jetty P, Komori K, Lavery L, Liang W, Lookstein R, Menard M, Misra S, Miyata T, Moneta G, JAM P, Munoz A, Paolini JE, Patel M, Pomposelli F, Powell R, Robless P, Rogers L, Schanzer A, Schneider P, Taylor S, Vega De Ceniga M, Veller M, Vermassen F, Wang J, Wang S. Global vascular guidelines on the management of chronic limb-threatening ischemia. J Vasc Surg. 2019;69:3S–125S.
22. CTCAE (2016). https://www.uptodate.com/contents/common-terminology-criteria-for-adverse-events
23. Dohmen A, Eder S, Euringer W, Zeller T, Beyersdorf F. Chronic critical limb ischemia. Dtsch Arztebl Int. 2012;109(6):95–101.
24. Dong Z, Chen B, Fu W, Wang Y, Guo D, Wei Z, Xu X, Mendelsohn FO. Transplantation of purified CD34+ cells in the treatment of critical limb ischemia. J Vasc Surg. 2013;58(2):404–411.e403.
25. Dormandy JA, Rutherford RB. Management of peripheral arterial disease (PAD). TASC Working Group. TransAtlantic Inter-Society Consensus (TASC). J Vasc Surg. 2000;31:1–296.

26. Dubois B, Massacrier C, Vanbervliet B, Fayette J, Briere F, Banchereau J, Caux C. Critical role of il-12 in dendritic cell-induced differentiation of naive b lymphocytes. J Immunol. 1998;161:2223–31.
27. Dubsky M, Jirkovska A, Bem R, Fejfarova V, Pagacova L, Sixta B, Varga M, Langkramer S, Sykova E, Jude EB. Both autologous bone marrow mononuclear cell and peripheral blood progenitor cell therapies similarly improve ischaemia in patients with diabetic foot in comparison with control treatment. Diabetes Metab Res Rev. 2013;29(5):369–76.
28. Fadini G, Agostini PC, Avogaro A. Autologous stem cell therapy for peripheral arterial disease meta-analysis and systematic review of the literature. Atherosclerosis. 2010;209(1):10–7.
29. Fadini GP, Schiavon M, Cantini M, Baesso I, Facco M, Miorin M, et al. Circulating progenitor cells are reduced in patients with severe lung disease. Stem Cells. 2006;24(7):1806–13. https://doi.org/10.1634/stemcells.2005-0440
30. Fernandez Pujol B, Lucibello FC, Zuzarte M, Lutjens P, Muller R, Havemann K. Dendritic cells derived from peripheral monocytes express endothelial markers and in the presence of angiogenic growth factors differentiate into endothelial-like cells. Eur J Cell Biol. 2001;80:99–110.
31. Fontaine R, Kim M, Kieny R. Surgical treatment of periph- eral circulation disorders. Helv Chir Acta. 1954;21:499–533.
32. Fujita R, Crist C. Translational control of the myogenic program in developing, regenerating, and diseased skeletal muscle. Curr Top Dev Biol. 2018;126:67–98.
33. Fuh E, Brinton TJ. Bone marrow stem cells for the treatment of ischemic heart disease: a clinical trial review. J Cardiovasc Transl Res. 2009;2(2):202–18. https://doi.org/10.1007/s12265-009-9095-8.
34. Gottrup F, Holstein P, Jørgensen B, Lohmann M, Karlsmar T. A new concept of a multidisciplinary wound healing center and a national expert function of wound healing. Arch Surg. 2001;136(7):765–72.
35. Gratwohl A. Thomas' hematopoietic cell transplantation. Eur J Haematol. 2010;84(1):95.
36. Gupta PK, Chullikana A, Parakh R, Desai S, Das A, Gottipamula S, Krishnamurthy S, Anthony N, Pherwani A, Majumdar AS. A double blind randomized placebo controlled phase I/II study assessing the safety and efficacy of allogeneic bone marrow derived mesenchymal stem cell in critical limb ischemia. J Transl Med. 2013;11:143.
37. Hardman R, Jazaeri O, Yi J, Smith M, Gupta R. Overview of classification systems in peripheral artery disease. Semin Interv Radiol. 2014;31(4):378–88.
38. Hicks CW, Canner JK, Mathioudakis N, Lippincott C, Sherman RL, Abularrage CJ. Incidence and risk factors associated with ulcer recurrence among patients with diabetic foot ulcers treated in a multidisciplinary setting. J Surg Res. 2019;246:243–50.
39. Hicks C, Canner JK, Mathioudakis N, Lippincott C. Incidence and risk factors associated with ulcer recurrence among patients with diabetic foot ulcers treated in a multidisciplinary. Setting J Surg Res. 2020;246:243–50.
40. Huang P, Li S, Han M, Xiao Z, Yang R, Han ZC. Autologous transplantation of granulocyte colony-stimulating factor-mobilized peripheral blood mononuclear cells improves critical limb ischemia in diabetes. Diabetes Care. 2005;28(9):2155–60.
41. Huang P, Yang XF, Li SZ, Wen JC, Zhang Y, Han ZC. Randomised comparison of G-CSF-mobilized peripheral blood mononuclear cells versus bone marrow-mononuclear cells for the treatment of patients with lower limb arteriosclerosis obliterans. Thromb Haemost. 2007;98(6):1335–42.
42. Jensen S, Vatten LJ, Myhre HO. The prevalence of chronic critical lower limb ischaemia in a population of 20,000 subjects 40–69 years of age. Vasc Endovasc Surg. 2006;32:60–5.
43. Kawamura A, Horie T, Tsuda I, Ikeda A, Egawa H, Imamura E, Iida J, Sakata H, Tamaki T, Kukita K, Meguro J, Yonekawa M, Kasai M. Prevention of limb amputation in patients with limbs ulcers by autologous peripheral blood mononuclear cell implantation. Ther Apher Dial. 2005;9(1):59–63.
44. Kawamura A, Horie T, Tsuda I, Abe Y, Yamada M, Egawa H, Iida J, Sakata H, Onodera K, Tamaki T, Furui H, Kukita K, Meguro J, Yonekawa M, Tanaka S. Clinical study of therapeutic

angiogenesis by autologous peripheral blood stem cell (PBSC) transplantation in 92 patients with critically ischemic limbs. J Artif Organs. 2006;9(4):226–33.

45. Kim SJ, Kim N, Kim EH, Roh YH, Song J, Park KH, Choi YS. Use of regional anesthesia for lower extremity amputation may reduce the need for perioperative vasopressors: a propensity score-matched observational study. Ther Clin Risk Manag. 2019;15:1163–71.

46. Kitrou P, Katsanos K, Karnabatidis D, Reppas L, Brountzos E, Spiliopoulos S. Current evidence and future perspectives on anti-platelet and statin pharmacotherapy for patients with symptomatic peripheral arterial disease. Curr Vasc Pharmacol. 2017;15(5):430–45.

47. Klepanec A, Mistrik M, Altaner C, Valachovicova M, Olejarova I, Slysko R, Balazs T, Urlandova T, Hladikova D, Liska B, Tomka J, Vulev I, Madaric J. No difference in intraarterial and intramuscular delivery of autologous bone marrow cells in patients with advanced critical limb ischemia. Cell Transplant. 2012;21(9):1909–18.

48. Krishna SM, Moxon J, Golledge J. A review of the pathophysiology and potential biomarkers for peripheral artery disease. Int J Mol Sci. 2015;16:11294–322.

49. Lawall H, Bramlage P, Amann B. Treatment of peripheral arterial disease using stem and progenitor cell therapy. J Vasc Surg. 2011;53(2):445–53.

50. Li M, Zhou H, Jin X, Wang M, Zhang S, Xu L. Autologous bone marrow mononuclear cells transplant in patients with critical leg ischemia: preliminary clinical results. Exp Clin Transplant. 2013;(5):435–9. https://doi.org/10.6002/ect.2012.0129

51. Losordo DW, Kibbe MR, Mendelsohn F, Marston W, Driver VR, Sharafuddin M, Teodorescu V, Wiechmann BN, Thompson C, Kraiss L, Carman T, Dohad S, Huang P, Junge CE, Story K, Weistroffer T, Thorne TM, Millay M, Runyon JP, Schainfeld R. A randomized, controlled pilot study of autologous CD34+ cell therapy for critical limb ischemia. Circ Cardiovasc Interv. 2012;5(6):821–30.

52. Lu D, Chen B, Liang Z, Deng W, Jiang Y, Li S, Xu J, Wu Q, Zhang Z, Xie B, Chen S. Comparison of bone marrow mesenchymal stem cells with bone marrow-derived mononuclear cells for treatment of diabetic critical limb ischemia and foot ulcer: a double-blind, randomized, controlled trial. Diabetes Res Clin Pract. 2011;92(1):26–36.

53. Lumsden A, Davies M, Peden E. Medical and endovascular management of critical limb ischemia. J Endovasc Ther. 2009;16(2):II31–62.

54. Mahnke K, Schmitt E, Bonifaz L, Enk AH, Jonuleit H. Immature, but not inactive: the tolerogenic function of immature dendritic cells. Immunol Cell Biol. 2002;80:477–83.

55. McDermott MM, Guralnik JM, Criqui MH, Liu K, Kibbe MR, Ferrucci L. Six-minute walk is a better outcome measure than treadmill walking tests in therapeutic trials of patients with peripheral artery disease. Circulation. 2014;130(1):61–8.

56. Mills J, Conte M, Armstrong D, Pomposelli F, Schanzer A, Sidawy A, Andros G. The Society for Vascular Surgery Lower Extremity Threatened Limb Classification System: risk stratification based on Wound, Ischemia, and foot Infection (WIfI). Vasc Surg. 2014;59:220–34.

57. Miyamoto M, Yasutake M, Takano H, Takagi H, Takagi G, Mizuno H, Kumita S, Takano T. Therapeutic angiogenesis by autologous bone marrow cell implantation for refractory chronic peripheral arterial disease using assessment of neovascularization by 99mTc-tetrofosmin (TF) perfusion scintigraphy. Cell Transplant. 2004;13(4):429–37.

58. Montoya M, Edwards MJ, Reid DM, Borrow P. Rapid activation of spleen dendritic cell subsets following lymphocytic choriomeningitis virus infection of mice: analysis of the involvement of type 1 ifn. J Immunol. 2005;174:1851–61.

59. Morgan MB, Crayford T, Murrin B, Fraser SC. Developing the vascular quality of life questionnaire: a new disease-specific quality of life measure for use in lower limb ischemia. J Vasc Surg. 2001;33(4):679–87.

60. Mutirangura P, Ruangsetakit C, Wongwanit C, Chinsakchai K, Porat Y, Belleli A, Czeiger D. Enhancing limb salvage by non-mobilized peripheral blood Angiogenic cell precursors therapy in patients with critical limb ischemia. J Med Assoc Thail. 2009;92(3):320–7.

61. Norgren L, Hiatt WR, Dormandy JA, Nehler MR, Harris KA, Fowkes FG, Rutherford RB. Inter-society consensus for the management of peripheral arterial disease. Int Angiol. 2007;26(2):81–157.

62. Olinic DM, Spinu M, Olinic M, Homorodean C, Tataru DA, Liew A, Schernthaner GH, Stanek A, Fowkes G, Catalano M. Epidemiology of peripheral artery disease in Europe: VAS educational paper. Int Angiol. 2018;37(4):327–34. https://doi.org/10.23736/S0392-9590.18.03996-2.
63. Perl L, Weissler A, Mekori YA, Mor A. Cellular therapy in 2010: focus on autoimmune and cardiac diseases. Isr Med Assoc J. 2010;12(2):110–5.
64. Perera S, Mody SH, Woodman RC, Studenski SA. Meaningful change and responsiveness in common physical performance measures in older adults. J Am Geriatr Soc. 2006;54:743–9.
65. Procházka V, Gumulec J, Jalůvka F, Šalounová D, Jonszta T, Czerný D, Krajča J, Urbanec R, Klement P, Martinek J, Klement GL. Cell therapy, a new standard in management of chronic critical limb ischemia and foot ulcer. Cell Transplant. 2010;19(11):1413–24.
66. Powell R, Comerota A, Berceli S, Guzman R, Henry T, Tzeng E, Velazquez O, Marston W, Bartel R, Longcore A, Stern T, Watling S. Interim analysis results from the RESTORE-CLI, a randomized, double-blind multicenter phase II trial comparing expanded autologous bone marrow-derived tissue repair cells and placebo in patients with critical limb ischemia. J Vasc Surg. 2011;54(4):1032–41.
67. Porat Y, Assa-Kunik E, Belkin M, Krakovsky M, Lamensdorf I, Duvdevani R, Sivak G, Niven M, Bulvik S. A novel potential therapy for vascular diseases: blood-derived stem/progenitor cells specifically activated by dendritic cells. Diabetes Metab Res Rev. 2014;30(7):623–34.
68. Porat Y, Abraham E, Karnieli O, Nahum S, Woda J, Zylberberg C. Critical elements in the development of cell therapy potency assays for ischemic conditions. Cytotherapy. 2015;17(7):817–31.
69. Powell RJ, Simons M, Mendelsohn FO, Daniel G, Henry TD, Koga M, et al. Results of a double-blind, placebo-controlled study to assess the safety of intramuscular injection of hepatocyte growth factor plasmid to improve limb perfusion in patients with critical limb ischemia. Circulation. 2008;118(1):58–65. https://doi.org/10.1161/CIRCULATIONAHA.107.727347
70. Raval AN, Schmuck EG, Tefera G, Leitzke C, Ark CV, Hei D, Centanni JM, de Silva R, Koch J, Chappell RG, Hematti P. Bilateral administration of autologous CD133+ cells in ambulatory patients with refractory critical limb ischemia: lessons learned from a pilot randomized, double-blind, placebo-controlled trial. Cytotherapy. 2014;16(12):1720–32. https://doi.org/10.1016/j.jcyt.2014.07.011
71. Raval AD, Vyas A. Trends in healthcare expenditures among individuals with arthritis in the United States from 2008 to 2014. J Rheumatol. 2018;45(5):705–16.
72. Rutherford R, Baker D, Ernst C, Johnston W, Porter J, Jones S, Darrell N. Recommended standards for reports dealing with lower extremity ischemia: revised version. J Vasc Surg. 1997;26(3):517–38.
73. Riboldi E, Musso T, Moroni E, Urbinati C, Bernasconi S, Rusnati M, Adorini L, Presta M, Sozzani S. Cutting edge: proangiogenic properties of alternatively activated dendritic cells. J Immunol. 2005;175(5):2788–92.
74. Rigato M, Monami M, Fadini GP. Autologous cell therapy for peripheral arterial disease: systematic review and meta-analysis of randomized, nonrandomized, and noncontrolled studies. Circ Res. 2017;120(8):1326–40.
75. Rivollier A, Perrin-Cocon L, Luche S, Diemer H, Strub JM, Hanau D, van Dorsselaer A, Lotteau V, Rabourdin-Combe C, Rabilloud T, Servet-Delprat C. High expression of antioxidant proteins in dendritic cells: possible implications in atherosclerosis. Mol Cell Proteomics. 2006;5:726–36.
76. Schanzer A, Conte MS. Critical limb ischemia. Curr Treat Options Cardiovasc Med. 2010;12(3):214–29.
77. Smith RB, Walker HK, Hall WD, Hurst JW, editors. Clinical methods: the history, physical, and laboratory examinations. 3rd ed. Boston: Butterworths; 1990. Chapter 13. PMID: 21250079.
78. Steinman RM, Cohn ZA. Identification of a novel cell type in peripheral lymphoid organs of mice. I. Morphology, quantitation, tissue distribution. J Exp Med. 1973;137:1142–62.
79. Steinman RM. Some interfaces of dendritic cell biology. APMIS. 2003;111:675–97.
80. Sozzani S, Rusnati M, Riboldi E, Mitola S, Presta M. Dendritic cell-endothelial cell cross-talk in angiogenesis. Trends Immunol. 2007;28:385–92.

81. Szabo GV, Kovesd Z, Cserepes J, Daroczy J, Belkin M, Acsady G. Peripheral blood-derived autologous stem cell therapy for the treatment of patients with late-stage peripheral artery disease-results of the short- and long-term follow-up. Cytotherapy. 2013;15(10):1245–52.
82. Tang H, Guo Z, Zhang M, Wang J, Chen G, Cao X. Endothelial stroma programs hematopoietic stem cells to differentiate into regulatory dendritic cells through il-10. Blood. 2006;108:1189–97.
83. Tateishi-Yuyama E, Matsubara H, Murohara T, Ikeda U, Shintani S, Masaki H, Amano K, Kishimoto Y, Yoshimoto K, Akashi H, Shimada K, Iwasaka T, Imaizumi T. Therapeutic angiogenesis for patients with limb ischaemia by autologous transplantation of bone-marrow cells: a pilot study and a randomised controlled trial. Lancet. 2002;360(9331):427–35.
84. Teraa M, Sprengers RW, Schutgens RE, Slaper-Cortenbach IC, van der Graaf Y, Algra A, van der Tweel I, Doevendans PA, Mali WP, Moll FL, Verhaar MC. Effect of repetitive intraarterial infusion of bone marrow mononuclear cells in patients with no-option limb ischemia: the randomized, double-blind, placebo-controlled Rejuvenating Endothelial Progenitor Cells via Transcutaneous Intra-arterial Supplementation (JUVENTAS) trial. Circulation. 2015;131(10):851–60.
85. Teraa M, Conte M, Moll F, Verhaar M. Critical limb ischemia: current trends and future directions. J Am Heart Assoc. 2016;5(2):2938.
86. Tongers J, Roncalli JG And Losordo DW. Therapeutic angiogenesis for critical limb ischemia: microvascular therapies coming of age. Circulation 2008;118(1):9–16.
87. Trinchieri G, Pflanz S, Kastelein RA. The il-12 family of heterodimeric cytokines: new players in the regulation of t cell responses. Immunity. 2003;19:641–4.
88. Veith FJ, Gupta SK, Wengerter KR, Samson RH, Scher LA, Fell SC, Weiss P, Janko G, Flores SW, Rifkin H, Bernstein G, Haimovici H, Gliedman ML, Sprayregen S. Progress in limb salvage by reconstructive arterial surgery combined with new or improved adjunctive procedures. Ann Surg. 1981;194(4):386–401.
89. Veith FJ, Gupta SK, Wengerter KR, Goldsmith J, Rivers SP, Bakal CW, Dietzek AM, Cynamon J, Sprayregen S, Gliedman M. Effects of metoprolol on rest and exercise cardiac function and plasma catecholamines in chronic congestive heart failure secondary to ischemic or idiopathic cardiomyopathy. Am J Cardiol. 1990;66(10):843–8.
90. Walter DH, Krankenberg H, Balzer JO, Kalka C, Baumgartner I, et al. Intraarterial Administration of Bone Marrow Mononuclear Cells in patients with critical limb ischemia: a randomized-start, placebo-controlled pilot trial (PROVASA). Circ Cardiovasc Interv. 2011;4(1):26–37. https://doi.org/10.1161/CIRCINTERVENTIONS.110.958348
91. Wang N, Yang BH, Wang G, Gao Y, Cao X, Zhang XF, Yan CC, Lian XT, Liu BH, Ju S. A meta-analysis of the relationship between foot local characteristics and major lower extremity amputation in diabetic foot patients. J Cell Biochem. 2019;120(6):9091–6.
92. Yu Z, Witmanb N, Wang W, Li D, Yan B, Deng M, Wang X, Wang H, Zhou G, Liu W, Sahara M, Cao Y, Fritsche-Danielsonf R, Zhanga W, Fud W, Chienb K. Cell-mediated delivery of VEGF modified mRNA enhances blood vessel regeneration and ameliorates murine critical limb ischemia. J Control Release. 2019;310:103–14.
93. Zhang Y, Zhang C. Role of dendritic cells in cardiovascular diseases. World J Cardiol. 2010;2:357–64.
94. Ziegler-Graham K, MacKenzie EJ, Ephraim PL, Travison TG, Brookmeyer R. Estimating the prevalence of limb loss in the United States: 2005 to 2050. Arch Phys Med Rehabil. 2008;89(3):422–9.

Chapter 13
Stem Cell Delivery for the Treatment of Arteriovenous Fistula Failure

Akshaar N. Brahmbhatt and Sanjay Misra

13.1 Introduction

Chronic kidney disease is associated with significant morbidity, mortality, and healthcare costs. The vast majority of patients with chronic kidney disease go on to develop end-stage renal disease (ESRD) [12]. There are several treatment options for patients with ESRD, including transplant and various forms of renal replacement therapy. However, the vast majority of patients rely on hemodialysis to survive.

Although hemodialysis has proven to be a lifeline for many patients, it requires a well-functioning vascular access. The maintenance and complications arising from vascular access are some of the most costly and often frustrating aspects of hemodialysis care for both the patients and providers. Over the past few decades, there has been progress in providing reliable vascular access, and more patients are receiving dialysis through the use of arteriovenous fistulas (AVFs). AVFs have fewer complications, namely, infection when compared with catheters [13, 14].

In addition to the decreased complication rate of AVFs, they can help preserve central access. However, arteriovenous fistulas often fail due to poor remodeling of the venous outflow. There are multiple factors implicated in AVF failure, including location, venous size, surgical technique, patient comorbidities, and others [13, 15].

Multiple studies examining fistula failure have shown that a majority of fistulas fail due to stenosis caused by venous neointimal hyperplasia (VNH). Venous neointimal hyperplasia occurs due to increased proliferation of smooth muscle cells, myofibroblasts, and inflammatory cells, which result in narrowing of the lumen of

A. N. Brahmbhatt
Diagnostic Radiology - Department of Imaging Sciences, University of Rochester, Rochester, NY, USA
e-mail: akshaar_brahmbhatt@urmc.rochester.edu

S. Misra (✉)
Department of Radiology, Mayo Clinic, Rochester, MN, USA
e-mail: misra.sanjay@mayo.edu

© Springer Nature Switzerland AG 2021
T. P. Navarro et al. (eds.), *Stem Cell Therapy for Vascular Diseases*,
https://doi.org/10.1007/978-3-030-56954-9_13

the vein. This negative remodeling can eventually result in clinically significant stenosis or thrombosis, leading to fistula failure [1].

There are multiple molecular pathways implicated in the development of VNH. As a whole, the process can be thought of as a stress response due to the inflammation and hypoxia during fistula placement. This coupled with the underlying uremic state of the patient with alterations in shear stress, actives multiple reactive cytokines. These, in turn, act on nearby fibroblasts, endothelial cells, smooth muscle cells, and macrophages. This runaway stress response leads to cellular proliferation, migration, and remodeling of the extracellular matrix, which ultimately narrows the lumen [16].

Many in vitro studies have demonstrated the capacity of stem cells, specifically mesenchymal stem cells (MSCs), to mitigate and counteract many of the mechanisms implicated in VNH. Preclinical in vivo studies have corroborated these findings demonstrating a reduction in inflammatory cytokines and VNH [11, 17, 18]. This chapter will explore the molecular mechanisms of VNH, the positive modulatory effects of stem cells), and the therapeutic potential of stem cells in the setting of arteriovenous fistula failure.

13.2   The Molecular Basis of Arteriovenous Fistula Failure

Pathological analysis of failed AVFs demonstrate thickening of the intima due to the presence of multiple cell types, including endothelial cells, fibroblasts, vascular smooth muscle cells, and macrophages [19, 20]. After the creation of the fistula, there is proliferation and migration of smooth muscle cells, derived from a combination of venous smooth muscle cells, arterial smooth muscle cells, adventitial fibroblasts and circulating progenitor cells. These changes are the result of multiple intertwined cellular signaling pathways [16, 20–22] (Fig. 13.1).

These pathways are complex and interwoven but can be grossly separated into several indistinct groups. One of the major drivers of fistula failure is hypoxia, which results from disruption of the vaso vasorum during fistula placement. Hypoxia increases the transcription of several key genes, including hypoxia-inducible factor-1 (HIF-1α) and radiation inducible immediate early gene (IEX-1). These activate multiple cascades resulting in upregulation of several downstream factors, including vascular endothelial growth factor A (VEGF-A), matrix metalloproteinase-2 (MMP-2), matrix metalloproteinase-9 (MMP-9), NADPH oxidase 2 (NOX-2), monocyte chemoattractant protein-1 (MCP-1), among others [23–27]. These downstream cytokines are responsible for a variety of functions, including angiogenesis, remodeling of the extracellular matrix and promoting inflammation. As a whole, these factors lay the groundwork for cellular proliferation and migration, discussed later in this section [26, 28, 29]. Several in vivo studies aimed at reducing hypoxia using hyperbaric oxygen and in vitro studies targeting these genes have shown decreased VNH and cellular proliferation, respectively. These studies provide further support for the multifactorial nature of VNH [30, 31].

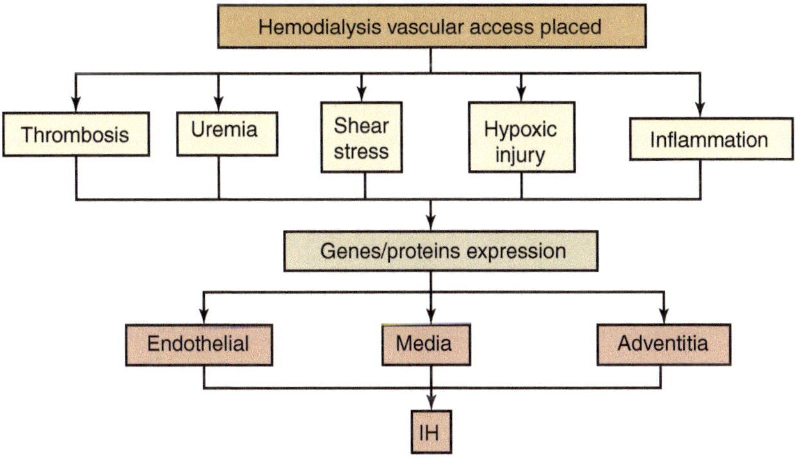

Fig. 13.1 Schematic of vascular injuries contributing to stenosis formation in hemodialysis vascular access. IH intimal hyperplasia. (Reprinted with permissions from Kidney International)

In addition to these factors activated secondary to hypoxia, there are many effects secondary to inflammation that occur during AVF placement. This inflammatory process drives macrophages which exacerbate cellular migration and proliferation [32]. These inflammatory factors share similar biochemical pathways with hypoxia response and both contributed to VNH [16].

One of the major drivers of this inflammatory phenomenon is MCP-1. In vitro and in vivo work has demonstrated that decreasing MCP-1 results in a decrease of proliferation and vein graft thickening [33]. Also, several clinical studies have linked higher levels of circulating MCP-1 with fistula failure [34]. MCP-1 has been shown to work through activation of transcription factors NF-κB implicated in immune responses and Activator Protein-1 (AP-1) implicated in the growth response. In addition to these, the cascade of pro-inflammatory markers includes plasminogen activator inhibitor-1 (PAI-1) and endothelin (ET)-1. ET-1 not only contributes to inflammation but also vasoconstriction [35]. Monocyte infiltration into the vascular wall has also been shown to increase transformative growth factor-beta 1 (TGF-β1), and tumor necrosis factor-alpha (TNF-α), and these are hypothesized to have a proliferative effect in the setting of fistula failure mediated through the NF-κB pathway [16].

In addition to the acute inflammatory response during fistula creation, there is an underlying heightened inflammatory state in patients with chronic kidney disease due to increased uremia [36]. In addition to uremia, patients with CKD often have other comorbidities, including diabetes, which also adds to dysregulation. Several clinical studies have shown that patients with an increased uremic burden have lower rates of fistula patency [34]. In vitro and animal work has also shown that uremia increases cellular proliferation [36–38]. For example, uremia has been shown to induce pro-inflammatory, M1 macrophages. This has been linked to multiple complex interactions [39]. One crucial factor is

Delta-like ligand 4 (DLL-4) release. DLL-4 is a Notch activating cytokine. Notch activation has been shown to increase cellular proliferation and migration. In addition, Notch activation can worsen the inflammatory response by transforming FSP-1-positive cells into macrophages [40, 41]. In vitro work has shown to suppress Notch activation and inhibit DLL-4 and reduce smooth muscle cell proliferation [42].

Uremia has also been linked to decreasing circulating endothelial progenitor cells (EPCs) and decreased proliferation of EPCs. These cells are important for vascular reparative functions and uremia negatively affects the number, which likely exacerbates vascular disease and fistula failure in CKD patients [43, 44].

In addition to hypoxia and inflammation, alterations in shear stress on the endoluminal endothelial cells also contribute to fistula failure [45–47] (Fig. 13.2). Sustained unidirectional wall shear stress (WSS) activates several transcription factors that maintain a quiescent phenotype, including NO and Kruppel-Like Factor-2 (KLF-1). KLF-2 downregulates inflammatory cytokines, including IL-8 and MCP-1 [48, 49]. NO acts as a vasodilator and modulates matrix metalloproteinases toward maintaining the vessel wall. In contrast to this, altered WSS, as in some AVFs, leads to a decrease in KLF-2 and NO resulting in decreased vasodilation as well as upregulation of inflammatory cytokines and several of which are involved in remodeling of the extracellular matrix (ECM) [50]. These include TGF-B1, MCP-1, and IL-8, among others [47]. Overall these alterations promote cellular proliferation and migration leading to VNH [16, 27, 46].

Beyond these, there are many other cytokines and molecular pathways implicated in fistula failure, but overall the mix of stressors leads to an environment that favors cellular proliferation, migration, and adverse remodeling of the vascular wall. As a result of this, multiple clinical studies examining AVF failure have tried to reduce these cellular processes.

There have been several clinical trials examining the role of paclitaxel via drug-coated balloons with promising but mixed results [51–56]. Brachytherapy trials using endovascular radiation did demonstrate some initial benefit, but they were not durable at 1 year, nor was external beam radiation [57–60]. Multiple studies examining the impact of Omega-3 PUF and aspirin have demonstrated no durable benefit [61, 62]. Several studies have also examined the possible benefits of statins, but these have resulted in mixed largely inconclusive results [63]. Other studies examining antiplatelet therapy have shown similar mixed results [64]. Transdermal glyceryl trinitrate does increase blood flow in the perioperative period but did not demonstrate any durable benefit [65, 66]. In addition to these and several other studies using chemical and medical therapies, there are numerous studies examining technique, patient-based factors, cannulation, etc. These are primarily outside the scope of this chapter, but should be considered in the greater context of vascular access failure and when designing studies.

Overall the majority of these prior studies have focused on one or several mechanisms of AVF failure. Additionally, many targeted downstream cellular functions, such as paclitaxel. Stem cell therapy is different from these prior therapies in several ways. Stem cells can modulate the microenvironment using multiple paracrine

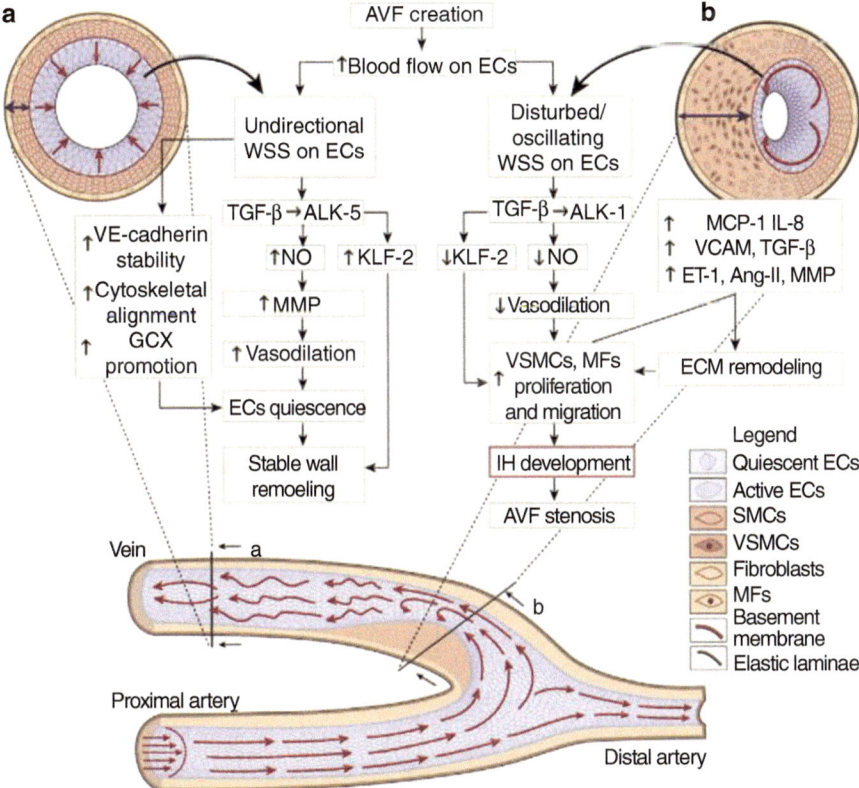

Fig. 13.2 Section of a side-to-end arteriovenous fistula (AVF). Laminar blood flow coming from the proximal artery stimulates the endothelial cells (ECs) with unidirectional wall shear stress (WSS) until the anastomosis level where the blood flow splits in two directions. At the vein curvature, the blood flow becomes unstable with disturbed and oscillating WSS and reverse flows at the inner curvature of the anastomosis. After the curvature, blood flow oscillations decrease and WSS returns to almost unidirectional. The different WSS patterns generated on the endothelium lead wall remodeling. At (a), the unidirectional WSS maintains vessel patency, while at (b) oscillating and reversing WSS impair ECs quiescence leading to intimal hyperplasia (IH). ALK-5 activin receptor-like kinases 1/5, Ang-II angiotensin II, ECM extracellular matrix, ET 1 endothelin 1, GCX glycocalyx, IL-8 interleukin 8, KLF-2 Krüppel-like factor 2, MCP-1 monocytes chemoattractant protein 1, MFs myofibroblasts, MMP metalloproteinase, NO nitric oxide, SMCs smooth muscle cells, TGF-β transforming growth factor β, VCAM vascular cell adhesion protein, VE vascular endothelial, VSMC vascular smooth muscle cells. (Reprinted with permissions from Kidney International)

effects to alter many pathways simultaneously and at higher levels of cellular signaling. These and other beneficial properties have allowed stem cells to be used in a variety of disease states with good results [3, 9, 10, 67–70]. Due to these properties, stem cells were hypothesized to serve as a potential treatment for AVF failure [2, 11, 17, 18].

13.3   Stem Cells

Several types of stem cells have been used in vascular applications. Earlier work involved adult stem cells derived from either tissue, blood, or bone marrow. These endothelial progenitor cells, such as blood outgrowth endothelial cells (BOECs), have multiple favorable vasculogenic properties and were used in several trials [7]. However, more recent work has incorporated the use of MSCs [9]. These cells have greater plasticity allowing for greater cellular differentiation. This along with several reliable methods of harvest and proliferation has made them a more desirable therapeutic option [7, 9].

MSCs are pluripotent and are able to differentiate themselves into several different cell types [71]. MSCs have several intrinsic properties, which have allowed them to serve as therapeutic agents in innumerable pathological diseases. The main therapeutic function of MSCs is through their paracrine immunomodulatory properties. There are multiple studies examining these proteins, transcription factors, and microRNA that induce a variety of responses. The signaling molecules and their effects depend on the existing environment [6, 67, 72]. However, in multiple studies, given a baseline inflammatory environment, MSCs serve an anti-inflammatory role. Overall, MSCs can drive differentiation of macrophages toward a M2 phenotype in the setting of inflammation. The M2 phenotype is associated with repair and anti-inflammatory cytokines, including TGF-B and IL-10. In contrast, M1 macrophages are associated with inflammation. These are tied linked to TNF-α, interferon-γ *(IFN-γ), MCP-1, IL-6, among others* [4].

Several studies have demonstrated decreased levels of TNF- α and IL-6 in models of acute kidney and lung injuries after administration of MSCs. This is likely being mediated through tumor necrosis factor receptor-1, which effectively neutralizes circulating TNF-α and subsequently reduces IL-6 and IFN-γ. Other studies have demonstrated that TNF-α induced protein 6 and high levels of prostaglandin 2 release, which acts on the EP2 and EP4 receptors of macrophages may be responsible. This concomitant decrease is also tied to the increased release of anti-inflammatory factors such as IL-10, which drive cells toward an M2 phenotype [68, 73–76]. In vivo studies using MSCs to treat fistula failure have demonstrated a reduction in inflammatory markers such as MCP-1 and CD-68. This reduction supports the anti-inflammatory properties of MSCs in the setting of fistula failure [11].

It is important to note that in several studies examining ischemia and damaged organs that MSCs have been shown to increase levels of angiogenesis and cellular proliferation [68]. Some of these factors may negatively impact fistula remodeling such as VEGF-A [77]. It is likely that the MSCs aid in a reparative process that varies based on the surrounding microenvironment. Thus in some cases, it may promote angiogenesis, while in others it may serve to attenuate the process [68, 78]. Overall, work in this area is limited with regard to MSCs in the setting of AVF failure. Future studies may shed light on these additional factors.

MSCs also migrate toward sites of inflammation, though several cytokines including parts of the complement cascade and chemokines including CXCR4 [5,

79, 80]. CXR4 is also implicated in multiple other downstream immunoregulatory pathways [81]. This migratory process has been tied to matrix metalloproteinases, immunoglobulins, and transcription factors several of which are implicated in fistula failure [82]. MSCs delivered to the adventitia migrate to the lumen in murine arteriovenous fistulae [11]. This intrinsic migratory propensity toward inflammation adds to their therapeutic value.

13.4 Isolation and Safety of Mesenchymal Stem Cells

MSCs can be derived from a number of different sources, including umbilical cord blood, bone marrow, and adipose tissue [8]. However, given the minimally invasive nature of adipose tissue extraction and the availability of reliable MSCs using good manufacturing practice compliant production, supported the use of adipose-derived MSCs in preclinical experiments. Additionally, using these established practices was thought to facilitate an easier transition to clinical trials [83, 84]. There are some challenges in harvesting stem cells from patients with renal dysfunction. Uremia, along with common comorbidities such as diabetes and cardiovascular disease, negatively affects MSCs. However, there are several preconditioning techniques and chemicals that can be used to increase the function of MSCs, including hypoxic preconditioning and statins. In the future, more robust techniques including epigenetic programming might be employed [70].

MSCs are also a safe therapeutic option. There have been multiple studies examining the safety of adipose-derived MSCs in multiple settings. Countless studies across many disciples have demonstrated the safety and therapeutic potential of stem cells [3, 9, 85]. Initially, given the pluripotency of MSCs, there was some concern that therapy with MSCs might lead to neoplasms or that these cells may undergo malignant transformation. Hover, several studies have not found any meaningful evidence to support this [86, 87].

13.5 Drug Delivery Technologies Applied to and Available for Fistula Failure

There are several drug delivery and treatment options that can be applied in the setting of fistulae and grafts. These can be broadly divided into two types, endovascular and perivascular.

The most commonly used endoluminal delivery device is a balloon. The standard of care to treat fistula failure is plain balloon angioplasty; however, balloons have also been used for cryotherapy, brachytherapy, and drug delivery via drug-coated balloons [59, 88, 89]. There have also been several animal studies delivering gene therapy into the lumen via infusion of viral vector and temporary clamping of the vessel to allow for transfection [90–92]. Similar techniques have been used with high-dose vitamin D [93]. Viral vectors and other therapies requiring endoluminal infusion and incubation have the potential to be used at the time of fistula placement or with the use of an occlusion balloon in an existing fistula. In addition to balloons, intraluminal delivery of drugs can be performed using micro infusion catheters. These devices, upon inflation, puncture the vessel with a small needle and can deliver a therapeutic agent into the vessel wall [94]. This latter method may be useful for the delivery of stem cells or cytokine containing exosomes in the future.

Stent placement is another commonly used endovascular treatment option for arteriovenous fistula failure. Overall stents have been less commonly used due to the risk of thrombosis, fracture, and migration. Additionally, stenting can limit further intervention in cases of in-stent restenosis [95–97]. Future developments, including drug eluting and bioabsorbable stents, may prove to be durable treatment options [96, 98]. Currently, there is limited technology to allow for the reliable intraluminal delivery of stem cells, which would allow them to integrate into the vascular lumen. Additionally, MSCs need to be kept viable in a suitable media. There is promising work with regard to stem cell impregnated stents [99]. However there are several challenges with stent-based delivery including the risk of washing cells away or damaging them during delivery with mechanical, immune, and chemical stressors [99–101]. Additionally, stem cell behavior can vary based on the surrounding structure and potential stent material. These effects should be considered when designing delivery methods and devices [102–104].

Perivascular treatment delivery can be used during fistula creation or after placement. This method avoids the need for endovascular instrumentation and predominantly treats the adventitial and medial vascular layers, thought to be the predominant source of cells leading to venous neointimal hyperplasia. One of the more well-studied perivascular delivery systems is the use of biodegradable gels. These can be altered or used with other technologies such as nanoparticles to optimize the release kinetics of the therapeutic agent [105]. Several in vivo studies have used gels to deliver paclitaxel, sirolimus, peptides, vitamin D, and stem cells, among others [30, 106–108].These studies have had promising results. In addition to gels, perivascular wraps have also been utilized in a variety of in vivo models and in several clinical trials [109–111].

MSCs can be grown in gels, and artificial matrices, which can be optimized for perivascular delivery, serve as a vascular wrap [69, 112]. These delivery mechanisms can be applied to the fistula under direct visualization or with the use of imaging guidance. Given the ease of use and the ability to easily deliver cells either at the time of fistula placement or afterward allows for therapeutic flexibility. Perivascular delivery of MSCs for AVF failure is the most feasible. Additionally, it does not necessitate the use of a durable implant and allows for greater flexibility, should the patient require future therapy or a revision.

Beyond these, there are several other treatment delivery methods, systemic, topical, etc. [113]. While these may be useful for other therapeutic agents, they are not particularly efficacious for stem cells, which require proximity to exert their paracrine effects. Although MSCs do have homing properties toward inflammation, a higher number might be needed to generate the desired effect especially in patients with multiple comorbidities. However, systemic treatment may be more feasible in the future [5, 79, 80].

13.6   Preclinical Work

Early in vitro work utilized BOECs. Although BOECs exhibit less plasticity than embryonic and induced pluripotent stem cells, they exert similar effects [2, 7]. When co-cultured with fibroblasts in a hypoxic environment, BOECs reduced angiogenic cytokine production and resulted in decreased conversion of fibroblasts to smooth muscle cells. This demonstrated the potential for blood endothelial out-growth cells to reduce angiogenesis, a major hypoxia driven response implicated in VNH (Fig. 13.3) [17, 23].

These findings were corroborated in a porcine model of fistula failure. In this model, uremia was induced by partial renal infarction and PTFE grafts were placed between the carotid and jugular to create a fistula. BOECs were delivered to the adventia with a polyglycolic acid scaffolding. Compared with controls fistulae which had been treated with BOEC, demonstrated reduced neointima (Fig. 13.4). There was also decrease in HIF-1α. Interestingly many of the BOEC cells had migrated to neointima of both the treated and contralateral control sides under-scoring the homing proprieties of these cells to seek out areas of tissue damage and hypoxia likely through factors like HIF-1α [18]. These studies eventually paved the way for more streamlined work using adipose-derived stem cells in a murine models.

Preclinical work using a murine carotid jugular model of AVF failure and human adipose-derived MSCs has demonstrated the feasibility and utility of treat-ing AVF failure with MSCs. In this study B6.Cg-*Foxn1^{nu}*/J mice (Charles River Laboratories, Wilmington, MA, USA) were used. These mice lack a thymus and

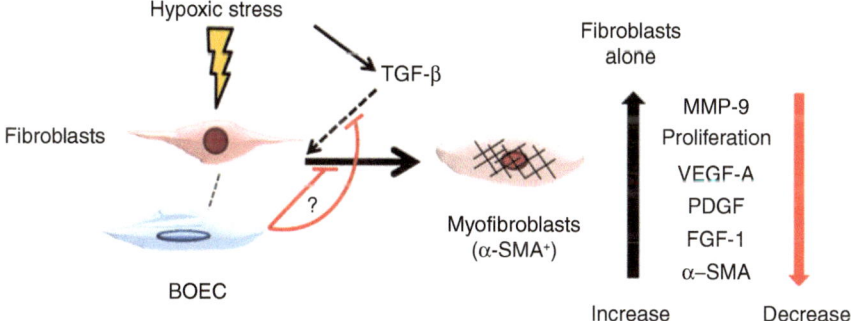

Fig. 13.3 Schematic of proposed interaction by BOEC under hypoxic conditions changes. (The final, published version of this article is available at http://www.karger.com/? doi/10.1159/0003699290)

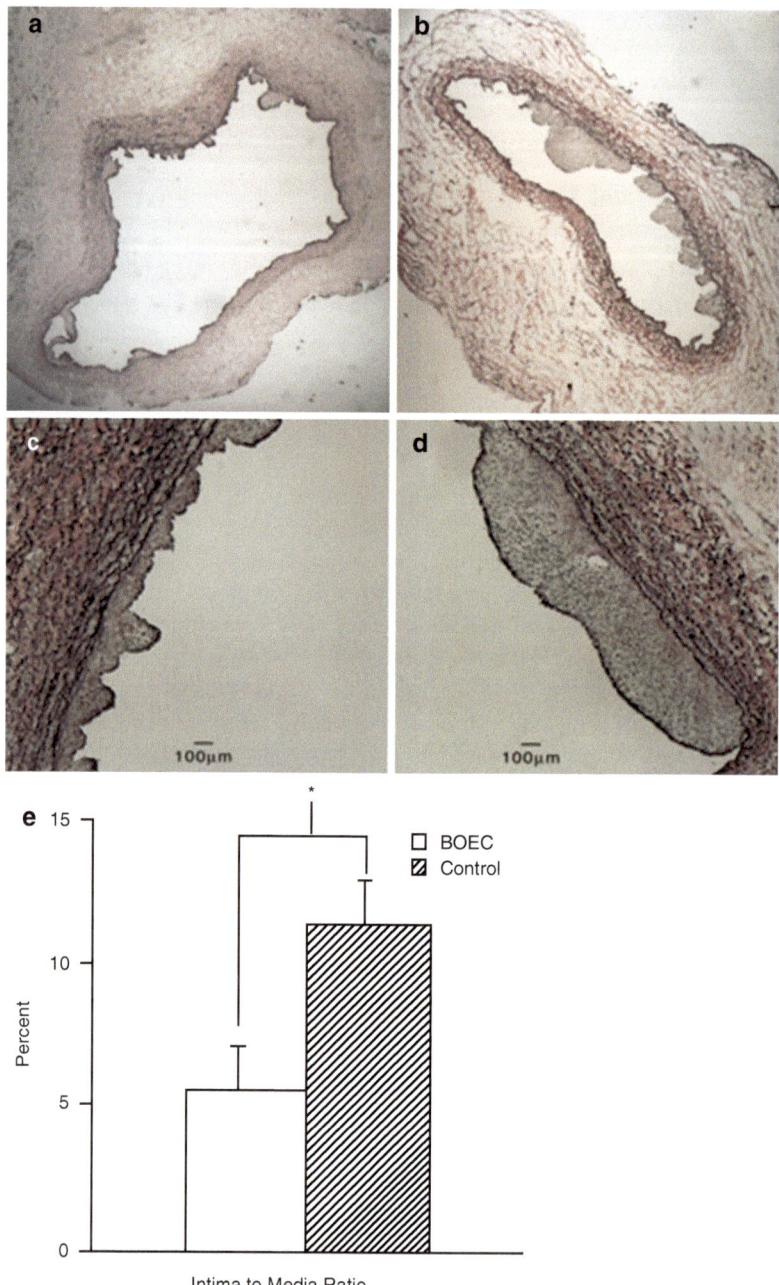

Fig. 13.4 Verhoeff's van Giesen staining was performed at the venous stenosis (section V1, see Figure Figure1C)1C) from the cushioning region of the BOEC-transplanted (**a, c**) and contralateral non-transplanted (control) veins (**b, d**). A and B are 5× and C and D are 40× magnification. The lower panel (**e**) shows that there was a 50% decrease in the intima-to-media ratio in the BOEC-transplanted samples when compared to controls ($P < 0.05$). Data are mean ± SD. (Reprinted with permissions from Nephrology Dialysis Transplantation)

thus cannot mount an immunogenic response to certain cells, namely, human-derived MSCs, which made them suitable for the xenograft study. Carotid-jugular AVFs were created in these mice. At the time of a creation, GFP and ^{89}Zr-labeled stem cells were delivered perivascularly to the adventitial of the outflow vein, in culture media. Approximately 250,000 cells from healthy adult donors were delivered. These cells were confirmed using several markers and used in several clinical trials [11].

These animals were followed to several weeks and sacrificed for genetic and histomorphological analysis. ^{89}Zr labeling was used to evaluate the retention of cells, approximately 90% of this tracer was present at the fistula site at 4 days, and this slowly translocated to the bones over the course of several weeks. GFP labeling was used to evaluate the local response and the majority of cells were present at the site, including a significant amount that had migrated toward the lumen. This confirmed that a majority of the cells delivered to the adventitia were retained at the site and locally migrated to the lumen. Genetic analysis also showed a decrease in MCP-1 and HIF-1α expression compared to controls at 7 days. Markers of fibroblasts and smooth muscle cells, FSP-1 and α-SMA, were also decreased at day seven and day 21 [11].

These findings were consistent with morphometric analysis at 7 and 21 days showed a decrease in neointimal area and cell density, compared with controls. Overall, these findings support an anti-inflammatory effect of the MSCs, resulting in decreased cellular proliferation and migration. Overall, these adipose-derived MSCs resulted in favorable remodeling [11]. This body of promising work, combined with our understanding of VNH and clinical use of these adipose-derived MSCs, make up the foundation for translation into clinical trials.

13.7 Conclusion

AVFs are an essential lifeline for patients with ESRD. In the past few decades, there has been an increased understanding of arteriovenous fistula failure and progress in improving AVF outcomes. However, a majority of AVFs still require repeated intervention due to stenosis. Multiple prior studies have identified out several intertwined mechanisms leading to fistula failure and possible targeted solutions. Stem cells, specifically MSCs, have been shown in multiple studies to modulate and counteract the mechanisms of fistula failure. This along with reliable methods of harvest and their use in multiple clinical paradigms supports the use of MSCs in the setting of AVF failure. Several animal models have confirmed the efficacy of MSCs to reduce venous neointimal hyperplasia. Overall, MSCs are a promising therapy with the potential to significantly reduce the number of interventions needed to maintain AVF function and improve the lives of those with ESRD.

References

1. Al-Jaishi AA, Oliver MJ, Thomas SM, et al. Patency rates of the arteriovenous fistula for hemodialysis: a systematic review and meta-analysis. Am J Kidney Dis. 2014;63(3):464–78.
2. Yoder MC. Endothelial progenitor cell: a blood cell by many other names may serve similar functions. J Mol Med (Berl). 2013;91(3):285–95.
3. Dave M, Mehta K, Luther J, Baruah A, Dietz AB, Faubion WA Jr. Mesenchymal stem cell therapy for inflammatory bowel disease: a systematic review and meta-analysis. Inflamm Bowel Dis. 2015;21(11):2696–707.
4. Redondo-Castro E, Cunningham C, Miller J, et al. Interleukin-1 primes human mesenchymal stem cells towards an anti-inflammatory and pro-trophic phenotype in vitro. Stem Cell Res Ther. 2017;8(1):79.
5. Ponte AL, Marais E, Gallay N, et al. The in vitro migration capacity of human bone marrow mesenchymal stem cells: comparison of chemokine and growth factor chemotactic activities. Stem Cells. 2007;25(7):1737–45.
6. Luz-Crawford P, Djouad F, Toupet K, et al. Mesenchymal stem cell-derived interleukin 1 receptor antagonist promotes macrophage polarization and inhibits B cell differentiation. Stem Cells. 2016;34(2):483–92.
7. Leeper NJ, Hunter AL, Cooke JP. Stem cell therapy for vascular regeneration: adult, embryonic, and induced pluripotent stem cells. Circulation. 2010;122(5):517–26.
8. Kern S, Eichler H, Stoeve J, Klüter H, Bieback K. Comparative analysis of mesenchymal stem cells from bone marrow, umbilical cord blood, or adipose tissue. Stem Cells. 2006;24(5):1294–301.
9. Gu W, Hong X, Potter C, Qu A, Xu Q. Mesenchymal stem cells and vascular regeneration. Microcirculation. 2017;24(1) https://doi.org/10.1111/micc.12324.
10. Ding DC, Shyu WC, Lin SZ. Mesenchymal stem cells. Cell Transplant. 2011;20(1):5–14.
11. Yang B, Brahmbhatt A, Nieves Torres E, et al. Tracking and therapeutic value of human adipose tissue-derived mesenchymal stem cell transplantation in reducing venous neointimal hyperplasia associated with arteriovenous fistula. Radiology. 2016;279(2):513–22.
12. Murphy D, McCulloch CE, Lin F, et al. Trends in prevalence of chronic kidney disease in the United States. Ann Intern Med. 2016;165(7):473–81.
13. Sequeira A, Naljayan M, Vachharajani TJ. Vascular access guidelines: summary, rationale, and controversies. Tech Vasc Interv Radiol. 2017;20(1):2–8.
14. Lok CE, Foley R. Vascular access morbidity and mortality: trends of the last decade. Clin J Am Soc Nephrol. 2013;8(7):1213–9.
15. Bashar K, Conlon PJ, Kheirelseid EA, Aherne T, Walsh SR, Leahy A. Arteriovenous fistula in dialysis patients: factors implicated in early and late AVF maturation failure. Surgeon : journal of the Royal Colleges of Surgeons of Edinburgh and Ireland. 2016;14(5):294–300.
16. Brahmbhatt A, Remuzzi A, Franzoni M, Misra S. The molecular mechanisms of hemodialysis vascular access failure. Kidney Int. 2016;89(2):303–16.
17. Nieves Torres EC, Yang B, Brahmbhatt A, Mukhopadhyay D, Misra S. Blood outgrowth endothelial cells reduce hypoxia-mediated fibroblast to myofibroblast conversion by decreasing proangiogenic cytokines. J Vasc Res. 2014;51(6):458–67.
18. Hughes D, Fu AA, Puggioni A, et al. Adventitial transplantation of blood outgrowth endothelial cells in porcine haemodialysis grafts alleviates hypoxia and decreases neointimal proliferation through a matrix metalloproteinase-9-mediated pathway--a pilot study. Nephrol Dial Transplant. 2009;24(1):85–96.
19. Rotmans JI, Bezhaeva T. The battlefield at arteriovenous crossroads: invading arterial smooth muscle cells occupy the outflow tract of fistulas. Kidney Int. 2015;88(3):431–3.
20. Lee T, Roy-Chaudhury P. Advances and new frontiers in the pathophysiology of venous neointimal hyperplasia and dialysis access stenosis. Adv Chronic Kidney Dis. 2009;16(5):329–38.

21. Brahmbhatt A, Misra S. The biology of hemodialysis vascular access failure. Semin Intervent Radiol. 2016;33(1):15–20.
22. Lee T, Ul Haq N. New developments in our understanding of neointimal hyperplasia. Adv Chronic Kidney Dis. 2015;22(6):431–7.
23. Misra S, Fu AA, Misra KD, Shergill UM, Leof EB, Mukhopadhyay D. Hypoxia-induced phenotypic switch of fibroblasts to myofibroblasts through a matrix metalloproteinase 2/tissue inhibitor of metalloproteinase-mediated pathway: implications for venous neointimal hyperplasia in hemodialysis access. J Vasc Interven Radiol. 2010;21(6):896–902.
24. Misra S, Doherty MG, Woodrum D, et al. Adventitial remodeling with increased matrix metalloproteinase-2 activity in a porcine arteriovenous polytetrafluoroethylene grafts. Kidney Int. 2005;68(6):2890–900.
25. Misra S, Fu AA, Rajan DK, et al. Expression of hypoxia inducible factor-1 alpha, macrophage migration inhibition factor, matrix metalloproteinase-2 and -9, and their inhibitors in hemodialysis grafts and arteriovenous fistulas. J Vasc Interv Radiol. 2008;19(2 Pt 1):252–9.
26. Misra S, Shergill U, Yang B, Janardhanan R, Misra KD. Increased expression of HIF-1alpha, VEGF-A and its receptors, MMP-2, TIMP-1, and ADAMTS-1 at the venous stenosis of arteriovenous fistula in a mouse model with renal insufficiency. J Vasc Interv Radiol. 2010;21(8):1255–61.
27. Misra S, Fu AA, Puggioni A, et al. Increased shear stress with upregulation of VEGF-A and its receptors and MMP-2, MMP-9, and TIMP-1 in venous stenosis of hemodialysis grafts. Am J Physiol Heart Circ Physiol. 2008;294(5):H2219–30.
28. Kilari S, Cai C, Zhao C, et al. The role of MicroRNA-21 in venous neointimal hyperplasia: implications for targeting miR-21 for VNH treatment. Mol Ther the journal of the American Society of Gene Therapy. 2019;27(9):1681–93.
29. Duque JC, Vazquez-Padron RI. Myofibroblasts: the ideal target to prevent arteriovenous fistula failure? Kidney Int. 2014;85(2):234–6.
30. Brahmbhatt A, NievesTorres E, Yang B, et al. The role of Iex-1 in the pathogenesis of venous neointimal hyperplasia associated with hemodialysis arteriovenous fistula. PLoS One. 2014;9(7):e102542.
31. Yang B, Janardhanan R, Vohra P, et al. Adventitial transduction of lentivirus-shRNA-VEGF-A in arteriovenous fistula reduces venous stenosis formation. Kidney Int. 2014;85(2):289–306.
32. Wong CY, de Vries MR, Wang Y, et al. Vascular remodeling and intimal hyperplasia in a novel murine model of arteriovenous fistula failure. J Vasc Surg. 2014;59(1):192–201.e191.
33. Schepers A, Eefting D, Bonta PI, et al. Anti-MCP-1 gene therapy inhibits vascular smooth muscle cells proliferation and attenuates vein graft thickening both in vitro and in vivo. Arterioscler Thromb Vasc Biol. 2006;26(9):2063–9.
34. De Marchi S, Falleti E, Giacomello R, et al. Risk factors for vascular disease and arteriovenous fistula dysfunction in hemodialysis patients. J Am Soc Nephrol. 1996;7(8):1169–77.
35. Nath KA, Kanakiriya SKR, Grande JP, Croatt AJ, Katusic ZS. Increased venous proinflammatory gene expression and intimal hyperplasia in an aorto-caval fistula model in the rat. Am J Pathol. 2003;162(6):2079–90.
36. Aitken E, Jackson A, Kong C, Coats P, Kingsmore D. Renal function, uraemia and early arteriovenous fistula failure. BMC Nephrol. 2014;15(1):179.
37. Weber CL, Djurdjev O, Levin A, Kiaii M. Outcomes of vascular access creation prior to dialysis: building the case for early referral. ASAIO J. 2009;55(4):355–60.
38. Langer S, Paulus N, Koeppel TA, et al. Cardiovascular remodeling during arteriovenous fistula maturation in a rodent uremia model. J Vasc Access. 2011;12(3):215–23.
39. Henaut L, Candellier A, Boudot C, et al. New insights into the roles of monocytes/macrophages in cardiovascular calcification associated with chronic kidney disease. Toxins. 2019;11(9):529.
40. Liang M, Guo Q, Huang F, et al. Notch signaling in bone marrow-derived FSP-1 cells initiates neointima formation in arteriovenous fistulas. Kidney Int. 2019;95(6):1347–58.

41. Liang M, Wang Y, Liang A, et al. Migration of smooth muscle cells from the arterial anastomosis of arteriovenous fistulas requires Notch activation to form neointima. Kidney Int. 2015;88(3):490–502.
42. Koga JI, Nakano T, Dahlman JE, et al. Macrophage Notch Ligand Delta-Like 4 promotes vein graft lesion development: implications for the treatment of vein graft failure. Arterioscler Thromb Vasc Biol. 2015;35(11):2343–53.
43. Pan L, Ye X, Ding J, Zhou Y. Antiproliferation effect of the uremic toxin paracresol on endothelial progenitor cells is related to its antioxidant activity. Mol Med Rep. 2017;15(4):2308–12.
44. Ozkok A, Yildiz A. Endothelial progenitor cells and kidney diseases. Kidney Blood Press Res. 2018;43(3):701–18.
45. Ballermann BJ, Dardik A, Eng E, Liu A. Shear stress and the endothelium. Kidney Int Suppl. 1998;67:S100–8.
46. Misra S, Fu AA, Misra KD, Glockner JF, Mukhopadyay D. Evolution of shear stress, protein expression, and vessel area in an animal model of arterial dilatation in hemodialysis grafts. J Vasc Interv Radiol. 2010;21(1):108–15.
47. Dardik A, Chen L, Frattini J, et al. Differential effects of orbital and laminar shear stress on endothelial cells. J Vasc Surg. 2005;41(5):869–80.
48. Zhang L, Coombes J, Pascoe EM, et al. The effect of pentoxifylline on oxidative stress in chronic kidney disease patients with erythropoiesis-stimulating agent hyporesponsiveness: sub-study of the HERO trial. Redox Rep. 2016;21(1):14–23.
49. Locatelli F, Canaud B, Eckardt KU, Stenvinkel P, Wanner C, Zoccali C. Oxidative stress in end-stage renal disease: an emerging threat to patient outcome. Nephrol Dial Transplant. 2003;18(7):1272–80.
50. Paniagua OA, Bryant MB, Panza JA. Role of endothelial nitric oxide in shear stress-induced vasodilation of human microvasculature: diminished activity in hypertensive and hypercholesterolemic patients. Circulation. 2001;103(13):1752–8.
51. Katsanos K, Karnabatidis D, Kitrou P, Spiliopoulos S, Christeas N, Siablis D. Paclitaxel-coated balloon angioplasty vs. plain balloon dilation for the treatment of failing dialysis access: 6-month interim results from a prospective randomized controlled trial. J Endovasc Ther. 2012;19(2):263–72.
52. Kitrou PM, Katsanos K, Spiliopoulos S, Karnabatidis D, Siablis D. Drug-eluting versus plain balloon angioplasty for the treatment of failing dialysis access: final results and cost-effectiveness analysis from a prospective randomized controlled trial (NCT01174472). Eur J Radiol. 2015;84(3):418–23.
53. Patanè D, Giuffrida S, Morale W, et al. Drug-eluting balloon for the treatment of failing hemodialytic radiocephalic arteriovenous fistulas: our experience in the treatment of juxta-anastomotic stenoses. J Vasc Access. 2014;15(5):338–43.
54. Björkman P, Weselius EM, Kokkonen T, Rauta V, Albäck A, Venermo M. Drug-coated versus plain balloon angioplasty in arteriovenous fistulas: a randomized, controlled study with 1-year follow-up (the Drecorest ii-study). Scand J Surg. 2019;108(1):61–6.
55. Lučev J, Breznik S, Dinevski D, Ekart R, Rupreht M. Endovascular treatment of Haemodialysis arteriovenous fistula with drug-coated balloon angioplasty: a single-centre study. Cardiovasc Intervent Radiol. 2018;41(6):882–9.
56. Phang CC, Tan RY, Pang SC, et al. Paclitaxel-coated balloon in the treatment of recurrent dysfunctional arteriovenous access, real-world experience and longitudinal follow up. Nephrology (Carlton). 2019;24(12):1290–5.
57. El Sharouni SY, Smits HF, Wüst AF, Battermann JJ, Blankestijn PJ. Endovascular brachytherapy in arteriovenous grafts for haemodialysis does not prevent development of stenosis. Radiother Oncol. 1998;49(2):199–200.
58. Misra S, Bonan R, Pflederer T, Roy-Chaudhury P, Investigators BI. BRAVO I: a pilot study of vascular brachytherapy in polytetrafluoroethylene dialysis access grafts. Kidney Int. 2006;70(11):2006–13.

59. Roy-Chaudhury P, Arnold P, Seigel J, Misra S. From basic biology to randomized clinical trial: the beta radiation for arteriovenous graft outflow stenosis (BRAVO II). Semin Dial. 2013;26(2):227–32.
60. van Tongeren RB, Levendag PC, Coen VL, et al. External beam radiation therapy to prevent anastomotic intimal hyperplasia in prosthetic arteriovenous fistulas: results of a randomized trial. Radiother Oncol. 2003;69(1):73–7.
61. Irish AB, Viecelli AK, Hawley CM, et al. Effect of fish oil supplementation and aspirin use on arteriovenous fistula failure in patients requiring hemodialysis: a randomized clinical trial. JAMA Intern Med. 2017;177(2):184–93.
62. Viecelli AK, Irish AB, Polkinghorne KR, et al. Omega-3 polyunsaturated fatty acid supplementation to prevent arteriovenous fistula and graft failure: a systematic review and meta-analysis of randomized controlled trials. Am J Kidney Dis. 2018;72(1):50–61.
63. Wan Q, Li L, Yang S, Chu F. Impact of statins on arteriovenous fistulas outcomes: a meta-analysis. Ther Apher Dial. 2018;22(1):67–72.
64. Tanner NC, Da Silva A. Medical adjuvant treatment to increase patency of arteriovenous fistulae and grafts. Cochrane Database Syst Rev. 2015;2015(7):Cd002786.
65. Akin EB, Topcu O, Ozcan H, Ersoz S, Aytac S, Anadol E. Hemodynamic effect of transdermal glyceryl trinitrate on newly constructed arteriovenous fistula. World J Surg. 2002;26(10):1256–9.
66. Field M, McGrogan D, Marie Y, et al. Randomized clinical trial of the use of glyceryl trinitrate patches to aid arteriovenous fistula maturation. Br J Surg. 2016;103(10):1269–75.
67. Poggi A, Zocchi MR. Immunomodulatory properties of mesenchymal stromal cells: still unresolved "Yin and Yang". Curr Stem Cell Res Ther. 2019;14(4):344–50.
68. Khubutiya MS, Vagabov AV, Temnov AA, Sklifas AN. Paracrine mechanisms of proliferative, anti-apoptotic and anti-inflammatory effects of mesenchymal stromal cells in models of acute organ injury. Cytotherapy. 2014;16(5):579–85.
69. Blázquez R, Sánchez-Margallo FM, Álvarez V, Usón A, Casado JG. Surgical meshes coated with mesenchymal stem cells provide an anti-inflammatory environment by a M2 macrophage polarization. Acta Biomater. 2016;31:221–30.
70. Hickson LJ, Eirin A, Lerman LO. Challenges and opportunities for stem cell therapy in patients with chronic kidney disease. Kidney Int. 2016;89(4):767–78.
71. Pittenger MF, Mackay AM, Beck SC, et al. Multilineage potential of adult human mesenchymal stem cells. Science (New York, NY). 1999;284(5411):143–7.
72. Wu Y, Hoogduijn MJ, Baan CC, et al. Adipose tissue-derived mesenchymal stem cells have a heterogenic cytokine secretion profile. Stem Cells Int. 2017;2017:4960831.
73. Yagi H, Soto-Gutierrez A, Navarro-Alvarez N, et al. Reactive bone marrow stromal cells attenuate systemic inflammation via sTNFR1. Mol Ther: the journal of the American Society of Gene Therapy. 2010;18(10):1857–64.
74. Eliopoulos N, Zhao J, Bouchentouf M, et al. Human marrow-derived mesenchymal stromal cells decrease cisplatin renotoxicity in vitro and in vivo and enhance survival of mice post-intraperitoneal injection. Am J Physiol Renal Physiol. 2010;299(6):F1288–98.
75. Maggini J, Mirkin G, Bognanni I, et al. Mouse bone marrow-derived mesenchymal stromal cells turn activated macrophages into a regulatory-like profile. PLoS One. 2010;5(2):–e9252.
76. Carelli S, Colli M, Vinci V, Caviggioli F, Klinger M, Gorio A. Mechanical activation of adipose tissue and derived mesenchymal stem cells: novel anti-inflammatory properties. Int J Mol Sci. 2018;19(1):267.
77. Janardhanan R, Yang B, Kilari S, Leof EB, Mukhopadhyay D, Misra S. The role of repeat administration of adventitial delivery of lentivirus-shRNA-Vegf-A in arteriovenous fistula to prevent venous stenosis formation. J Vasc interv Radiol. 2016;27(4):576–83.
78. Valledor AF, Comalada M, Santamaría-Babi LF, Lloberas J, Celada A. Macrophage proinflammatory activation and deactivation: a question of balance. Adv Immunol. 2010;108:1–20.

79. Sasaki M, Abe R, Fujita Y, Ando S, Inokuma D, Shimizu H. Mesenchymal stem cells are recruited into wounded skin and contribute to wound repair by transdifferentiation into multiple skin cell type. J Immunol. 2008;180(4):2581–7.
80. Mousawi F, Peng H, Li J, et al. Chemical activation of the Piezo1 channel drives mesenchymal stem cell migration via inducing ATP release and activation of P2 receptor purinergic signalling. 2019.
81. Mousavi A. CXCL12/CXCR4 signal transduction in diseases and its molecular approaches in targeted-therapy. Immunol Lett. 2019;217:91.
82. Nitzsche F, Muller C, Lukomska B, Jolkkonen J, Deten A, Boltze J. Concise review: MSC adhesion cascade-insights into homing and transendothelial migration. Stem Cells. 2017;35(6):1446–60.
83. Camilleri ET, Gustafson MP, Dudakovic A, et al. Identification and validation of multiple cell surface markers of clinical-grade adipose-derived mesenchymal stromal cells as novel release criteria for good manufacturing practice-compliant production. Stem Cell Res Ther. 2016;7(1):107.
84. Riester SM, Denbeigh JM, Lin Y, et al. Safety studies for use of adipose tissue-derived mesenchymal stromal/stem cells in a rabbit model for osteoarthritis to support a phase I clinical trial. Stem Cells Transl Med. 2017;6(3):910–22.
85. Im GI. Clinical use of stem cells in orthopaedics. Eur Cell Mater. 2017;33:183–96.
86. Centeno CJ, Schultz JR, Cheever M, et al. Safety and complications reporting update on the re-implantation of culture-expanded mesenchymal stem cells using autologous platelet lysate technique. Curr Stem Cell Res Ther. 2011;6(4):368–78.
87. Pak J, Chang J-J, Lee JH, Lee SH. Safety reporting on implantation of autologous adipose tissue-derived stem cells with platelet-rich plasma into human articular joints. BMC Musculoskelet Disord. 2013;14:337.
88. Rifkin BS, Brewster UC, Aruny JE, Perazella MA. Percutaneous balloon cryoplasty: a new therapy for rapidly recurrent anastomotic venous stenoses of hemodialysis grafts? Am J Kidney Dis. 2005;45(2):e27–32.
89. Kitrou PM, Spiliopoulos S, Papadimatos P, et al. Paclitaxel-coated balloons for the treatment of dysfunctional dialysis access. Results from a single-center, retrospective analysis. Cardiovasc Intervent Radiol. 2017;40(1):50–4.
90. Eslami MH, Gangadharan SP, Sui X, Rhynhart KK, Snyder RO, Conte MS. Gene delivery to in situ veins: differential effects of adenovirus and adeno-associated viral vectors. J Vasc Surg. 2000;31(6):1149–59.
91. Hashimoto T, Yamamoto K, Foster T, Bai H, Shigematsu K, Dardik A. Intraluminal drug delivery to the mouse arteriovenous fistula endothelium. J Vis Exp. 2016;(109):e53905-e53905.
92. Globerman AS, Chaouat M, Shlomai Z, Galun E, Zeira E, Zamir G. Efficient transgene expression from naked DNA delivered into an arterio-venous fistula model for kidney dialysis. J Gene Med. 2011;13(11):611–21.
93. Sato T, Iwasaki Y, Kikkawa Y, Fukagawa M. An efficacy of intensive vitamin D delivery to neointimal hyperplasia in recurrent vascular access stenosis. J Vasc Access. 2016;17(1):72–7.
94. Gasper WJ, Jimenez CA, Walker J, Conte MS, Seward K, Owens CD. Adventitial nab-rapamycin injection reduces porcine femoral artery luminal stenosis induced by balloon angioplasty via inhibition of medial proliferation and adventitial inflammation. Circ Cardiovasc Interv. 2013;6(6):701–9.
95. Bakken AM, Protack CD, Saad WE, Lee DE, Waldman DL, Davies MG. Long-term outcomes of primary angioplasty and primary stenting of central venous stenosis in hemodialysis patients. J Vasc Surg. 2007;45(4):776–83.
96. McLennan G. Stent and stent-graft use in arteriovenous dialysis access. Semin Intervent Radiol. 2016;33(1):10–4.
97. Anaya-Ayala JE, Smolock CJ, Colvard BD, et al. Efficacy of covered stent placement for central venous occlusive disease in hemodialysis patients. J Vasc Surg. 2011;54(3):754–9.
98. Dinh K, Thomas SD, Cho T, Swinnen J, Crowe P, Varcoe RL. Use of paclitaxel eluting stents in arteriovenous fistulas: a pilot study. Vasc Specialist Int. 2019;35(4):225–31.

99. Hwang CW, Johnston PV, Gerstenblith G, et al. Stem cell impregnated nanofiber stent sleeve for on-stent production and intravascular delivery of paracrine factors. Biomaterials. 2015;52:318–26.
100. Delattre C, Velazquez D, Roques C, et al. In vitro and in vivo evaluation of a dextran-graft-polybutylmethacrylate copolymer coated on CoCr metallic stent. Bioimpacts. 2019;9(1):25–36.
101. Johnston PV, Hwang CW, Bogdan V, et al. Intravascular stem cell bioreactor for prevention of adverse remodeling after myocardial infarction. J Am Heart Assoc. 2019;8(15):e012351.
102. Carter K, Lee HJ, Na KS, et al. Characterizing the impact of 2D and 3D culture conditions on the therapeutic effects of human mesenchymal stem cell secretome on corneal wound healing in vitro and ex vivo. Acta Biomater. 2019;99:247–57.
103. Zhang P, Zhang C, Li J, Han J, Liu X, Yang H. The physical microenvironment of hemato poietic stem cells and its emerging roles in engineering applications. Stem Cell Res Ther. 2019;10(1):327.
104. Dubey SK, Alexander A, Sivaram M, et al. Uncovering the diversification of tissue engineering on the emergent areas of stem cells, nanotechnology and biomaterials. Curr Stem Cell Res Ther. 2020;15:187.
105. Flores AM, Ye J, Jarr K-U, Hosseini-Nassab N, Smith BR, Leeper NJ. Nanoparticle therapy for vascular diseases. Arterioscler Thromb Vasc Biol. 2019;39(4):635–46.
106. Kuji T, Masaki T, Goteti K, et al. Efficacy of local dipyridamole therapy in a porcine model of arteriovenous graft stenosis. Kidney Int. 2006;69(12):2179–85.
107. Masaki T, Rathi R, Zentner G, et al. Inhibition of neointimal hyperplasia in vascular grafts by sustained perivascular delivery of paclitaxel. Kidney Int. 2004;66(5):2061–9.
108. Rotmans JI, Verhagen HJM, Velema E, et al. Local overexpression of C-type natri-uretic peptide ameliorates vascular adaptation of porcine hemodialysis grafts. Kidney Int. 2004;65(5):1897–905.
109. Paulson WD, Kipshidze N, Kipiani K, et al. Safety and efficacy of local periadventi-tial delivery of sirolimus for improving hemodialysis graft patency: first human experi-ence with a sirolimus-eluting collagen membrane (Coll-R). Nephrol Dial Transplant. 2012;27(3):1219–24.
110. Kelly B, Melhem M, Zhang J, et al. Perivascular paclitaxel wraps block arteriovenous graft stenosis in a pig model. Nephrol Dial Transplant. 2006;21(9):2425–31.
111. Yang B, Kilari S, Brahmbhatt A, et al. CorMatrix wrapped around the adventitia of the arteriovenous fistula outflow vein attenuates venous neointimal hyperplasia. Sci Rep. 2017;7(1):–14298.
112. Huang Q, Zou Y, Arno MC, et al. Hydrogel scaffolds for differentiation of adipose-derived stem cells. Chem Soc Rev. 2017;46(20):6255–75.
113. Terry CM, Dember LM. Novel therapies for hemodialysis vascular access dysfunction: myth or reality? Clin J Am Soc Nephrol. 2013;8(12):2202–12.

Chapter 14
Stem Cell Therapy to Improve Acute Myocardial Infarction Remodeling

Jolanta Gorecka and Alan Dardik

Abbreviations

3D	Three dimensional
ADSC	Adipose-derived stem cell
AMI	Acute myocardial infarction
Ang-1α	Angiopoietin-1α
BM	Bone marrow
BM-MNC	Bone marrow-derived mononuclear cell
BM-SC	Bone marrow stem cells
CABG	Coronary artery bypass grafting
CDC	Cardiosphere-derived cells
CSC	Cardiac stem cell
CVD	Cardiovascular disease
ECM	Extracellular matrix
EDV	End-diastolic volume
EF	Ejection fraction
EHT	Engineered heart tissue
EPC	Endothelial progenitor cell
ESC	Embryonic stem cell
ESV	End-systolic volume
FGF	Fibroblast growth factor
Flk1	Fetal liver kinase 1
GCP	Glycolytic cardiac progenitor
GCSF	Granulocyte colony-stimulating factor
HF	Heart failure
HGF	Hepatocyte growth factor
IC	Intracoronary
IGF	Insulin-like growth factor

J. Gorecka · A. Dardik (✉)
Vascular Biology and Therapeutics Program and the Departments of Surgery and Cellular and Molecular Physiology, Yale University School of Medicine, New Haven, CT, USA
e-mail: alan.dardik@yale.edu

© Springer Nature Switzerland AG 2021
T. P. Navarro et al. (eds.), *Stem Cell Therapy for Vascular Diseases*,
https://doi.org/10.1007/978-3-030-56954-9_14

ILK	Integrin-linked kinase
IM	Intramyocardial
iPSC	Induced pluripotent stem cell
Isl1	Insulin gene enhancer protein-1
IV	Intravenous injection
LV	Left ventricular
LVEDV	Left ventricular end-diastolic volume
LVEF	Left ventricular ejection fraction
LVESV	Left ventricular end-systolic volume
MI	Myocardial infarction
MMP	Matrix metalloproteinase
MSC	Mesenchymal stem cell
NSTEMI	Non-ST segment elevation myocardial infarction
PCI	Percutaneous coronary intervention
PEU	Polyester urethane
PEUU	Polyester urethane urea
PGS	Polyglycerol sebacate
PU	Polyurethane
SC	Stem cell
Sca1	Stem cell antigen-1
SDF1	Stromal cell-derived factor 1
SMC	Skeletal myoblast cell
SP	Side population
SSEA	Stage-specific embryonic antigen 1
STEMI	ST-segment elevation myocardial infarction
VEGF	Vascular endothelial growth factor

14.1 Introduction

14.1.1 *General Considerations for Myocardial Infarction*

Ischemic heart disease remains the leading cause of death worldwide [1]. According to the American Heart Association, 720,000 Americans experienced a new coronary artery event in 2018, with the median survival after a first myocardial infarction (MI) being 8.4, 5.6, 7, and 5.5 years, respectively, for white males, white females, Black males, and Black females [2]. The burden of cardiovascular disease (CVD) and MI affects low- and middle-income countries disproportionately, where 80% of CVD-related deaths occur [3]. While a large majority of the risk factors associated with ischemic heart disease such as high serum cholesterol, hypertension, diabetes, obesity, and smoking are modifiable, family history, age, male sex, and female sex associated with postmenopausal status cannot be altered [4].

Myocardial infarction is broadly defined as myocardial death secondary to prolonged ischemia and can result from multiple etiologies including coronary artery occlusion, supply/demand imbalance, MI related to percutaneous coronary intervention (PCI), stent thrombosis, MI associated with coronary artery bypass grafting (CABG), and others [5]. Rupture or erosion of an atherosclerotic coronary plaque, with resultant exposure of highly thrombogenic material, is the most common inciting factor for coronary occlusion [6]. While a completely occlusive thrombus in the coronary circulation results in an ST-segment elevation MI (STEMI), incomplete thrombosis, or occlusion in the presence of well-established collaterals, results in a non-ST elevation MI (NSTEMI) or unstable angina [7, 8].

14.1.2 Current Myocardial Infarction Standard of Care

Patients with a suspected acute coronary syndrome should be immediately evaluated with an electrocardiogram and cardiac troponin testing. These diagnostic tests, along with history of symptoms, group patients into those suffering from STEMI, NSTEMI, or nonischemic chest pain, distinctions that dictate further care [7, 8]. Initial medical care of patients with STEMI and NSTEMI includes oxygen, analgesics, nitrates, beta-blockers, antiplatelet, and anticoagulation therapy [7, 8]. Urgent reperfusion of ischemic myocardium is the primary therapeutic goal in both groups. All patients with a STEMI should undergo percutaneous coronary intervention within 90 minutes of presentation, while those suffering from NSTEMI undergo immediate, early, and elective PCI depending on time of symptom onset [7, 8]. Diagnostic angiography delineates the extent of disease and dictates reperfusion strategies including stenting, fibrinolysis, or CABG.

Despite urgent reperfusion, life-threatening post-MI complications arise depending on the amount and location of lost myocardium. These complications can be grouped into five subtypes including ischemic, mechanical, arrhythmic, embolic, and inflammatory [9]. Coronary artery disease, including MI, is the number one cause for development of heart failure (HF) in the United States [10]. With improved medical and interventional care, patients are living longer post MI, resulting in a projected increase of HF from six to over eight million by 2030 [11].

14.1.3 Post-Myocardial Infarction Cardiac Remodeling

Following an MI, the injured myocardium and surrounding tissue undergo a series of early and late remodeling changes in an attempt to compensate for the ischemia-induced damage [12]. The early remodeling phase occurs hours to days post MI and includes myonecrosis-induced inflammation, matrix metalloproteinase (MMP)-driven collagen matrix breakdown, thinning and dilation of ventricular walls, as well as fibroblast-induced scar formation [13, 14]. Over the subsequent weeks to months, uninjured myocardium hypertrophies eccentrically overcompensate for increased stress, further contributing to ventricular dilation. As preload increases without resultant change in ventricular contractility, the ejection fraction (EF) decreases, and dilated cardiomyopathy and resultant HF ensue, worsened by the adult myocardium's limited ability to recover after ischemia [15].

Unfortunately, current therapies aimed at decreasing pathologic post-MI remodeling and HF are limited and include pharmacological treatments to decrease scarring and tissue ischemia, devices and implants aimed at restoring heart function, as well as transplantation [16]. Mammalian myocardium has traditionally been viewed as a non-regenerative organ, and although resident cardiac stem cells (CSC) contribute to cardiac regeneration and some evidence of mammalian heart regeneration exists in animal models, resident stem cells lack the capacity to regenerate all of the myocardium lost after an MI [17, 18]. Furthermore, the contribution of CSC to cardiac regeneration remains highly controversial. Reports of cardiomyocyte exchange in humans range from 50 to 100% during a normal life span, with many such reports having been retracted secondary to lack of reproducibility [19, 20]. Delivery of endogenous and exogenous cardiac progenitor cells to increase myocardial regeneration post MI and in ischemic cardiomyopathy has recently been explored in animal and human studies, with promising results [21].

14.2 Stem Cells in Cardiac Regeneration

14.2.1 Exogenous Cellular Sources

Although cellular transfer for treatment of ischemic heart disease is a relatively new field, with the first clinical trial occurring in 2000, a multitude of cellular sources have been trialed to date in preclinical and clinical models of MI and HF, with relatively few cellular types remaining unexplored [22].

Exogenous cardiac progenitor and stem cells of clinical interest include skeletal myoblast cells (SMC), bone marrow-derived mononuclear cells (BM-MNC), bone marrow-derived populations including lin-c-kit+, CD133+, CD133-/CD34+, c-kit+, and Sca1+, mesenchymal stem cells (MSC), adipose-derived stem cells (ADSC), endothelial progenitor cells (EPC), induced pluripotent stem cells (iPSC), as well as embryonic stem cells (ESC) including early cardiovascular (Isl1+/SSEA1+) cells. Although exogenous stem cell therapy demonstrates some improvement of cardiac function post MI, direct cardiomyogenic differentiation from these cells is rare [23].

Non-satellite CD34-/CD45-/Sca1- stem cells isolated from skeletal muscle have demonstrated rhythmic beating similar to cardiomyocytes and when transplanted into adult mice differentiate into cardiac tissue, while C-kit+Sca1- cells improved survival, enhanced cardiac function, reduced regional strain, and attenuated remodeling in mice [24].

In rodent studies, embryonic stem cell-derived cardiomyocytes attenuated progression of HF after acute myocardial infarction (AMI) by reducing ventricular dilation and improving global left ventricular (LV) function. Subsequent studies established that human embryonic cell cardiomyocytes can limit AMI size and preserve LV contractility [25]. Further, xenotransplantation of cardiac-committed mouse embryonic cells into ovine models has shown that ESC are immune privileged and cardiomyocytes from human ESC are capable of repopulating rat hearts [24].

MSC can be derived from adult peripheral blood, adipose tissue, bone marrow, and neonatal umbilical cord, amnion, cord blood, and placenta [26]. They are potent stimulators of angiogenesis and cardiac regeneration and have been shown to be superior than hematopoietic stem cells in rodent post-MI models [27, 28]. Although they improve tissue regeneration predominantly via paracrine mechanisms, some porcine studies have shown that MSC injected intramyocardially can differentiate into vascular smooth muscle or endothelial cells. Furthermore, human umbilical cord blood-derived MSC preconditioned with 5-aza transdifferentiated into cardiomyocytes, when transplanted into mouse models of MI, preventing infarct expansion and improving heart function [24].

The groundbreaking discovery of iPSC generation via in vitro reprogramming of adult cells into a pluripotent state, and subsequent differentiation into any lineage, transformed the field of regenerative medicine [29]. Although their use in humans remains limited, cardiomyocytes, endothelial cells, and smooth muscle cells derived from iPSC have been tested on porcine infarct models with resultant reduction in infarct size, ventricular wall stress, and apoptosis [30].

14.2.2   Endogenous Cellular Sources

The concept of resident cardiac stem cells is not very well established, with reports quoting vastly different cardiomyocyte renewal capacity [19, 20]. At best, CSC account for approximately 1/30,000 cells in the human heart, although this number increases post injury, likely secondary to migration from bone marrow [31]. The hallmark of CSC is their ability to differentiate into every cardiac lineage including myocytes, fibroblasts, smooth muscle, and endothelial cells. Multiple previous studies have shown their contribution to cardiac regeneration [18, 32]. Specific subtypes of CSC implicated in cardiac regeneration include cardiosphere-derived cells, c-Kit+ cells, insulin gene enhancer protein 1 (Isl1+) progenitor cells, fetal liver kinase 1 (Flk1+) progenitor cells, glycolytic cardiac progenitors (GCP), stage-specific embryonic antigen1 (SSEA1+) progenitors, side population (SP) progenitors, as well as stem cell antigen-1 (Sca1+) progenitors [21]. CSC are localized mainly in the atria of the heart, including the right atrial appendage, and are more numerous in the subepicardium compared to the myocardium [33].

CSC have greater potential to differentiate into cardiomyocytes compared to MSC and in animal studies show potential to reduce post-MI scar size and vascular overload [18, 34]. Other studies have shown their ability to engraft in the myocardium, recruit endogenous stem cells, and attenuate myocyte apoptosis, via release of growth factors and promotion of angiogenesis [25]. Lastly, administration of human W8B2+ CSC into rat hearts 1 week post MI improved cardiac function and reduced scar tissue formation [35].

SP progenitor cells differentiate into cells expressing sarcomeric proteins including troponin and cardiac α-actinin [36]. Flk-1+ cells can give rise to myocardial, endothelial, and smooth muscle lineages, and their concentration in the circulation increases in humans during an MI [37, 38]. Although Isl1+ cells are capable of differentiating into mature cardiomyocytes, they can only be extracted from neonatal tissue [39]. C-kit+ cells migrate through infarcted myocardium, give rise to cardiomyocytes, and reduce oxidative stress and apoptosis in cardiac and noncardiac cell populations [40, 41]. Sca1+ progenitors are found in myocardial stromal tissue, can be differentiated into myocardium, smooth muscle, and endothelial cells, and their absence leads to myocardial contractile dysfunction in rodents [42–44]. Rodent SSEA+ cells express surface markers which signal cardiomyogenic differentiation potential, form beating colonies when co-cultured with primary cardiomyocytes, and induce myocardial regeneration and functional improvement post MI in animal studies [45]. GCP are isolated from the epicardial/subepicardial hypoxic environment; they express all cardiac stem cells markers and differentiate into endothelial, smooth muscle, and cardiac lineages [46].

In the clinics, skeletal myoblasts were the first cell type to be transferred to human hearts. Early clinical trials focused mainly on bone marrow-derived cells including unselected progenitor/stromal/hematopoietic cells, with a gradual transition to more specific cellular populations including hematopoietic stem and progenitor (CD34+, CD133+) cells and later MSC. More recently, the focus of trials has shifted to various cardiac-committed cell types, including C-kit+ and cardiosphere-derived cells, especially given their increased preclinical success. Embryonic-derived early cardiovascular cells are the most recent cellular type to be examined, and the first trial using iPSC-derived cardiomyocytes is in the early planning phase [22, 47]. Treatment and delivery models for post-acute MI myocardial salvage and ischemic cardiomyopathy regeneration overlap, mononuclear cells have seen a larger success in post-MI studies, while CSC and embryonic-derived early myocardial progenitors have been more extensively studied in ischemic cardiomyopathy trials. This chapter will focus on the specific results of clinical trials in early post-MI patients.

14.2.3 Paracrine Factors, Exosomes, and Direct Cellular Reprogramming

Despite showing some clinical efficacy, stem cell therapy is associated with several important limitations including immune rejection, tumorigenicity, and arrhythmogenicity. In addition, few cells survive after transplantation despite improved myocardial function, suggesting that the mechanism of their action is predominantly paracrine in nature [48]. A recent study of ischemia/reperfusion injury in rodents showed that intracardiac injection of two separate adult-derived stem cells improved cardiac function without altering the number of new cardiomyocytes. The proposed mechanism for this improvement was selective induction of CCR2+ and CX3CR1+ macrophages, resulting in altered fibroblast activity, extracellular matrix (ECM) content, and enhanced mechanical properties [49]. In order to circumvent these obstacles, researchers have begun to study stem cell-derived paracrine factors, exosomes, and cells directly reprogrammed into cardiac progenitors, although no such studies have yet entered clinical trials, despite animal studies showing promising results.

MSC-derived growth factors and cytokines derived from cell culture supernatants have been shown to decrease inflammation, decrease myocyte apoptosis, recruit endogenous stem cells, and decrease infarct size [25]. In further animal and in vitro studies, MSC-conditioned medium increased neovascularization and fibrosis while improving cardiomyocyte contractility [50].

Exosomes are 40–100-micron vesicles released from cells by fusion with cellular membranes and carry mRNA, miRNA, as well as antiapoptotic and proangiogenic proteins. Exosomes are involved in cell signaling, mediate stem cell paracrine effects, and improve resident cardiac stem cell function without the downsides associated with direct cellular use [48]. In murine models, ESC-derived exosomes increased cardiomyocyte proliferation, upregulated the number of cardiac progenitor cells, and increased cardiac repair following ischemic injury. MSC-derived exosomes also reduced the size of postischemic infarcts, in animal models, via increased cardiac progenitor cell proliferation and decreased fibroblast proliferation [51, 52]. In addition, MSC-derived exosomal miRNA upregulated angiogenesis in postinfarct ischemia [48].

One of the major challenges associated with iPSC use in clinical trials include their tumorigenic potential in an undifferentiated state. Accordingly, new protocols have been designed to directly reprogram cells via induction of lineage-specific factors, without passage through a pluripotent and tumorigenic state [53]. For example, three factors including Gata4, Mef2c, and Tbx5 reprogram cardiac fibroblasts into induced cardiomyocytes. Further addition or modification of reprogramming factors microRNAs has been shown to promote reprogramming efficiency and maturation [54]. In vivo reprogramming of cells following acute MI in animal models has been reported and resulted in improved cardiac function and reduced fibrosis [55]. Most recently, direct in vivo reprogramming has been achieved without genomic integration of viral DNA with the use of a *Sendai virus* vector, which remains outside of the nucleus [56].

14.2.4   Lineage-Specific Considerations

The advantages and drawbacks of specific cellular subtypes in post-MI regenerative therapy are summarized in Table 14.1. Skeletal muscle cells are easier to obtain although likely only provide structural benefits, as opposed to forming new cardiac

Table 14.1 Advantages and drawbacks of lineage-specific cell therapy in myocardial regeneration

Cellular Source	Advantages	Disadvantages
Skeletal muscle cells	1. Less invasive harvest 2. Large source pool 3. Provide structural support	1. No transdifferentiation into cardiomyocytes 2. Low survival 3. Arrhythmogenic in large quantities
MSC	1. Minimally invasive harvest 2. Multiple source pools 3. Differentiation into osteoblasts, chondrocytes, myocytes, and adipocytes 4. High self-renewal, proliferative, and differentiation capacity 5. Beneficial paracrine signaling 6. Immunomodulatory	1. Relatively low yield in peripheral blood and bone marrow 2. Source-dependent variation in quality and yield
Hematopoietic stem cells	1. Minimally invasive harvest 2. Multiple source pools 3. Differentiation into cardiomyocytes and endothelial cells 4. Simultaneously capable of myogenesis and angiogenesis	1. Relatively low yield 2. Difficult in vitro maintenance 3. Unknown signaling pathways
Embryonic stem cells	1. Pluripotent 2. Genomic stability 3. Large differentiation and proliferation potential	1. Derived from human blastocysts, ethical dilemmas 2. Tumorigenic when undifferentiated 3. Immunogenic
iPSC	1. Pluripotent 2. In vitro reprogramming from adult cells 3. Minimally invasive harvest 4. No ethical dilemmas	1. Inefficient differentiation 2. Tumorigenic when undifferentiated 3. Often require viral transfection resulting in genomic instability
Adult-derived stem cells	1. No ethical dilemmas 2. Low risk of immune rejection	1. Limited source 2. Invasive harvesting technique 3. Unclear regeneration potential

Summary of advantages and drawbacks of specific cells used in post-MI regenerative therapy
MSC mesenchymal stem cells, *iPSC* induced pluripotent stem cells

tissue, secondary to lack of transdifferentiation. In addition, 90% of injected cells die within a few days, and higher cellular counts are arrhythmogenic [24].

Stem cell sources can be divided into three main groups: embryonic, induced, and adult. Embryonic stem cells are pluripotent and can differentiate into all three germ layers and have genomic stability and good differentiation and proliferative capacity [57]. They are, however, derived from human blastocysts and require the destruction of embryos to attain, raising ethical dilemmas, in addition to having tumorigenic and immunogenic potential [58, 59]. In human and rodent studies, it was noted that transplanted embryonic stem cells generated small numbers of cardiomyocytes [60]. As they are reprogrammed in vitro from adult cells, iPSC avoid the ethical dilemmas associated with embryonic stem cells. Differentiation of iPSC into adult cells is at times inefficient, and they are teratogenic in their undifferentiated states. Furthermore, cells that are derived via viral transfection suffer from genomic instability [61]. Adult-derived cardiac stem cells also avoid ethical dilemmas associated with embryonic stem cells, and they carry a lower risk of immune rejection. However, they are obtained via invasive techniques and have a limited regeneration potential [62].

Mesenchymal stem cells are adult fibroblast-like cells and can differentiate into osteoblasts, adipocytes, and cardiomyocytes, among others [63]. Mesenchymal stem cells can be extracted from peripheral blood, bone marrow, dental pulp, placenta, umbilical cord, or adipose tissue with minimally invasive biopsy. They can self-renew, proliferate, and differentiate, as well as promote growth of adjacent tissue via strong paracrine signaling pathways [64]. MSC have immunosuppressive properties; they decrease the immune response by inhibiting T-cell proliferation and cytotoxicity while increasing the production of regulatory T cells. Drawbacks of MSC include small number in bone marrow and blood, as well as source-dependent variation [25].

Hematopoietic stem cells are multipotent cells, with capacity to differentiate into multiple lineages including cardiomyocytes and endothelial cells [65]. Although they can be harvested from peripheral blood and bone marrow, bone marrow yields are higher [66]. Hematopoietic stem cells are perfect regenerative candidates as they can achieve myogenesis and angiogenesis concomitantly, although their low numbers, difficult in vitro maintenance, and unknown signaling pathways need to be improved [66]. Endothelial progenitor cells are also found in the bone marrow and peripheral blood although in very low concentrations. They can differentiate into endothelial cells and participate in angiogenesis [67]. The number of circulating EPC increases with myocardial ischemia and cytokine release, infiltrating the injured myocardium and possibly differentiating into myocytes [68, 69].

14.3   Stem Cell Delivery Methods

14.3.1   Delivery Methods in Humans

The ideal delivery platform for stem cell therapy in cardiac regeneration should use a noninvasive technique that directly delivers cells to the site of infarct, to prevent cellular loss via aberrant homing. The carrier vehicle for cells should promote survival in the ischemic environment, facilitate retention and promote stem cell differentiation, augment paracrine effects, and protect native myocardium from scarring and arrhythmias [70]. Despite continued studies predominantly in animal studies, no such vehicle exists for use in clinical trials. At present, stem cell delivery can be accomplished via intravenous injection, intracoronary infusion, direct epicardial and endocardial injection, as well as topical application at the time of surgery [24]. Peripheral intravenous (IV) injection is by far the least invasive, though studies examining homing of radioactively labeled bone marrow cells into infarcted myocardium did not reveal any signal in the heart [71]. Intracoronary and intramyocardial delivery is by far the most commonly used methods reported in clinical trials [72]. Intracoronary (IC) infusion is less invasive than intramyocardial injection and can be achieved in an antegrade or retrograde fashion. IC delivery is also less arrhythmogenic and has been associated with a modest improvement in EF and infarcted area size [72]. Despite these benefits, IC delivery results in delivery of only 1.3–2.6% of cells into the infarcted myocardium, with the majority of cells circulating to the liver or spleen [71]. In addition, IC injection depends on patency of coronary arteries and is associated with a small risk of embolization [73, 74]. Intramyocardial delivery (IM) of cells facilitates their delivery to target tissues and can be accomplished via transepicardial, transendocardial, or transcoronary routes [57]. Transepicardial injection requires direct exposure of the heart, and all intramuscular injections are associated with ventricular arrhythmias [75].

14.3.2 Implantable and Injectable Systems

Cellular scaffolds and hydrogels enhance stem cell survival, and while hydrogels can retain cells at desired locations, scaffolds provide mechanical support to adjacent structures; unfortunately, both require invasive topical application [76, 77]. In rodent studies, human bone marrow CD133+ cells delivered in collagen patches increased local angiogenesis, though the cells themselves failed to differentiate into cardiomyocytes [78]. In addition to collagen, multiple other substrates mimic the ECM of the heart, including polyurethane (PU), poly(ester urethane) (PEU), polyester urethane urea (PEUU), and poly(glycerol sebacate) (PGS) [24]. Animal studies of biodegradable PU patches promoted the contractile phenotype of smooth muscle cells and improved cardiac remodeling [79].

Hydrogels composed of materials such as fibrin, Matrigel, alginate, and polyethylene glycol can all be modified to resemble the physical properties of cardiac tissue [24]. ECM and collagen containing hydrogels allowed for differentiation of human ESC into functional cardiomyocytes in vitro, and cell-impregnated alginate hydrogels delivered to murine hearts reduced left ventricular remodeling [80, 81]. Engineered heart tissue (EHT) has been developed from type I collagen and neonatal heart tissue. When sutured onto rat hearts in vivo, this tissue becomes electrically integrated and perfused [82, 83]. Finally, engineered heart muscle has been developed by ESC-derived cardiomyocytes onto EHT [84].

To overcome the invasive methods required for scaffold and hydrogel delivery, gelling systems based on materials including fibrin glue, collagen, Matrigel, hyaluronic acid, and alginate have been developed that undergo a fluid-to-solid transition when in vivo, allowing catheter-based delivery [24]. Self-assembling RAD16-II scaffolds induced angiogenesis, retained myocytes, and promoted ESC differentiation into MHC-positive cells [85]. Catheter-delivered, collagen-encapsulated bone marrow cells showed improved LV function, and vascularization and self-assembling peptides loaded with insulin-like growth factor (IGF) allowed for sustained release of paracrine factors [86, 87]. Acellular alginate is undergoing clinical trials to prevent ventricular remodeling [24].

14.4 Clinical Trials of Post-MI Regeneration

14.4.1 Trial Design

A query of completed clinical trials in post-acute MI stem cell therapy shows that approximately 28 studies have been completed thus far (Table 14.2) [88–119]. The number of patients randomized varied from 20 to 250 in each trial. The intracoronary route of cell delivery after initial diagnostic and therapeutic PCI, used in 25 out of 29 trials, was the most widely used method of cell delivery. One study delivered cells both via the intracoronary and intramyocardial routes concomitantly, one study injected cells intramyocardially at the time of CABG, and two studies delivered cells peripherally via intravenous injection.

Autologous, rather than allogenic, cells were most commonly used, with just five studies employing allogenic sources (Table 14.2). Autologous bone marrow (BM)-derived mononuclear cells were the most commonly studied, followed by autologous bone marrow-derived unselected progenitor cells. Several studies further sorted out autologous bone marrow-derived hematopoietic, endothelial, endothelial/cardiac, and early progenitor cells based on differential expression of various combinations of cell surface markers including CD34, CD45, CD133, CXCR4, among others. Less common cell sources included autologous bone marrow-derived MSC from commercially available products, allogenic Wharton's jelly-derived MSC, and autologous peripheral blood stem cells. Although more extensively studied in the context of heart failure, as compared with acute MI, autologous cardiosphere-derived stem cells and allogenic cardiac stem cells have also been examined.

The timing of cell delivery and number of cells varied widely across studies. Despite all being acute post-MI models, therapy was delivered anywhere from less than 24 hours to several months post-initial therapeutic PCI. Although the ideal timing of cell delivery has not yet been standardized, the majority of studies implemented the therapeutic intervention within 10 days of PCI. Comparison of early (3–6 weeks) versus late (3–4 months) delivery did not change the primary outcome, increased left ventricular ejection fraction (LVEF), and decreased infarct size [94]. Final cell count delivered differed significantly between and often within studies; all studies used a magnitude of cells on the order of millions, in the range of 1.9–1300 million cells. Although the majority of studies used a fixed number across participants, several studies used weight-based dosing of 0.5–five million cells/kg. In preparations containing mixed cell subtypes, such as nucleated and mononuclear cells, the percentage of cells between subjects varied to a small degree.

Table 14.2 Clinical trials in post-myocardial infarction stem cell therapy

Study	Cell type	Cell number	Route	N	Time	Outcome
TIME (2012) [89]	Autologous BM-MNC	100 million	IC	40	3–10 days post MI	No change in LVEF Decreased LVEDV
Late TIME (2010) [119]	Autologous BM-MNC	150 million	IC	120	3–7 days post MI	No change in LVEF or LV function
SWISS-AMI (2013) [91]	Autologous BM-MNC	50–500 million	IC	200	5–7 days or 3–4 weeks post MI	No change in LVEF
MYSTAR (2009) [94]	Autologous BM-MNC	Intramyocardial (E/L): 200.3/194.8 million Intracoronary (E/L): 1300/1290 million	IC + IM	60	3–6 weeks or 3–4 months post MI	Increased LVEF and decreased infarct size in E/L groups
SCAMI (2013) [100]	Autologous BM-MNC	381 million	IC	42	5–7 days post MI	No change in EF, infarct size, EDV, and ESV
MI3 (2015) [103]	Autologous BM-MNC	558 million	IC	250	Median 15 days post MI	No change in LVEF
BONAMI (2011) [114]	Autologous BM-MNC	98.3 million	IC	100	9.3 days post MI	No change in LVEF or myocardial viability
ASTAMI (2006) [109]	Autologous BM-MNC	Median 68 million	IC	100	Median 6 days post MI	No change in LVEF
FINCELL (2008) [106]	Autologous BM-MNC	Mononuclear: Mean 402 million	IC	80	2–6 days post MI	Improved LVEF
TECAM (2015) [104]	Autologous BM-MNC ± GCSF	BM-MNC: 83 million BM-MNC + GCSF: 560 million	IC	120	3–5 days post MI	No change in LVEF/ LVESV Reduced infarct size
COMPARE CPM-RMI (2018) [102]	Autologous BM-MNC v CD133+ cells	BM-MNC: 564.63 million CD133+: 8.19 million	IM	77	26.5–30 days post MI	Improved LVEF and decreased wall thickening in both groups Decreased nonviable segments in CD133+ group

Study	Cell type	Cell dose	Route	N	Timing	Outcome
REGENT (2009) [118]	Autologous BM-MNC v CD34+/CXCR4+ cells	BM-MNC: Median 178 million CD34+/CXCR4+: Median 1.9 million	IC	200	Median 7 days post MI	Improved LVEF in both cellular groups only in baseline EF < 37%
NCT00264316 (2006) [93]	Autologous BM-SC	304 million nucleated and 172 million mononuclear	IC	67	24 hours post MI	Reduced infarct size Improved regional systolic function No change in LVEF
REPAIR-AMI (2006) [97]	Autologous BM-SC	CD34+/CD45+: Mean 3.6 million CD34+/CD133+/CD45+: Mean 2.5 million	IC	204	3–7 days post MI	Improved LVEF Reduced death, MI, revascularization
REGENERATE-AMI (2016) [101]	Autologous BM-SC	Mononuclear: 59.8 million CD34+: 1.9 million	IC	100	<24 hours post MI	Improved myocardial salvage index No change in LVEF
BOOST (2004) [108]	Autologous BM-SC	Nucleated: 24.6 million CD34+: 9.5 million Hematopoietic colony forming: 3.6 million	IC	60	Mean 4.8 days post MI	Improved LVEF
NCT00363324 (2010) [113]	Autologous BM-SC	402 million	IC	78	2–6 days post MI	Improved LVEF in patients with baseline below average EF
TOPCARE-AMI (2004) [95]	Autologous BM-CD34+/CD45+ cells ± circulating progenitor cells	BM-CD34+/CD45+: 213 million CPC: 16 million	IC	59	3–7 days post MI	Improved LVEF in both groups Decreased ESV in both groups

(continued)

Table 14.2 (continued)

Study	Cell type	Cell number	Route	N	Time	Outcome
AMR1 (2011) [105]	Autologous BM-CD34+ cells	5, 10, 15 million	IC	31	Median 8.3 days post MI	Reduced infarct size and perfusion with increasing cellular doses
PreSERVE AMI (2017) [111]	Autologous BM-CD34+ cells	Mean 14.9 million	IC	161	Mean 9.3 days post MI	No change in resting myocardial perfusion
SEED-MSC (2014) [98]	Autologous BM-MSC	72 million	IC	60	1 month post MI	Improved LVEF
IRB SCH2011-006 (2018) [116]	Autologous BM-MSC	7.2x107 cells	IC	26	1 month post MI	Improved LVEF
NCT00114452 (2009) [92]	Allogenic BM-MSC	0.5, 1.6, 5 million cells/kg	IV	53	1–10 days post MI	Improved LVEF Improved global symptoms score
NCT00883727 (2015) [107]	Allogenic BM-MSC	2 million cells/kg	IV	20	2 days post MI	No change in EF No change in perfusion
NCT01291329 (2015) [99]	Allogenic Wharton's jelly MSC	6 million	IC	116	5–7 days post MI	Improved LVEF Decreased ESV/EDV Increased myocardial viability and perfusion
MAGIC Cell (2004) [110]	Autologous peripheral blood SC mobilized with GCSF	100 million	IC	27	2–270 days post MI	Improved exercise capacity, perfusion, systolic function Increased stent stenosis with GCSF

CADUCEUS (2012) [88]	Autologous CDSC *	12.5, 17.3, 25 million	IC	31	1.5–3 months post MI	Reduced scar mass Increased viable heart mass and regional contractility Increased regional systolic wall thickening No change in LVEF/ESV/EDS
CAREMI (2018) [115]	Allogenic CSC *	35 million	IC	49	5–7 days post MI	No change in infarct size or LV remodeling

Summary table of design and outcomes of current post-MI stem cell therapy clinical trials

N number of participants randomized, *BM-MNC* bone marrow mononuclear cells, *IC* intracoronary, *MI* myocardial infarction, *LVEF* left ventricular ejection fraction, *LVEDV* left ventricular end-diastolic volume, *LV* left ventricular, *E/L* early/late, *IM* intramyocardial, *EF* ejection fraction, *EDV* end-diastolic volume, *ESV* end-systolic volume, *GCSF* granulocyte colony-stimulating factor, *LVESV* left ventricular end-systolic volume, *BM-SC* bone marrow stem cells, *BM-MSC* bone marrow mesenchymal stem cells, *IV* intravascular, *MSC* mesenchymal stem cells, *SC* stem cells, *CDSC* cardiosphere-derived stem cells, *CSC* cardiac stem cell, *endogenous stem cell source

14.4.2 Trial Outcomes

Comparison of outcomes across studies is difficult due to the lack of standardization of timing, inclusion criteria, cell number, and type. Despite these limitations, a generalization can be made that stem cell treatment is associated with only a modest improvement in outcome, as only 64% of the studies examined showed efficacy. Autologous bone marrow-derived mononuclear cells, although most studied, were associated with the least favorable outcomes. Six out of 12 patient cohorts treated with mononuclear cells did not have any significant improvement in any outcome. Three studies showed improvement in LVEF. One study showed decreased left ventricular end-diastolic volume (LVEDV), and one study showed reduced infarct size. Mononuclear cell treatment was also associated with decreased infarct size regardless of treatment timing (3–6 weeks versus 3–4 months) in one study and decreased systolic wall thickening in another. LVEF improved in one study only in a subset of patients with initial EF < 37%.

Autologous BM-derived stem cells, including hematopoietic, endothelial, cardiac/hematopoietic, and early progenitor cells, showed by far the highest efficacy rates with 90% of studies showing a significant increase in various outcome parameters. Six studies reported increased LVEF, up to as much as 18 months after treatment. Perhaps most notably, treatment with a combination of CD34+/CD45+ and CD34+/CD133+/CD45+ cells reduced combined death, recurrent MI, and any revascularization procedures at 1 year. Other outcomes associated with BM-derived stem cell treatment included reduced myocardial infarct size, recovery of regional systolic function and myocardial deformation, improved perfusion, decrease in end-systolic volume (ESV), improved myocardial salvage index, decreased systolic wall thickening and nonviable segments, as well as increased LVEF in patients with baseline EF < 37%.

Autologous BM-MSC improved LVEF in two studies, while allogenic BM-MSC were only efficacious 50% of the time, though they were only used in two studies. They increased LVEF and global symptom score in patients at 6 months in one cohort, although no change in LVEF or perfusion was observed in another study at the same time point. Wharton's jelly-derived MSC were associated with a higher absolute increase in myocardial viability and perfusion at 4 months, as well as increased LVEF and decreased end-systolic and diastolic volumes at 18 months.

Autologous cardiosphere-derived stem cells reduced scar mass and increased viable heart mass, regional contractility, and regional systolic wall thickening, though there was no appreciable change in LVEF at 12 months. Interestingly, allogenic cardiac stem cells were not associated with a change in infarct size or LV remodeling. Peripheral blood stem cells mobilized with granulocyte colony-stimulating factor (GCSF) increased exercise capacity, myocardial perfusion, and systolic function, although the use of GCSF was associated with a higher rate of in-stent stenosis at 6 months. Beneficial effects based on cellular type are summarized in Table 14.3 and Fig. 14.1.

Table 14.3 Benefits after acute MI-based on cell type

Cellular subtype	Improvements seen
Autologous BM-MNC	Increased LVEF Decreased LVEDV Decreased infarct size Decreased systolic wall thickening
Autologous CD133+ cells	Increased LVEF Decreased nonviable segments Decreased systolic wall thickening
Autologous CD34+/CXCR4+ cells	Increased LVEF in patients with EF < 37%
Autologous BM-SC	Increased LVEF Reduced myocardial infarct size Improved recovery of regional function Reduced combined death, recurrence of MI, and need for revascularization Improved myocardial salvage index Improved regional myocardial deformation
Autologous BM-CD34+ cells	Reduced infarct size Improved perfusion
Autologous BM-CD34+/CD45+ cells	Increased LVEF Decreased ESV
Autologous circulating peripheral blood stem cells	Increased LVEF Decreased ESV Increased exercise capacity Improved myocardial perfusion Improved systolic function
Autologous BM-MSC	Increased LVEF
Allogenic BM-MSC	Improved LVEF Improved global symptoms score
Allogenic Wharton's jelly MSC	Increased LVEF Improved infarct perfusion Increased myocardial viability Decreased ESV/EDV
Autologous CDSC	Reduced scar mass Increased viable heart mass Increased regional contractility Increased regional systolic wall thickening

Summary of advantageous post-acute MI outcomes based on cell source
BM-MNC bone marrow-derived mononuclear cell, *LVEF* left ventricular ejection fraction, *LVEDV* left ventricular end-diastolic volume, *EF* ejection fraction, *BM-SC* bone marrow-derived stem cells, *MI* myocardial infarction, *ESV* end-systolic volume, *BM-MSC* bone marrow mesenchymal stem cells, *MSC* mesenchymal stem cell, *EDV* end-diastolic volume, *CDSC* cardiosphere-derived stem cell

14.4.3 Stem Cell Therapy in Ischemic Cardiomyopathy

Although the primary focus of stem cell therapy remains to prevent myocardial loss and allow for regeneration of tissue immediately after an MI, clinical trials are also underway to evaluate the ability of stem cells to remuscularize and reactivate innate

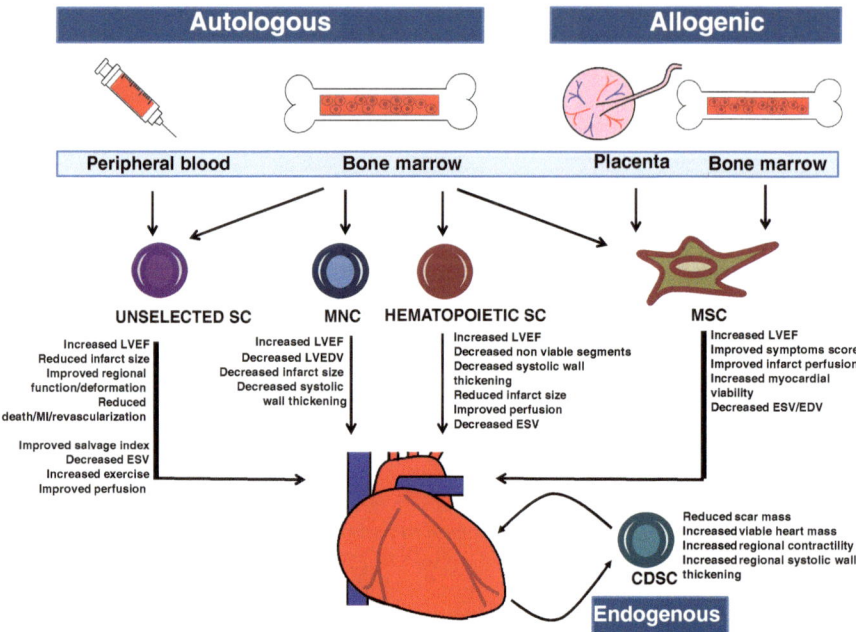

Fig. 14.1 Stem cell types and benefits in treatment after MI. SC, stem cell; MNC, mononuclear cell; MSC, mesenchymal stem cell; LVEF, left ventricular ejection fraction; MI, myocardial infarction; ESV, end-systolic volume; LVEDV, left ventricular end-diastolic volume; EDV, end diastolic volume; CDSC, cardiosphere-derived stem cell

cardiac regeneration pathways in models of heart failure secondary to chronic cardiomyopathy [22]. Similar to studies targeting treatment of acute MI, cells evaluated in ischemic cardiomyopathy include skeletal myoblasts, bone marrow-derived unselected and selected stem cells, MSC, embryonic stem cells, and cardiac-committed progenitor cells [22].

Skeletal myoblasts do not appear to improve LVEF [120]. Unselected bone marrow stem cells are less commonly used in HF models although appear to have as little efficacy as when used in acute MI trials [121–125]. Bone marrow-derived hematopoietic stem and progenitor cells appear to improve unstable angina, but their efficacy in HF is less established [126–129]. Similar to post-MI studies, MSC appear to be among the most efficacious in HF models [130–133]. Cardiac stem cells including KIT+ and cardiosphere-derived cells (CDC) both appear to show some efficacy in clinical trials [134, 135]. Transplantation of embryonic stem cell-derived cardiac progenitor cells appears to confer a symptomatic benefit, although a very small number of patients have been evaluated thus far, necessitating further trials [136]. Analysis of completed clinical trials in chronic HF suggests MSC and CSC as the most promising cell types, and although some efficacy has been established, many more clinical trials and optimal delivery vehicles are needed before stem cell therapy becomes standard of care.

14.5 Limitations of Stem Cells Therapy

A substantial limitation of stem cell therapy post-MI is the low homing, retention, and differentiation rate of cells in the ischemic microenvironment of the infarcted heart [137]. Human studies have shown a 39% cellular retention rate just 1 hour following transplantation that is attributable to high rates of apoptosis [71]. The high rate of cell death after transplantation can be attributed to inflammation, mechanical injury, hypoxia, and reperfusion injury [138]. Furthermore, loss of matrix attachment during cell preparation and following injection contributes to programmed cell death [139]. Ischemia is a major hurdle for stem cell populations to differentiate into cardiomyocytes, particularly ones that become electromechanically integrated [24].

Although most clinical trials demonstrate safety following stem cell transfer, with only a few complications reported, animal studies have shown increased risk of ventricular arrhythmias following human cardiomyocyte transfer into guinea pigs and nonhuman primates [140, 141]. In addition, isolation of adequate quantity of stem cells, expansion, and optimal delivery methods that allow for cell retention and differentiation are lacking [28]. Although peripheral and bone marrow stem cells are easier to harvest, attaining adequate number of organ-derived cells, such as cardiac stem cells, is invasive and often low yield [28]. Several clinical trials have also shown that transplanted cells may not be capable of integration and electrochemical coupling, suggesting that their effects are predominantly paracrine in nature and may not add directly to myocyte mass [142].

Meaningful decisions and meta-analyses of clinical trial data are difficult to interpret and synthesize in light of heterogeneity of trial design and reporting. Clinical trials completed thus far have varying, though usually low, number of participants. Primary outcomes measured vary from study to study, and some lack diverse clinical assessment tools. Inclusion criteria, stem cell type and number, delivery methods, and timing vary greatly across trials. Some studies lack placebo groups, making them prone to observation bias, while others evaluate safety only without efficacy. Variable outcomes across studies can easily be attributed to the heterogeneous number and quality of cells used [143].

14.5.1 Modifications to Enhance Cell Function

Multiple strategies including in vitro cellular preconditioning or reprogramming via environmental, pharmacological, and genetic means have been explored in order to increase in vivo cell survival [137]. These strategies include culturing cells under ischemic conditions, supplementing culture medium with growth factors, as well as transfecting cells with proangiogenic and anti-apoptotic factors [57]. Culturing MSC in low oxygen conditions prior to transplant activates survival pathways, upregulates pro-survival genes, increases anti-apoptotic genes including Akt and eNOS, and upregulates pro-angiogenic cytokines including vascular endothelial growth factor (VEGF) [144]. Additionally, hypoxia allows cells to preserve stemness and promote differentiation and proliferation in vivo [145]. In vitro burst exposure of cells to low levels of oxidative stress and thermal shock treatment also improves cell viability and functional outcomes [146, 147].

Preconditioning of cells with several therapeutic drugs increased secretion of growth factors, including vascular endothelial growth factor (VEGF), angiopoietin-1α (Ang-1α), stromal cell-derived factor-1 (SDF-1), hepatocyte growth factor (HGF), and IGF [148]. Several mitochondrial potassium channel opening drugs, including pinacidil and diazoxide, suppress apoptosis and increase cell survival in ischemic conditions [149, 150]. In one study, treatment of cardiac stem cells with hydrogen peroxide increased endothelial and vascular smooth muscle gene expression and angiogenesis [25]. In vivo treatment with statins increased cell survival and differentiation, while in vitro treatment improved function of endothelial progenitor cells [151, 152]. Pre-treatment of several cell lines with oxytocin improves their response to oxidative stress and differentiation into cardiomyocytes and vascular cells [153, 154]. Multiple other drug classes including trimetazine, β-mercaptoethanol, caspase inhibitors, 5-Azacytidine, and the kinase inhibitor Imatinib have been used in vitro to increase cell viability, confer resistance to oxidative injury, increase cellular engraftment, and prime cellular differentiation toward a cardiac fate, respectively [155–157].

Genetic manipulation of stem cells prior to transfer is another strategy used to improve efficacy, as transgenes can be targeted to release pro-angiogenic and chemoattractant factors, as well as anti-apoptotic proteins. For example, insertion of the pro-survival gene Pim-1 kinase into cardiac stem cells decreased infarct scar mass in a pig model [25]. Transformation of stem cells with IGF-1, which induces expression of survival genes, enhanced survival, engraftment, and differentiation [158]. IGF-1-transformed MSC showed efficacy in improving ejection fraction in animal studies. Overexpression of Ang-1, HGF, VEGF, and MyoD in post-MI studies have consistently shown improved cellular retention, likely secondary to increased angiogenic potential of pre-treated cells [159–161]. Akt-modified bone marrow-derived MSC survival is upregulated via secretion of numerous growth factors, including bFGF, HGF, IFG-1, and VEGF [162].

Because adhesion to an extracellular matrix is important for the survival of several stem cells, notably MSC, injection of cells and lack of healthy ECM in infarcted hearts potentiate apoptosis. To address this, overexpression of tissue transglutaminase in MSC increased survival leading to improved restoration of cardiac function [163]. Transfection of integrin-linked kinase (ILK), which contributed to cell adhesion and ECM assembly, improves cellular survival in hypoxic conditions and reduces infarct size in animal studies [164].

Resident stem cells become senescent and lose their regenerative capacity with age, resulting in reduced proliferation, differentiation, and metabolic activity [165]. These changes are driven by telomere shortening and upregulation of p53 genes [166]. For example, MSC derived from older patients are not as efficacious in post-MI models as those derived from younger patients [167]. Strategies to combat senescence have been examined and include modification of human cardiac progenitor cells with Pim-1 and upregulation of the WNT/β-catenin signaling pathway, both of which result in improved cellular function [168, 169].

14.6 Future Directions

Although stem cell therapy after MI is gaining momentum with promising initial results, multiple limitations must be overcome to realize the full potential that cellular therapy has to offer. The optimal cell source for use in clinical trials must be determined. Although embryonic stem cells confer immune privilege, they are associated with ethical dilemmas and are teratogenic in undifferentiated forms. While embryonic stem cell-derived cardiac precursors eliminate teratogenic potential, their differentiation protocols currently produce low yields and must be improved. Resident cardiac stem cells are difficult to harvest and are low in number. Bioreactors and devices to standardize and improve differentiation yields are on the horizon, although further research needs to be accomplished [170].

iPSC are an ideal cell candidate for clinical translation since they are derived from adult somatic cells via noninvasive techniques and can repopulate any cardiac lineage. Although the first iPSC clinical trial is currently being planned, nonviral transfection protocols to derive iPSC cells must be optimized to prevent genomic instability. Furthermore, differentiation protocols and elimination of undifferentiated cells via induced cell apoptosis must ensure patient safety. Paracrine effects of cell therapy must be defined more clearly, and the potential of exosomes must be studied, as use of exosomes alone without cellular transfer could realize the full potential of iPSC cells.

Cell survival and homing, particularly with intravenous and intracoronary routes, are extremely low, with cell loss being exacerbated by the ischemic post-infarct environment. Preconditioning of cells prior to transfer via genetic modifications and drug treatments, as well as improved homing mechanisms, must be developed to improve the number of cells participating in repair. In addition, methods of preventing resident stem cell senescence and improve mobilization must be elucidated.

Optimal delivery methods for stem cell treatment must be redesigned. Although intramyocardial injections deliver cells directly to infarcted areas, they are invasive and associated with generating pro-arrhythmogenic foci. Intracoronary and intravenous injections suffer from poor cellular homing. While patches and scaffolds afford the added benefit of maintaining an optimal scaffold, they can only be delivered at the time of surgery. Gelling systems loaded with cytokines and pro-survival proteins must be refined to allow for noninvasive delivery. In addition, three-dimensional (3D) and bioprinted cellularized vascular constructs are currently being developed.

Currently, protocols for clinical trials of stem cell therapy vary greatly and lack standardization. In order to make meaningful comparisons and interpretations across trials cell type, delivery methods and timing, as well as measured outcomes, must be standardized.

14.7 Conclusion

Myocardial infarction and ischemic cardiomyopathy confer significant morbidity and mortality, yet despite best medical care, many patients who suffer from an MI go on to develop heart failure, secondary to myocardial necrosis and pathologic myocardial remodeling. The population of resident cardiac stem cells available to replenish lost cells is low and easily overwhelmed by ischemia. Although the design of clinical trials is not uniform, and comparisons cannot be easily made, delivery of both endogenous and exogenous stem cells to ischemic myocardium has shown some efficacy at reducing infarct size and improving long-term function.

Several issues are currently being addressed in order to optimize stem cell efficacy. In addition to standardizing cellular type, delivery method, and timing, clinical trials must focus on similar outcomes. The optimal cell type and differentiation methods are being determined, with iPSC and exosomes holding great promise. The most direct, least invasive delivery method and improvement of cell homing and survival are yet to be overcome. Despite all of these obstacles, stem cell therapy holds great promise in post-MI regeneration.

References

1. Smit M, Coetzee AR, Lochner A. The pathophysiology of myocardial ischemia and perioperative myocardial infarction. J Cardiothorac Vasc Anesth. 2019. https://doi.org/10.1053/j.jvca.2019.10.005.
2. Benjamin Emelia J, Virani Salim S, Callaway Clifton W, et al. Heart disease and stroke statistics—2018 update: a report from the American Heart Association. Circulation. 2018;137(12):e67–e492.
3. Dalys GBD, Collaborators H, Murray CJL, et al. Global, regional, and national disability-adjusted life years (DALYs) for 306 diseases and injuries and healthy life expectancy (HALE) for 188 countries, 1990-2013: quantifying the epidemiological transition. Lancet (London, England). 2015;386(10009):2145–91.
4. Mahmood SS, Levy D, Vasan RS, Wang TJ. The Framingham heart study and the epidemiology of cardiovascular disease: a historical perspective. Lancet (London, England). 2014;383(9921):999–1008.
5. White H, Thygesen K, Alpert JS, Jaffe A. Universal MI definition update for cardiovascular disease. Curr Cardiol Rep. 2014;16(6):492.
6. Libby P. Mechanisms of acute coronary syndromes and their implications for therapy. N Engl J Med. 2013;368(21):2004–13.
7. 2013 ACCF/AHA Guideline for the Management of ST-Elevation Myocardial Infarction. Executive summary: a report of the American College of Cardiology Foundation/American Heart Association task force on practice guidelines. Catheter Cardiovasc Interv. 2013;82(1):E1–E27.
8. Amsterdam EA, Wenger NK, Brindis RG, et al. 2014 AHA/ACC guideline for the Management of Patients with non–ST-elevation acute coronary syndromes: a report of the American College of Cardiology/American Heart Association task force on practice guidelines. J Am Coll Cardiol. 2014;64(24):e139–228.

9. Stephens NR, Restrepo CS, Saboo SS, Baxi AJ. Overview of complications of acute and chronic myocardial infarctions: revisiting pathogenesis and cross-sectional imaging. Postgrad Med J. 2019;95(1126):439.
10. Mozaffarian D, Benjamin Emelia J, Go Alan S, et al. Executive summary: heart disease and stroke statistics—2015 update. Circulation. 2015;131(4):434–41.
11. Heidenreich PA, Albert NM, Allen LA, et al. Forecasting the impact of heart failure in the United States: a policy statement from the American Heart Association. Circ Heart Fail. 2013;6(3):606–19.
12. Pfeffer MA, Braunwald E. Ventricular remodeling after myocardial infarction. Experimental observations and clinical implications. Circulation. 1990;81(4):1161–72.
13. Cleutjens JPM, Kandala JC, Guarda E, Guntaka RV, Weber KT. Regulation of collagen degradation in the rat myocardium after infarction. J Mol Cell Cardiol. 1995;27(6):1281–92.
14. Warren SE, Royal HD, Markis JE, Grossman W, Mckay RG. Time course of left ventricular dilation after myocardial infarction: influence of infarct-related artery and success of coronary thrombolysis. J Am Coll Cardiol. 1988;11(1):12–9.
15. Mckay RG, Pfeffer MA, Pasternak RC, et al. Left ventricular remodeling after myocardial infarction: a corollary to infarct expansion. Circulation. 1986;74(4):693–702.
16. Qasim M, Arunkumar P, Powell HM, Khan M. Current research trends and challenges in tissue engineering for mending broken hearts. Life Sci. 2019;229:233–50.
17. Kajstura J, Urbanek K, Perl S, et al. Cardiomyogenesis in the adult human heart. Circ Res. 2010;107(2):305–15.
18. Beltrami AP, Barlucchi L, Torella D, et al. Adult cardiac stem cells are multipotent and support myocardial regeneration. Cell. 2003;114(6):763–76.
19. Bergmann O, Bhardwaj RD, Bernard S, et al. Evidence for cardiomyocyte renewal in humans. Science. 2009;324(5923):98.
20. Kajstura J, Rota M, Cappetta D, et al. Cardiomyogenesis in the aging and failing human heart. Circulation. 2012;126(15):1869–81.
21. Arbatlı S, Aslan GS, Kocabaş F. Stem cells in regenerative cardiology. In: Turksen K, editor. Cell biology and translational medicine, Volume 1: Stem cells in regenerative medicine: advances and challenges. Cham: Springer International Publishing; 2018. p. 37–53.
22. Menasché P. Cell therapy trials for heart regeneration — lessons learned and future directions. Nat Rev Cardiol. 2018;15(11):659–71.
23. Wang WE, Chen X, Houser SR, Zeng C. Potential of cardiac stem/progenitor cells and induced pluripotent stem cells for cardiac repair in ischaemic heart disease. Clinical science (London, England : 1979). 2013;125(7):319–27.
24. Carvalho E, Verma P, Hourigan K, Banerjee R. Myocardial infarction: stem cell transplantation for cardiac regeneration. Regen Med. 2015;10(8):1025–43.
25. Henning RJ. Current status of stem cells in cardiac repair. Futur Cardiol. 2018;14(2):181–92.
26. Hass R, Kasper C, Böhm S, Jacobs R. Different populations and sources of human mesenchymal stem cells (MSC): a comparison of adult and neonatal tissue-derived MSC. Cell Commun Signal. 2011;9:12.
27. Armiñán A, Gandía C, García-Verdugo JM, et al. Mesenchymal stem cells provide better results than hematopoietic precursors for the treatment of myocardial infarction. J Am Coll Cardiol. 2010;55(20):2244–53.
28. Sun Q, Zhang Z, Sun Z. The potential and challenges of using stem cells for cardiovascular repair and regeneration. Genes Dis. 2014;1(1):113–9.
29. Takahashi K, Yamanaka S. Induction of pluripotent stem cells from mouse embryonic and adult fibroblast cultures by defined factors. Cell. 2006;126(4):663–76.
30. Ye L, Chang Y-H, Xiong Q, et al. Cardiac repair in a porcine model of acute myocardial infarction with human induced pluripotent stem cell-derived cardiovascular cells. Cell Stem Cell. 2014;15(6):750–61.
31. Bearzi C, Rota M, Hosoda T, et al. Human cardiac stem cells. Proc Natl Acad Sci. 2007;104(35):14068.

32. Hosoda T, D'amario D, Cabral-Da-Silva MC, et al. Clonality of mouse and human cardiomyogenesis in vivo. Proc Natl Acad Sci U S A. 2009;106(40):17169–74.
33. Castaldo C, Di Meglio F, Nurzynska D, et al. CD117-positive cells in adult human heart are localized in the subepicardium, and their activation is associated with Laminin-1 and α6 integrin expression. Stem Cells. 2008;26(7):1723–31.
34. Oskouei BN, Lamirault G, Joseph C, et al. Increased potency of cardiac stem cells compared with bone marrow mesenchymal stem cells in cardiac repair. Stem Cells Transl Med. 2012;1(2):116–24.
35. Zhang Y, Sivakumaran P, Newcomb AE, et al. Cardiac repair with a novel population of mesenchymal stem cells resident in the human heart. Stem Cells. 2015;33(10):3100–13.
36. Liang SX, Tan TYL, Gaudry L, Chong B. Differentiation and migration of Sca1+/CD31− cardiac side population cells in a murine myocardial ischemic model. Int J Cardiol. 2010;138(1):40–9.
37. Kattman SJ, Huber TL, Gordon m K. Multipotent Flk-1+ cardiovascular progenitor cells give rise to the cardiomyocyte, endothelial, and vascular smooth muscle lineages. Dev Cell. 2006;11(5):723–32.
38. Suresh R, Chiriac A, Goel K, et al. CXCR4+ and FLK-1+ identify circulating cells associated with improved cardiac function in patients following myocardial infarction. J Cardiovasc Transl Res. 2013;6(5):787–97.
39. Laugwitz K-L, Moretti A, Lam J, et al. Postnatal isl1+ cardioblasts enter fully differentiated cardiomyocyte lineages. Nature. 2005;433(7026):647–53.
40. Kazakov A, Meier T, Werner C, et al. C-kit+ resident cardiac stem cells improve left ventricular fibrosis in pressure overload. Stem Cell Res. 2015;15(3):700–11.
41. Sullivan KE, Burns LJ, Black LD. An in vitro model for the assessment of stem cell fate following implantation within the infarct microenvironment identifies ISL-1 expression as the strongest predictor of c-kit+ cardiac progenitor cells' therapeutic potential. J Mol Cell Cardiol. 2015;88:91–100.
42. Bailey B, Fransioli J, Gude NA, et al. Sca-1 knockout impairs myocardial and cardiac progenitor cell function. Circ Res. 2012;111(6):750–60.
43. Linke A, Müller P, Nurzynska D, et al. Stem cells in the dog heart are self-renewing, clonogenic, and multipotent and regenerate infarcted myocardium, improving cardiac function. Proc Natl Acad Sci U S A. 2005;102(25):8966–71.
44. Uchida S, De Gaspari P, Kostin S, et al. Sca1-derived cells are a source of myocardial renewal in the murine adult heart. Stem Cell Rep. 2013;1(5):397–410.
45. Ott HC, Matthiesen TS, Brechtken J, et al. The adult human heart as a source for stem cells: repair strategies with embryonic-like progenitor cells. Nat Clin Pract Cardiovasc Med. 2007;4(1):S27–39.
46. Kocabas F, Mahmoud AI, Sosic D, et al. The hypoxic Epicardial and Subepicardial microenvironment. J Cardiovasc Transl Res. 2012;5(5):654–65.
47. Sadahiro T. Cardiac regeneration with pluripotent stem cell-derived cardiomyocytes and direct cardiac reprogramming. Regenerat Therap. 2019;11:95–100.
48. Moghaddam AS, Afshari JT, Esmaeili S-A, Saburi E, Joneidi Z, Momtazi-Borojeni AA. Cardioprotective microRNAs: lessons from stem cell-derived exosomal microRNAs to treat cardiovascular disease. Atherosclerosis. 2019;285:1–9.
49. Vagnozzi RJ, Maillet M, Sargent MA, et al. An acute immune response underlies the benefit of cardiac stem-cell therapy. Nature. 2019; https://doi.org/10.1038/s41586-019-1802-2.
50. Burchfield JS, Dimmeler S. Role of paracrine factors in stem and progenitor cell mediated cardiac repair and tissue fibrosis. Fibrogenesis Tissue Repair. 2008;1(1):4–4.
51. Lai RC, Arslan F, Lee MM, et al. Exosome secreted by MSC reduces myocardial ischemia/reperfusion injury. Stem Cell Res. 2010;4(3):214–22.
52. Arslan F, Lai RC, Smeets MB, et al. Mesenchymal stem cell-derived exosomes increase ATP levels, decrease oxidative stress and activate PI3K/Akt pathway to enhance myocardial viability and prevent adverse remodeling after myocardial ischemia/reperfusion injury. Stem Cell Res. 2013;10(3):301–12.

53. Fu X, Khalil H, Kanisicak O, et al. Specialized fibroblast differentiated states underlie scar formation in the infarcted mouse heart. J Clin Invest. 2018;128(5):2127–43.
54. Ieda M, Fu J-D, Delgado-Olguin P, et al. Direct reprogramming of fibroblasts into functional cardiomyocytes by defined factors. Cell. 2010;142(3):375–86.
55. Jayawardena TM, Egemnazarov B, Finch EA, et al. MicroRNA-mediated in vitro and in vivo direct reprogramming of cardiac fibroblasts to cardiomyocytes. Circ Res. 2012;110(11):1465–73.
56. Miyamoto K, Akiyama M, Tamura F, et al. Direct in vivo reprogramming with sendai virus vectors improves cardiac function after myocardial infarction. Cell Stem Cell. 2018;22(1):91–103.e105.
57. Parizadeh SM, Jafarzadeh-Esfehani R, Ghandehari M, et al. Stem cell therapy: a novel approach for myocardial infarction. J Cell Physiol. 2019;234(10):16904–12.
58. Lev S, Kehat I, Gepstein L. Differentiation pathways in human embryonic stem cell-derived cardiomyocytes. Ann N Y Acad Sci. 2005;1047(1):50–65.
59. Evans MJ, Kaufman MH. Establishment in culture of pluripotential cells from mouse embryos. Nature. 1981;292(5819):154–6.
60. Amit M, Carpenter MK, Inokuma MS, et al. Clonally derived human embryonic stem cell lines maintain pluripotency and proliferative potential for prolonged periods of culture. Dev Biol. 2000;227(2):271–8.
61. Gorecka J, Kostiuk V, Fereydooni A, et al. The potential and limitations of induced pluripotent stem cells to achieve wound healing. Stem Cell Res Ther. 2019;10(1):87.
62. Abbott JD, Giordano FJ. Stem cells and cardiovascular disease. J Nucl Cardiol. 2003;10(4):403–12.
63. Thakker R, Yang P. Mesenchymal stem cell therapy for cardiac repair. Curr Treat Options Cardiovasc Med. 2014;16(7):323.
64. Caplan AI. Why are MSCs therapeutic? New data: new insight. J Pathol. 2009;217(2):318–24.
65. Krause K, Schneider C, Kuck K-H, Jaquet K. REVIEW: stem cell therapy in cardiovascular disorders. Cardiovasc Ther. 2010;28(5):e101–10.
66. Asahara T, Kalka C, Isner JM. Stem cell therapy and gene transfer for regeneration. Gene Ther. 2000;7(6):451–7.
67. Urbich C, Dimmeler S. Endothelial progenitor cells: characterization and role in vascular biology. Circ Res. 2004;95(4):343–53.
68. Shintani S, Murohara T, Ikeda H, et al. Mobilization of endothelial progenitor cells in patients with acute myocardial infarction. Circulation. 2001;103(23):2776–9.
69. Badorff C, Brandes RP, Popp R, et al. Transdifferentiation of blood-derived human adult endothelial progenitor cells into functionally active cardiomyocytes. Circulation. 2003;107(7):1024–32.
70. Perin EC, López J. Methods of stem cell delivery in cardiac diseases. Nat Clin Pract Cardiovasc Med. 2006;3(1):S110–3.
71. Hofmann M, Wollert Kai C, Meyer Gerd P, et al. Monitoring of bone marrow cell homing into the infarcted human myocardium. Circulation. 2005;111(17):2198–202.
72. Campbell NG, Suzuki K. Cell delivery routes for stem cell therapy to the heart: current and future approaches. J Cardiovasc Transl Res. 2012;5(5):713–26.
73. Moreira RDC, Haddad AF, Silva SA, et al. Injeção intracoronariana de células tronco após infarto do miocárdio: subestudo da microcirculação. Arq Bras Cardiol. 2011;97:420–6.
74. Vulliet PR, Greeley M, Halloran SM, Macdonald KA, Kittleson MD. Intra-coronary arterial injection of mesenchymal stromal cells and microinfarction in dogs. Lancet. 2004;363(9411):783–4.
75. Fukushima S, Varela-Carver A, Coppen Steven R, et al. Direct Intramyocardial but not intracoronary injection of bone marrow cells induces ventricular arrhythmias in a rat chronic ischemic heart failure model. Circulation. 2007;115(17):2254–61.
76. Christman KL, Vardanian AJ, Fang Q, Sievers RE, Fok HH, Lee RJ. Injectable fibrin scaffold improves cell transplant survival, reduces infarct expansion, and induces Neovasculature formation in ischemic myocardium. J Am Coll Cardiol. 2004;44(3):654–60.

77. Suuronen Erik J, Veinot John P, Wong S, et al. Tissue-engineered injectable collagen-based matrices for improved cell delivery and vascularization of ischemic tissue using CD133+ progenitors expanded from the peripheral blood. Circulation. 2006;114(1_supplement):I-138-I-144.
78. Pozzobon M, Bollini S, Iop L, et al. Human bone marrow-derived CD133+ cells delivered to a collagen patch on Cryoinjured rat heart promote angiogenesis and Arteriogenesis. Cell Transplant. 2010;19(10):1247–60.
79. Fujimoto KL, Tobita K, Merryman WD, et al. An elastic, biodegradable cardiac patch induces contractile smooth muscle and improves cardiac remodeling and function in subacute myocardial infarction. J Am Coll Cardiol. 2007;49(23):2292–300.
80. Duan Y, Liu Z, O'neill J, Wan LQ, Freytes DO, Vunjak-Novakovic G. Hybrid gel composed of native heart matrix and collagen induces cardiac differentiation of human embryonic stem cells without supplemental growth factors. J Cardiovasc Transl Res. 2011;4(5):605–15.
81. Leor J, Aboulafia-Etzion S, Dar A, et al. Bioengineered cardiac grafts. Circulation. 2000;102(suppl_3):Iii-56-Iii-61.
82. Naito H, Melnychenko I, Didié M, et al. Optimizing engineered heart tissue for therapeutic applications as surrogate heart muscle. Circulation. 2006;114(1_supplement):I-72-I-78.
83. Zimmermann W-H, Didié M, Wasmeier Gerald H, et al. Cardiac grafting of engineered heart tissue in Syngenic rats. Circulation. 2002;106(12_suppl_1):I-151-I-157.
84. Soong PL, Tiburcy M, Zimmermann W-H. Cardiac differentiation of human embryonic stem cells and their assembly into engineered heart muscle. Curr Protoc Cell Biol. 2012;55(1):–23.28.21.
85. Davis ME, Motion JPM, Narmoneva DA, et al. Injectable self-assembling peptide nanofibers create intramyocardial microenvironments for endothelial cells. Circulation. 2005;111(4):442–50.
86. Huang NF, Yu J, Sievers R, Li S, Lee RJ. Injectable biopolymers enhance angiogenesis after myocardial infarction. Tissue Eng. 2005;11(11–12):1860–6.
87. Davis ME, Hsieh PCH, Takahashi T, et al. Local myocardial insulin-like growth factor 1 (IGF-1) delivery with biotinylated peptide nanofibers improves cell therapy for myocardial infarction. Proc Natl Acad Sci U S A. 2006;103(21):8155–60.
88. Makkar RR, Smith RR, Cheng K, et al. Intracoronary cardiosphere-derived cells for heart regeneration after myocardial infarction (CADUCEUS): a prospective, randomised phase 1 trial. Lancet (London, England). 2012;379(9819):895–904.
89. Traverse JH, Henry TD, Pepine CJ, et al. Effect of the use and timing of bone marrow mononuclear cell delivery on left ventricular function after acute myocardial infarction: the TIME randomized trial. JAMA. 2012;308(22):2380–9.
90. Traverse JH, Mckenna DH, Harvey K, et al. Results of a phase 1, randomized, double-blind, placebo-controlled trial of bone marrow mononuclear stem cell administration in patients following ST-elevation myocardial infarction. Am Heart J. 2010;160(3):428–34.
91. Sürder D, Manka R, Lo Cicero V, et al. Intracoronary injection of bone marrow–derived mononuclear cells early or late after acute myocardial infarction. Circulation. 2013;127(19):1968–79.
92. Hare JM, Traverse JH, Henry TD, et al. A randomized, double-blind, placebo-controlled, dose-escalation study of intravenous adult human mesenchymal stem cells (prochymal) after acute myocardial infarction. J Am Coll Cardiol. 2009;54(24):2277–86.
93. Janssens S, Dubois C, Bogaert J, et al. Autologous bone marrow-derived stem-cell transfer in patients with ST-segment elevation myocardial infarction: double-blind, randomised controlled trial. Lancet. 2006;367(9505):113–21.
94. Gyöngyösi M, Lang I, Dettke M, et al. Combined delivery approach of bone marrow mononuclear stem cells early and late after myocardial infarction: the MYSTAR prospective, randomized study. Nat Clin Pract Cardiovasc Med. 2009;6(1):70–81.

95. Schächinger V, Assmus B, Britten MB, et al. Transplantation of progenitor cells and regeneration enhancement in acute myocardial infarction: final one-year results of the TOPCARE-AMI trial. J Am Coll Cardiol. 2004;44(8):1690–9.

96. Schächinger V, Erbs S, Elsässer A, et al. Intracoronary bone marrow–derived progenitor cells in acute myocardial infarction. N Engl J Med. 2006;355(12):1210–21.

97. Schächinger V, Erbs S, Elsässer A, et al. Improved clinical outcome after intracoronary administration of bone-marrow-derived progenitor cells in acute myocardial infarction: final 1-year results of the REPAIR-AMI trial. Eur Heart J. 2006;27(23):2775–83.

98. Lee J-W, Lee S-H, Youn Y-J, et al. A randomized, open-label, multicenter trial for the safety and efficacy of adult mesenchymal stem cells after acute myocardial infarction. J Korean Med Sci. 2014;29(1):23–31.

99. Gao LR, Chen Y, Zhang NK, et al. Intracoronary infusion of Wharton's jelly-derived mesenchymal stem cells in acute myocardial infarction: double-blind, randomized controlled trial. BMC Med. 2015;13:162.

100. Wöhrle J, Von Scheidt F, Schauwecker P, et al. Impact of cell number and microvascular obstruction in patients with bone-marrow derived cell therapy: final results from the randomized, double-blind, placebo controlled intracoronary stem cell therapy in patients with acute myocardial infarction (SCAMI) trial. Clin Res Cardiol. 2013;102(10):765–70.

101. Choudry F, Hamshere S, Saunders N, et al. A randomized double-blind control study of early intra-coronary autologous bone marrow cell infusion in acute myocardial infarction: the REGENERATE-AMI clinical trial. Eur Heart J. 2016;37(3):256–63.

102. Naseri MH, Madani H, Ahmadi Tafti SH, et al. COMPARE CPM-RMI trial: Intramyocardial transplantation of autologous bone marrow-derived CD133+ cells and MNCs during CABG in patients with recent MI: a phase II/III, multicenter, placebo-controlled, randomized, double-blind clinical trial. Cell J. 2018;20(2):267–77.

103. Nair V, Madan H, Sofat S, et al. Efficacy of stem cell in improvement of left ventricular function in acute myocardial infarction--MI3 trial. Indian J Med Res. 2015;142(2):165–74.

104. San Roman JA, Sánchez PL, Villa A, et al. Comparison of different bone marrow–derived stem cell approaches in Reperfused STEMI: a multicenter, prospective, randomized, open-labeled TECAM trial. J Am Coll Cardiol. 2015;65(22):2372–82.

105. Quyyumi AA, Waller EK, Murrow J, et al. CD34+ cell infusion after ST elevation myocardial infarction is associated with improved perfusion and is dose dependent. Am Heart J. 2011;161(1):98–105.

106. Huikuri HV, Kervinen K, Niemelä M, et al. Effects of intracoronary injection of mononuclear bone marrow cells on left ventricular function, arrhythmia risk profile, and restenosis after thrombolytic therapy of acute myocardial infarction. Eur Heart J. 2008;29(22):2723–32.

107. Chullikana A, Majumdar AS, Gottipamula S, et al. Randomized, double-blind, phase I/II study of intravenous allogeneic mesenchymal stromal cells in acute myocardial infarction. Cytotherapy. 2015;17(3):250–61.

108. Wollert KC, Meyer GP, Lotz J, et al. Intracoronary autologous bone-marrow cell trans fer after myocardial infarction: the BOOST randomised controlled clinical trial. Lancet. 2004;364(9429):141–8.

109. Lunde K, Solheim S, Aakhus S, et al. Intracoronary injection of mononuclear bone marrow cells in acute myocardial infarction. N Engl J Med. 2006;355(12):1199–209.

110. Kang H-J, Kim H-S, Zhang S-Y, et al. Effects of intracoronary infusion of peripheral blood stem-cells mobilised with granulocyte-colony stimulating factor on left ventricular systolic function and restenosis after coronary stenting in myocardial infarction: the MAGIC cell randomised clinical trial. Lancet. 2004;363(9411):751–6.

111. Quyyumi AA, Vasquez A, Kereiakes DJ, et al. PreSERVE-AMI: a randomized, double-blind, placebo-controlled clinical trial of intracoronary administration of autologous CD34+ cells in patients with left ventricular dysfunction post STEMI. Circ Res. 2017;120(2):324–31.

112. Miettinen JA, Ylitalo K, Hedberg P, et al. Determinants of functional recovery after myocardial infarction of patients treated with bone marrow-derived stem cells after thrombolytic therapy. Heart. 2010;96(5):362.
113. Miettinen JA, Salonen RJ, Niemelä M, et al. Effects of intracoronary infusion of bone marrow-derived stem cells on pulmonary artery pressure and diastolic function after myocardial infarction. Int J Cardiol. 2010;145(3):631–3.
114. Roncalli J, Mouquet F, Piot C, et al. Intracoronary autologous mononucleated bone marrow cell infusion for acute myocardial infarction: results of the randomized multicenter BONAMI trial. Eur Heart J. 2011;32(14):1748–57.
115. Fernández-Avilés F, Sanz-Ruiz R, Bogaert J, et al. Safety and efficacy of intracoronary infusion of allogeneic human cardiac stem cells in patients with ST-segment elevation myocardial infarction and left ventricular dysfunction. Circ Res. 2018;123(5):579–89.
116. Kim SH, Cho JH, Lee YH, et al. Improvement in left ventricular function with intracoronary mesenchymal stem cell therapy in a patient with Anterior Wall ST-segment elevation myocardial infarction. Cardiovasc Drugs Ther. 2018;32(4):329–38.
117. Herbots L, D'hooge J, Eroglu E, et al. Improved regional function after autologous bone marrow-derived stem cell transfer in patients with acute myocardial infarction: a randomized, double-blind strain rate imaging study. Eur Heart J. 2008;30(6):662–70.
118. Tendera M, Wojakowski W, Rużyłło W, et al. Intracoronary infusion of bone marrow-derived selected CD34+CXCR4+ cells and non-selected mononuclear cells in patients with acute STEMI and reduced left ventricular ejection fraction: results of randomized, multicentre myocardial regeneration by intracoronary infusion of selected population of stem cells in acute myocardial infarction (REGENT) trial. Eur Heart J. 2009;30(11):1313–21.
119. Traverse JH, Henry TD, Vaughan DE, et al. LateTIME: a phase-II, randomized, double-blinded, placebo-controlled, pilot trial evaluating the safety and effect of administration of bone marrow mononuclear cells 2 to 3 weeks after acute myocardial infarction. Tex Heart Inst J. 2010;37(4):412–20.
120. Menasché P, Alfieri O, Janssens S, et al. The myoblast autologous grafting in ischemic cardiomyopathy (MAGIC) trial. Circulation. 2008;117(9):1189–200.
121. Hendrikx M, Hensen K, Clijsters C, et al. Recovery of regional but not global contractile function by the direct Intramyocardial autologous bone marrow transplantation. Circulation. 2006;114(1_supplement):I-101-I-107.
122. Ang K-L, Chin D, Leyva F, et al. Randomized, controlled trial of intramuscular or intracoronary injection of autologous bone marrow cells into scarred myocardium during CABG versus CABG alone. Nat Clin Pract Cardiovasc Med. 2008;5(10):663–70.
123. Pätilä T, Lehtinen M, Vento A, et al. Autologous bone marrow mononuclear cell transplantation in ischemic heart failure: a prospective, controlled, randomized, double-blind study of cell transplantation combined with coronary bypass. J Heart Lung Transplant. 2014;33(6):567–74.
124. Perin EC, Willerson JT, Pepine CJ, et al. Effect of Transendocardial delivery of autologous bone marrow mononuclear cells on functional capacity, left ventricular function, and perfusion in chronic heart failure: the FOCUS-CCTRN trial. JAMA. 2012;307(16)
125. Heldman AW, Difede DL, Fishman JE, et al. Transendocardial mesenchymal stem cells and mononuclear bone marrow cells for ischemic cardiomyopathy: the TAC-HFT randomized trial. JAMA. 2014;311(1):62–73.
126. Povsic TJ, Henry TD, Traverse JH, et al. The RENEW trial: efficacy and safety of Intramyocardial autologous CD34+ cell administration in patients with refractory angina. J Am Coll Cardiol Intv. 2016;9(15):1576–85.
127. Stamm C, Kleine H-D, Choi Y-H, et al. Intramyocardial delivery of CD133+ bone marrow cells and coronary artery bypass grafting for chronic ischemic heart disease: safety and efficacy studies. J Thorac Cardiovasc Surg. 2007;133(3):717–25.e715.
128. Nasseri BA, Ebell W, Dandel M, et al. Autologous CD133+ bone marrow cells and bypass grafting for regeneration of ischaemic myocardium: the Cardio133 trial. Eur Heart J. 2014;35(19):1263–74.

129. Noiseux N, Mansour S, Weisel R et al., The IMPACT-CABG trial: a multicenter, randomized clinical trial of CD133+ stem cell therapy during coronary artery bypass grafting for ischemic cardiomyopathy. J Thorac Cardiovasc Surg. 2016;152(6):1582–8.e1582.
130. Mathiasen AB, Qayyum AA, Jørgensen E, et al. Bone marrow-derived mesenchymal stromal cell treatment in patients with severe ischaemic heart failure: a randomized placebo-controlled trial (MSC-HF trial). Eur Heart J. 2015;36(27):1744–53.
131. Bartunek J, Terzic A, Davison BA, et al. Cardiopoietic cell therapy for advanced ischaemic heart failure: results at 39 weeks of the prospective, randomized, double blind, sham-controlled CHART-1 clinical trial. Eur Heart J. 2017;38(9):648–60.
132. Butler J, Epstein Stephen E, Greene Stephen J, et al. Intravenous allogeneic mesenchymal stem cells for nonischemic cardiomyopathy. Circ Res. 2017;120(2):332–40.
133. Perin Emerson C, Borow Kenneth M, Silva Guilherme V, et al. A phase II dose-escalation study of allogeneic mesenchymal precursor cells in patients with ischemic or nonischemic heart failure. Circ Res. 2015;117(6):576–84.
134. Chugh AR, Beache GM, Loughran JH, et al. Administration of cardiac stem cells in patients with ischemic cardiomyopathy: the SCIPIO trial: surgical aspects and interim analysis of myocardial function and viability by magnetic resonance. Circulation. 2012;126(11 Suppl 1):S54–64.
135. Malliaras K, Makkar RR, Smith RR, et al. Intracoronary Cardiosphere-derived cells after myocardial infarction: evidence of therapeutic regeneration in the final 1-year results of the CADUCEUS trial (CArdiosphere-derived aUtologous stem CElls to reverse ventricUlar dySfunction). J Am Coll Cardiol. 2014;63(2):110–22.
136. Menasché P, Vanneaux V, Hagège A, et al. Transplantation of human embryonic stem cell–derived cardiovascular progenitors for severe ischemic left ventricular dysfunction. J Am Coll Cardiol. 2018;71(4):429–38.
137. Der Sarkissian S, Lévesque T, Noiseux N. Optimizing stem cells for cardiac repair: current status and new frontiers in regenerative cardiology. World J Stem Cells. 2017;9(1):9–25.
138. Hodgetts SI, Beilharz MW, Scalzo AA, Grounds MD. Why do cultured transplanted myoblasts die in vivo? DNA quantification shows enhanced survival of donor male myoblasts in host mice depleted of CD4+ and CD8+ cells or NK1.1+ cells. Cell Transplant. 2000;9(4):489–502.
139. Chiarugi P, Giannoni E. Anoikis: a necessary death program for anchorage-dependent cells. Biochem Pharmacol. 2008;76(11):1352–64.
140. Chong JJH, Yang X, Don CW, et al. Human embryonic-stem-cell-derived cardiomyocytes regenerate non-human primate hearts. Nature. 2014;510(7504):273–7.
141. Shiba Y, Filice D, Fernandes S, et al. Electrical integration of human embryonic stem cell-derived cardiomyocytes in a Guinea pig chronic infarct model. J Cardiovasc Pharmacol Ther. 2014;19(4):368–81.
142. Leri A, Kajstura J, Anversa P, Frishman WH. Myocardial regeneration and stem cell repair. Curr Probl Cardiol. 2008;33(3):91–153.
143. Singh A, Singh A, Sen D. Mesenchymal stem cells in cardiac regeneration: a detailed progress report of the last 6 years (2010-2015). Stem Cell Res Ther. 2016;7(1):82.
144. Tang YL, Zhu W, Cheng M, et al. Hypoxic preconditioning enhances the benefit of cardiac progenitor cell therapy for treatment of myocardial infarction by inducing CXCR4 expression. Circ Res. 2009;104(10):1209–16.
145. Theus MH, Wei L, Cui L, et al. In vitro hypoxic preconditioning of embryonic stem cells as a strategy of promoting cell survival and functional benefits after transplantation into the ischemic rat brain. Exp Neurol. 2008;210(2):656–70.
146. Zhang J, Chen G-H, Wang Y-W, et al. Hydrogen peroxide preconditioning enhances the therapeutic efficacy of Wharton's Jelly mesenchymal stem cells after myocardial infarction. Chin Med J. 2012;125(19):3472–8.
147. Su C-Y, Chong K-Y, Chen J, Ryter S, Khardori R, Lai C-C. A physiologically relevant hyperthermia selectively activates constitutive hsp70 in H9c2 cardiac myoblasts and confers oxidative protection. J Mol Cell Cardiol. 1999;31(4):845–55.

148. Haider KH, Ashraf M. Chapter 15 – preconditioning approach in stem cell therapy for the treatment of infarcted heart. In: Tang Y, editor. Progress in molecular biology and translational science. Cambridge, MA: Academic Press. 2012. p. 323–56.

149. Sato T, Li Y, Saito T, Nakaya H. Minoxidil opens mitochondrial K(ATP) channels and confers cardioprotection. Br J Pharmacol. 2004;141(2):360–6.

150. Niagara Muhammad I, Haider Husnain K, Jiang S, Ashraf M. Pharmacologically preconditioned skeletal myoblasts are resistant to oxidative stress and promote Angiomyogenesis via release of paracrine factors in the infarcted heart. Circ Res. 2007;100(4):545–55.

151. Yang Y-J, Qian H-Y, Huang J, et al. Atorvastatin treatment improves survival and effects of implanted mesenchymal stem cells in post-infarct swine hearts. Eur Heart J. 2008;29(12):1578–90.

152. Assmus B, Urbich C, Aicher A, et al. HMG-CoA reductase inhibitors reduce senescence and increase proliferation of endothelial progenitor cells via regulation of cell cycle regulatory genes. Circ Res. 2003;92(9):1049–55.

153. Szeto A, Nation DA, Mendez AJ, et al. Oxytocin attenuates NADPH-dependent superoxide activity and IL-6 secretion in macrophages and vascular cells. Am J Physiol Endocrinol Metab. 2008;295(6):E1495–501.

154. Cattaneo MG, Lucci G, Vicentini LM. Oxytocin stimulates in vitro angiogenesis via a Pyk-2/Src-dependent mechanism. Exp Cell Res. 2009;315(18):3210–9.

155. Wisel S, Khan M, Kuppusamy ML, et al. Pharmacological preconditioning of mesenchymal stem cells with trimetazidine (1-[2,3,4-trimethoxybenzyl]piperazine) protects hypoxic cells against oxidative stress and enhances recovery of myocardial function in infarcted heart through Bcl-2 expression. J Pharmacol Exp Ther. 2009;329(2):543–50.

156. Čížková D, Rosocha J, Vanický I, Radonák J, Gálik J, Čížek M. Induction of mesenchymal stem cells leads to HSP72 synthesis and higher resistance to oxidative stress. Neurochem Res. 2006;31(8):1011–20.

157. Imai Y, Adachi Y, Shi M, et al. Caspase inhibitor ZVAD-fmk facilitates engraftment of donor hematopoietic stem cells in intra–bone marrow–bone marrow transplantation. Stem Cells Dev. 2009;19(4):461–8.

158. Kanemitsu N, Tambara K, Premaratne GU, et al. Insulin-like growth Factor-1 enhances the efficacy of myoblast transplantation with its multiple functions in the chronic myocardial infarction rat model. J Heart Lung Transplant. 2006;25(10):1253–62.

159. Duan H-F, Wu C-T, Wu D-L, et al. Treatment of myocardial ischemia with bone marrow-derived mesenchymal stem cells overexpressing hepatocyte growth factor. Mol Ther. 2003;8(3):467–74.

160. Murry CE, Kay MA, Bartosek T, Hauschka SD, Schwartz SM. Muscle differentiation during repair of myocardial necrosis in rats via gene transfer with MyoD. J Clin Invest. 1996;98(10):2209–17.

161. Payne TR, Oshima H, Okada M, et al. A relationship between vascular endothelial growth factor, angiogenesis, and cardiac repair after muscle stem cell transplantation into ischemic hearts. J Am Coll Cardiol. 2007;50(17):1677–84.

162. Gnecchi M, He H, Noiseux N, et al. Evidence supporting paracrine hypothesis for Akt-modified mesenchymal stem cell-mediated cardiac protection and functional improvement. FASEB J. 2006;20(6):661–9.

163. Song H, Chang W, Lim S, et al. Tissue transglutaminase is essential for integrin-mediated survival of bone marrow-derived mesenchymal stem cells. Stem Cells. 2007;25(6):1431–8.

164. Cho H-J, Youn S-W, Cheon S-I, et al. Regulation of endothelial cell and endothelial progenitor cell survival and vasculogenesis by integrin-linked kinase. Arterioscler Thromb Vasc Biol. 2005;25(6):1154–60.

165. Conboy IM, Conboy MJ, Wagers AJ, Girma ER, Weissman IL, Rando TA. Rejuvenation of aged progenitor cells by exposure to a young systemic environment. Nature. 2005;433(7027):760–4.

166. Chimenti C, Kajstura J, Torella D, et al. Senescence and death of primitive cells and myocytes Lead to premature cardiac aging and heart failure. Circ Res. 2003;93(7):604–13.
167. Fan M, Chen W, Liu W, et al. The effect of age on the efficacy of human mesenchymal stem cell transplantation after a myocardial infarction. Rejuvenation Res. 2010;13(4):429–38.
168. Muraski JA, Rota M, Misao Y, et al. Pim-1 regulates cardiomyocyte survival downstream of Akt. Nat Med. 2007;13(12):1467–75.
169. Brunt KR, Zhang Y, Mihic A, et al. Role of WNT/β-catenin signaling in rejuvenating myogenic differentiation of aged mesenchymal stem cells from cardiac patients. Am J Pathol. 2012;181(6):2067–78.
170. Cameron CM, Hu W-S, Kaufman DS. Improved development of human embryonic stem cell-derived embryoid bodies by stirred vessel cultivation. Biotechnol Bioeng. 2006;94(5):938–48.

Chapter 15
Stem Cell Therapy for Stroke

S. M. Robert and C. Matouk

15.1 Introduction

Stroke is a leading cause of death and disability worldwide. In recent years, the mortality rate of ischemic stroke has sharply decreased as a result of significant treatment advances. However, the incidence of this disease has not declined at the same pace; therefore, there exists a growing stroke burden in terms of disability and economic costs, as more patients are living with the physical sequelae of stroke [23].

Ischemic stroke comprises over 80% of the total number of strokes and occurs when blood supply to the brain is interrupted. This phenomenon is typically caused by thrombosis within a blood vessel, which interrupts normal blood flow supplying a region of brain tissue. Underlying medical conditions such as hypertension, atrial fibrillation, and diabetes, among others, all increase the risk of ischemic stroke. Acute strokes, if brought to medical attention quickly, can be treated by administration of tissue plasminogen activator (tPA) to dissolve the blood clot in the vessel and/or by direct removal of the clot through mechanical thrombectomy. Unfortunately, many patients do not receive these interventions as they do not reach medical attention within the required time frame, there is ambiguity of timing of symptom onset, or the medical center to which they present is not capable of performing the more advanced, invasive therapy of clot retrieval. As expected, these patients tend to have significant disability post-stroke. Of the patients that are fully revascularized (the blood clot is fully removed from the vessel and normal flow is restored), many still have significant disability as a result of the damage the brain endures prior to restoration of blood flow [38].

Common disabilities from stroke include hemiparesis or hemiplegia (weakness or paralysis of one side of the body) contralateral to the side of the stroke, problems with attention, learning, judgment, and/or memory. Damage to the dominant side

S. M. Robert · C. Matouk (✉)
Department of Neurosurgery, Yale University School of Medicine, New Haven, CT, USA
e-mail: stephanie.robert@yale.edu; charles.matouk@yale.edu

© Springer Nature Switzerland AG 2021
T. P. Navarro et al. (eds.), *Stem Cell Therapy for Vascular Diseases*,
https://doi.org/10.1007/978-3-030-56954-9_15

of the brain (most often the left side) can cause significant difficulties with speech and language. For patients with the largest territory strokes, a decreased level of consciousness and a coma-like state may require the placement of tracheostomies and permanent feeding tubes and permanent placement in long-term nursing facilities.

Although advances in acute stroke care and post-stroke neurorehabilitation have proven effective in improving some neurological function, no approved therapies currently exist to reliably reverse residual deficits in stroke patients. Significant research efforts are focused on developing new approaches to restore damaged brain tissue and improve function in this patient population. One of the most promising avenues of current research is in cell-based therapies, specifically administration of stem cells to the post-stroke brain. This therapeutic approach is attractive due to stem cells multipotent, neuroprotective, and immunomodulatory potential. Preclinical and clinical studies are promising, with evidence of functional improvement in animal models and patients. Although a fast-growing area of investigation, many questions regarding the safety, efficacy, and appropriate clinical application in humans remain. This chapter reviews the most common stem cell-based therapies being investigated for ischemic stroke, describes the recent preclinical and clinical studies being performed, and discusses the current and future applications of this therapy for treatment of stroke patients.

15.2   Stem Cell-Based Therapies for Ischemic Stroke

Ischemic stroke causes extensive damage to multiple types of brain cells, as well as neuronal and vascular networks. Current treatments are effective in restoring blood flow through undamaged blood vessels; however, they are not effective at reversing the damage incurred during the period of ischemia before revascularization. Without further medical intervention, many stroke patients are able to gain some degree of functional recovery over time, suggesting that innate compensatory plasticity or remodeling may occur in the post-ischemic brain. Stem cell-based approaches gained momentum with the objective of enhancing this assumed endogenous repair mechanism or, as initially hypothesized, to replace injured cells in the ischemic core. However, current studies are beginning to suggest that several different mechanisms play a role in the neuroregeneration seen with stem cell therapies, including acting in a neuroprotective manner and by inducing angiogenesis, neurogenesis, and axonal sprouting [26], among others.

Over the past decade, cell-based regenerative therapies have been developed using different types of stem/progenitor cells in the attempt to restore lost brain tissue and function. Several types of stem cells have been investigated for use in this therapy, mainly mesenchymal (MSC), neural (NSC), embryonic (ESC), and induced pluripotent stem cells (iPSCs). Although data on these stem cell-based therapies in animal models and human patients are conflicting, many studies suggest an important role for cellular-based therapy for stroke.

15.2.1   Mesenchymal Stem Cells

Mesenchymal stem cells (MSCs) are pluripotent progenitor cells that give rise to a variety of tissues, including muscle, bone, cartilage, and adipose. The most widely studied source of MSCs in stroke therapy is bone marrow-derived cells, as it was hypothesized early on that these MSCs could differentiate into brain cells. Studies have confirmed that bone marrow-derived mesenchymal stem cells (BMSCs) are capable of differentiating into neural cell lineages and have been shown to express neuronal and glial markers upon differentiation [26, 40, 53]. BMSCs promote synaptogenesis, stimulate nerve regeneration, and improve motor function in animal models of ischemia [29, 40]. Furthermore, it is hypothesized that the more important mechanisms underlying the functional recovery observed is due to the effect of transplanted cells on neuroprotection, stimulation of regeneration, expression of cytokines and/or growth factors, and angiogenesis, rather than direct integration of the transplanted cells into damaged host networks [40].

15.2.2   Neural Stem Cells

Neural stem cells (NSCs) persist in the adult brain in the subgranular zone of the dentate gyrus of the hippocampus and subventricular zone of the third ventricle. They are multipotent cells that give rise to neurons and glial cells. In rodent models of hypoxia, NSCs are able to establish functional connections with innate neurons, develop into mature neurons and glial cells, and demonstrate some functional recovery in the animals observed [30, 52]. Furthermore, neuroimaging studies in rats have shown reduction of infarct volume which corresponds to improvements in behavioral testing [49]. These effects have been shown to occur through several mechanisms, including neuronal replacement, modulation of synaptic plasticity, enhanced neuroprotection, changes in inflammatory mediated processes, and stimulation of angiogenesis.

Although NSCs have shown promise for stroke therapy, their use has significant limitations in human therapies. Human stem cells are needed for implantation into stroke patients, and the main source of these cells is from fetal tissue. In addition to a limited availability of cells, this approach raises important and difficult ethical issues, which has impacted the ability to translate this research to human application. Studies have shown successful in vitro propagation of human fetal NSCs for an extended period of time with successful implantation and differentiation into the ischemic cortex of rats [18], requiring fewer human cells; regardless, much debate still surrounds the use of fetal tissue for medical therapies.

Interestingly, some of the functional recovery observed in post-stroke patients may be, in part, due to stimulation of innate adult NSCs after ischemic stroke. A few studies in rodents, primates, and humans suggest generation of new neurons from persistent host NSCs [4, 32, 54, 55] and hypothesize that they may play an important role in the post-ischemic brain. The functional significance of this neurogenesis remains unclear; however, these findings raise new possibilities for development of stem cell stimulation therapies and even potential transplantation of adult NSCs in stroke patients.

15.2.3 Embryonic Stem Cells

Embryonic stem cells are pluripotent cells derived from blastocysts 4–5 days after fertilization. These cells are valuable in that they are capable of unlimited and undifferentiated proliferation [51]. They readily differentiate into neuronal and glial elements, including astrocytes and oligodendrocytes. In vivo studies have shown that implanted rodent ESCs survive, migrate into ischemic tissue and can restore synaptic connections with improvement in behavioral deficits [11, 50, 58].

Similar to NSCs, however, production and use of ESCs raise challenging issues. Isolation of human ESCs requires destruction of a blastocyst and therefore again raises ethical issues as discussed above; however, cells can be captured from unused fertilized embryos from in vitro fertilization procedures and maintained in culture for use, potentially lessening the controversy surrounding their origination. However, as a result of their robust ability to propagate and transform, this risk of tumor formation after implantation is high [42]. One method developed to decrease this risk is the pre-differentiation of ESCs into NPCs that are restricted to neural cell lines upon differentiation, which has some efficacy once implanted into rodent models [17].

15.2.4 Induced Pluripotent Stem Cells

An important and recent advancement in this field has been the development of human-induced pluripotent stem cells (iPSCs). This technology allows pluripotent cells to be created by reprogramming a host patient's own somatic cells, which are easily obtained from a blood sample or connective tissue biopsy. The use of a patient's own tissue sample for this therapy alleviates much of the ethical concerns surrounding the previously discussed stem cell-based treatments. Using specific transcriptional factors, cells can be reprogrammed [48] and induced to form specific cell types, including induced pluripotent stem cell-derived neural stem cells (iNSCs) [28]. As a distinct advantage, these cells exhibit the properties of ESCs and NSC and are less likely to undergo immune system rejection [3].

Given their capacity for proliferation and differentiation, tumorigenicity is a significant concern with iPSCs. To address this issue, researchers have developed induced pluripotent stem cell-derived neural stem cells (iNSCs), which retain their ability to differentiate into neural cells, with significantly decreased tumorigenicity compared to iPSCs. These iNSCs are showing promise in neuroprotection and regeneration after stroke [12]. A recent paper using an ischemic pig stroke model demonstrated reduced white matter, cerebral perfusion, and metabolism changes on magnetic resonance imaging (MRI) in animals implanted with iNSC implantation after induced stroke. The implanted cells differentiated into neurons, astrocytes, and oligodendrocytes, demonstrated long-term integration, promoted decreased microglial activation, and stimulated neurogenesis [7, 36]. Other studies using rodent models demonstrate similar findings [39, 41, 56].

15.3 Stem Cell Therapy Mechanisms of Action

The mechanism by which transplanted stem cells exert therapeutic effects is an area of active research. Initially, the hypothesis was that the engrafted cells would replace the lost cells in the ischemic core of the infarcted brain tissue and restore function. However, as research in this area continues to shed light on the interactions of these stem cells and the damaged brain, it is becoming clear that the interactions are much more complicated than initially imagined.

Neuronal replacement remains one of the main focuses of stem cell-based therapies, and many studies demonstrate synaptic connections between host and implanted cells, as well as functional integration of grafted neurons. The establishment of axial projections and synaptic connections in unaffected animal models has been demonstrated in multiple studies. Steinbeck et al. recently demonstrated that after implantation of ESCs into the motor cortex of the normal adult rodent brain, axons of donor neurons extended via the external and internal capsule to the cervical spinal cord and through the corpus callosum into the contralateral cortex, where they made functional synaptic connections with host neurons [47]. A recent study in a rodent stroke model using iPSCs showed motor improvement after transplantation of cells into stroke-damaged cortex. The cells differentiated into mature neurons, sent axonal projections to unaffected brain tissue, and exhibited appropriate electrophysiological and synaptic input signals from host neurons [39].

Interestingly, Oki et al. argue that the initial motor improvements observed in their animal model post-transplantation was likely due to increased vascular endothelial growth factor (VEGF) levels and resulting improvement in endogenous plasticity rather than neuronal replacement. Further studies corroborate VEGF as an important growth factor, stimulating neovascularization, enhanced integrity of the blood-brain barrier, axonal plasticity, and suppression of the inflammatory response, glial scar formation, and neuronal apoptosis [2, 5, 16, 27].

Preclinical studies of NSC implantation support the immunomodulatory effects of stem cells as a significant mechanism contributing to the beneficial effects seen with this therapy. In the ischemic brain, activation of microglia, the resident immune cells of the brain, causes a robust inflammatory response. Minutes after the onset of ischemia, many pro-inflammatory cytokines are produced. These cytokines also induce opening of the blood-brain barrier and infiltration of peripheral macrophages, further exacerbating the immune response and resulting injury [14]. NSCs dampen this inflammatory response by the release of neurotrophic factors such as brain-derived neurotrophic factor (BDNF) and glial-derived neurotrophic factor [40]. Minimizing the immune response in the post-stroke brain has been shown to correlate with decreased infarct volume and improved functional recovery [14, 40].

Although most evidence for stem cell-mediated effects come from studies of direct implantation of cells into the post-infarcted brain, a few studies have found NSC culture-conditioned media alone may provide a neuroprotective effect and resulting behavioral improvements in animals [19, 57, 61]. Webb et al. demonstrated extracellular vesicles from NSC conditioned media were sufficient to alter the immune response, reduce lesion size, and improve motor outcomes in mice [57]. The advantage of NSC extracellular vesicle-based therapy is largely due to their limited tumorigenicity and enhanced biodistribution. However, further data are needed to determine if this type of acellular therapy will be effective in stroke patients.

15.4 Stem Cell Therapy in Experimental Stroke Models

Preclinical research on cell therapy for stroke began in the 1980s, when Mampalam et al. demonstrated the ability to graft cells from a fetal rat cortex to be successfully implanted into the ischemic cortex of an adult rat [37]. The study not only showed survival of the fetal cells but also demonstrated integration of these cells into the damaged host brain. As animal studies advanced, further evidence suggested implanted cells survived and integrated into ischemic brain tissue and, in some cases, stimulated anatomical reconstruction and behavioral recovery in the post-stroke brain.

Early on in this field, given their capacity to differentiate into a variety of neural cell types, the use of NCS and ESC quickly gained momentum. However, advancement to clinical application slowed after the recognition that allogenic transplantation (i.e., implanting stem cells from the same species) is safer and likely more effective. Difficulties in obtaining human-derived (fetal and embryonic) cells, confounded by the ethical challenges surrounding their harvesting, significantly slowed translation of preclinical research to patient trials. The late 1990s ban placed on the use of federal funds for research on embryonic tissue further discouraged the translation of preclinical advancements to clinical studies using human-derived embryonic and neural stem cells.

Given these constraints, adult stem cells became the focus of most studies, and specifically bone marrow-derived MSCs emerged as the commonly used adult source of these cells. BMSCs promote synaptogenesis, stimulate nerve regeneration, and improve motor function in animal models of ischemia [29, 40]. The use of MSCs has been widely studied in stroke, and although these studies vary in the source (human, rodent), route of administration (intracerebral, intraarterial, intrathecal), and timing of introduction (in relationship to the stroke onset), most of the published data show some positive effect on infarct volume or behavioral testing, or at the molecular level with changes associated with positive neurological benefits [62].

The most recent and significant advancement in the stem cell field has been the development of iPSC technology. Although in its infancy, there is significant focus on using iPSC as well as neuronal stem cells derived from iPSCs (iNSC) for stroke therapies. This technology appears to be a promising alternative that provides cells with the differentiation capability of NCS/ESC, with fewer ethical issues and minimal difficulty with harvesting. Recent studies have found implantation of iPSCs/iNSCs into infarcted tissue leads to reduction in infarct volume and improvement in functional recovery in animal models. Some studies attribute these effects to these cells' ability to differentiate into adult stem cells after implantation [31, 56]. Human iPSCs implanted into ischemic cortex of rodents also show differentiation to neurons of different subtypes and exhibit electrophysiological properties of mature neurons [39]. Studies in a pig ischemic stroke model using iPSCs and iNSC have demonstrated decreased immune response, enhanced neuroprotection, increased neurogenesis, and functional recovery in treated animals [6, 7, 36].

15.4.1 Preclinical Models

Most preclinical studies on stroke pathology and treatment have relied on small animal models, specifically using rodents, given the ease of use and cost-effectiveness of these models. Although much of the field has advanced using these small animals, there has been difficulty translating novel therapeutics to the development of beneficial clinical treatments. Some propose this translational gap can be better addressed by a greater emphasis on the use of large animal models, specifically pigs, and sheep, and nonhuman primates. These animals have large gyrencephalic brains, which are more similar to the structure of human brains compared to the small lissencephalic brains of rodents. The lack of gyri and sulci in the brains of mice and rats, and therefore more simplified cortical structure and functional organization, as well as vascular anatomy, likely confounds the response of these animals to ischemic stroke and their response to the studied therapeutics. Larger animal models with more human-like brain structures are now being used more readily and often are becoming a key step of verification prior to introduction of novel therapies into humans [46]. Used in combination with initial studies in rodents, a greater use of large animal models will likely contribute to advancing therapeutic interventions and better predicting which therapies will likely have a clinical impact prior to testing in humans.

15.5 Clinical Studies on Stem Cell Implantation

Although hundreds of preclinical studies have been published over the past few decades showing positive results for stem cell-based therapies in animal models, many unique challenges exist in the translation of this therapy into human studies.

In addition to the high cost and extended timelines for such studies, the harvesting and/or production of stem cells remains difficult and limited. Furthermore, preclinical studies have not successfully answered important questions including ideal route of administration and most effective source of stem cells to be used; therefore, these questions are being addressed by the clinical trials, in addition to safety and effectiveness. Importantly, although initial studies support the safety profile of this therapy, the potential adverse outcomes, specifically tumor formation and/or immune rejection, are significant and must be addressed [34].

Most clinical studies involve MSCs due to their well-studied and beneficial effects in in vitro *and* in vivo models. Initial trials using bone marrow MSCs (BMSCs) have also proven safe for human use. The first pilot study to introduce MSCs in stroke patients was in 2005 by Bang et al., and although a small study, they found improved functional recovery in the treated group [8]. The InVeST trial, which did not show a beneficial treatment effect, provided valuable evidence that intravenous infusion of BMSCs is safe and well tolerated in humans [43]. Similarly, the MASTERS trial, a phase 2, randomized, double-blinded, placebo-controlled study, showed no dose-limiting toxicity but also showed no significant improvement after 90 days [24]. The first clinical trial to investigate the intracranial implantation of neural stem cells, called PISCES, also supported the safety profile of stem cell transplants in patients and, furthermore, showed some neurological improvement in treated patients [33]. More recent studies being published continue to show safety and improvement in neurological function in patients [38].

A recent systematic review and meta-analysis of the literature regarding stem cell transplantation in patients after brain ischemia determined the therapy significantly improved neurological deficits and quality of life without serious adverse events [13]. However, although initial data are encouraging, larger studies are still needed to further investigate the safety and effectiveness of this treatment before it becomes widely used in the clinical setting.

15.6 Endogenous Stem Cell Therapy

Although most studies looking at stem cells in stroke are focused on implanting cells into the post-stroke brain, a few groups are exploring options to take advantage of the capacity of the adult brain for self-repair. Neurogenesis in the adult brain is located mainly in the subventricular zone (SVZ) of the lateral ventricles and the subgranular zone (SGZ) of the dentate gyrus, as well as the olfactory bulb [20]. Pathological processes, such as ischemia, that cause neuronal death have been found to stimulate new neuronal formation in these areas. Arvidsson et al. found that these newly developed endogenous neurons from the SVZ are able to migrate into damaged striatum in rodent models. However, they also noted that the majority of the new neurons died within 2 weeks after stroke, likely indicating an unfavorable environment to support these new cells in the post-ischemic brain [4]. In two studies, Tonchev et al. demonstrated increased proliferation of neuronal progenitor cells in the dentate gyrus, subventricular zone, and hippocampus in post-ischemic monkey brains [54, 55]. These results were translated to the human brain by Jin et al., when they demonstrated similar findings in human brain biopsies of ischemic strokes [32]. Immunohistochemical staining of these specimens showed new neurons with a migratory phenotype in the ischemic penumbra. They also demonstrated that in the stroke brain tissue, new neurons tended to cluster near blood vessels, suggesting vascular endothelial cells promote neurogenesis [32]. However, it appears from these studies that the number of newly generated neurons is low and does not represent a large enough population of cells to induce a significant therapeutic response. Factors that stimulate production as well as induce a supportive and protective brain environment for growth and survival of these cells are an active area of research. Granulocyte-colony stimulating factor (G-CSF) is one of these mechanisms and has been shown to reduce infarct volume in experimental models of ischemia, act as a neuroprotective mechanism by reducing glutamate release, inflammation, and apoptosis activation, among others. Administration of G-CSF immediately after middle cerebral artery occlusion in a rodent model immediately after and in the subacute period both showed increase in proliferation of endogenous stem cells in the post-stroke brain [1]. Studies are also investigating the effect of transplanted NSCs on endogenous neurogenic behavior, with some evidence suggesting enhancement of neurogenesis through secretion of neurotrophic and regenerative growth factors [6].

15.7   Important Considerations for Stem Cell-Based Therapies

Although much of the data from completed and ongoing clinical trials appear promising, most of the trials remain small, and many questions remain unanswered. Specifically, the most effective stem cell type, ideal route of administration, and timing of administration are active areas of research. Furthermore, important considerations with this therapy also include consideration of potential adverse events, including malignant potential and immunogenicity, as well as beneficial adjuvant treatments that may enhance the therapeutic effect of this therapy.

15.7.1   Selection of Stem Cell Type

Of the main types of stem cells investigated for use in stroke therapy, MSCs have been the most widely studied, in both preclinical and clinical trials. Given the ethical and sourcing issues of ESCs and NSCs, research using these cell types has lagged behind MSCs, and with the introduction of iPSCs, much of this research is being replaced given the advantages of this new technology. iPSCs have shown promise and ease of use, especially with the ability to differentiate them into iNSCs prior to transplantation. As the field advances and new technologies are introduced, a standardized type and readily available source will likely be developed for use in clinical therapies.

15.7.2 Route of Administration

Different routes of stem cell administration have been used, with the most common being intravascular (venous and arterial) and intraparenchymal routes [34]. Less common routes investigated include intracerebroventricular, intracisternal, intrathecal, and intraperitoneal routes [59]. The intravascular route has been mostly used for administration of MSCs. It is the least invasive and allows the introduction of a large number of cells. However, the delivery is non-specific, and although cells are able to migrate into ischemic regions, the number that were deposited in the brain was significantly less than the number of injected cells, and cells have been found to distribute into multiple other peripheral organs [15, 35]. Newer technologies are addressing this issue using mechanisms such as magnets and fibrin glue to target cells to the ischemic brain regions [14, 45]. Song et al. (2015) demonstrated that intravenously delivered, magnetically targeted NSCs accumulated in the ischemic brain and correlated to decreased infarct size compared to non-targeted NSCs, suggesting that targeting cells into the damaged tissue may be advantageous.

Intraparenchymal transplantation is more invasive and requires injecting a cell suspension directly into the brain tissue. However, this route allows precise control over cell placement and avoids the issue of cells distributing into peripheral organs. Some studies suggest better functional improvement with this technique [25]. Further consideration must also be given to the timing of cell therapy in determining the most effective route of administration. In subacute and chronic strokes, the blood-brain barrier is less permeable than in acute stroke [22], which would likely render intravenous therapies less effective. Although different routes have been investigated and compared, no optimal route of administration has yet been determined [44, 59], and there is little evidence for a specific route having a positive effect on patient outcome.

15.7.3 Malignant Potential

One of the most important considerations regarding the use of stem cells for any therapy is the potential for the cells to undergo malignant transformation and allow tumor formation in the host. Overall MSCs appear to be safe upon implantation into animal models and humans; however, several studies have shown the potential for tumorigenic transformation of iPSCs. Teratomas were found to develop in mice brains after implantation, and it is suggested that specific transcription factors contribute to the tumorigenic potential of iPSCs. The presence of undifferentiated cells may trigger tumor formation [21, 38, 60]. Given the ability for iPSCs to be transformed further into multipotent cells, researchers have found that differentiating them into neural stem cells (iNSCs) decreases the tumorigenicity significantly while maintaining their therapeutic potential [12].

15.7.4 Adjuvant Therapies

Biomaterials are being investigated for enhancing delivery of cells and improving post-implantation survival. This technology provides a scaffold for transplanted cells, as well as growth factors and other biochemical signals that could stimulate tissue restoration and neuronal differentiation. Although preclinical studies suggest improved survival and differentiation of implanted cells, it remains unclear if there is any benefit in functional outcome using this technology, and further studies are need to understand what adverse effects may be caused by introduction of these biomaterials in humans [9].

15.7.5 Neurorehabilitation

Neurorehabilitation is an important component of post-stroke therapy and can significantly improve the neurological function of patients. This is important to consider when designing clinical trials. Many initial studies, especially preclinical, did not take into account the potential benefits of patient improvement with rehabilitation. However, more attention is being drawn to this issue, and it is being encouraged in the literature and at the recent Stem Cell Therapeutics as an Emerging Paradigm for Stroke (STEP3) meeting to include rehabilitation therapy as part of clinical trials using stem cell therapy [10].

15.8 Conclusion

Much of the data from preclinical and clinical trials appears promising for stem cell therapy in stroke patients. However, it is important to acknowledge that most trials are, in general, small cohorts of patients, and therefore results should be interpreted conservatively. Larger and more conclusive studies are needed to show clear patient benefit before stem cell-based therapies become widely used clinically. Furthermore, as a recently developed technology, the transition from preclinical to clinical trials for iPSCs has not occurred. Many questions remain regarding their potential benefit for stroke treatment in a clinical setting. Stem cell therapy is a promising technology that continues to advance and will likely offer new treatment paradigms in the future.

Bibliography

1. Abe K, Yamashita T, Takizawa S, Kuroda S, Kinouchi H, Kawahara N. Stem cell therapy for cerebral ischemia: from basic science to clinical applications. J Cereb Blood Flow Metab. 2012;32(7):1317–31.
2. Andres RH, Horie N, Slikker W, Keren-Gill H, Zhan K, Sun G, Manley NC, Pereira MP, Sheikh LA, McMillan EL, Schaar BT, Svendsen CN, Bliss TM, Steinberg GK. Human neural stem cells enhance structural plasticity and axonal transport in the ischaemic brain. Brain J Neurol. 2011;134(Pt 6):1777–89.
3. Araki R, Uda M, Hoki Y, Sunayama M, Nakamura M, Ando S, Sugiura M, Ideno H, Shimada A, Nifuji A, Abe M. Negligible immunogenicity of terminally differentiated cells derived from induced pluripotent or embryonic stem cells. Nature. 2013;494(7435):100–4.
4. Arvidsson A, Collin T, Kirik D, Kokaia Z, Lindvall O. Neuronal replacement from endogenous precursors in the adult brain after stroke. Nat Med. 2002;8(9):963–70.
5. Bacigaluppi M, Pluchino S, Peruzzotti-Jametti L, Kilic E, Kilic U, Salani G, Brambilla E, West MJ, Comi G, Martino G, Hermann DM. Delayed post-ischaemic neuroprotection following systemic neural stem cell transplantation involves multiple mechanisms. Brain J Neurol. 2009;132(Pt 8):2239–51.
6. Baker EW, Kinder HA, West FD. Neural stem cell therapy for stroke: a multimechanistic approach to restoring neurological function. Brain Behav. 2019;9(3):e01214.
7. Baker EW, Platt SR, Lau VW, Grace HE, Holmes SP, Wang L, Duberstein KJ, Howerth EW, Kinder HA, Stice SL, Hess DC, Mao H, West FD. Induced pluripotent stem cell-derived neural stem cell therapy enhances recovery in an ischemic stroke Pig Model. Sci Rep. 2017;7(1):10075.
8. Bang OY, Lee JS, Lee PH, Lee G. Autologous mesenchymal stem cell transplantation in stroke patients. Ann Neurol. 2005;57(6):874–82.
9. Boltze J, Modo MM, Mays RW, Taguchi A, Jolkkonen J, Savitz SI, STEPS 4 Consortium. Stem cells as an emerging paradigm in stroke 4: advancing and accelerating preclinical research. Stroke. 2019;50(11):3299–306.
10. Borlongan CV, Jolkkonen J, Detante O. The future of stem cell therapy for stroke rehabilitation. Future Neurol. 2015;10:313.
11. Bühnemann C, Scholz A, Bernreuther C, Malik CY, Braun H, Schachner M, Reymann KG, Dihné M. Neuronal differentiation of transplanted embryonic stem cell-derived precursors in stroke lesions of adult rats. Brain J Neurol. 2006;129(Pt 12):3238–48.
12. Chang D-J, Lee N, Park I-H, Choi C, Jeon I, Kwon J, Oh S-H, Shin DA, Do JT, Lee DR, Lee H, Moon H, Hong KS, Daley GQ, Song J. Therapeutic potential of human induced pluripotent stem cells in experimental stroke. Cell Transplant. 2013;22(8):1427–40.
13. Chen L, Zhang G, Khan AA, Guo X, Gu Y. Clinical efficacy and meta-analysis of stem cell therapies for patients with brain ischemia. Stem Cells Int. 2016;2016:1–8.
14. Chen S-J, Chang C-M, Tsai S-K, Chang Y-L, Chou S-J, Huang S-S, Tai L-K, Chen Y-C, Ku H-H, Li H-Y, Chiou S-H. Functional improvement of focal cerebral ischemia injury by subdural transplantation of induced pluripotent stem cells with fibrin glue. Stem Cells Dev. 2010;19(11):1757–67.
15. Chu K, Kim M, Chae S-H, Jeong S-W, Kang K-S, Jung K-H, Kim J, Kim Y-J, Kang L, Kim SU, Yoon B-W. Distribution and in situ proliferation patterns of intravenously injected immortalized human neural stem-like cells in rats with focal cerebral ischemia. Neurosci Res. 2004;50(4):459–65.
16. Daadi MM, Davis AS, Arac A, Li Z, Maag A-L, Bhatnagar R, Jiang K, Sun G, Wu JC, Steinberg GK. Human neural stem cell grafts modify microglial response and enhance axonal sprouting in neonatal hypoxic-ischemic brain injury. Stroke. 2010;41(3):516–23.
17. Daadi MM, Maag A-L, Steinberg GK. Adherent self-renewable human embryonic stem cell-derived neural stem cell line: functional engraftment in experimental stroke model. PLoS One. 2008;3(2):e1644.

18. Darsalia V, Kallur T, Kokaia Z. Survival, migration and neuronal differentiation of human fetal striatal and cortical neural stem cells grafted in stroke-damaged rat striatum. Eur J Neurosci. 2007;26(3):605–14.

19. Delaloy C, Liu L, Lee J-A, Su H, Shen F, Yang G-Y, Young WL, Ivey KN, Gao F-B. MicroRNA-9 coordinates proliferation and migration of human embryonic stem cell-derived neural progenitors. Cell Stem Cell. 2010;6(4):323–35.

20. Eriksson PS, Perfilieva E, Björk-Eriksson T, Alborn AM, Nordborg C, Peterson DA, Gage FH. Neurogenesis in the adult human hippocampus. Nat Med. 1998;4(11):1313–7.

21. Fu W, Wang SJ, Zhou GD, Liu W, Cao Y, Zhang WJ. Residual undifferentiated cells during differentiation of induced pluripotent stem cells in vitro and in vivo. Stem Cells Dev. 2012;21(4):521–9.

22. Garbuzova-Davis S, Haller E, Williams SN, Haim ED, Tajiri N, Hernandez-Ontiveros DG, Frisina-Deyo A, Boffeli SM, Sanberg PR, Borlongan CV. Compromised blood-brain barrier competence in remote brain areas in ischemic stroke rats at chronic stage. J Comp Neurol. 2014;522:3120.

23. GBD 2016 Stroke Collaborators 2019. Global, regional, and national burden of stroke, 1990-2016: a systematic analysis for the Global Burden of Disease Study. Lancet Neurol. 2016;18(5):439–58.

24. Hess DC, Wechsler LR, Clark WM, Savitz SI, Ford GA, Chiu D, Yavagal DR, Uchino K, Liebeskind DS, Auchus AP, Sen S, Sila CA, Vest JD, Mays RW. Safety and efficacy of multipotent adult progenitor cells in acute ischaemic stroke (MASTERS): a randomised, double-blind, placebo-controlled, phase 2 trial. Lancet Neurol. 2017;16(5):360–8.

25. Hicks AU, Lappalainen RS, Narkilahti S, Suuronen R, Corbett D, Sivenius J, Hovatta O, Jolkkonen J. Transplantation of human embryonic stem cell-derived neural precursor cells and enriched environment after cortical stroke in rats: cell survival and functional recovery. Eur J Neurosci. 2009;29(3):562–74.

26. Honmou O, Onodera R, Sasaki M, Waxman SG, Kocsis JD. Mesenchymal stem cells: therapeutic outlook for stroke. Trends Mol Med. 2012;18(5):292–7.

27. Horie N, Pereira MP, Niizuma K, Sun G, Keren-Gill H, Encarnacion A, Shamloo M, Hamilton SA, Jiang K, Huhn S, Palmer TD, Bliss TM, Steinberg GK. Transplanted stem cell-secreted vascular endothelial growth factor effects poststroke recovery, inflammation, and vascular repair. Stem Cells. 2011;29(2):274–85.

28. Hu B-Y, Weick JP, Yu J, Ma L-X, Zhang X-Q, Thomson JA, Zhang S-C. Neural differentiation of human induced pluripotent stem cells follows developmental principles but with variable potency. Proc Natl Acad Sci U S A. 2010;107(9):4335–40.

29. Huang W, Mo X, Qin C, Zheng J, Liang Z, Zhang C. Transplantation of differentiated bone marrow stromal cells promotes motor functional recovery in rats with stroke. Neurol Res. 2013;35(3):320–8.

30. Ishibashi S, Sakaguchi M, Kuroiwa T, Yamasaki M, Kanemura Y, Shizuko I, Shimazaki T, Onodera M, Okano H, Mizusawa H. Human neural stem/progenitor cells, expanded in long-term neurosphere culture, promote functional recovery after focal ischemia in Mongolian gerbils. J Neurosci Res. 2004;78(2):215–23.

31. Jiang M, Lv L, Ji H, Yang X, Zhu W, Cai L, Gu X, Chai C, Huang S, Sun J, Dong Q. Induction of pluripotent stem cells transplantation therapy for ischemic stroke. Mol Cell Biochem. 2011;354(1–2):67–75.

32. Jin K, Wang X, Xie L, Mao XO, Zhu W, Wang Y, Shen J, Mao Y, Banwait S, Greenberg DA. Evidence for stroke-induced neurogenesis in the human brain. Proc Natl Acad Sci U S A. 2006;103(35):13198–202.

33. Kalladka D, Sinden J, Pollock K, Haig C, McLean J, Smith W, McConnachie A, Santosh C, Bath PM, Dunn L, Muir KW. Human neural stem cells in patients with chronic ischaemic stroke (PISCES): a phase 1, first-in-man study. Lancet. 2016;388(10046):787–96.

34. Krause M, Phan TG, Ma H, Sobey CG, Lim R. Cell-based therapies for stroke: are we there yet? Front Neurol. 2019;10:656.

35. Lappalainen RS, Narkilahti S, Huhtala T, Liimatainen T, Suuronen T, Närvänen A, Suuronen R, Hovatta O, Jolkkonen J. The SPECT imaging shows the accumulation of neural progenitor cells into internal organs after systemic administration in middle cerebral artery occlusion rats. Neurosci Lett. 2008;440(3):246–50.

36. Lau VW, Platt SR, Grace HE, Baker EW, West FD. Human iNPC therapy leads to improvement in functional neurologic outcomes in a pig ischemic stroke model. Brain Behav. 2018;8(5):e00972.

37. Mampalam TJ, Gonzalez MF, Weinstein P, Sharp FR. Neuronal changes in fetal cortex transplanted to ischemic adult rat cortex. J Neurosurg. 1988;69(6):904–12.

38. Marei HE, Hasan A, Rizzi R, Althani A, Afifi N, Cenciarelli C, Caceci T, Shuaib A. Potential of stem cell-based therapy for ischemic stroke. Front Neurol. 2018;9:34.

39. Oki K, Tatarishvili J, Wood J, Koch P, Wattananit S, Mine Y, Monni E, Tornero D, Ahlenius H, Ladewig J, Brüstle O, Lindvall O, Kokaia Z. Human-induced pluripotent stem cells form functional neurons and improve recovery after grafting in stroke-damaged brain. Stem Cells. 2012;30(6):1120–33.

40. Parr AM, Tator CH, Keating A. Bone marrow-derived mesenchymal stromal cells for the repair of central nervous system injury. Bone Marrow Transplant. 2007;40(7):609–19.

41. Polentes J, Jendelova P, Cailleret M, Braun H, Romanyuk N, Tropel P, Brenot M, Itier V, Seminatore C, Baldauf K, Turnovcova K, Jirak D, Teletin M, Côme J, Tournois J, Reymann K, Sykova E, Viville S, Onteniente B. Human induced pluripotent stem cells improve stroke outcome and reduce secondary degeneration in the recipient brain. Cell Transplant. 2012;21(12):2587–602.

42. Pomper MG, Hammond H, Yu X, Ye Z, Foss CA, Lin DD, Fox JJ, Cheng L. Serial imaging of human embryonic stem-cell engraftment and teratoma formation in live mouse models. Cell Res. 2009;19(3):370–9.

43. Prasad K, Sharma A, Garg A, Mohanty S, Bhatnagar S, Johri S, Singh KK, Nair V, Sarkar RS, Gorthi SP, Hassan KM, Prabhakar S, Marwaha N, Khandelwal N, Misra UK, Kalita J, Nityanand S, InveST Study Group. Intravenous autologous bone marrow mononuclear stem cell therapy for ischemic stroke: a multicentric, randomized trial. Stroke. 2014;45(12):3618–24.

44. Rodríguez-Frutos B, Otero-Ortega L, Gutiérrez-Fernández M, Fuentes B, Ramos-Cejudo J, Díez-Tejedor E. Stem cell therapy and administration routes after stroke. Transl Stroke Res. 2016;7(5):378–87.

45. Song M, Kim Y-J, Kim Y, Roh J, Kim SU, Yoon B-W. Using a neodymium magnet to target delivery of ferumoxide-labeled human neural stem cells in a rat model of focal cerebral ischemia. Hum Gene Ther. 2010;21(5):603–10.

46. Sorby-Adams AJ, Vink R, Turner RJ. Large animal models of stroke and traumatic brain injury as translational tools. Am J Physiol Regul Integr Comp Physiol. 2018;315(2):R165–90.

47. Steinbeck JA, Koch P, Derouiche A, Brüstle O. Human embryonic stem cell-derived neurons establish region-specific, long-range projections in the adult brain. Cell Mol Life Sci. 2012;69(3):461–70.

48. Takahashi K, Yamanaka S. Induction of pluripotent stem cells from mouse embryonic and adult fibroblast cultures by defined factors. Cell. 2006;126(4):663–76.

49. Takahashi K, Yasuhara T, Shingo T, Muraoka K, Kameda M, Takeuchi A, Yano A, Kurozumi K, Agari T, Miyoshi Y, Kinugasa K, Date I. Embryonic neural stem cells transplanted in middle cerebral artery occlusion model of rats demonstrated potent therapeutic effects, compared to adult neural stem cells. Brain Res. 2008;1234:172–82.

50. Theus MH, Wei L, Cui L, Francis K, Hu X, Keogh C, Yu SP. In vitro hypoxic preconditioning of embryonic stem cells as a strategy of promoting cell survival and functional benefits after transplantation into the ischemic rat brain. Exp Neurol. 2008;210(2):656–70.

51. Thomson JA, Itskovitz-Eldor J, Shapiro SS, Waknitz MA, Swiergiel JJ, Marshall VS, Jones JM. Embryonic stem cell lines derived from human blastocysts. Science. 1998;282(5391):1145–7.

52. Toda H, Takahashi J, Iwakami N, Kimura T, Hoki S, Mozumi-Kitamura K, Ono S, Hashimoto N. Grafting neural stem cells improved the impaired spatial recognition in ischemic rats. Neurosci Lett. 2001;316(1):9–12.
53. Tohill M, Mantovani C, Wiberg M, Terenghi G. Rat bone marrow mesenchymal stem cells express glial markers and stimulate nerve regeneration. Neurosci Lett. 2004;362(3):200–3.
54. Tonchev AB, Yamashima T, Zhao L, Okano H. Differential proliferative response in the post-ischemic hippocampus, temporal cortex, and olfactory bulb of young adult macaque monkeys. Glia. 2003a;42(3):209–24.
55. Tonchev AB, Yamashima T, Zhao L, Okano HJ, Okano H. Proliferation of neural and neuronal progenitors after global brain ischemia in young adult macaque monkeys. Mol Cell Neurosci. 2003b;23(2):292–301.
56. Tornero D, Wattananit S, Grønning Madsen M, Koch P, Wood J, Tatarishvili J, Mine Y, Gc R, Monni E, Devaraju K, Hevner RF, Brüstle O, Lindvall O, Kokaia Z. Human induced pluripotent stem cell-derived cortical neurons integrate in stroke-injured cortex and improve functional recovery. Brain J Neurol. 2013;136(Pt 12):3561–77.
57. Webb RL, Kaiser EE, Scoville SL, Thompson TA, Fatima S, Pandya C, Sriram K, Swetenburg RL, Vaibhav K, Arbab AS, Baban B, Dhandapani KM, Hess DC, Hoda MN, Stice SL. Human neural stem cell extracellular vesicles improve tissue and functional recovery in the murine thromboembolic stroke model. Transl Stroke Res. 2018;9(5):530–9.
58. Wichterle H, Lieberam I, Porter JA, Jessell TM. Directed differentiation of embryonic stem cells into motor neurons. Cell. 2002;110(3):385–97.
59. Willing AE, Shahaduzzaman M. Delivery routes for cell therapy in stroke. In: Jolkkonen J, Walczak P, editors. Cell-based therapies in stroke. Vienna: Springer Vienna; 2013. p. 15–28.
60. Yamashita T, Kawai H, Tian F, Ohta Y, Abe K. Tumorigenic development of induced pluripotent stem cells in ischemic mouse brain. Cell Transplant. 2011;20(6):883–91.
61. Yang H, Wang C, Chen H, Li L, Ma S, Wang H, Fu Y, Qu T. Neural stem cell-conditioned medium ameliorated cerebral ischemia-reperfusion injury in rats. Stem Cells Int. 2018;2018:4659159.
62. Zheng H, Zhang B, Chhatbar PY, Dong Y, Alawieh A, Lowe F, Hu X, Feng W. Mesenchymal stem cell therapy in stroke: a systematic review of literature in pre-clinical and clinical research. Cell Transplant. 2018;27(12):1723–30.

Chapter 16
Use of Stem Cells in the Treatment of Erectile Dysfunction

Benjamin Press and Stanton C. Honig

16.1 Incidence and Risk Factors for Erectile Dysfunction

Erectile dysfunction (ED) is the consistent or recurrent inability of a man to attain and/or maintain a penile erection sufficient for sexual performance. ED has a high prevalence in the general population, with incidence increasing with age. In a large cross-sectional, community-based study, among men between the ages of 40 and 49 years, the prevalence of complete or severe erectile dysfunction was 5% and the prevalence of moderate erectile dysfunction was 17% [1]. Selvin et al. analyzed data from 2126 adult male participants in the 2001–2002 National Health and Nutrition Examination Survey (NHANES). From this study, ED was estimated to be 18.4%. Incidence increased from 5.1% to 14.8% to 43.8% to 70.2% in age groups 20–39, 40–59, 60–69, and 70+ years old, respectively [2]. The MALES study was an international study involving 27, 839 men in eight countries (the United States, the United Kingdom, Germany, France, Italy, Spain, Mexico, and Brazil) aged 20–75. Overall prevalence of ED was 16% overall, with a high of 22% in the United States and a low of 10% in Spain [3].

Erectile dysfunction has been associated with cardiovascular conditions (i.e., hypertension, hypercholesterolemia) diabetes mellitus, and metabolic syndrome [4–6]. Lower urinary tract symptoms (LUTS) and depression have also been implicated as risk factors for erectile dysfunction [7–9]. Lifestyle factors, including smoking and obesity, are also significant predictors of erectile dysfunction [4, 10, 11]. A prospective randomized controlled trial demonstrated that lowering body mass index and increased physical activity were independently associated with changes in

B. Press
Yale School of Medicine, New Haven, CT, USA
e-mail: Benjamin.press@yale.edu

S. C. Honig (✉)
Department of Urology, Yale School of Medicine, New Haven, CT, USA
e-mail: Stanton.honig@yale.edu

© Springer Nature Switzerland AG 2021
T. P. Navarro et al. (eds.), *Stem Cell Therapy for Vascular Diseases*,
https://doi.org/10.1007/978-3-030-56954-9_16

International Index of Erectile Function (IIEF) score [12], suggesting that improve-ments in general health status is associated with improved erectile function.

Erectile dysfunction has substantial impact on quality of life. In addition to the impact on the sexual experience in many men, erectile dysfunction creates psychological distress that affects their relationships with family and friends [13]. In a study of a general measure of health-related quality of life, men with erectile dysfunction reported significantly worse results than normal respondents on measures of social function, role limitations due to emotional problems, and emotional well-being [14]. In another study, men with erectile dysfunction reported significantly lower physical and emotional satisfaction and lower general happiness than men in the study without ED. [15]

16.2   Anatomy and Physiology of Normal Erection

The penis is composed of three cylindrical structures: the paired vascular corpora cavernosa and the corpus spongiosum (which houses the urethra), covered by a loose subcutaneous layer and skin. (Fig. 16.1) The tunica albuginea is the fibrous envelope that surrounds the two corpora cavernosa. Within the corpora, interconnected sinusoids are enveloped by trabeculae of smooth muscle, collagen, and elastin. The smooth muscle is closely associated with the cavernous nerves and helicine arteries. In the flaccid state, intracavernosal blood gas levels are similar to those of mixed venous blood due to the low rate of arterial blood flow. During erection, the rapid entry of arterial blood into the sinusoids causes the blood gas levels in the corpora cavernosa to be more similar to that of arterial blood [16].

The smooth musculature of both the cavernosa and the vasculature plays key role in the erectile process. In the flaccid state, smooth muscles are contracted, restricting the amount of blood flow to the corpora. Relaxation of the smooth musculature results from the release of the neurotransmitter, nitric oxide (NO), from the cavernous nerve terminals following sexual stimulation. With the smooth muscle relaxed, it triggers a cascade of physiologic changes resulting in erection. Relaxation of the smooth muscle results in the dilatation of the arterioles and arteries by increased blood flow. This causes blood to collect in the sinusoids. The trapping of blood in the sinusoids causes a compression of the venous plexuses between the tunica albuginea and the peripheral sinusoids, reducing the venous outflow. Eventually the tunica becomes stretched to capacity, subsequently reducing the venous outflow to a minimum. The increase in PO2 with increased arterial blood flow coupled with increased intracavernosal pressure raises the penis from flaccid to erect state [17, 18].

The penis receives neural innervation from both the autonomic and somatic pathways. The sympathetic pathway originates from the 11th thoracic to the 2nd lumbar spinal segments. The parasympathetic pathway arises from neurons in the intermediolateral cell columns of the second, third, and fourth sacral spinal cord segments. Parasympathetic and sympathetic nerve fibers meet in the pelvic plexus. The branches that innervate the penis from the plexus are the cavernous nerves [19, 20].

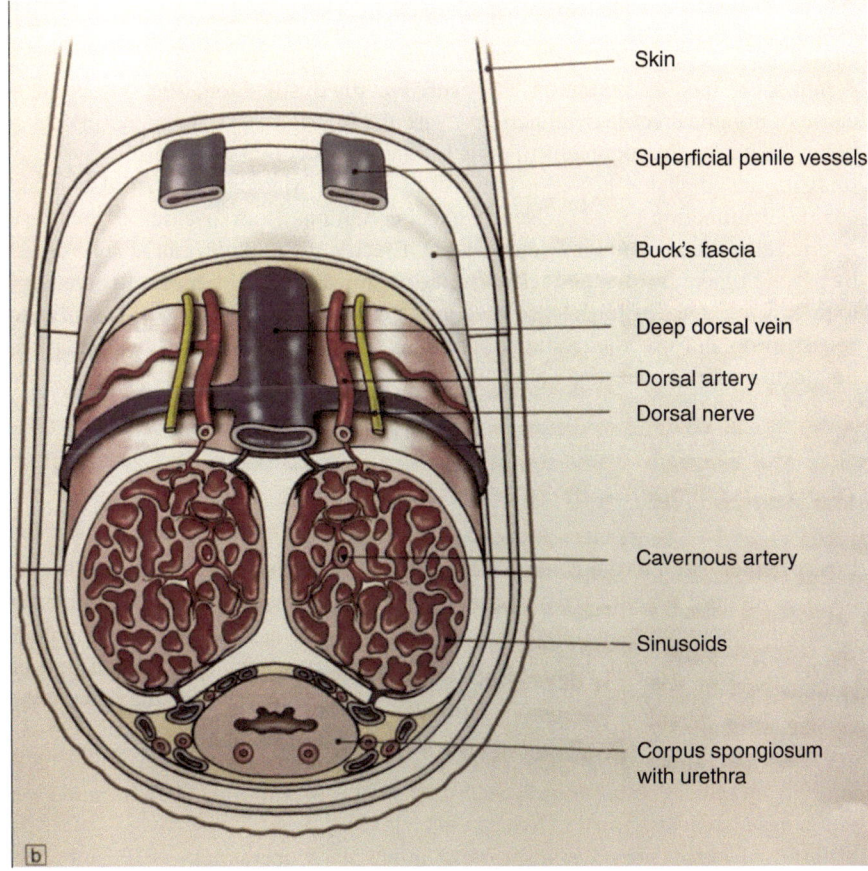

Fig. 16.1 Cross-sectional anatomy of the penis showing the three vascular chambers with sinusoidal tissue with endothelial cells. (Reprinted with permission: Carson et al. [117])

Somatic input comes from abundant free nerve endings [21] in the glans penis, as well as sensory receptors in the penile skin, urethra, and within the corpus cavernosum. The nerve fibers from the receptors converge to form bundles of the dorsal nerve of the penis, which joins other nerves to become the pudendal nerve, which enters the spinal cord at the S2-S4 level [22].

Numerous neurotransmitters have been implicated in normal erectile function, principally nitric oxide (NO). General consensus is that NO is the principal neurotransmitter mediating penile erection. NO stimulates cGMP production, one of the major second messengers in smooth muscle relaxation. Production of cGMP in turn relaxes cavernous smooth muscle [23, 24]. NO derived from neuronal nitric oxide synthase (nNOS) in the non-adrenergic, non-cholinergic (NANC) nerves is responsible for the initiation, whereby NO from endothelial nitric oxide synthase (eNOS) contributes to the maintenance of smooth muscle relaxation and erection [25].

16.3 Primary Etiologies of Erectile Dysfunction

A number of medical conditions can cause erectile dysfunction. The most common cause of organic erectile dysfunction is vascular in origin. Certain endocrine conditions, including hypogonadism, hyperprolactinemia, hypothyroidism, hyperthyroidism, and diabetes [26–29], may result in ED. Medications can also induce erectile dysfunction [30, 31]. Neurological conditions from disease or from nerve injuries also are a significant cause of ED. Erectile dysfunction can also be caused by psychological factors, and result from overstimulation, and increased adrenergic tone causing smooth muscle contraction of erectile tissue [1, 15]. The primary causes of organic erectile dysfunction implicated in the use of stem cell therapy for treatment so far are neurogenic and vascular in etiology.

16.3.1 Neurogenic Erectile Dysfunction

Loss of innervation to the corpora cavernosa is the mechanism of neurogenic erectile dysfunction. Without the nerve input, the smooth muscle in the corpora cavernosa is unable to relax, limiting the blood flow to the penis. Long-term morphologic changes can occur with loss of corporal innervations, including smooth muscle apoptosis and fibrosis [32, 33]. The insult causing this denervation can occur either at the central nervous system level including the spinal cord [34] and brain [35–37] or the peripheral nervous system including the pelvic ganglia and cavernous nerve injury from radical pelvic surgery such as radical prostatectomy . Penile tactile sensation has also been shown to reduce with age [38].

Rates of iatrogenic cavernosal nerve injury have decreased significantly with improved understanding of the neuroanatomy of pelvic nerves. Historically, outcomes following pelvic surgery (i.e., radical prostatectomy, abdominal perianal resection) reported ED rates at above 80% [39–41]. More contemporary literature in the era of emphasis on nerve sparing pelvic surgery have caused those rates to be reduced by over 50% [42–48] depending on how erectile dysfunction is defined, nerve sparing status of procedures, pre-op erectile status, and age [49]. In diabetic patients, autonomic neuropathy by progressive demyelination may cause erectile dysfunction [50].

16.3.2 Vascular Erectile Dysfunction

Erectile and flaccid states are regulated by relaxation and contraction of vascular smooth muscle. Atherosclerotic or rarely traumatic arterial occlusive disease of the penile arteries can decrease the perfusion pressure and arterial flow and cause an imbalance of relaxation and contractile factors, causing erectile dysfunction.

Common risk factors associated with arterial insufficiency include coronary artery disease, hypertension, hyperlipidemia, cigarette smoking, diabetes mellitus, pelvic irradiation, and rarely blunt perineal trauma [4–6, 51, 52]. Age-related vascular changes resulting in erectile dysfunction include increased tone of cavernous smooth muscle [53] as well as endothelial dysfunction [54], causing a reduced ability of vascular smooth muscle to relax.

16.4   Overview of Current Therapy for Erectile Dysfunction

In many cases, erectile dysfunction is a manifestation of systemic vascular disease. Because of this, lifestyle modifications designed to optimize a patient's cardiovascular health have been shown to stabilize and sometimes improve erectile dysfunction [55, 56]. Modifications include dietary improvement [57], increased exercise [58, 59], decrease in signs of metabolic syndrome or adjusting medications if appropriate.

The standard of care first-line therapy for erectile dysfunction is oral phosphodiesterase type 5 inhibitors (PDE5i) [60–62]. PDE5 inhibitors work to block the catalytic action of the PDE5, the enzyme that degrades cGMP, the downstream effector of the erection mediator nitric oxide [63–65]. These medications serve to augment the erectile response, not induce an erection. In the United States, sildenafil (Viagra, Pfizer) was brought to market in 1998. Two additional PDE5i, vardenafil (Levitra®, GSK) and tadalafil (Cialis®, Lilly), were released in the United States in 2003. A fourth PDE5i, avanafil (Stendra®, Auxilium), was approved in 2013. Lodenafil, mirodenafil, and udenafil have been approved outside of the United States. PDE5is have been demonstrated to be superior to placebo in the treatment of erectile dysfunction of all etiologies despite success rates with placebo of about 30% in most studies [61, 66]. Typically success rates with first time prescription is 60–75% [67–70]. However, these success rates are lower in men following radical pelvic surgery (35–41%) [71–73] and autonomic neuropathy from diabetes (48–54%) [60, 74–76]. The use of nitrite medications (i.e., sublingual nitroglycerin, isosorbide mononitrate, or dinitrate) is the only absolute contraindication to taking PDE5is [77]. Side effects observed with PDE5i therapy include headache (7–16%), dyspepsia (4–10%), flushing (4–10%), myalgia/back pain (typically tadalafil only) (0–3%), nasal congestion (3–4%), and visual disturbances (0–3%) [78].

If oral pharmaceutical agents fail to treat erectile dysfunction, other excellent treatment options are available. Intracavernosal injections (ICI) involves directly injecting a vasoactive agent directly into the corpora cavernosa resulting in penile erection by relaxation of vascular smooth muscle and increased arterial flow into the penis [79]. Prostaglandin E1 (PGE_1) is the only FDA-approved agent for penile injection monotherapy. PGE_1 is a direct cyclic AMP stimulator, which in turn induces tissue relaxation through a second messenger system [80]. Trimix, a mixture of papaverine, phentolamine, and PGE_1, has been used as an alternative for PGE_1 injection monotherapy due to lack of clinical response or for issues of cost

[81]. ICI has been demonstrated to be more efficacious than other second-line therapies, including vacuum erection devices [82] and intraurethral suppositories of PGE₁ [83, 84]. In a study of 296 men who received alprostadil ICI, penile pain was the most commonly reported side effect. While usually mild, penile pain occurred in 50% of the men at any point. Prolonged erections occurred in 5% of the men, priapism in 1%, penile fibrotic complications in 2%, and hematoma or ecchymosis in 8% [85].

Vacuum erection devices are a high satisfaction, low-cost treatment option for erectile dysfunction. It should be noted that the majority of the studies that evaluated patient and partner satisfaction using vacuum devices predate the widespread availability of oral PDE5is [86]. Vacuum devices have been proven to be effective, and adverse events are largely minor, like bruising [87]. Intraurethral alprostadil is a treatment option for men for whom PDE5i are contraindicated (i.e., men taking nitrates) or for men with an aversion to the needles required for IC injections [86]. In a randomized, double-blind placebo controlled trial, IU alprostadil significantly improved sexual function compared to placebo [88]. However, efficacy in widespread use is lower than intracavernosal therapy or vacuum erection devices. Adverse events are relatively frequent with the use of IU alprostadil but often minor. The most common adverse events reported in the literature were genital pain (6.5–34.7%), minor urethral trauma (1–5.1%), urethral pain or burning (0–29%), and dizziness (0–7.0%) [86].

A penile prosthesis (IPP) is a device that is surgically implanted into the corpora cavernosa. Penile implants are used in patients who have failed nonoperative management or who find minimally invasive options to be suboptimal. The operation is generally highly successful with very high satisfaction rates both from the patient and their partners [86, 89–91]. The most worrisome complication of IPP placement is infection, which will often require device removal. Improvements in surgical technique and devices have reduced the rates of infection of device infection to 1–2% in large modern series [92, 93]. Device malfunction may occur in 20% of patients over 10–15 years requiring removal and replacement [94].

16.5 Rationale for Stem Cell Therapy

The use of stem cell therapy for various diseases has long been the subject of significant clinical interest and research. Stem cells are defined by their ability to self-renew and differentiate into various types of cells and tissues [95]. They have been repeatedly shown to have the ability to regenerate and restore functional status to damaged tissues [96]. Mesenchymal stem cells (MSCs) are attractive cells due to their capacity for proliferation, multilineage differentiation, and immunomodulatory properties [97]. These cells were first identified and isolated from bone marrow and have played an important role in regeneration therapy by multiple cellular mechanisms [98]. The impact of using MSCs is not primarily due to cell differentiation and direct integration within the target tissues. Rather, a paracrine effect is the proposed method of immunomodulation, whereby secretion of cytokines and growth factors decrease inflammation and promote healing [99–101]. In the scope of erectile dysfunction, while oral therapy and intracavernosal injection have proven to be effective therapies, they treat the symptoms of erectile dysfunction, and not the cause. Stem cell therapy provides the potential for curative treatment.

16.6   Stem Cell Studies in Animals

Several studies have evaluated the use of stem cells for the treatment of erectile dysfunction in animal models, and these studies are listed in Table 16.1 [102]. The use of stem cells as treatment for erectile dysfunction was first described in 2004 by Bochinski et al. [103] Rats were divided into four groups: a sham operation; bilateral cavernosal nerve crush injury (BCNCI) and injection of stem cell culture medium into the corpora cavernosa; injection of neural embryonic stem (NES) cells into the major pelvic ganglion (MPG) following BCNCI; and injection of NES cells into the corpora cavernosa following BCNCI. Erectile response was assessed at

Table 16.1 Animal studies

Author	Year	Country	Stem cell type	ED model	N	Control	Results
Bocinski, et al.	2004	United States	Neural embryonic	Neurogenic	26	Yes	Higher ICP and improved neurofilament staining in treatment group compared to controls
Kendrici, et al.	2010	United States	Bone marrow	Neurogenic	32	Yes	Higher mean ICP/MAP and total ICP in treatment compared to control
Ryu, et al.	2014	Korea	Bone marrow	Neurogenic	24	Yes	Significantly restored cavernous endothelial and smooth muscle content, and penile nNOS and neurofilament
Xu, et al.	2014	China	Adipose tissue	Neurogenic	80	Yes	Partial but significant recovery of erectile response, nNOS expression and smooth muscle cells
Liu, et al.	2016	China	Adipose tissue	Neurogenic	64	No	Improved retention of stem cells in erectile tissue when cultured with NanoShuttle
Ouyang, et al.	2014	China	Urine	Diabetic	65	Yes	Significantly raised ICP, ICP/MAP, increased expression of endothelial and smooth muscle markers ratio in treatment compared to control

3 months. No significant difference in return of erectile function was noted between the two experimental groups (injection of stem cells in MPG vs. cavernous body). The groups injected with NES cells into the MPG and corpora cavernosa following BCNCI had significantly higher intracavernosal pressures than the group without stem cell injection following BCNCI. Neurofilament staining was significantly improved in the experimental groups injected with NES cells compared with control group. ICP remained significantly lower in experimental groups compared with the rats which underwent a sham operation, indicating only a partial return of erectile function.

Kendirici et al. investigated the effects of transplanting bone marrow-derived multipotent stromal cells (BMSC) in a rat model of BCNCI [104]. They tested the effects of multipotent stromal cells as well cells activated by antibodies against p75 nerve growth factor receptor. Thirty-two rats underwent BCNCI procedure. Immediately following the surgery, 8 rats each were injected intracavernously with either phosphate-buffered saline, fibroblasts, rat MSC, or p75-activated MSC. Another eight rats underwent sham operation and were injected with phosphate-buffered saline. Mean intracavernosal pressure (ICP)/mean arterial pressure (MAP) and total ICP were measured to assess erectile function 4 weeks after BCNCI and treatment. At that time cavernous nerve stimulation was done at 2.5, 5.0, and 7.5 V. At 5 V of cavernous nerve stimulation, rats that received BMSC injection had significantly improved erectile function (higher intracavernosal pressure) compared to rats that received PBS or fibroblasts. Rats that received p75-activated rat stem cells after BCNCI) had significantly higher mean ICP/MAP and total ICP than rats that received saline, fibroblasts, or nonactivated MSCs. The investigators also found that in rats who received p75-activated stem cells, a higher concentration of ß-fibroblast growth factor was expressed. This growth factor has been identified as a neurotrophic factor in the penis [105].

Ryu et al. also investigated the effectiveness of bone marrow-derived stem cells to restore erectile function in mice following BCNCI [106]. Mice were divided into four groups: a sham operation group, BCNCI group receiving a single intracavernosal injection of saline or clonal mesenchymal bone marrow-derived stem cells, and a BCNCI receiving a single intraperitoneal injection of clonal stem cells. A single IC injection of clonal BMSCs induced recovery of erectile function (determined by the ratios max ICP and total ICP to mean systolic blood pressure) compared with that in saline-treated BCNCI mice, which reached 90–100% of sham control values. A single IP injection of clonal BMSCs significantly improved erectile function based on maximum intracavernosal pressures compared to saline-treated groups, but the response was not as robust as the IC injection. Increases in cavernosal endothelial and smooth muscle content, as well as penile nNOS and neurofilament content, were seen in mice who received injections of BMSCs.

In another study investigating the restoration of erectile function following BCNCI, Xu and colleagues investigated the effects of both adipose-derived stem cells (ADSC) and adipose-derived stem cells-based microtissues (MT, formed after culturing ADSC for 3 days) [107]. Ten rats underwent sham surgery and intracavernosal injection of saline. Another 70 rats underwent BCNCI and were then treated with either saline, dissociated ADSCs, or microtissues. Erectile function was measured 4 weeks after treatment. Partial but significant recovery of erectile response was seen both in the ADSCs group and the MTs group. However, the recovery in function was significantly higher in the MT group compared to the ADSC group. Partially but significant recovery of the nNOS expression and smooth muscle cells was observed both in the ADSCs group and the MTs group, but more nNOS-positive nerves and smooth muscle cells were found in the MTs group compared to the ADSCs group. Of note, there was no significant difference between the sham-operated group and the MTs group with respect to smooth muscle content. The results of this study indicate that IC-injected ADSC plus MTs resulted in a better restoration of erectile function than traditional single-cell strategy.

Changes in the single-cell strategy were further tested by Lin and colleagues, who investigated NanoShuttle™ magnetic nanoparticles as a vehicle to maintain stem cells in the corpus cavernosum after IC injection [108]. Four weeks following BCNCI, rats which have received an injection of ADSCs cultured and magnetized with NanoShuttle had a significantly higher ICP/MAP compared to ADSCs cultured with NanoShuttle as well as ADSCs without NanoShuttle. The latter two groups exhibited a statistically similar response in erectile recovery. Similar findings were observed with respect to endothelial cell and smooth muscle cell recovery. Cell tracking showed that ADSCs cultured and magnetized with NanoShuttle were successfully retained in the corpus cavernosum for up to 3 days while most ADSCs in other groups were washed out in other by day 1.

Additionally, human urine-derived stem cells (USC) has been tested in rat models. Ouyang et al. [109] evaluated human USC or human USC genetically modified with a fibroblast growth factors (FGF2) to improve erectile dysfunction in the diabetic model. A control group of normal rats were compared with three treatment groups in rats with induced type II diabetes: saline USC, lentivirus-FGF2, and USCs-FGF2. Erectile function was evaluated at 4 weeks following treatment. After treatment with USCs-FGF2, a partial but significant increase in ICP and the ICP/MAP ratios was demonstrated in diabetic rats. The ICP in USC and lentivirus-FGF2-treated rats was also significantly higher than saline-treated rats but significantly lower than that in the USC-FGF2 rats. Cavernosal endothelial content was significantly restored after USC-FGF2 injection compared to USC or lentivirus-FGF2 injection alone. USC or lentivirus-FGF2-treated ED rats also showed a significant increase of VEGF, eNOS expression, and cell/collagen ratio when compared to PBS-treated rats, but results were lower than in USC-FGF2 treated rats.

16.7   Stem Cell Studies in Humans

A PubMed review revealed that only four human clinical trials exist for evaluating stem cells as treatment for erectile dysfunction. At the time of writing, the Sexual Medicine Society of North America (SMSNA) has released a position statement on treatment of erectile dysfunction with restorative therapies such as stem cells. It reads as follows:

> Thus, given the current lack of regulatory agency approval for any restorative (regenerative) therapies for the treatment of ED and until such time as approval is granted, SMSNA believes that the use of shock waves or stem cells or platelet rich plasma is experimental and should be conducted under research protocols in compliance with Institutional Review Board approval. [110]

Herein, we review the published literature to date with stem cells in the treatment of erectile dysfunction in humans and are summarized in Table 16.2.

Table 16.2 Human studies

Author	Year	Country	Stem cell type	ED model	N	Control	Results	Comments
Bahk, et al.	2010	Korea	Umbilical cord	Diabetic	10	Yes	Improvements in the libido, erectile dysfunction, and blood glucose	
Yiou, et al	2015	France	Bone marrow	Neurogenic	12	No	Sexual function improved significantly at 6 months compared to baseline (using IIEF-15 and EHS)	Findings confirmed with additional 6 patients in phase II trial
Haahr, et al.	2016	Denmark	Adipose tissue	Neurogenic	21	No	Sexual function improved significantly at 12 months compared to baseline (using IIEF-15)	Correlation of improvement in sexual function with urinary continence at inclusion
Levy, et al.	2015	United States	Placenta	n/a	8	No	Between 6 weeks and 3 months and 6 months PSV significantly increased	Changes in measured end diastolic velocity, stretched penile length, penile width, and IIEF-15 scores were not statistically significant

The first trial was a single-blind study of ten men with type II diabetes with erectile dysfunction. All patients had proven unresponsive to previous medical therapies for more than 6 months, and all were awaiting penile prostheses [111]. Seven men received injections of human umbilical cord blood stem cells into both corpus cavernosa. Three men received injections of saline into both corpus cavernosa. Patients were followed for 11 months and were instructed to use a PDE5 inhibitor when they wished to engage in sexual activity. Among the seven men, who had no erections in the morning or during sexual activity prior to the study, three experienced morning erections by 1 month after treatment, and all but one regained morning erections by the second month. With the addition of sildenafil, two patients could achieve penetration, maintenance, and orgasm. Two patients opted for penile prosthesis during the follow-up period (11 months) and one returned to non-erectile status. Three of the seven subjects agreed that stem cell therapy applied alone had some effect on erectile dysfunction, and five of the seven subjects regarded stem cell therapy as effective for erectile dysfunction when combined with a PDE5 inhibitor. Only one patient reported confidence in the effects of stem cell therapy without a PDE5 inhibitor on erectile dysfunction, and one other patient expressed confidence in the effects of stem cell therapy with a PDE5 inhibitor on erectile dysfunction. Although data was collected, there was no statistical analysis done using standard validated questionnaires for erectile dysfunction(IIEF).

The INSTIN Clinical Trial tested four doses of intracavernosal injection of autologous bone marrow mononuclear cells in men with post-radical prostatectomy erectile dysfunction [112]. Twelve patients with localized prostate cancer and post-prostatectomy ED refractory to medical therapy were divided equally into four groups receiving escalating doses of bone marrow mononuclear cells. Erectile function was evaluated at 1, 3, 6, and 12 months post-injection using the International Index of Erectile Function-15 and Erection Hardness Scale questionnaires. Using ultrasound, systolic velocity in cavernous arteries was assessed, and endothelial function was determined using the penile nitric oxide release test. Overall, sexual function improved significantly at 6 months compared to baseline. Mean improvements were $+1.3 \pm 1$ for on-medication EHS, $+0.8 \pm 1.2$ for off-medication EHS, and $+10.1 \pm 8.6$ for the International Index of Erectile Function-15 erectile function subscore. Nine of the 12 patients reported successful intercourse with the assistance of medication. The groups with the two highest doses of stem cell therapy demonstrated greater increase for off-medication EHS at 6 months when compared to the groups with the lowest two doses of stem cell therapy. Sexual function scores at 12 months were not significantly different from those at 6 months. Basal and 20-min peak systolic velocity increased significantly after BM-MNC injection. 20-min PSV was normal in 7 of the 11 patients with baseline arterial insufficiency at 6 months. Investigators also found that there was a significant increase in the proportion of patients with normal endothelial function at 6 months after treatment compared with baseline (8/11 vs 2/11, $p = 0.032$). A second underpowered stage II study of six patients showed similar findings [113].

Haahr et al. tested the efficacy of intracavernosal injection ADSCs to treat post-radical prostatectomy erectile dysfunction. Twenty-one men with medication refractory erectile dysfunction following radical prostatectomy were given a single intracavernosal injection of autologous ADSC. Sexual function was evaluated at 1, 3, 6, and 12 months. Baseline median IIEF-5 scores (6.0; IQR 3) were unchanged 1 month after the treatment but increased after 6 months to 7 (IQR 17, $P = .002$). After 1 year, the improvements in erectile function was found to be maintained at IIEF-5 scores (median 8; IQR 14, $P = .004$). Eight out of 21 participants could attain an erection sufficient for intercourse in the 12 month follow-up. After treatment, three men could complete intercourse with additional medications, and the other five men could complete with additional medications at 12 months after treatment. When comparing men having nerve-sparing prostatectomy to men with non-nerve-sparing prostatectomy, no difference in IIEF-5 score was observed. Interestingly, an apparent association with refractory ED and urine continence was found during post hoc stratification according to urine continence at inclusion. Among men who were continent of urine, IIEF-5 scores were unchanged 1 month after the treatment (median 6; IQR 4) but significantly increased after 6 months to a median of 11 (IQR17; $P = .002$) and at 12 months to a median of 9 (IQR 13, $P = .012$). IIEF-5 scores were similar after 1, 3, 6, and 12 months and not different from the score at the time of inclusion (median 5; IQR 4; $P > .99$) among men who were incontinent of urine.

Levy et al. evaluated the efficacy of placental matrix-derived mesenchymal stem cells as treatment of erectile dysfunction in eight men in an IRB-approved prospective, observational cohort study [114]. Each patient received an injection of placental matrix-derived mesenchymal stem cells. Erectile function was assessed by assess peak systolic velocity (PSV), end diastolic velocity, stretched penile length, penile width, and erectile function status based on the International Index of Erectile Function (IIEF) questionnaire at 6 weeks, 3 months, and 6 months. Between 6 weeks and 3 months, PSV significantly increased from a range of 25.5 cm/s–56.5 cm/s to 32.5 cm/s–66.7 cm/s. PSV ranged from 50.7 cm/s to 73.9 cm/s at 6 months which was a statistically significant increase from the 3 month values. Changes in measured end diastolic velocity, stretched penile length, penile width, and International Index of Erectile Function scores were not statistically significant. At the 6-week follow-up, two patients for whom previous oral therapies failed had the ability to sustain erections on their own. At the 3-month follow-up, one additional patient was able to achieve erections on his own.

16.8 Conclusions and Future Implications

Stem cell therapy is an exciting new possible treatment alternative for men with erectile dysfunction. While studies and humans and animals have demonstrated promising results in safety and efficacy, long-term data is lacking. While stem cell therapy holds promise for other disease states, data on erectile dysfunction is scant. However, stem cell treatment centers are offering this treatment throughout the United States and the world without significant evidence-based data.

Standardization of this treatment modality is also necessary [115]. Because of this, the FDA has warned that "unapproved stem cell therapies can be harmful and may be illegal and unproven" and has started to regular therapies [116]. The Sexual Medicine Society of North America has developed a position statement on regenerative therapies that includes stem cell therapy [110]. Enclosed here are some important paraphrases:

> The SMSNA strongly supports the development of novel erectogenic therapies, given that many men with ED either fail currently available treatments or find them unpalatable. The society, however, recognizes the need for adequately powered, multicenter, randomized, sham/placebo-controlled trials in well-characterized patient populations to ensure that efficacy and safety are demonstrated for any novel ED therapy [110].
>
> The SMSNA both advocates for and supports the application of high quality research, both pre-clinical and clinical, aimed at better understanding the mechanisms involved, the magnitude and durability of benefit and the long-term safety of restorative therapies. Thus, given the current lack of regulatory agency approval for any restorative (regenerative) therapies for the treatment of ED and until such time as approval is granted, SMSNA believes that the use of shock waves or stem cells or platelet rich plasma is experimental and should be conducted under research protocols in compliance with Institutional Review Board approval. Patients considering such therapies should be fully informed and consented regarding the potential benefits and risks. Finally, the SMSNA advocates that patients involved in these clinical trials should not incur more than basic research costs for their participation. [110]

No optimal concentration of stem cell solution has been identified for intracavernosal injection nor has there been any optimal dosing or treatment protocol developed. Clinical efforts will need to be standardized. Prior to implementation of large-scale clinical trials, agreed-upon validated measures must be selected. The debate between allogenic and autologous stem cells is still ongoing. While autologous stem cells would reduce the rate of immunogenic complications of stem cell treatment, obtaining them requires more invasive procedures. Ethical concerns about the use of stem cell therapy have jeopardized therapeutic use of stem cells in all possible medical conditions. Further scientific investigation is required in order to advance the promising early results of stem cell therapy in the treatment of erectile dysfunction.

References

1. Feldman HA, Goldstein I, Hatzichristou DG, Krane RJ, McKinlay JB. Impotence and its medical and psychosocial correlates: results of the Massachusetts male aging study. J Urol. 1994;151(1):54–61.
2. Selvin E, Burnett AL, Platz EA. Prevalence and risk factors for erectile dysfunction in the US. Am J Med. 2007;120(2):151–7.
3. Rosen RC, Fisher WA, Eardley I, Niederberger C, Nadel A, Sand M. The multinational Men's Attitudes to Life Events and Sexuality (MALES) study: I. Prevalence of erectile dysfunction and related health concerns in the general population. Curr Med Res Opin. 2004;20(5):607–17.

4. Bacon CG, Mittleman MA, Kawachi I, Giovannucci E, Glasser DB, Rimm EB. Sexual function in men older than 50 years of age: results from the health professionals follow-up study. Ann Intern Med. 2003;139(3):161–8.
5. Braun M, Wassmer G, Klotz T, Reifenrath B, Mathers M, Engelmann U. Epidemiology of erectile dysfunction: results of the 'Cologne Male Survey'. Int J Impot Res. 2000;12(6):305–11.
6. Schulster ML, Liang SE, Najari BB. Metabolic syndrome and sexual dysfunction. Curr Opin Urol. 2017;27(5):435–40.
7. Blanker MH, Bohnen AM, Groeneveld FP, Bernsen RM, Prins A, Thomas S, et al. Correlates for erectile and ejaculatory dysfunction in older Dutch men: a community-based study. J Am Geriatr Soc. 2001;49(4):436–42.
8. Rosen R, Altwein J, Boyle P, Kirby RS, Lukacs B, Meuleman E, et al. Lower urinary tract symptoms and male sexual dysfunction: the multinational survey of the aging male (MSAM-7). Eur Urol. 2003;44(6):637–49.
9. Rosen RC, Seidman SN, Menza MA, Shabsigh R, Roose SP, Tseng LJ, et al. Quality of life, mood, and sexual function: a path analytic model of treatment effects in men with erectile dysfunction and depressive symptoms. Int J Impot Res. 2004;16(4):334–40.
10. Nicolosi A, Glasser DB, Moreira ED, Villa M. Prevalence of erectile dysfunction and associated factors among men without concomitant diseases: a population study. Int J Impot Res. 2003;15(4):253–7.
11. Rosen RC, Wing R, Schneider S, Gendrano N. Epidemiology of erectile dysfunction: the role of medical comorbidities and lifestyle factors. Urol Clin N Am. 2005;32(4):403–17.
12. Esposito K, Giugliano F, Di Palo C, Giugliano G, Marfella R, D'Andrea F, et al. Effect of lifestyle changes on erectile dysfunction in obese men: a randomized controlled trial. JAMA. 2004;291(24):2978–84.
13. Impotence: NIH Consensus Development Panel on Impotence. JAMA. 1993;270(1):83–90.
14. Litwin MS, Nied RJ, Dhanani N. Health-related quality of life in men with erectile dysfunction. J Gen Intern Med. 1998;13(3):159–66.
15. Laumann EO, Paik A, Rosen RC. Sexual dysfunction in the United States prevalence and predictors. JAMA. 1999;281(6):537–44.
16. Sattar AA, Wespes E, Schulman CC. Computerized measurement of penile elastic fibres in potent and impotent men. Eur Urol. 1994;25(2):142–4.
17. Dean RC, Lue TF. Physiology of penile erection and pathophysiology of erectile dysfunction. Urol Clin North Am. 2005;32(4):379.
18. Lue TF. Physiology of penile erection and pathophysiology of erectile dysfunction. In: Wein AJK, Louis R, Partin AW, Peters CA, editors. Campbell-Walsh urology. Philadelphia, PA, USA: Elsevier. 2016. p. 612–42.e9.
19. de Groat WC, Booth A. Neural control of penile erection. In: Maggi C, editor. The autonomic nervous system. London, UK: Academic Publishers; 1993. p. 465–513.
20. Giuliano F. Neurophysiology of erection and ejaculation. J Sex Med. 2011;8:310–5.
21. Halata Z, Munger BL. The neuroanatomical basis for the protopathic sensibility of the human glans penis. Brain Res. 1986;371(2):205–30.
22. McKenna KE. Central control of penile erection. Int J Impot Res. 1998;10(Suppl 1):S25–34.
23. Ignarro LJ, Bush PA, Buga GM, Wood KS, Fukuto JM, Rajfer J. Nitric oxide and cyclic GMP formation upon electrical field stimulation cause relaxation of corpus cavernosum smooth muscle. Biochem Biophys Res Commun. 1990;170(2):843–50.
24. Kim N, Azadzoi KM, Goldstein I, Saenz de Tejada I. A nitric oxide-like factor mediates nonadrenergic-noncholinergic neurogenic relaxation of penile corpus cavernosum smooth muscle. J Clin Invest. 1991;88(1):112–8.
25. Hurt KJ, Musicki B, Palese MA, Crone JK, Becker RE, Moriarity JL, et al. Akt-dependent phosphorylation of endothelial nitric-oxide synthase mediates penile erection. Proc Natl Acad Sci U S A. 2002;99(6):4061–6.
26. Bhasin S, Enzlin P, Coviello A, Basson R. Sexual dysfunction in men and women with endocrine disorders. Lancet (London, England). 2007;369(9561):597–611.
27. Buvat J, Lemaire A. Endocrine screening in 1,022 men with erectile dysfunction: clinical significance and cost-effective strategy. J Urol. 1997;158(5):1764–7.

28. Corona G, Mannucci E, Fisher AD, Lotti F, Ricca V, Balercia G, et al. Effect of hyperprolactinemia in male patients consulting for sexual dysfunction. J Sex Med. 2007;4(5):1485–93.
29. Guay AT, Traish A. Testosterone deficiency and risk factors in the metabolic syndrome: implications for erectile dysfunction. Urol Clin North Am. 2011;38(2):175–83.
30. Francis ME, Kusek JW, Nyberg LM, Eggers PW. The contribution of common medical conditions and drug exposures to erectile dysfunction in adult males. J Urol. 2007;178(2):591–6.
31. Keene LC, Davies PH. Drug-related erectile dysfunction. Adverse Drug React Toxicol Rev. 1999;18(1):5–24.
32. Leungwattanakij S, Bivalacqua TJ, Usta MF, Yang DY, Hyun JS, Champion HC, et al. Cavernous neurotomy causes hypoxia and fibrosis in rat corpus cavernosum. J Androl. 2003;24(2):239–45.
33. User HM, Hairston JH, Zelner DJ, McKenna KE, McVary KT. Penile weight and cell subtype specific changes in a post-radical prostatectomy model of erectile dysfunction. J Urol. 2003;169(3):1175–9.
34. Biering-Sorensen F, Sonksen J. Sexual function in spinal cord lesioned men. Spinal Cord. 2001;39(9):455–70.
35. Chaudhuri KR, Schapira AH. Non-motor symptoms of Parkinson's disease: dopaminergic pathophysiology and treatment. Lancet Neurol. 2009;8(5):464–74.
36. Jeon SW, Yoo KH, Kim TH, Kim JI, Lee CH. Correlation of the erectile dysfunction with lesions of cerebrovascular accidents. J Sex Med. 2009;6(1):251–6.
37. Jung JH, Kam SC, Choi SM, Jae SU, Lee SH, Hyun JS. Sexual dysfunction in male stroke patients: correlation between brain lesions and sexual function. Urology. 2008;71(1):99–103.
38. Rowland DL, Greenleaf W, Mas M, Myers L, Davidson JM. Penile and finger sensory thresholds in young, aging, and diabetic males. Arch Sex Behav. 1989;18(1):1–12.
39. Borchers H, Brehmer B, Kirschner-Hermanns R, Reineke T, Tietze L, Jakse G. Erectile function after non-nerve-sparing radical prostatectomy: fact or fiction? Urol Int. 2006;76(3):213–6.
40. Walsh PC, Donker PJ. Impotence following radical prostatectomy: insight into etiology and prevention. J Urol. 1982;128(3):492–7.
41. Weinstein M, Roberts M. Sexual potency following surgery for rectal carcinoma. A followup of 44 patients. Ann Surg. 1977;185(3):295–300.
42. Catalona WJ, Bigg SW. Nerve-sparing radical prostatectomy: evaluation of results after 250 patients. J Urol. 1990;143(3):538–43; discussion 44.
43. Kendirci M, Hellstrom WJ. Current concepts in the management of erectile dysfunction in men with prostate cancer. Clin Prostate Cancer. 2004;3(2):87–92.
44. Liang J-T, Lai H-S, Lee P-H, Chang K-J. Laparoscopic pelvic autonomic nerve-preserving surgery for sigmoid colon cancer. Ann Surg Oncol. 2008;15(6):1609–16.
45. Quinlan DM, Epstein JI, Carter BS, Walsh PC. Sexual function following radical prostatectomy: influence of preservation of neurovascular bundles. J Urol. 1991;145(5):998–1002.
46. Tal R, Valenzuela R, Aviv N, Parker M, Waters WB, Flanigan RC, et al. Persistent erectile dysfunction following radical prostatectomy: the association between nerve-sparing status and the prevalence and chronology of venous leak. J Sex Med. 2009;6(10):2813–9.
47. Vale J. Erectile dysfunction following radical therapy for prostate cancer. Radiother Oncol. 2000;57(3):301–5.
48. Walsh PC, Brendler CB, Chang T, Marshall FF, Mostwin JI, Stutzman R, et al. Preservation of sexual function in men during radical pelvic surgery. Maryland Med J (Baltimore, Md : 1985). 1990;39(4):389–93.
49. Nelson CJ, Scardino PT, Eastham JA, Mulhall JP. Back to baseline: erectile function recovery after radical prostatectomy from the patients' perspective. J Sex Med. 2013;10(6):1636–43.
50. Ziegler D. Diagnosis and treatment of diabetic autonomic neuropathy. Curr Diab Rep. 2001;1(3):216–27.
51. Martin-Morales A, Sanchez-Cruz JJ, Saenz de Tejada I, Rodriguez-Vela L, Jimenez-Cruz JF, Burgos-Rodriguez R. Prevalence and independent risk factors for erectile dysfunction in Spain: results of the Epidemiologia de la Disfuncion Erectil Masculina Study. J Urol. 2001;166(2):569–74; discussion 74-5.
52. Shabsigh R, Fishman IJ, Schum C, Dunn JK. Cigarette smoking and other vascular risk factors in vasculogenic impotence. Urology. 1991;38(3):227–31.

53. Christ GJ, Maayani S, Valcic M, Melman A. Pharmacological studies of human erectile tissue: characteristics of spontaneous contractions and alterations in alpha-adrenoceptor responsiveness with age and disease in isolated tissues. Br J Pharmacol. 1990;101(2):375–81.
54. Toda N. Age-related changes in endothelial function and blood flow regulation. Pharmacol Ther. 2012;133(2):159–76.
55. Derby CA, Mohr BA, Goldstein I, Feldman HA, Johannes CB, McKinlay JB. Modifiable risk factors and erectile dysfunction: can lifestyle changes modify risk? Urology. 2000;56(2):302–6.
56. Esposito K, Ciotola M, Giugliano F, Maiorino MI, Autorino R, De Sio M, et al. Effects of intensive lifestyle changes on erectile dysfunction in men. J Sex Med. 2009;6(1):243–50.
57. Esposito K, Giugliano F, De Sio M, Carleo D, Di Palo C, D'Armiento M, et al. Dietary factors in erectile dysfunction. Int J Impot Res. 2006;18(4):370–4.
58. Belardinelli R, Lacalaprice F, Faccenda E, Purcaro A, Perna G. Effects of short-term moderate exercise training on sexual function in male patients with chronic stable heart failure. Int J Cardiol. 2005;101(1):83–90.
59. Kolotkin RL, Binks M, Crosby RD, Ostbye T, Mitchell JE, Hartley G. Improvements in sexual quality of life after moderate weight loss. Int J Impot Res. 2008;20(5):487–92.
60. Goldstein I, Lue TF, Padma-Nathan H, Rosen RC, Steers WD, Wicker PA. Oral Sildenafil in the treatment of erectile dysfunction. N Engl J Med. 1998;338(20):1397–404.
61. Yuan J, Zhang R, Yang Z, Lee J, Liu Y, Tian J, et al. Comparative effectiveness and safety of oral phosphodiesterase type 5 inhibitors for erectile dysfunction: a systematic review and network meta-analysis. Eur Urol. 2013;63(5):902–12.
62. Giuliano F, Jackson G, Montorsi F, Martin-Morales A, Raillard P. Safety of sildenafil citrate: review of 67 double-blind placebo-controlled trials and the postmarketing safety database. Int J Clin Pract. 2010;64(2):240–55.
63. Card GL, England BP, Suzuki Y, Fong D, Powell B, Lee B, et al. Structural basis for the activity of drugs that inhibit Phosphodiesterases. Structure. 2004;12(12):2233–47.
64. Corbin JD. Mechanisms of action of PDE5 inhibition in erectile dysfunction. Int J Impot Res. 2004;16(Suppl 1):S4–7.
65. Jeon YH, Heo YS, Kim CM, Hyun YL, Lee TG, Ro S, et al. Phosphodiesterase: overview of protein structures, potential therapeutic applications and recent progress in drug development. Cell Mol Life Sci. 2005;62(11):1198–220.
66. Porst H, Burnett A, Brock G, Ghanem H, Giuliano F, Glina S, et al. SOP conservative (medical and mechanical) treatment of erectile dysfunction. J Sex Med. 2013;10(1):130–71.
67. Brock GB, McMahon CG, Chen KK, Costigan T, Shen W, Watkins V, et al. Efficacy and safety of Tadalafil for the treatment of erectile dysfunction: results of integrated analyses. J Urol. 2002;168(4 Part 1):1332–6.
68. Hellstrom WJ, Gittelman M, Karlin G, Segerson T, Thibonnier M, Taylor T, et al. Vardenafil for treatment of men with erectile dysfunction: efficacy and safety in a randomized, double-blind, placebo-controlled trial. J Androl. 2002;23(6):763–71.
69. Porst H, Rosen R, Padma-Nathan H, Goldstein I, Giuliano F, Ulbrich E, et al. The efficacy and tolerability of vardenafil, a new, oral, selective phosphodiesterase type 5 inhibitor, in patients with erectile dysfunction: the first at-home clinical trial. Int J Impot Res. 2001;13(4):192–9.
70. Smith WB, McCaslin IR, Gokce A, Mandava SH, Trost L, Hellstrom WJ. PDE5 inhibitors: considerations for preference and long-term adherence. Int J Clin Pract. 2013;67(8):768–80.
71. Brock G, Nehra A, Lipshultz LI, Karlin GS, Gleave M, Seger M, et al. Safety and efficacy of Vardenafil for the treatment of men with erectile dysfunction after radical Retropubic prostatectomy. J Urol. 2003;170(4 Part 1):1278–83.
72. Montorsi F, McCullough A. Efficacy of sildenafil citrate in men with erectile dysfunction following radical prostatectomy: a systematic review of clinical data. J Sex Med. 2005;2(5):658–67.
73. Montorsi F, Nathan HP, Mccullough A, Brock GB, Broderick G, Ahuja S, et al. Tadalafil in the treatment of erectile dysfunction following bilateral nerve sparing radical retropubic prostatectomy: a randomized, double-blind, placebo controlled trial. J Urol. 2004;172(3):1036–41.

74. Rendell MS, Rajfer J, Wicker PA, Smith MD. Sildenafil for treatment of erectile dysfunction in men with diabetes: a randomized controlled trial. Sildenafil Diabetes Study Group. JAMA. 1999;281(5):421–6.
75. Kang SG, Kim JJ. Udenafil: efficacy and tolerability in the management of erectile dysfunction. Ther Adv Urol. 2013;5(2):101–10.
76. Kedia GT, Uckert S, Assadi-Pour F, Kuczyk MA, Albrecht K. Avanafil for the treatment of erectile dysfunction: initial data and clinical key properties. Ther Adv Urol. 2013;5(1):35–41.
77. Corona G, Razzoli E, Forti G, Maggi M. The use of phosphodiesterase 5 inhibitors with concomitant medications. J Endocrinol Investig. 2008;31(9):799–808.
78. Burnett A. Evaluation and management of erectile dysfunction. In: Wein AJK, Louis R, Partin AW, Peters CA, editors. Campbell-Walsh urology. Philadelphia, PA, USA: Elsevier. 2016. p. 643–68.e7.
79. Virag R. Intracavernous injection of papaverine for erectile failure. 1982. J Urol. 2002;167(2 Pt 2):1196.
80. Palmer LS, Valcic M, Melman A, Giraldi A, Wagner G, Christ GJ. Characterization of cyclic AMP accumulation in cultured human corpus cavernosum smooth muscle cells. J Urol. 1994;152(4):1308–14.
81. Seyam R, Mohamed K, Akhras AA, Rashwan H. A prospective randomized study to optimize the dosage of trimix ingredients and compare its efficacy and safety with prostaglandin E1. Int J Impot Res. 2005;17(4):346–53.
82. Soderdahl DW, Thrasher JB, Hansberry KL. Intracavernosal drug-induced erection therapy versus external vacuum devices in the treatment of erectile dysfunction. Br J Urol. 1997;79(6):952–7.
83. Shabsigh R, Padma-Nathan H, Gittleman M, McMurray J, Kaufman J, Goldstein I. Intracavernous alprostadil alfadex is more efficacious, better tolerated, and preferred over intraurethral alprostadil plus optional actis: a comparative, randomized, crossover, multi-center study. Urology. 2000;55(1):109–13.
84. Shokeir AA, Alserafi MA, Mutabagani H. Intracavernosal versus intraurethral alprostadil: a prospective randomized study. BJU Int. 1999;83(7):812–5.
85. Linet OI, Ogrinc FG. Efficacy and safety of intracavernosal alprostadil in men with erectile dysfunction. The Alprostadil Study Group. N Engl J Med. 1996;334(14):873–7.
86. Burnett AL, Nehra A, Breau RH, Culkin DJ, Faraday MM, Hakim LS, et al. Erectile dysfunction: AUA guideline. J Urol. 2018;200(3):633–41.
87. Brison D, Seftel A, Sadeghi-Nejad H. The resurgence of the Vacuum Erection Device (VED) for treatment of erectile dysfunction. J Sex Med. 2013;10(4):1124–35.
88. Williams G, Abbou CC, Amar ET, Desvaux P, Flam TA, Lycklama a Nijeholt GA, et al. Efficacy and safety of transurethral alprostadil therapy in men with erectile dysfunction. MUSE Study Group. Br J Urol. 1998;81(6):889–94.
89. Akdemir F, Okulu E, Kayigil O. Long-term outcomes of AMS Spectra(R) penile prosthesis implantation and satisfaction rates. Int J Impot Res. 2017;29(5):184–8.
90. Akakpo W, Pineda MA, Burnett AL. Critical analysis of satisfaction assessment after penile prosthesis surgery. Sex Med Rev. 2017;5(2):244–51.
91. Levine LA, Becher EF, Bella AJ, Brant WO, Kohler TS, Martinez-Salamanca JI, et al. Penile prosthesis surgery: current recommendations from the international consultation on sexual medicine. J Sex Med. 2016;13(4):489–518.
92. Carson CC 3rd, Mulcahy JJ, Harsch MR. Long-term infection outcomes after original antibiotic impregnated inflatable penile prosthesis implants: up to 7.7 years of followup. J Urol. 2011;185(2):614–8.
93. Serefoglu EC, Mandava SH, Gokce A, Chouhan JD, Wilson SK, Hellstrom WJ. Long-term revision rate due to infection in hydrophilic-coated inflatable penile prostheses: 11-year follow-up. J Sex Med. 2012;9(8):2182–6.
94. Enemchukwu EA, Kaufman MR, Whittam BM, Milam DF. Comparative revision rates of inflatable penile prostheses using woven Dacron(R) fabric cylinders. J Urol. 2013;190(6):2189–93.

95. Zhang H, Albersen M, Jin X, Lin G. Stem cells: novel players in the treatment of erectile dysfunction. Asian J Androl. 2012;14(1):145–55.
96. Mahla RS. Stem cells applications in regenerative medicine and disease therapeutics. Int J Cell Biol. 2016;2016:24.
97. Ding D-C, Chang Y-H, Shyu W-C, Lin S-Z. Human umbilical cord mesenchymal stem cells: a new era for stem cell therapy. Cell Transplant. 2015;24(3):339–47.
98. Pittenger MF, Mackay AM, Beck SC, Jaiswal RK, Douglas R, Mosca JD, et al. Multilineage potential of adult human mesenchymal stem cells. Science. 1999;284(5411):143–7.
99. Lin C, Shih D, editors. Green consumption attitudes of the tourists lodging in the resort hotel. 2010 4th international conference on bioinformatics and biomedical engineering, 2010, 18–20 June.
100. Peak TC, Anaissie J, Hellstrom WJG. Current perspectives on stem cell therapy for erectile dysfunction. Sex Med Rev. 2016;4(3):247–56.
101. Xin Z-C, Xu Y-D, Lin G, Lue T, Guo Y-L. Recruiting endogenous stem cells: a novel therapeutic approach for erectile dysfunction. Asian J Androl. 2016;18(1):10–5.
102. Shan H, Chen F, Zhang T, He S, Xu L, Wei A. Stem cell therapy for erectile dysfunction of cavernous nerve injury rats: a systematic review and meta-analysis. PLoS One. 2015;10(4):e0121428-e.
103. Bochinski D, Lin GT, Nunes L, Carrion R, Rahman N, Lin CS, et al. The effect of neural embryonic stem cell therapy in a rat model of cavernosal nerve injury. BJU Int. 2004;94(6):904–9.
104. Kendirci M, Trost L, Bakondi B, Whitney MJ, Hellstrom WJG, Spees JL. Transplantation of nonhematopoietic adult bone marrow stem/progenitor cells isolated by p75 nerve growth factor receptor into the penis rescues erectile function in a Rat Model of cavernous nerve injury. J Urol. 2010;184(4):1560–6.
105. Te AE, Santarosa RP, Koo HP, Buttyan R, Greene LA, Kaplan SA, et al. Neurotrophic factors in the rat penis. J Urol. 1994;152(6 Pt 1):2167–72.
106. Ryu JK, Kim DH, Song KM, Yi T, Suh JK, Song SU. Intracavernous delivery of clonal mesenchymal stem cells restores erectile function in a Mouse Model of cavernous nerve injury. J Sex Med. 2014;11(2):411–23.
107. Xu Y, Guan R, Lei H, Li H, Wang L, Gao Z, et al. Therapeutic potential of adipose-derived stem cells-based micro-tissues in a rat model of postprostatectomy erectile dysfunction. J Sex Med. 2014;11(10):2439–48.
108. Lin H, Dhanani N, Tseng H, Souza GR, Wang G, Cao Y, et al. Nanoparticle improved stem cell therapy for erectile dysfunction in a Rat Model of cavernous nerve injury. J Urol. 2016;195(3):788–95.
109. Ouyang B, Sun X, Han D, Chen S, Yao B, Gao Y, et al. Human urine-derived stem cells alone or genetically-modified with FGF2 improve type 2 diabetic erectile dysfunction in a Rat Model. PLoS One. 2014;9(3):e92825.
110. Position statement: ED restorative (regenerative) therapies (shock waves, autologous platelet rich plasma, and stem cells). Available from: https://www.smsna.org/V1/resources/position-statements.
111. Bahk JY, Jung JH, Han H, Min SK, Lee YS. Treatment of diabetic impotence with umbilical cord blood stem cell intracavernosal transplant: preliminary report of 7 cases. Exp Clin Transplant. 2010;8(2):150–60.
112. Yiou R, Hamidou L, Birebent B, Bitari D, Lecorvoisier P, Contremoulins I, et al. Safety of intracavernous bone marrow-mononuclear cells for postradical prostatectomy erectile dysfunction: an open dose-escalation pilot study. Eur Urol. 2016;69(6):988–91.
113. Yiou R, Hamidou L, Birebent B, Bitari D, Le Corvoisier P, Contremoulins I, et al. Intracavernous injections of bone marrow mononucleated cells for postradical prostatectomy erectile dysfunction: final results of the INSTIN clinical trial. Eur Urol Focus. 2017;3(6):643–5.

114. Levy JA, Marchand M, Iorio L, Cassini W, Zahalsky MP. Determining the feasibility of managing erectile dysfunction in humans with placental-derived stem cells. J Am Osteopath Assoc. 2016;116(1):e1–5.
115. Lin CS, Xin ZC, Wang Z, Deng C, Huang YC, Lin G, et al. Stem cell therapy for erectile dysfunction: a critical review. Stem Cells Dev. 2012;21(3):343–51.
116. FDA warns about stem cell therapies. [Available from: https://www.fda.gov/consumers/consumer-updates/fda-warns-about-stem-cell-therapies.
117. Carson CC, Kirby R, Goldstein I. Textbook of erectile dysfunction. Oxford, UK: Isis Medical Media Ltd; 1999. p. 26.

Chapter 17
Stem Cell Therapy for Ophthalmic Vascular Disease

Caio Vinicius Regatieri, Augusto Vieira, and Marcio Bittar Nehemy

17.1 Introduction

Scientists have desired for many years to cure blindness. Achieving this endeavor has been challenging, as many of the diseases associated with irreversible loss of vision involve retinal neurons, and most mammalian neurons do not regenerate [1]. Since many retinal and neurodegenerative diseases progress slowly, it may be possible to use stem cell-derived cells to prevent visual loss if such therapy is performed at an early stage of the disease. Advances in stem cell technology and tissue engineering in the last several years have opened the possibility of replacing lost retinal neurons and restoring vision. As a result of these advances, as well as a challenge involving multiple stakeholders, the National Eye Institute (NEI) launched its Audacious Goals Initiative (AGI) in 2013 with the aim "to restore vision through the regeneration of neurons and neural connections in the eye and visual system" [1]. Additional information are available at www.nei.nih.gov/audacious. The majority of diseases that lead to vision loss, such as age-related macular degeneration, diabetic retinopathy, and inherited retinal degenerations, do so at least in part as a result of abnormalities in the retinal or choroidal vasculature.

The eye has unique advantages as a target organ for cell transplantation [2]. The intraocular environment is relatively protected against systemic immune responses that threaten allograft survival. The compartmentalized structure of the globe

C. V. Regatieri
Department of Ophthalmology, Federal University of São Paulo, São Paulo, Brazil

Department of ophthalmology, Tufts Medical School, Boston, MA, USA

A. Vieira
Department of Ophthalmology, Federal University of São Paulo, São Paulo, Brazil

M. B. Nehemy (✉)
Department of Ophthalmology, Federal University of Minas Gerais,
Belo Horizonte, MG, Brazil

© Springer Nature Switzerland AG 2021
T. P. Navarro et al. (eds.), *Stem Cell Therapy for Vascular Diseases*,
https://doi.org/10.1007/978-3-030-56954-9_17

367

restricts potential dissemination locally and systemically. The retina is an extension of the brain that is readily accessible to surgical intervention under direct observation. Retinal microstructure can be observed in detail in the living eye noninvasively owing to the optical transparency of ocular media, which allows its evaluation by high-resolution fundus photography, fundus angiography, and optic coherence tomography. In addition, retinal function can be mapped topographically, by microperimetry, or multifocal eletroretinography [3]. The impact of intervention within a defined target region of the retina can be determined with confidence by comparison with untreated regions within the same eye and in the contralateral eye, which offer invaluable intraocular and intraindividual controls for the natural history of the condition and variability in performance [2].

17.1.1   Retina Development

The development of both the sensory retina and the RPE begins with the invagination of the optic vesicle [4, 5]. This invagination of neural-epithelial cells forms a bilayered cup; the inner layer of the optic cup will become the sensory retina; and the outer layer will give rise to the RPE. At this stage, the primordial retina is composed of these two layers separated by a lumen. As the retina continues to develop, these two layers begin to come closer together, closing the lumen that will become the subretinal space. This shrinking lumen is filled with a new material called the interphotoreceptor matrix (IPM) that will become the interface of communication between the mature photoreceptors and the mature RPE. The presence of the IPM triggers the outer layer of the optic cup to begin its differentiation into the RPE. It is thought that the maturation of the RPE includes the production of a variety of factors that trigger the differentiation of the inner layer of the optic cup [6, 7].

Maturation of the putative sensory retina is a series of carefully orchestrated events, in which all seven cell types of the mature retina are derived from a set of common retinal progenitor cells (RPC). The RPCs of the inner layer of the optic cup proliferate to form the inner marginal and outer nuclear zones. Next, the nuclear zone invades the marginal zone forming the inner and outer neuroblastic zones [8, 9]. Of the seven cell types in the mature sensory retina, there are six types of neurons and one glial cell type. Despite there being some overlap, the differentiation of these cell types occurs according to the following temporal sequence: retinal ganglion cell, cone photoreceptors, amacrine cells, horizontal cells, rod photoreceptors, bipolar cells, and finally Müller glial cells [5, 10]. Once these cells have matured, they organize into the iconic retinal layers. As an aside, Müller cells are not the only glial cells in the retina: there are also astrocytes at the inner retinal surface and oligodendrocytes that envelop the optic nerve. These cells, however, form in the brain and migrate to the retina later in development [4, 6, 8].

This well-organized neuronal layering, in addition to the close anatomical proximity of the PR and RPE, must be maintained in order for the light we perceive as vision to reach the brain. In its simplest circuit, light that enters the eye passes through the cornea and lens which focuses it on the retina. This focused light passes through the inner retinal layers and reaches the photoreceptors. In the photoreceptor outer segments, photonic energy activates visual pigments, generating electrical impulses. In turn, the photoreceptors release neurotransmitters to the bipolar cells that transmit signals to the ganglion cells. The ganglion cells axons come together and form the innermost layer of the retina, the nerve fiber layer. As the signal is passed along the nerve fiber layer, the axons of the retinal ganglion cells cluster and form the optic nerve. The optic nerve then transmits neuronal signals to the lateral geniculate body. Next, the optic radiations carry the impulses to occipital cortex where they are processed for vision [10, 11].

Before the sensory retina attains its fully functional state, each of the retinal neurons must differentiate. An important step in the maturation of the sensory retina occurs when the primordial photoreceptor extends its outer segment into the subretinal space. When this happens, the PR outer segment comes in contact with the apical surface of the nearly mature RPE. Subsequently, a myriad of biochemical communication ensues, which has been reported to coincide with development and differentiation of both these cell types [7, 12].

17.1.2 Target Diseases

In diseases such as age-related macular degeneration (AMD) and retinitis pigmentosa (RP), it is clear that areas of RPE atrophy are associated with degeneration of the adjacent photoreceptors. Two major strategies have emerged that aim to regenerate the degenerating retina. The first aims to restore the photoreceptors themselves, while the second attempts to replace the RPE. A number of cellular sources have been studied with the hope of finding an ideal donor cell. This list includes embryonic stem cells (ESCs), fetal tissue, progenitor cells, induced pluripotent stem (iPS) cells, and adult tissue-specific stem cells [12, 13].

There are multiple retinal diseases that are targets for regenerative therapies. Two of the most relevant to cell-replacement therapy are AMD and inherited retinal degenerations, such as RP. AMD and RP are common degenerative retinal diseases that are characterized by the progressive loss of retinal photoreceptor cells (PR). Current estimates suggest that, in the United States, more than 1.75 million people are living with AMD [14], and there are 80,000 people who are affected with RP. As recently as 30 years ago, there were no therapeutic options for people who suffered from photoreceptor-specific degenerative retinal diseases. Today, there are a wide variety of treatment options for neovascular degenerative processes, including anti-angiogenic drugs, conventional laser therapies, and photodynamic therapies. Despite these advances, treatment options for atrophic macular disease are currently limited to dietary supplements. Although AMD does not result in complete blindness, it is the most important cause of legal blindness in developed countries. The involvement of the central retina reduces significantly the quality of life of patients with this disease. In addition, there are patients who lose vision as result of either fibrovascular scarring from neovascular macular degeneration, or from advanced non-neovascular AMD, or geographic atrophy. These patients would be candidates for restoration of vision targeted to the macula [1].

A second group of retinal diseases are the inherited retinal degenerations, such as Stargardt disease and RP. Stargardt disease (STGD1) is the most common cause of macular degeneration in children and young adults. Retinal degeneration in STGD1 typically advances progressively by expansion from the macula [2]. The visual loss in patients with RP typically progress over years, beginning in the periphery and eventually involving central vision. Ultimately, complete blindness can occur. A third group are diseases where trophic factor-mediated cell rescue may be particularly effective in the early stages, e.g., diabetic retinopathy or acute retinal detachment [1]. Fortunately, both of these diseases can present good outcomes with conventional treatments, and, therefore, at present, they are not preferred targets for stem cell therapy.

On the other hand, for AMD and retinal degenerations, the currently available therapies merely attenuate vision loss. Therefore, the ideal treatment regime for individuals that suffer from photoreceptor-specific degenerations would simultaneously mitigate disease progression and restore visual potential. Retinal regeneration, using stem cells, has emerged as a promising therapeutic option because it offers the possibility of restoring sight. Currently, photoreceptors (PR) and retinal pigment epithelium (RPE) cells are targets to be replaced in order to regenerate the retina. Because stem cells can generate the types of cells lost in disease, it is possible that they might someday restore vision by replacing dead photoreceptors and retinal pigment epithelium (RPE) cells in atrophic age-related macular degeneration (AMD), inherited retinal degenerations, and dying retinal ganglion cells (RGCs) in glaucoma and other optic nerve atrophies. Thus, because stem cells can produce nearly unlimited quantities of retinal cells, stem cell regenerative therapies—in theory—represent a plausible approach to address the significant unmet needs associated with these disorders [15–17].

17.2   Background and Cell Types

In a recent paper, Rao et al. [15] summarized the key concepts and the main sources of stem cells currently used for chorioretinal diseases. Stem cells are precursor cell types that remain undifferentiated and have the capacity to self-renew by proliferation while in the precursor state. When in contact with specific cytokines, stem cells can differentiate into specialized cell types such as retinal cells. Because stem cells can proliferate in an immature state, clinically relevant amounts of differentiated retinal tissue (e.g., RPE) can be produced for transplantation. Progenitor cells are similar to stem cells but are considered to have a more limited ability to proliferate and/or a narrower spectrum of mature cell types into which they can differentiate [15]. Progenitor cells are isolated from developing tissue and exist in more advanced ontogenetic stages than those of ESCs. This means that progenitor cells are committed to the eye field, and, therefore, progenitor cell differentiation potential is intrinsically more robust. Despite tremendous promise, both ESC and progenitor cell research have been hindered by both ethical and immunologic concerns [13].

For retinal diseases most studies use three sources of cells: pluripotent, fetal, and postnatal ("adult stem cells") [15]. Pluripotent stem cells (PSCs) can differentiate into any tissue in the body. Two types of PSCs are currently employed for the treatment of retinal diseases: human embryonic stem cells (hESCs) [15, 18, 19] and induced pluripotent stem cells (iPSCs) [15, 20, 21]. Embryonic stem cells are pluripotent cells cultivated from the inner cell mass of a 5-day-old blastocyst. These cells are characterized by their properties of unlimited self-renewal and the ability to give rise to the body's three germ layers (endoderm, mesoderm, ectoderm), and therefore, when given the appropriate cues, ESCs can potentially differentiate into any of the body's over 200 cell types. Driving ESCs toward a fully differentiated postmitotic RPE or photoreceptor cell fate in vitro has been studied by a number of groups. However, posttransplantation complications have given rise to investigations using more mature progenitor cell retinal transplants [13, 22].

iPSCs are pluripotent cells derived from differentiated but reprogrammed somatic cells, such as adult skin fibroblasts or white blood cells. Induced pluripotent stem cells are adult somatic cells that have had pluripotent factors introduced into the adult genome, a process referred to as reprogramming. Therefore, iPSC cells represent an autologous pluripotent cell population that is widely available and mitigates the ethical concerns that have plagued embryonic stem cell research. However, altering donor cell DNA (which often includes the introduction of well-known oncogenes) carries a number of translational concerns, specifically tumorigenicity. Whereas an in-depth review of these cell types is beyond the scope of this paper, it is important to point out that these cells types have been the focus of retinal regeneration investigations because of their in vitro proliferative capacity, multipotent properties, and differentiation potential [23–25].

hESCs and iPSCs can then be converted to neural retinal or RPE cells [15]. Other classes of stem/progenitor cells being used in trials for retinal diseases are those derived from the fetal central nervous system, such as cells derived from the developing brain, spinal cord, and retina [26]. Fetal retinal stem/progenitor cells build the retina during embryonic development, through limited self-renewal and tissue-specific differentiation [27]. Adult stem/progenitor cells are nonpluripotent postnatal cells that can generate some, or all, of the cell types comprising the organs from which they originate. Bone marrow-derived cells, umbilical tissue-derived cells, mesenchymal stem cells, and adipose (fat) cells have been proposed for use or are being used in various interventions for a variety of retinal disorders [15]. A novel cell-based potential therapy – palucorcel (CNTO-2476) – has been evaluated for the treatment of AMD. Palucorcel comprises human umbilical tissue-derived cells (hUTCs) in a proprietary cryopreserved formulation. hUTCs are derived from extraembryonic mesoderm. These hUTCs do not meet the US National Institutes of Health definition of a stem cell for two major reasons. First, these cells cannot grow for indefinite generations in culture; they senesce at approximately 40–60 population doublings. Second, these cells are not rare and do not spontaneously differentiate in vitro, or when transplanted in vivo, into other cell types of the umbilical cord (endothelial cells or epithelial cells) [28].

For delivery of stem/progenitor cells to the retina, various methods have been used, cells including intravitreous injection, vitrectomy with subretinal transplantation, (internal), and "external" subretinal delivery across the sclera and choroid [15]. Polymeric constructs and the cell delivery systems based on them are being geared toward retinal tissue engineering. They have substantial capability to promote and ameliorate the current strategies applied for cell-based treatments in the eye.

Perhaps the most promising of these potential therapeutic options involves the injection of progenitor cells into the eye. This strategy came to fruition because of the failure of ectopic retinal transplantation studies and the simultaneous success of studies that have demonstrated the integration of neural stem cells and retinal progenitor cells [8]. One of the first of these studies involved injection of adult rat hippocampal-derived stem cells into the vitreous of rats with degenerative retinal disease. These progenitor cells demonstrated robust integration and the expression of neuronal markers; however, they did not produce photoreceptor-specific markers [6].

Subsequently, it was hypothesized that isolated multipotent neuroretinal stem cells, already committed to a retinal cell fate, would be more likely to differentiate into photoreceptors. More recent transplant studies have confirmed this hypothesis using mouse models. McLaren et al. demonstrated that retinal progenitor cells (a cell at a more advanced ontogenetic stage than a retinal stem cell) that were injected to the eye were able to integrate into host retinas and differentiate and express photoreceptor-specific proteins. This study suggested that the injected RPCs created functional synaptic connections within the host retina because mice that were exposed to light after RPC transplantation demonstrated moderate improvements in pupillary responses. Because only a small fraction of donor cells was able to penetrate the outer retinal barrier, functional improvements were limited. This study, as well as others, has shown the potential of retinal progenitor cell transplantation, and this field of research has demonstrated two things: (1) cell-based therapies are capable of regenerating degenerating retinas; and (2) in order for RPC transplantation to be an effective therapeutic option, new techniques must be explored that promote RPC survival after transplantation, integration into host retinas, and photoreceptor-specific differentiation [23, 24].

Adult mouse fibroblasts were first converted into pluripotent stem cells in 2006 by Takahashi and Yamanaka (Fig. 17.1). The resulting cells were named induced pluripotent stem cells (iPSC). Four transcription factors were used first: sex-determining region Y-box 2 (Sox2), Myc proto-oncogene protein (c-Myc), POU domain, class 5 transcription factor 1, also kwon as Oct ¾, and Kruppel-like factor 4 (Klf4) [29–31]. In 2007, the same team performed the conversion of human fibroblasts into iPSCs using the aforementioned method [32, 33]. Thompson's group achieved similar results using different reprogramming factors, OCT4, SOX2, Nanog homeobox (NANOG), and Lin-28 homolog A (LIN28) [21, 34–36]. By successfully reprogramming these patient-extracted cells, the scientists were able to create a pivotal in vitro model for analyzing and creating protocols geared toward

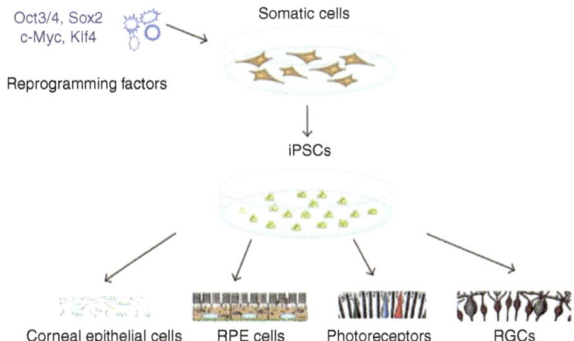

Fig. 17.1 Schematic illustration of iPSC induction and reprogramming into ocular cells. iPS cells are generated by reprogramming adult somatic cells. In the ophthalmic field, iPSCs have been successfully differentiated into a variety of the ocular cells, including corneal epithelial cells, RPE, photoreceptors, and RGCs. (Figure and legend adapted from Retinal stem cell transplantation: Balancing safety and potential. Singh MS, et al. Prog Retin Eye Res. 2019)

new approaches for the treatment of several genetic diseases. iPSCs are able to differentiate themselves into all three lineages, mesodermal, endodermal, and ectodermal. Human-induced pluripotent cells are fully functional, self-renewable, and expandable cells that preserve the exclusive genomic information of each individual and can be acquired in a practically infinite fashion from its donor (Fig. 17.1). This method also provides the studies a bypass to an ethically disputed subject, because it does not involve embryos and are an autologous cell source, thereby most likely negating immunological problems intrinsically related to human embryonic stem cell treatments [36–39].

Successful cell therapy requires well-characterized cell lineages at very specific differentiation stages. The cellular original in vivo configuration has to be gradually recapitulated until anterior neuroblast composition is achieved. Then, this cell line has to be transformed into eye field cells, then specifically into retinal pigment epithelium (RPE), or, for instance, into retinal ganglion cells (RGC) [32, 40, 41] (Fig. 17.2). Safety and efficiency are paramount when it comes to new therapies. Improving these cornerstones is an ongoing challenge, and some groups proposed using different pluripotency induction factors from those previously described by Takahashi and Yamanaka. MicroRNA, valproic acid, and SV40 large T antigen are some of the newly proposed factors. Myc transcription factor is an active oncogene and was a major concern until 2008, when it was demonstrated that iPSC could be generated without its use. Adenoviruses, *Sendai virus*, plasmids, microRNAs, mRNA transfections, and episomal vectors are some examples of methods that do not require the use of retroviral vectors, thereby diminishing the risk of creating a tumorigenic state [34, 35, 37, 38, 42–44]. Generation of RPE and its replacement in degenerated retinas have been the primary focus of the most recent and robust scientific endeavors that gave rise to current human clinical trials. RPE and RGC transplantation has already occurred successfully [20, 45, 46].

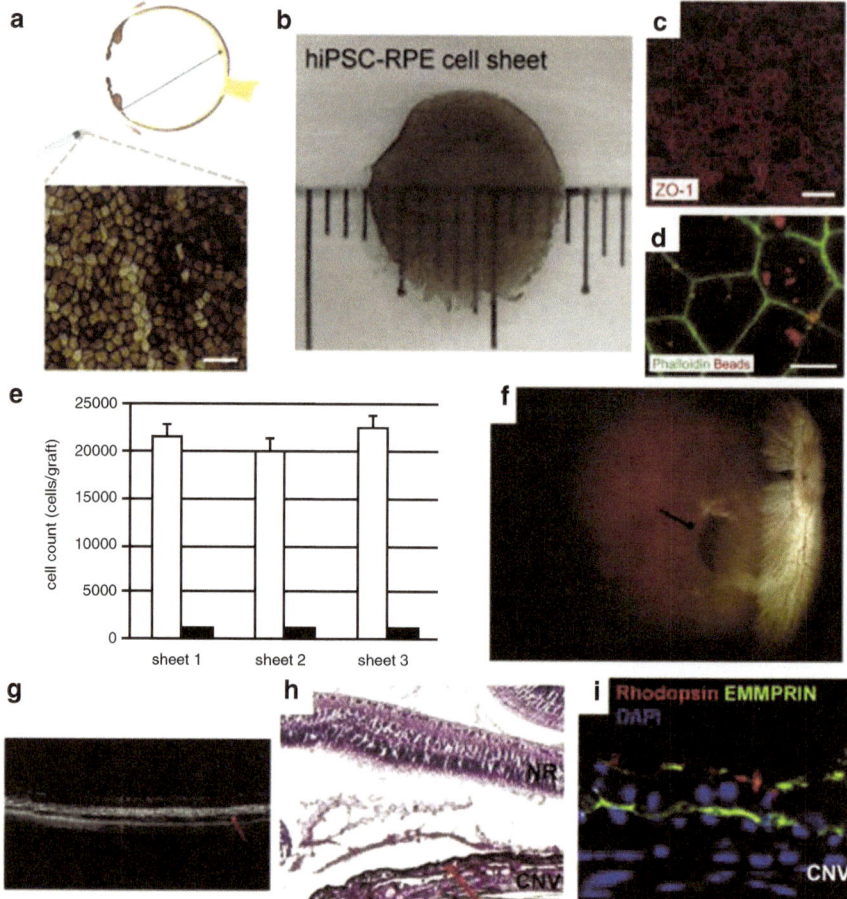

Fig. 17.2 Stem cell-based differentiation of light-sensitive photoreceptor cells in three-dimensional culture. (**a, b**) Human-induced pluripotent stem cells differentiating in adherent conditions formed neural retinal (NR) domains expressing VSX2 that were surrounded by a retinal pigment epithelium (RPE) domain expressing MITF. (**c**) These NR domains were isolated and cultured in suspension to yield three-dimensional (3D) retinal cups containing NR and retinal pigment epithelium (RPE) cells. (**d**) Higher magnification of a retinal cup showing the NR and RPE cells that typically formed adjacent to each other. (**e**) Over time, 3D retinal cups acquired the characteristic retinal lamination containing the precursors of most of the major neuronal cell types, including ganglion, amacrine and horizontal cells (PAX6), and photoreceptors (OTX2). (**f–i**) Relatively advanced differentiation of photoreceptors occurred in culture, with morphological and molecular differentiation of rods and cones, including expression of rod opsin (**f–g**), S-opsin (**h**), and L/M-opsin (**i**) in individual cells. (**j**) As further evidence of relatively advanced differentiation, transmission electron microscopy showed presence of inner segments containing centriole (C), basal bodies (BB), and connecting cilia (CC); an outer limiting membrane (*) was also observed. (**k**) Laminated outer segments discs (arrowheads) also grew in culture, indicating specific and relatively advanced photoreceptor ultrastructural differentiation. (**i**) Perforated-patch electrophysiological recordings showed a flash-triggered response from light-sensitive photoreceptors. Scale bars: 100μm (**a–c** and **e**), 50 μm (**d**), 10 μm (**f**), 0.05 μm (**j, k**). (Figure and legend adapted from Retinal stem cell transplantation: Balancing safety and potential. (From: Singh MS, et al. Prog Retin Eye Res. 2019)

Currently, lymphocytes, peripheral blood mononuclear cells, and keratinocytes are also used and even more readily available than fibroblasts for iPSC and can be equally differentiated into RPE using distinctive methods. Four distinguished methods are currently adopted to differentiate iPSCs into RPE cells: serum-free embryoid body (SFEB), stromal cell-derived-inducing activity (SDIA), spontaneous continuously adherent culture (SCAC), and the directed differentiation method (DDM).

SCAC method: if iPSC is applied into media specific for expansion such as E8, RPE cell lines will be found after 1–2 months. Unfortunately, this simpler method is not efficient because its differentiation rate is 1% and it is very time-consuming.

SDIA operates with a stromal cell medium to induce RPE cells. PA6, a bone marrow stromal cell line, is responsible for presenting unknown factors to the iPSCs colonies co-cultured with them. Pax6, paired box 6, is a transcription factor encountered in the RPE that is found in approximately 9% of the iPSCs colonies after 21 days of culture. Using Sertoli cells, Yue and Okamoto were able to obtain RPE cells in just 14 days; when Okamoto used the PA6 cell line, it took 30 days to acquire RPE cells [47].

In the SFEB method, embryonic bodies are prepared with various types of media. For retinogenesis to be complete, several growth factors are essential. For example, nodal signaling, Wnt signaling, and bmp signaling antagonists are used to assist iPSCs to develop into RPE. Embryonic growth naturally presents the three fundamental lineages, endo-, meso-, and ectoderm. Primeval endoderm is then found in the external part of these embryonic bodies and can be stimulated to grow into eye lineages.

The SFEB method and the directed differentiation method (DDM) are very similar. DDM is generally more appropriate when the aim is to proliferate RPE cells. Molecules and growth factors are used and added to the media. Factors such as nicotinamide, ROCK inhibitors, and dorsomorphin can optimize the cell line production and are very effective, reaching results of up to 97% of differentiation [47–53].

Cell regeneration is a daunting challenge. Retinal ganglion cells (RGCs) are neurons that have their function tightly connected to their inherent ability to form synapses, integrate to other cell types and other RGCs, to develop axons able to connect to the optic nerve and brain, and to link to the retinal ganglion cell layer in the retina. These cells are the first lineage of neurons to be developed in the vertebrate retina. RGCs have been transplanted to the vitreous chamber and retina of rodents. Parameswaran et al. found that the transplanted cell could link and form functional connections to the host RGC layer. By contrast, Chen et al. was not able to show the same results, as in their case, an irrelevant number of cells were able to successfully migrate and integrate to the host retina. In vitro studies demonstrated the ability of transplanted RGCs to form synapses when compared to host RGCs. Guidance molecules were also found in these transplanted cells and were able to direct the newly formed axons in the right path through the retina and optic chiasm [54–57].

Transcription factors such as Math5, Six6, Sox4, Notch, Ath5, Sox11, and Brn3 are critical for correct development of RGCs. In the absence or mutation of one or more of these factors, RGCs fail to successfully integrate with bipolar and amacrine cells, and or they form hypoplastic optic nerves; they fail to differentiate from retinal progenitors; and they suffer rapid and massive apoptosis and ultimately fail to link its original and pertinent destinations that are at the lateral geniculate nucleus, pretectal nuclei, suprachiasmatic nuclei, and superior colliculi. RGCs are larger than average retinal neurons. They act as integrating bridges communicating the input they receive from other retinal neurons, usually centimeters away from the output main source in the eye and the optic nerve. They are able of doing so by presenting a complex array of sophisticated dendritic axonal structures, ultimately directing information to the brain.

Deteriorated surroundings in the host retina may be highly toxic to transplanted cells. These incoming RGCs have to survive, proliferate, integrate, and eventually regenerate axonal paths toward the optic nerve and brain; all of these arduous processes have to function in a damaged environment. Venugopalan et al. found in a preclinical model of RGC transplantation that these cells were able to grow a significant number of axons that were functional and formed synapses, promoting local integration and having positive and proper responsiveness to light. In that study, cones were also found to thrive in further sites inside the degenerated retina. RGCs rely on their capability of being guided by proper molecules and transcription factors so as to form proper connections with the optic chiasm and brain (58) (58)[58](58). Teotia et al. found that hIPSC-derived RGCs were able to be accurately guided, forming dendritic axonal nets with the RGC layer; accordingly, Parameswaran et al. found that transplanted RGCs are connected to host cells and did not form any tumors [58–65].

The RPE is a monolayer structure of hexagonal individual non-regenerative cells. It is seated between the choroid and the photoreceptors (cones and rods). The RPE is crucially important to survival and precise activity of photoreceptors. Its main functions are as follows: formation and maintenance of the blood-retinal barrier (tight junctions); transportation of both nutrients (water, ions, glucose, fatty acids) and waste products required and produced by the photoreceptors; phagocytosis of outer rod segments; secretion of vascular endothelial growth factor and ultimately its use by choroidal circulation; vitamin a-rhodopsin conversion cycle; and promote free-radical scavenging, mainly by the use of melanin [66].

The California Project to Cure Blindness-Retinal Pigment Epithelium 1 is a clinical trial based on a platform designed by Kashani et al. The product is a synthetic parylene scaffold manufactured to imitate the Bruch membrane. The safety and efficacy of this device and its human embryonic stem cell-derived RPE were analyzed in four patients. Optical coherence tomography demonstrated hESC-RPE host integration and implantation. In one eye, an improvement of 17 letters was observed. No eye suffered negative alterations regarding its visual acuity [45, 46, 67].

Ocata/Advanced Cell Technology is now known as the Astellas Institute for Regenerative Medicine; its phase I/IIa clinical trial focuses on the treatment of Stargardt disease using transplanted hESCs RPE. The initial aforementioned study was carried out at the Jules Stein Eye Institute (UCLA) and included 13 patients. Profound deficit in visual acuity was defined as best-corrected vision worse than 20/400. Ten patients with this criterion received a subretinal injection of hESCs-RPE cells, 50,000 RPE cells (3 patients), 100,000 RPE cells (3 patients), 150,000 RPE cells (3 patients), and 200,000 RPE cells in 1 patient. Three patients with best-corrected visual acuity of ≤20/100 received 100,000 hESCs-RPE cells. Best-corrected visual acuity improved in ten eyes, worsened in one eye, and improved or sustained the same in seven eyes. In 72% of subjects (13/18), RPE patches were observed in areas where there was no pigment prior to the injection. In the course of the first 4 months, no aberrant growth, signs of oncogenesis, or immune-related reactions were identified [18].

Large numbers (approximately 60,000) of hIPSC-RPE cells are required for proper migration and assimilation to form accurate synapses. This is considered a challenge because transplanted cell proliferation in the host may be prone to tumorigenicity; oncogenic mutations have been found during expansion and proliferation. A study conducted by the Riken Institute in Japan found chromosomal abnormalities in iPSC cells injected into patients, and they had to pause the study. Uncontrolled cell proliferation is therefore a major concern. Preclinical studies must analyze this risk. Kokkinaki proposed that only the first lineages of acquired cells should be used. Molecular markers can now show us the differentiation status of the hIPSC-derived RPE cells, and that simpler differentiation protocols should be prioritized. Whenever IPSC cells are put through multiple proliferation cycles, telomere shortening and accelerated senescence are found, and these phenomena may lead to tumor growth. Even after transplantation, these cells continue to mature and differentiate depending on the environment of the host retinal niche in which it was injected. These cells pose a noteworthy affinity to cancer cells, regarding their inclination to suffer from chromosomal abnormalities and their innate ability to proliferate in a potentially anarchic fashion. Immunodeficient mice and rats with dystrophic RPE layer received injections with iPSC-derived RPE cells in sheets in their subcutaneous tissue and in their subretinal space; no tumor growth was observed after more than 15 months [68–70].

Although remote, the possibility of tumorigenesis is real, and its consequences are life-threatening. Organoid differentiation by-products, genomic changes, and chromosomal abnormalities have to be checked in the stem cell bank; furthermore, only low-passage hIPSC cell lines should be used; and these lineages have to be previous and rigorously tested in the subretinal space of mammals. The chances of tumorigenicity are augmented when the niche contains immature cells and/or the iPSC line is not test-proven for aberrant genome [67].

In 1988, the National Science Foundation defined tissue engineering term as "the application of principles and methods of engineering and life sciences toward the fundamental understanding of structure-function relationships in normal and pathological mammalian tissues and the development of biological substitutes to restore, maintain or improve tissue function." Dendrimers, natural, synthetic, and or semi-synthetic polymers are now key biological surrogates for delivering cells and ultimately rebuilding injured tissues into novel and functional ones. Cells use scaffolds as structural and functional frameworks in which their development, proliferation, and differentiation thrive. Studies showed success in using these cell-seeded or cell-populated structures for tissue repair in a variety of unrelated tissues, including cartilage, skin, bones, muscles, and nerves [71].

Age-related macular disease, Stargardt's disease, and glaucoma are all potential targets for the use of 3D-printed scaffold-based therapies. Most scaffolds serve as bioactive biomaterials responsible for underpinning structures that are fundamentally safe microenvironments for novel and fragile cell formations. These cells are expected to populate the scaffold template. Ultimately, this cell-scaffold structure ought to simulate the microenvironment in which they are going to be seeded and are supposed to flourish, including the ones found in the Bruch membrane and RPE layer. Poly lactic-co-glycolic acid seed hiPSC RGCs have been minimally invasively transplanted to the retinal external layers of rhesus monkeys and rabbits. New operative neurite web arrangements, axons, and dendritic arbors were shown to have functional electric and anatomical features.

17.2.1 Adjuvant Strategies

Safe and steady scaffolds hold their mechanical and biochemical properties before, during, and after its surgical implantation. Most scaffolds are made of biomaterials such as gelatin, alginate, chitosan, collagen, poly e-caprolectone, poly-lactic acid, poly-glycerol-sebacate, and poly lactic-co-glycolic acid [72–75] (Fig. 17.3).

The most straightforward method for transposing cells into the eye, especially to the retina layers, is to implant a highly populated cell suspension directly to the desired site, e.g., the vitreous humor, choroid, or retina. This is a classic example of a scaffold-free strategy. Sadly, this procedure produces unsuitable and haphazard cell suspensions and incompetent grafts, mostly with inaccurate localization into the tissue, or massive apoptosis of the transplanted cell populations. Natural outer and inner retinal barriers are taunting challenges for the transplanted cells to overcome, allowing only a small portion of the transplanted cells to be in the originally aimed host site. Subretinal injections are both more logical and more conceivable. Homologous and autologous RPEs have been injected in this fashion. Autologous cells transplantation showed more encouraging and consistent results regarding cell survival and increasing visual acuity [76–83].

Consonant and steady secretion of extracellular matrix by cells seeded in cell sheets leads to an alternative approach in which their own matrix is used to promote better cell adhesion and a safer microenvironment for them before, during, and after host integration. This conclusively rendered superior survival rates and greater functionality in the host tissue [84–86].

Intricate 3D bioprinted scaffolds and cell sheets foreshadowed the next generation of the bioengineered devices aimed at restoring vision and its complex relationship between biomaterials, cell-based therapies, and surgical techniques. Patient-specific hiPSCs and their autologous transplantation using the aforementioned devices or the use of progenitor cells/donor cells attached to biodegradable platforms are the keystones to circumvent immune-related issues and tumorigenic aspects of these cell lineages. Tailor-made stem cell therapies, although still expensive and sophisticated, are now a reality, and its proof of concept has been positively demonstrated and replicated [6, 87–90].

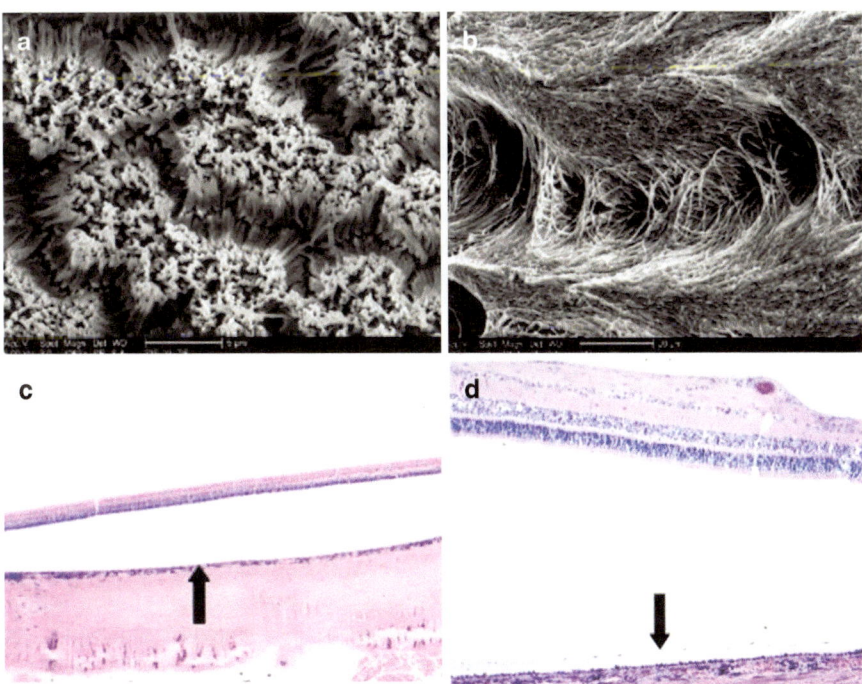

Fig. 17.3 PCL with incorporated nanowire. Scanning electron micrographs show the PCL polymers with short (**a**) and long (**b**) incorporated nanowires [47]. This PCL polymer is the thinnest polymer to be used in retinal tissue engineering to date. In both the histologic images (**c**, **d**), the detachment of the neural retina from the RPE is an artifactual by-product of the fixation process. The arrow on the left panel indicates the position on the polymer in the subretinal space. The inverted arrow on the right panel is demonstrating an example of a healthy retinal pigment epithelium, further suggesting the innocuous nature of the PCL polymer. (From Trese et al. [91])

Polymeric constructs and the cell delivery systems based on them are being geared toward retinal tissue engineering. They have substantial capability to promote and ameliorate the current strategies applied for cell-based treatments in the eye. This has generated a tangible clinical application capable of conveying cell differentiation, survival, and assimilation to host tissue. Multispecialty teams are key to develop such devices and, consequently accomplish the desired, but as yet unmet, challenge of promoting safe, cost-effective, and long-lasting vision restoration.

17.3 Current and Future Applications

Currently there are no FDA-approved stem cell therapies for retinal disease.

Most stem cell-based interventions for the retina seek to indirectly promote survival of the host's retinal cells through "trophic" effects. These interventions do not seek to replace dying cells. To date, there is only one class of stem cell trials in which transplanted cells are intended to replace dying cells. This involves the use of PSCs (embryonic or induced) that are differentiated to RPE and then transplanted subretinally in eyes with AMD and Stargardt disease [15]. Schwartz et al. in 2012 provided the first description of hESC-derived cells transplanted into human patients. The hESC-derived RPE cells showed no signs of hyperproliferation, tumorigenicity, ectopic tissue formation, or apparent rejection after 4 months. Best-corrected visual acuity improved from hand motions to 20/800 in the study eye of the patient with Stargardt's macular dystrophy, and vision also seemed to improve in the patient with dry age-related macular degeneration [18]. In 2015 Schwartz et al. reported the medium-term to long-term safety of cells derived from human embryonic stem cells (hESC) transplanted in nine patients with Stargardt's macular dystrophy and nine patients with atrophic age-related macular degeneration. Best-corrected visual acuity, monitored as part of the safety protocol, improved in ten eyes, improved or remained the same in seven eyes, and decreased by more than ten letters in one eye, whereas the untreated fellow eyes did not show similar improvements in visual acuity [19]. Mandai et al. assessed the feasibility of transplanting a sheet of retinal pigment epithelial (RPE) cells differentiated from induced pluripotent stem cells (iPSCs) in a patient with neovascular age-related macular degeneration. At 1 year after surgery, the transplanted sheet remained intact, but there was no change in visual acuity [20].

Ho et al. injected hUTCs via an ab externo approach to treat patients with geographic atrophy secondary to age-related macular degeneration and observed that at month 12, the median (range) change in BCVA from baseline was 4.5 (41 to 32) letters in the intervention eye and −0.5 (30 to 15) letters in the fellow eye. In this study, however, they observed significant procedure-related complications including retinal perforation (37.1%), retinal detachment (17.1%), and retinal hemorrhage (14.3%) [28].

In conclusion stem/progenitor cell-based therapy shows great promise to address blinding retinal diseases that currently have no curative treatment, including age-related macular degeneration, inherited retinal degenerations, and glaucoma. Although significant progresses have been made, additional studies in basic science, as well as well-controlled clinical trials, are needed, before the stem cell therapy can be widely applied in humans.

References

1. Levin LA, Miller JW, Zack DJ, Friedlander M, Smith LEH. Special commentary: early clinical development of cell replacement therapy: considerations for the National eye Institute audacious goals initiative. Ophthalmology. 2017;124(7):926–34.
2. Mehat MS, Sundaram V, Ripamonti C, Robson AG, Smith AJ, Borooah S, et al. Transplantation of human embryonic stem cell-derived retinal pigment epithelial cells in macular degeneration. Ophthalmology. 2018;125(11):1765–75.
3. Krohne TU, Westenskow PD, Kurihara T, Friedlander DF, Lehmann M, Dorsey AL, et al. Generation of retina pigment epithelial cells from small molecules and OCT4 reprogrammed human induced pluripotent stem cells. Stem Cells Transl Med. 2012;1(2):96–109.

4. Zahir T, Klassen H, Young MJ. Effects of ciliary neurotrophic factor on differentiation of late retinal progenitor cells. Stem Cells. 2005;23(3):424–32.
5. Osakada F, Jin ZB, Hirami Y, Ikeda H, Danjyo T, Watanabe K, et al. In vitro differentiation of retinal cells from human pluripotent stem cells by small-molecule induction. J Cell Sci. 2009;122(Pt 17):3169–79.
6. Young MJ, Ray J, Whiteley SJ, Klassen H, Gage FH. Neuronal differentiation and morphological integration of hippocampal progenitor cells transplanted to the retina of immature and mature dystrophic rats. Mol Cell Neurosci. 2000;16(3):197–205.
7. Strauss O. The retinal pigment epithelium in visual function. Physiol Rev. 2005;85(3):845–81.
8. Young MJ. Stem cells in the mammalian eye: a tool for retinal repair. APMIS. 2005;113(11–12):845–57.
9. Schmitt S, Aftab U, Jiang C, Redenti S, Klassen H, Miljan E, et al. Molecular characterization of human retinal progenitor cells. Invest Ophthalmol Vis Sci. 2009;50(12):5901–8.
10. Artero Castro A, Rodríguez Jimenez FJ, Jendelova P, Erceg S. Deciphering retinal diseases through the generation of three dimensional stem cell-derived organoids. Stem Cells. 2019;37:1496.
11. Mazzilli JL, Domozhirov AY, Mueller-Ortiz SL, Garcia CA, Wetsel RA, Zsigmond EM. Derivation and characterization of the human embryonic stem cell line CR-4: differentiation to human retinal pigment epithelial cells. Stem Cell Res. 2017;18:37–40.
12. Royall AH, Frankenberg S, Pask AJ, Holland PWH. Of eyes and embryos: subfunctionalization of the CRX homeobox gene in mammalian evolution. Proc Biol Sci. 2019;286(1907):20190830.
13. Garita-Hernandez M, Lampič M, Chaffiol A, Guibbal L, Routet F, Santos-Ferreira T, et al. Restoration of visual function by transplantation of optogenetically engineered photoreceptors. Nat Commun. 2019;10(1):4524.
14. Friedman DS, O'Colmain BJ, Munoz B, Tomany SC, McCarty C, de Jong PT, et al. Prevalence of age-related macular degeneration in the United States. Arch Ophthalmol. 2004;122(4):564–72.
15. Rao RC, Dedania VS, Johnson MW. Stem cells for retinal disease: a perspective on the promise and perils. Am J Ophthalmol. 2017;179:32–8.
16. Nakano T, Ando S, Takata N, Kawada M, Muguruma K, Sekiguchi K, et al. Self-formation of optic cups and storable stratified neural retina from human ESCs. Cell Stem Cell. 2012;10(6):771–85.
17. Kuwahara A, Ozone C, Nakano T, Saito K, Eiraku M, Sasai Y. Generation of a ciliary margin-like stem cell niche from self-organizing human retinal tissue. Nat Commun. 2015;6:6286.
18. Schwartz SD, Hubschman JP, Heilwell G, Franco-Cardenas V, Pan CK, Ostrick RM, et al. Embryonic stem cell trials for macular degeneration: a preliminary report. Lancet. 2012;379(9817):713–20.
19. Schwartz SD, Regillo CD, Lam BL, Eliott D, Rosenfeld PJ, Gregori NZ, et al. Human embryonic stem cell-derived retinal pigment epithelium in patients with age-related macular degeneration and Stargardt's macular dystrophy: follow-up of two open-label phase 1/2 studies. Lancet. 2015;385(9967):509–16.
20. Mandai M, Kurimoto Y, Takahashi M. Autologous induced stem-cell-derived retinal cells for macular degeneration. N Engl J Med. 2017;377(8):792–3.
21. Yu J, Vodyanik MA, Smuga-Otto K, Antosiewicz-Bourget J, Frane JL, Tian S, et al. Induced pluripotent stem cell lines derived from human somatic cells. Science. 2007;318(5858):1917–20.
22. Bertelli PM, Pedrini F, Guduric-Fuchs J, Peixoto E, Pathak V, Stitt AW, et al. Vascular regeneration for ischemic retinopathies: Hope from cell therapies. Curr Eye Res. 2019;45:372.
23. MacLaren RE, Buch PK, Smith AJ, Balaggan KS, MacNeil A, Taylor JS, et al. CNTF gene transfer protects ganglion cells in rat retinae undergoing focal injury and branch vessel occlusion. Exp Eye Res. 2006;83(5):1118–27.
24. MacLaren RE, Pearson RA, MacNeil A, Douglas RH, Salt TE, Akimoto M, et al. Retinal repair by transplantation of photoreceptor precursors. Nature. 2006;444(7116):203–7.
25. Gonzalez-Cordero A, West EL, Pearson RA, Duran Y, Carvalho LS, Chu CJ, et al. Photoreceptor precursors derived from three-dimensional embryonic stem cell cultures integrate and mature within adult degenerate retina. Nat Biotechnol. 2013;31(8):741–7.

26. Uchida N, Buck DW, He D, Reitsma MJ, Masek M, Phan TV, et al. Direct isolation of human central nervous system stem cells. Proc Natl Acad Sci U S A. 2000;97(26):14720–5.
27. Yang P, Seiler MJ, Aramant RB, Whittemore SR. In vitro isolation and expansion of human retinal progenitor cells. Exp Neurol. 2002;177(1):326–31.
28. Ho AC, Chang TS, Samuel M, Williamson P, Willenbucher RF, Malone T. Experience with a subretinal cell-based therapy in patients with geographic atrophy secondary to age-related macular degeneration. Am J Ophthalmol. 2017;179:67–80.
29. Yamanaka S, Takahashi K. Induction of pluripotent stem cells from mouse fibroblast cultures. Tanpakushitsu Kakusan Koso. 2006;51(15):2346–51.
30. Takahashi K, Yamanaka S. Induction of pluripotent stem cells from mouse embryonic and adult fibroblast cultures by defined factors. Cell. 2006;126(4):663–76.
31. Ji SL, Tang SB. Differentiation of retinal ganglion cells from induced pluripotent stem cells: a review. Int J Ophthalmol. 2019;12(1):152–60.
32. Jayakody SA, Gonzalez-Cordero A, Ali RR, Pearson RA. Cellular strategies for retinal repair by photoreceptor replacement. Prog Retin Eye Res. 2015;46:31–66.
33. Takahashi K, Tanabe K, Ohnuki M, Narita M, Ichisaka T, Tomoda K, et al. Induction of pluripotent stem cells from adult human fibroblasts by defined factors. Cell. 2007;131(5):861–72.
34. Fusaki N, Ban H, Nishiyama A, Saeki K, Hasegawa M. Efficient induction of transgene-free human pluripotent stem cells using a vector based on Sendai virus, an RNA virus that does not integrate into the host genome. Proc Jpn Acad Ser B Phys Biol Sci. 2009;85(8):348–62.
35. Yu J, Hu K, Smuga-Otto K, Tian S, Stewart R, Slukvin II, et al. Human induced pluripotent stem cells free of vector and transgene sequences. Science. 2009;324(5928):797–801.
36. Rabesandratana O, Goureau O, Orieux G. Pluripotent stem cell-based approaches to explore and treat optic neuropathies. Front Neurosci. 2018;12:651.
37. Woltjen K, Michael IP, Mohseni P, Desai R, Mileikovsky M, Hämäläinen R, et al. piggyBac transposition reprograms fibroblasts to induced pluripotent stem cells. Nature. 2009;458(7239):766–70.
38. Kaji K, Norrby K, Paca A, Mileikovsky M, Mohseni P, Woltjen K. Virus-free induction of pluripotency and subsequent excision of reprogramming factors. Nature. 2009;458(7239):771–5.
39. Bracha P, Moore NA, Ciulla TA. Induced pluripotent stem cell-based therapy for age-related macular degeneration. Expert Opin Biol Ther. 2017;17(9):1113–26.
40. Graw J. Eye development. Curr Top Dev Biol. 2010;90:343–86.
41. Rathod R, Surendran H, Battu R, Desai J, Pal R. Induced pluripotent stem cells (iPSC)-derived retinal cells in disease modeling and regenerative medicine. J Chem Neuroanat. 2019;95:81–8.
42. Stadtfeld M, Nagaya M, Utikal J, Weir G, Hochedlinger K. Induced pluripotent stem cells generated without viral integration. Science. 2008;322(5903):945–9.
43. Huangfu D, Osafune K, Maehr R, Guo W, Eijkelenboom A, Chen S, et al. Induction of pluripotent stem cells from primary human fibroblasts with only Oct4 and Sox2. Nat Biotechnol. 2008;26(11):1269–75.
44. Malik N, Rao MS. A review of the methods for human iPSC derivation. Methods Mol Biol. 2013;997:23–33.
45. Kashani AH, Lebkowski JS, Rahhal FM, Avery RL, Salehi-Had H, Dang W, et al. A bioengineered retinal pigment epithelial monolayer for advanced, dry age-related macular degeneration. Sci Transl Med. 2018;10(435):eaao4097.
46. da Cruz L, Fynes K, Georgiadis O, Kerby J, Luo YH, Ahmado A, et al. Phase 1 clinical study of an embryonic stem cell-derived retinal pigment epithelium patch in age-related macular degeneration. Nat Biotechnol. 2018;36(4):328–37.
47. Yue F, Johkura K, Shirasawa S, Yokoyama T, Inoue Y, Tomotsune D, et al. Differentiation of primate ES cells into retinal cells induced by ES cell-derived pigmented cells. Biochem Biophys Res Commun. 2010;394(4):877–83.
48. Buchholz DE, Pennington BO, Croze RH, Hinman CR, Coffey PJ, Clegg DO. Rapid and efficient directed differentiation of human pluripotent stem cells into retinal pigmented epithelium. Stem Cells Transl Med. 2013;2(5):384–93.

49. Buchholz DE, Hikita ST, Rowland TJ, Friedrich AM, Hinman CR, Johnson LV, et al. Derivation of functional retinal pigmented epithelium from induced pluripotent stem cells. Stem Cells. 2009;27(10):2427–34.
50. Iwasaki Y, Sugita S, Mandai M, Yonemura S, Onishi A, Ito S, et al. Differentiation/purification protocol for retinal pigment epithelium from mouse induced pluripotent stem cells as a research tool. PLoS One. 2016;11(7):e0158282.
51. Muñiz A, Ramesh KR, Greene WA, Choi JH, Wang HC. Deriving retinal pigment epithelium (RPE) from induced pluripotent stem (iPS) cells by different sizes of embryoid bodies. J Vis Exp. 2015;(96):52262.
52. Leach LL, Croze RH, Hu Q, Nadar VP, Clevenger TN, Pennington BO, et al. Induced pluripotent stem cell-derived retinal pigmented epithelium: a comparative study between cell lines and differentiation methods. J Ocul Pharmacol Ther. 2016;32(5):317–30.
53. Zahabi A, Shahbazi E, Ahmadieh H, Hassani SN, Totonchi M, Taei A, et al. A new efficient protocol for directed differentiation of retinal pigmented epithelial cells from normal and retinal disease induced pluripotent stem cells. Stem Cells Dev. 2012;21(12):2262–72.
54. Brown NL, Patel S, Brzezinski J, Glaser T. Math5 is required for retinal ganglion cell and optic nerve formation. Development. 2001;128(13):2497–508.
55. Schneider ML, Turner DL, Vetter ML. Notch signaling can inhibit Xath5 function in the neural plate and developing retina. Mol Cell Neurosci. 2001;18(5):458–72.
56. Pan L, Deng M, Xie X, Gan L. ISL1 and BRN3B co-regulate the differentiation of murine retinal ganglion cells. Development. 2008;135(11):1981–90.
57. Parameswaran S, Dravid SM, Teotia P, Krishnamoorthy RR, Qiu F, Toris C, et al. Continuous non-cell autonomous reprogramming to generate retinal ganglion cells for glaucomatous neuropathy. Stem Cells. 2015;33(6):1743–58.
58. Venugopalan P, Wang Y, Nguyen T, Huang A, Muller KJ, Goldberg JL. Transplanted neurons integrate into adult retinas and respond to light. Nat Commun. 2016;7:10472.
59. Teotia P, Chopra DA, Dravid SM, Van Hook MJ, Qiu F, Morrison J, et al. Generation of functional human retinal ganglion cells with target specificity from pluripotent stem cells by chemically defined recapitulation of developmental mechanism. Stem Cells. 2017;35(3):572–85.
60. Trakhtenberg EF, Li Y, Feng Q, Tso J, Rosenberg PA, Goldberg JL, et al. Zinc chelation and Klf9 knockdown cooperatively promote axon regeneration after optic nerve injury. Exp Neurol. 2018;300:22–9.
61. Benowitz LI, He Z, Goldberg JL. Reaching the brain: advances in optic nerve regeneration. Exp Neurol. 2017;287(Pt 3):365–73.
62. Stern JH, Tian Y, Funderburgh J, Pellegrini G, Zhang K, Goldberg JL, et al. Regenerating eye tissues to preserve and restore vision. Cell Stem Cell. 2018;23(3):453.
63. Stern JH, Tian Y, Funderburgh J, Pellegrini G, Zhang K, Goldberg JL, et al. Regenerating eye tissues to preserve and restore vision. Cell Stem Cell. 2018;22(6):834–49.
64. Miltner AM, La Torre A. Retinal ganglion cell replacement: current status and challenges ahead. Dev Dyn. 2019;248(1):118–28.
65. Dhande OS, Huberman AD. Retinal ganglion cell maps in the brain: implications for visual processing. Curr Opin Neurobiol. 2014;24(1):133–42.
66. Lu B, Malcuit C, Wang S, Girman S, Francis P, Lemieux L, et al. Long-term safety and function of RPE from human embryonic stem cells in preclinical models of macular degeneration. Stem Cells. 2009;27(9):2126–35.
67. Li Y, Tsai YT, Hsu CW, Erol D, Yang J, Wu WH, et al. Long-term safety and efficacy of human-induced pluripotent stem cell (iPS) grafts in a preclinical model of retinitis pigmentosa. Mol Med. 2012;18:1312–9.
68. Shirai H, Mandai M, Matsushita K, Kuwahara A, Yonemura S, Nakano T, et al. Transplantation of human embryonic stem cell-derived retinal tissue in two primate models of retinal degeneration. Proc Natl Acad Sci U S A. 2016;113(1):E81–90.
69. Assawachananont J, Mandai M, Okamoto S, Yamada C, Eiraku M, Yonemura S, et al. Transplantation of embryonic and induced pluripotent stem cell-derived 3D retinal sheets into retinal degenerative mice. Stem Cell Rep. 2014;2(5):662–74.

70. Seiler MJ, Aramant RB, Seeliger MW, Bragadottir R, Mahoney M, Narfstrom K. Functional and structural assessment of retinal sheet allograft transplantation in feline hereditary retinal degeneration. Vet Ophthalmol. 2009;12(3):158–69.
71. Zarbin M. Cell-based therapy for retinal disease: the new frontier. Methods Mol Biol. 2019;1834:367–81.
72. Hynes SR, Lavik EB. A tissue-engineered approach towards retinal repair: scaffolds for cell transplantation to the subretinal space. Graefes Arch Clin Exp Ophthalmol. 2010;248(6): 763–78.
73. Thomson HA, Treharne AJ, Walker P, Grossel MC, Lotery AJ. Optimisation of polymer scaffolds for retinal pigment epithelium (RPE) cell transplantation. Br J Ophthalmol. 2011;95(4):563–8.
74. Langer R. Biomaterials in drug delivery and tissue engineering: one laboratory's experience. Acc Chem Res. 2000;33(2):94–101.
75. Radtke ND, Aramant RB, Seiler MJ, Petry HM, Pidwell D. Vision change after sheet transplant of fetal retina with retinal pigment epithelium to a patient with retinitis pigmentosa. Arch Ophthalmol. 2004;122(8):1159–65.
76. Seras-Franzoso J, Díez-Gil C, Vazquez E, García-Fruitós E, Cubarsi R, Ratera I, et al. Bioadhesiveness and efficient mechanotransduction stimuli synergistically provided by bacterial inclusion bodies as scaffolds for tissue engineering. Nanomedicine (Lond). 2012;7(1):79–93.
77. Jain NK, Gupta U. Application of dendrimer-drug complexation in the enhancement of drug solubility and bioavailability. Expert Opin Drug Metab Toxicol. 2008;4(8):1035–52.
78. Jain A, Bansal R. Applications of regenerative medicine in organ transplantation. J Pharm Bioallied Sci. 2015;7(3):188–94.
79. Chen H, Fan X, Xia J, Chen P, Zhou X, Huang J, et al. Electrospun chitosan-graft-poly (ε-caprolactone)/poly (ε-caprolactone) nanofibrous scaffolds for retinal tissue engineering. Int J Nanomedicine. 2011;6:453–61.
80. Binder S, Krebs I, Hilgers RD, Abri A, Stolba U, Assadoulina A, et al. Outcome of transplantation of autologous retinal pigment epithelium in age-related macular degeneration: a prospective trial. Invest Ophthalmol Vis Sci. 2004;45(11):4151–60.
81. Binder S, Stolba U, Krebs I, Kellner L, Jahn C, Feichtinger H, et al. Transplantation of autologous retinal pigment epithelium in eyes with foveal neovascularization resulting from age-related macular degeneration: a pilot study. Am J Ophthalmol. 2002;133(2):215–25.
82. Lund RD, Wang S, Klimanskaya I, Holmes T, Ramos-Kelsey R, Lu B, et al. Human embryonic stem cell-derived cells rescue visual function in dystrophic RCS rats. Cloning Stem Cells. 2006;8(3):189–99.
83. Vugler A, Carr AJ, Lawrence J, Chen LL, Burrell K, Wright A, et al. Elucidating the phenomenon of HESC-derived RPE: anatomy of cell genesis, expansion and retinal transplantation. Exp Neurol. 2008;214(2):347–61.
84. Abedin Zadeh M, Khoder M, Al-Kinani AA, Younes HM, Alany RG. Retinal cell regeneration using tissue engineered polymeric scaffolds. Drug Discov Today. 2019;24(8):1669–78.
85. Takahashi H, Okano T. Thermally-triggered fabrication of cell sheets for tissue engineering and regenerative medicine. Adv Drug Deliv Rev. 2019;138:276–92.
86. Kubota A, Nishida K, Yamato M, Yang J, Kikuchi A, Okano T, et al. Transplantable retinal pigment epithelial cell sheets for tissue engineering. Biomaterials. 2006;27(19):3639–44.
87. Kong B, Mi S. Electrospun Scaffolds for corneal tissue engineering: a review. Materials (Basel). 2016;9(8):614.
88. Xu Y, Guan J. Biomaterial property-controlled stem cell fates for cardiac regeneration. Bioact Mater. 2016;1(1):18–28.
89. Lu T, Li Y, Chen T. Techniques for fabrication and construction of three-dimensional scaffolds for tissue engineering. Int J Nanomedicine. 2013;8:337–50.
90. Luo H, Cha R, Li J, Hao W, Zhang Y, Zhou F. Advances in tissue engineering of nanocellulose-based scaffolds: a review. Carbohydr Polym. 2019;224:115144.
91. Trese M, Regatieri C, Yong M. Advances in retinal tissue engineering. Materials (Basel). 2012;5(1):108–120. Published online 2012 Jan 5. https://doi.org/10.3390/ma5010108.

Chapter 18
Stem Cell Therapy Delivery in Liver Disease

John Langford and Gregory T. Tietjen

18.1 Introduction

18.1.1 Normal Liver Function and the Unique Capacity for Regeneration

The liver performs a wide array of physiologic functions including detoxification, synthesis of serum proteins, production of bile to facilitate digestion of fats, and nutrient absorption from the small intestine. Performing these myriad functions requires an equally diverse array of cell types. Hepatocytes, the main functional cell of the liver, constitute ~60% of total liver mass [1]. These specialized epithelial cells are the primary functional cells responsible for hepatic metabolism, protein synthesis, detoxification, and bile production. The hepatocytes are complemented by several additional specialized cell types that support and facilitate the various hepatic functions. Cholangiocytes are another specialized epithelial cell type that line the bile duct and facilitate collection and transport of bile from the hepatocytes to the small intestine [2]. Sinusoidal endothelial cells form a permeable barrier between the circulation and hepatocytes [3]. Fenestrations within the sinusoidal endothelial cells, combined with the absence of a basement membrane, allow hepatocytes direct access to the circulation. In addition to barrier function, sinusoidal endothelial cells also regulate several homeostatic processes including vascular tone, angiogenesis, and maintenance of stellate cell quiescence.

J. Langford
Department of Surgery, Yale University School of Medicine, New Haven, CT, USA

G. T. Tietjen (✉)
Department of Surgery, Yale University School of Medicine, New Haven, CT, USA

Department of Biomedical Engineering, Yale University, New Haven, CT, USA

Department of Surgery – Transplant Section, Yale School of Medicine, New Haven, CT, USA
e-mail: Gregory.tietjen@yale.edu

© Springer Nature Switzerland AG 2021   385
T. P. Navarro et al. (eds.), *Stem Cell Therapy for Vascular Diseases*,
https://doi.org/10.1007/978-3-030-56954-9_18

The functional role of quiescent stellate cells is not fully understood, outside of the observation that they store depots of vitamin A [4]. However, extensive research has now demonstrated that these cells play a critical role in response to liver injury and fibrotic liver disease [4]. Stellate cells are positioned in the space of Disse, i.e., the space between the sinusoidal endothelial cells and the hepatocytes [3]. Here they seem to act as sentinel cells that can sense and respond to liver injury by becoming "activated," whereupon they differentiate into myofibroblasts and gain new function [5]. One of these new functions is the production of extracellular matrix proteins. Under chronic injury conditions, this process can become dysregulated and can eventually lead to the fibrillar scarring that ultimately culminates in cirrhosis. Similar to stellate cells, Kupffer cells become activated upon liver injury and gain new functions that guide the response to liver injury. Moreover, there is evidence to suggest that cross-talk between Kupffer and stellate cells is integral to repair following liver injury [6].

In light of this rich diversity of hepatic cell types and physiologic functions, the regenerative capacity of mammalian livers after injury seems particularly extraordinary. However, the actual functional unit of the liver (i.e., the lobule) is a relatively simple, repeating anatomic structure [7]. Regeneration is then the process of replacing these functional units, not the regrowing of an exact liver replica. Depending on the nature and extent of the damage, this can be accomplished simply through hypertrophy and/or proliferation of existing hepatocytes. Even in instances of more extensive injury—as in partial hepatectomy—regeneration is generally believed to occur through proliferation of the various mature, differentiated cell types of the liver [8]. At the cellular level, periportal hepatocytes are the first cells to proliferate, followed by expansion of more centrally located hepatocytes. These proliferating hepatocytes then initiate signals to other liver cell types to trigger their subsequent proliferation. The initial clusters of hepatocytes organize with the other proliferating cells into normal lobular architecture [8]. In otherwise healthy livers, this process can enable as little as 25% of the initial liver mass to regenerate to near original size within 7–10 days [9, 10]. In instances of more severe liver disease, however, the proliferative capacity of terminally differentiated hepatocytes can become exhausted. Here, both endogenous and bone marrow-derived stem cells are believed to provide an alternative source of regenerative potential.

Stem cells are cells with the capacity to differentiate into other cell types. Perhaps the most canonical example is the fertilized egg or zygote. Beginning as a single totipotent cell, the zygote will eventually differentiate into all of the diverse cell types of the body. Stem cells are not, however, restricted to early development. Adults also have stem cells, but these have a more limited capacity for differentiation and are thought to be largely tissue specific [11, 12]. Endogenous liver stem cells, often called oval cells or hepatic progenitor cells, were first described in 1944 and were initially thought to be precursors of malignancy [13]. In 1995, oval cells were shown to be capable of differentiation into hepatocytes after native hepatocytes were rendered unable to proliferate due to treatment with acetylaminofluorene [14]. It is now known that these cells are located in the canals of herring and are capable of differentiating into either hepatocytes or cholangiocytes [15–22].

In addition to these endogenous liver stem cells, bone marrow-derived stem cells have also been shown to be involved in hepatocyte regeneration from mismatched-sex bone marrow transplants and liver transplants [23, 24]. Post-transplant biopsy of liver donated from a female donor to a male recipient revealed hepatocytes with a Y chromosome. A similar observation was made in a female patient who had received a bone marrow transplant from a male donor. These findings suggest that stem cells produced in the bone marrow of the males had trafficked to the female liver and differentiated into hepatocytes. This further suggests that stem cell therapies may be a viable treatment option in instances of liver disease.

18.1.2   Liver Disease, Cirrhosis, and Current Treatments

Cirrhosis is a late stage of liver disease characterized by progressive loss of liver function driven by fibrotic scarring throughout the liver parenchyma. There are many diverse etiologies that can result in cirrhosis. Worldwide almost 80% of cirrhosis is caused by hepatitis B (HBV), hepatitis C (HCV), and alcohol, while the remaining 20% are from other etiologies such as NAFLD and autoimmune diseases [25]. Regardless of the underlying mechanistic cause, cirrhosis typically progresses to end-stage liver disease (ESLD) following 'decompensation' or the point at which the remaining functioning liver parenchyma can no longer support the body's physiologic needs (i.e., liver failure). The only curative treatment for cirrhosis and ESLD at present is orthotropic liver transplant. Unfortunately, due to the severe shortage of donor organs, one million people each year will die due to complications of cirrhosis [26].

The only alternative therapy for the 90% of patients that do not receive liver transplants is supportive care [26]. This entails treating the numerous complications and symptoms that occur due to venous congestion and limited hepatocyte function [27]. Portal hypertension leads to a buildup of ascites which is managed with fluid restriction, sodium restriction, and diuretics. If this is unsuccessful, a paracentesis can be performed to drain ascites from the abdomen. Unfortunately, patients with excessive ascites are susceptible to spontaneous bacterial peritonitis, which must be urgently treated with antibiotics. Portal venous congestion can also lead to gastroesophageal varices, a condition with a high propensity to result in life-threating internal bleeding. To prevent bleeding, patients are treated with beta-blockers or if they do bleed can be treated with endoscopic ligation. In severe cases of portal hypertension, patients will undergo a transjugular intrahepatic portosystemic shunt (TIPS) procedure to decrease the portal venous pressure by connecting the inflow (portal vein) to the outflow (hepatic vein) [28]. Unfortunately, this can lead to worsening hepatic encephalopathy because the blood passes by the hepatocytes which would remove toxins such as ammonia.

This myriad of complications from liver disease can be debilitating and can further progress to disease states that will prevent otherwise eligible patients from being healthy enough to undergo organ transplantation. Contraindications that can develop in untreated patients include extrahepatic malignancy, sepsis, and severe hepatopulmonary or hepatorenal syndrome [29]. There is also the tragic reality that thousands of patients die on the liver waitlist each year. These complications are a daily reality for the 90% of patients that are unable to receive the liver transplant they need [26]. For this population of patients, stem cells have the potential to treat the associated symptoms or possibly even reverse cirrhosis by decreasing inflammation, replacing damaged cells, and degrading the fibrosis present in the injured liver [30–32].

18.2   Does Stem Cell Type Matter for Treating Liver Disease?

18.2.1   Origins of Stem Cell Therapy for Liver Disease

Informed by the regenerative capacity of the liver, cell-based therapies try to capitalize on the liver's natural regenerative properties [33]. Initially, research into cell-based therapies to treat liver disease focused on simply replacing hepatocytes via direct hepatocyte transplantation [34]. This method—first developed in the 1980s—is still in use today, but several limitations have been identified. First, the hepatocytes used for this approach derive from liver tissue collected from donor organs that have not been used for transplantation [35]. This represents an even more limited pool of organs than is available for orthotopic transplant, thereby severely restricting access to this treatment. Even if hepatocytes are available, there are additional difficulties associated with culturing these cells in vitro. Hepatocytes must be co-cultured with other liver cells and often require complex extracellular matrices for effective growth [36]. Furthermore, hepatocytes do not appear to function long term when grown in cell culture, thereby creating further logistical challenges [36]. Finally, after hepatocyte transplantation, patients typically need to be placed on lifelong immunosuppression [35, 37]. By contrast stem cell therapy can circumvent these challenges. Stem cells can be easily isolated from a number of sources including a patient's own bone marrow. Once harvested they are easily cultured and in some cases can be maintained indefinitely. Finally, when using autologous stem cells, patients do not require systemic immunosuppression [38–47].

Though these positive attributes make stem cells much more attractive as cellular therapy, many challenges to successful implementation remain. One of the key challenges is to identify the optimal stem cell type to use (Fig. 18.1). Stem cells of potential therapeutic relevance can generally be classified into one of three broad groups: embryonic, fetal, or adult stem cells. Embryonic stem cells derive from the inner cell mass of blastocyst and are totipotent (i.e., able to differentiate into all cell types of the body), but because of the source of these cells, their use in research is limited [48]. Fetal stem cells are derived from different fetal tissue such as liver and are referred to as fetal hepatic progenitor cells (FHPC). There is the belief that fetal stem cells may be better at homing and engraftment to the targeted tissue than their "adult" stem cell counterparts [49]. "Adult" stem cells do not refer to the age of the individual they are harvested from but their differentiation potential. They are tissue specific and have a more limited capacity for differentiation than embryonic and fetal stem cells [49]. The adult stem cells of relevance to treating liver disease

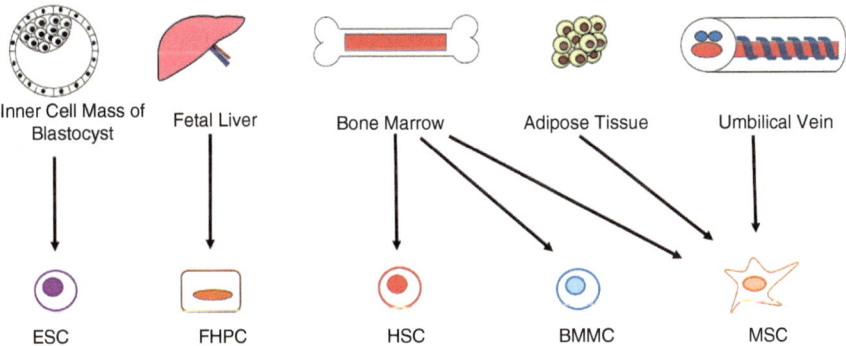

Fig. 18.1 Types of stem cells used in liver disease and where they originate from. ESC embryonic stem cells, FHPC fetal hepatic progenitor cells, HSC hematopoietic stem cells, BMMC bone marrow mononuclear cells, MSC mesenchymal stem cells

include endothelial progenitor cells (EPC), bone marrow mononuclear cells (BMMC), hematopoietic stem cells (HSC), and mesenchymal stem cells (MSC) [50, 51]. It is with the group of "adult" stem cells that the vast majority of preclinical and clinical research is being performed.

18.2.2 Embryonic Stem Cells

Embryonic stem cells (ESC) are derived from the inner cell mass of a blastocyst and are phenotypically characterized by the presence of markers such as SSEA-3, SSEA-4, TRA-1-60, and TRA-1-81 [48]. There are several benefits of ESC, which include the ability to give rise to any cell and a capacity for essentially indefinite self-renew [48]. However, the use of ESC in either a clinical or preclinical setting remains a controversial topic. Indeed, the ethical dilemmas associated with the use of ESC have prevented the study of these cells in clinical trials to date. However, ESC have been evaluated in preclinical animal research [52–55]. In one such study, Moriya et al. demonstrated that ESC could be found in mouse livers after injury by CCL₄; these ESC were able to differentiate into hepatocyte-like cells, and less fibrosis was seen 30 days after transplantation [54]. However, the profound proliferative capacity of ESC carries a potential risk of tumorigenicity that may be related to the time which embryonic stem cells are allowed to differentiate in culture prior to transplantation [56].

18.2.3 Fetal Hepatic Progenitor Cells

Fetal hepatic progenitor cells (FHPC) are highly proliferative cells capable of differentiating into either hepatocytes or cholangiocytes [57]. FHPC are distinguished by the expression of markers such as epithelial cell adhesion molecule (EpCAM), neural cell adhesion molecule (N-CAM), CK-19, and Dlk-1 [57–59]. These cells can be collected from fetuses in a rat model at 14 days and in humans at 16–20 weeks and can then be used to repopulate injured adult livers to restore normal function [57, 60]. Initially, these cells were believed to only be of benefit in liver regeneration after hepatectomy. However, they have also been shown to have the capacity to reduce fibrosis in cirrhotic livers. This benefit occurred through reduced activation of alpha-SMA-positive stellate cells and a decreased expression of fibrogenesis genes [61]. One clinical trial of 25 patients with cirrhosis demonstrated a significant decrease in MELD at 6 months after treatment with FHPC [59].

18.2.4   Hematopoietic Stem Cells

Hematopoietic stem cells (HSC) arise from the bone marrow and were first demonstrated to be able to differentiate into hepatocytes in 2000 [62]. HSC can be identified by CD34+/CD38- and CD133+/c-kit+/bcrp-1+. G-CSF is a mobilizing agent used to induce HSC to migrate out from the bone marrow and into circulation. This mobilization is dependent on the dose of G-CSF, and Lorenzini et al. found that a dose of 15ug/kg/day was optimal for patients with cirrhosis [63]. While G-CSF does appear to induce more circulating HSC, it was found that only a small number of these cells actually implant into the liver and subsequently differentiate into hepatocytes. Despite the low percent of HSC that implant in the liver, a decrease in fibrosis was still observed, perhaps arising from paracrine cell-signaling effects that modulate local inflammation [30]. When HSC are maintained in the liver via S-1-P agonist, there is further decrease in fibrosis [64]. This evidence to date suggests that these paracrine effects, even from a small number of HSC, are the main regenerative force as opposed to HSC repopulating the liver as hepatocytes.

18.2.5   Mesenchymal Stem Cells

Mesenchymal stem cells (MSC) are classically known to differentiate into bone, cartilage, and fat but have also been shown to differentiate into hepatocytes [65]. MSC surface markers include CD44, CD90, CD105, CD106, CD166, and Stro-1, and they lack hematopoietic markers such as CD11b, CD14, CD31, and CD45 [66, 67]. They can be found in and isolated from bone marrow, adipose tissue, placenta, amniotic fluid, and other fetal tissues [67]. The tissue of origin apperas to play role in the functional capabilities of MSC, and the surface markers have different levels of expression depending on the original location [66]. MSC are easy to harvest and remain phenotypically stable in culture which makes them a very attractive source for research; this is likely also one of the reasons MSC are the most frequently used cell in clinical studies [68]. MSC also have a strong immunomodulatory effect and can suppress the immune system. This property has led to extensive use of MSC in immune-mediated disease such as graft-versus-host disease and autoimmune disorders [69]. MSC are believed to be capable of evading the innate immune system due to low levels of HLA-I expression and no expression of HLA-II. This may contribute to the ability of MSC to implant into injured liver even in allogenic donors and would further enable the use of universal donor cells [67, 68]. Animal models have demonstrated the ability of MSC to improve biochemical markers of liver injury (albumin, AST) and decrease fibrosis [70, 71]. In human trials, MSC have demonstrated improvement in Child-Pugh score, MELD score, and histological evidence of fibrosis [41, 43, 46, 72–76].

18.2.6 Endothelial Progenitor Cells

Endothelial progenitor cells (EPC) arise from the bone marrow and are in involved in neovascularization of damaged tissue [77]. EPC express CD45, Thy-1, CD31, and fetal liver kinase-1 (FLK-1) [31]. They have only been used in animal studies so far but have shown promise in mice and rat models. EPC are able to enhance vascularization of livers after acute liver injury. In chronic injury to the liver, they can reduce fibrosis by modulating expression of matrix metalloproteinase (MMP) while inactivating hepatic stellate cells and inducing hepatocyte proliferation [31, 78].

18.2.7 Summary

From current research, it appears that the origin of the stem cells used for treatment is likely an important variable in treatment efficacy. Given the multitude of different ways stem cells are able to act on the injured liver, be it through paracrine effects or differentiating into hepatocytes, it seems fair to assume each type could be optimally selected for different applications. This is likely also true for the different etiologies of liver injury. Each etiology will have a different mechanism of liver injury, and certain stem cell types may prove superior to others in tailoring therapies to these underlying mechanisms.

18.3 Does the Etiology of Liver Disease Matter?

18.3.1 Current View of Liver Disease Etiology and Stem Cell Therapy

As previously described, cirrhosis is the progression of fibrosis from an underlying disease process that drives chronic liver injury. While the endpoint may be the same, how an underlying injury causes fibrosis can vary significantly between different disease etiologies. Thus, a key question to address is whether a standardized stem cell regimen can be used to treat cirrhosis regardless of the underlying cause or if the regimen should be tailored to the underlying disease etiology. Rodent animal models used for preclinical study of stem cell therapies typically focus on treatment of cirrhosis as an endpoint because it is difficult (or impossible) to faithfully replicate the various human etiologies. Thus, these models are more relevant to treatment of patients that have progressed to cirrhosis regardless of etiology. However, in the clinical research setting, the importance of etiology as a modulator of response to a given stem cell therapy has begun to be addressed. Multiple studies have attempted to isolate therapeutic response in specific disease processes such as HBV-, HCV-, or alcohol-induced cirrhosis. In this section, we describe the generally positive results in preclinical animal models and the more mixed results observed in clinical trials.

18.3.2 Animal Model

As mentioned above, commonly used animal models lack the ability to evaluate different mechanism of liver injury. But these can be used for evaluation of liver injury at different stages of fibrotic progression (Fig. 18.2). Liver fibrosis is typically induced through chemical injury via treatment with either carbon tetrachloride (CCL$_4$) or thioacetamide (TAA). CCL$_4$, the most frequently used method, causes fulminant fibrosis within 6 weeks [79]. TAA induces a slower progressing model of injury with mild cirrhosis at 6 weeks and severe cirrhosis by 3 months [61]. This variable kinetics of disease progression has been used to assess the impact of

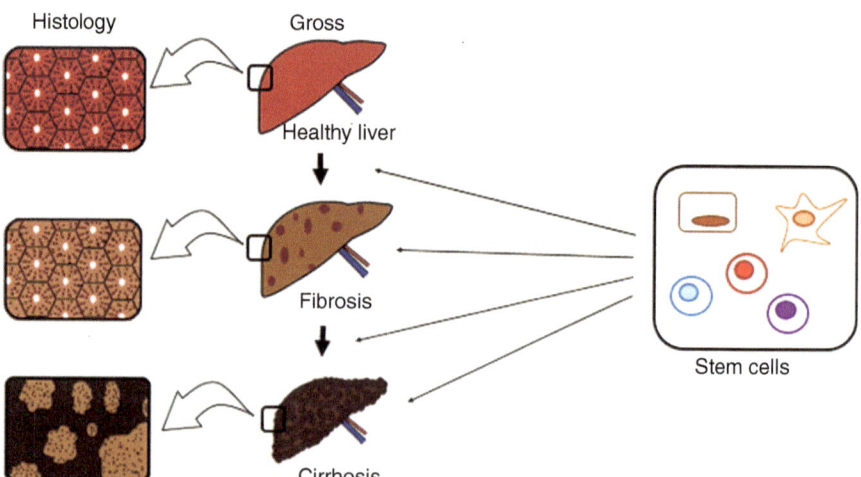

Fig. 18.2 Stem cell therapy delivered at different times in the progression of liver disease. Stem cells can be delivered prior to fibrosis forming, after fibrosis has developed, prior to progression to cirrhosis, or after cirrhosis has developed

treating animals with stem cells either at the onset of injury or after fibrosis has developed. Additional work has also evaluated the efficacy of stem cells in the context of ongoing liver injury or after the insult has been removed.

Treating with stem cells at the onset of liver injury tests for the capacity to slow or prevent fibrosis. In two separate mouse studies, G-CSF or plerixafor (a combination G-CSF and CXCR4 receptor agonist) was given at the same time as chemical injury. Both treatments lead to an increase of HSC in circulation and in the liver concomitant with a reduction in fibrosis [30, 80]. Another mouse study where ESC were given at the same time as CCL_4 administration also found a reduction in subsequent fibrosis [54]. These studies suggest that stem cells can have a protective effect in acute injury and can limit the resulting amount of fibrosis when delivered in close proximity to the initiating injury.

Several different studies first established fibrosis with chemical injury and then removed the insulting agent prior to stem cell transfusion. This allows evaluation of stem cells effects on established fibrosis. One such study evaluated the benefits of MSC in this setting and found a reduction in fibrosis and improvement in liver function at 4 weeks [70]. In another study of previously established fibrosis, Tang et al. evaluated the additional effects of splenectomy prior to MSC infusion, as splenectomy has been previously shown to enhance liver regeneration in patients with cirrhosis [81]. They demonstrated that both groups of animals (i.e., with and without splenectomy) had improvement in fibrosis and the splenectomy group had more substantial improvement [71]. Collectively, these studies demonstrate that stem cell therapy dose have potential to reverse established fibrosis in the absence of ongoing injury.

Finally, animals with established fibrosis and continued injury after stem cell infusion have also been evaluated. This model allows for evaluation of stem cells ability to not only correct underlying cirrhosis but also prevent further deterioration from continued insult. Yovchev et al. compared FHPC to mature hepatocyte injections in a continuous TAA injury model. Both populations of cells repopulated injured livers and reduced fibrogenesis, but FPHC did so to a greater extent [61]. In another study using CCL_4 as the mediator of injury, Sakaida et al. found that mice treated with BMMC had significantly less fibrosis as assessed by hydroxyproline content [32]. Finally, King et al. evaluated the benefit of enhancing the retention of stem cells in a chronic liver injury model using an S-1-P agonist which prevented HSC egress. This approach significantly reduced the amount of fibrosis in spite of the consistent presence of insult [64]. These findings support the fact that stem cells may be able to slow or reverse progression of liver injury even while the underlying cause of injury is still present.

18.3.3 Treating Cirrhosis and ESLD with Stem Cells

Most clinical studies have evaluated cohorts of patients with cirrhosis and end-stage liver disease (ESLD) irrespective of the underlying etiologies. Further complicating matters, the types of etiologies included in the patient cohorts are often heterogeneous between different studies [38, 39, 47, 59, 63, 72, 82, 83]. These patients are either treated with G-CSF to mobilize their own stem cells from the bone marrow, or they receive injections of stem cells. Multiple early pilot/phase I trials have evaluated the safety of these therapeutic techniques in patients with end-stage liver disease [47, 59, 63, 72, 82, 84]. In two example pilot studies of 10–18 patients with ESLD from various etiologies, no adverse events were recorded [63, 84]. However, one recent larger study of 81 patents performed by Newsome et al. in 2018 did report more serious adverse events. This cohort included patients with compensated cirrhosis from NAFLD, PBC, cryptogenic, or mixed causes who were treated with either G-CSF alone, G-CSF followed by leukapheresis to isolate and enrich autologous CD133+ HSC for readministration in the same patient, or standard of care. One-year follow-up revealed increased incidence of adverse events in the G-CSF followed by HSC enrichment and readministration group. These included diarrhea, sepsis, ascites, encephalopathy, acute kidney injury, and edema. Thus, while the safety of these stem cell therapies in cirrhotic patients from multiple etiologies is supported by pilot studies, more work needs to be done in larger patient populations to definitively establish safety across all etiologies and treatment modalities.

With respect to efficacy, several studies that evaluated the effect of stem cell therapies in cirrhotic patients at early time points have observed positive benefits. In one such study, improvements in bilirubin levels were seen as early as 1 week and in albumin levels at 1 month [82]. Three additional studies that followed patients to 6 months found a significant improvement in the Child-Pugh or the MELD scores [72, 85, 86]. However, two other studies that evaluated effects at 12 months found no difference in Child-Pugh or MELD scores [82, 83]. Overall these studies are heterogeneous in design with between 8 and 48 patients and using different types of stem cells injected through different routes. Thus, it is difficult to draw a specific conclusion, and there is a clear need for a more systematic approach.

18.3.4 Treating a Specific Cause of Cirrhosis

In an attempt to reduce potential confounding variables, some studies have evaluated if the etiology of cirrhosis can play a role in the effectiveness of a given stem cell therapy [42, 43, 45, 46, 73–76, 86]. These studies have evaluated the variable effects of HCV, HBV, and alcohol as mediators of liver injury as each of these disease processes damages the liver in different ways. In addition to the differences in injury, these etiologies each have different established treatment modalities. In the case of HBV, therapies are used to slow damage but the insulting virus remains. For both HCV and alcohol cirrhosis, the insulting agent can be removed; HCV can now be eradicated with antivirals, and patients can stop consuming alcohol. The following sections provide more details of each etiology and describe the clinical findings to date.

Hepatitis B Virus HBV is a DNA virus which infects hepatocytes where it replicates and then propagates. Hepatocytes infected with HBV undergo oxidative stress from the production of the viral proteins leading to inflammation and eventual cell death [87]. There is currently a vaccination for HBV, but worldwide there are still ~350 million people infected with HBV [46]. Two studies that specifically evaluated cirrhosis from HBV-infected patients demonstrated improvements after stem cell therapy. Peng et al. infused autologous bone marrow cells through the hepatic artery and found improved liver function at 2–3 weeks and an improved MELD score at 36 weeks [46]. Similarly, Zhang et al. demonstrated significantly improved ascites and Na-MELD scores at 50 weeks for patients that received MSC [75].

Hepatitis C Virus HCV is a RNA virus and is one of the world's most common causes of cirrhosis. The destruction of infected cells leads to chronic inflammation and eventually cirrhosis [88]. There are currently medications which can cure HCV infection, but there is still no treatment for the underlying cirrhosis that the infection causes. It is in this population of patients with HCV cirrhosis that stem cell therapy has been evaluated. Two studies that delivered stem cells to patients with HCV cirrhosis found significant reductions in Child-Pugh score and MELD score 6 months after receiving stem cell therapy [43, 76]. In a similar study, Salama et al. found improvements in liver enzymes and synthetic function in patients after stem cell therapy [86].

Alcohol Alcohol consumption is ubiquitous around the world with extensive use leading to cirrhosis. Multiple studies evaluated patients with cirrhosis from alcohol use with differing results. Two studies showed a benefit in liver function for patients that received stem cell therapy. Saito et al. injected autologous bone marrow cells through peripheral IV and found at 6 months that the five patients classified as Child-Pugh B had a decrease in their Child-Pugh score, while those that were classified as Child-Pugh A remained stable [45]. Suk et al. evaluated patients with biopsy-proven alcoholic cirrhosis. They received MSC trough the hepatic artery, and at 1 year the Child-Pugh score was significantly improved in the patients which received MSC therapy. They also found a reduction in fibrosis at a 6-month biopsy [74]. Spahr et al. evaluated a cohort of cirrhotic patients that also had alcoholic steatohepatitis at baseline; these patients were treated with BMMC. Contrary to the two previously mentioned studies, the authors did not find any improvement in liver function labs. Spahr also performed a liver biopsy at 4 weeks and evaluated for steatosis and the number of proliferating HPC. Neither analysis showed any difference between the stem cell-treated group and the standard medical therapy [42].

18.3.5 Summary

Stem cell therapy appears to have potential for benefit in all causes of cirrhosis, but grouping all etiologies together likely adds confounding variables that may mask the benefit of one treatment regimen over another for a given etiology. Relatedly, the design of an appropriate treatment regimen (e.g., stem cell type, timing related to disease progression, and frequency of treatment) should likely be informed by whether the stimulus of injury remains. For example, in diseases such as HBV where the underlying cause of injury is still present, it could be beneficial for multiple treatments compared to HCV or alcohol where the source of injury can be removed.

18.4 Stem Cell Delivery Methods

18.4.1 Number of Injections

It is unclear whether a single injection of stem cells or multiple injections of stem cells is superior, though this may depend on etiology as described in the preceding section. Suk et al. compared one-time and two-time injections of MSC via the hepatic artery in patients with alcoholic cirrhosis. These injections were done either 1 month (single injection) after bone marrow aspiration or 1 and 2 months (two injections) after bone marrow aspiration [74]. When evaluating reduction in fibrosis, patients that received one injection had a 25% reduction in fibrosis, while patients that received two injections had a 37% reduction. These were both significantly better than the untreated control group but were not significantly different compared to one another. Both groups had a decrease in Child-Pugh score [7.6 to 6.3 and 7.8 to 6.8, respectively], but only the group which received one injection was statistically significant from the control [8.1 to 7.4]. Clearly, further studies are needed to understand the impact of treatment frequency on efficacy.

18.4.2 Consideration of Injection Route

The liver receives both venous and arterial blood via the portal vein and hepatic artery. 80% of the volume of blood to the liver comes through the portal vein, which carries nutrients from the gastrointestinal tract. The hepatic artery accounts for only 20% of the total blood volume, but it provides half of the required oxygen [89]. Both of these blood supplies come together in liver lobules where it then flows through sinusoids before entering the central vein and dumping into the IVC. This unique blood flow can allow for direct delivery through the portal vein or hepatic artery to ensure direct liver access, but these are more invasive procedures. Alternatively, peripheral injections are simply done by injecting cells through a peripheral vein (e.g., in the arm). Though less invasive, this less direct route can allow stem cells to be inadvertently lost to other sites in the body. Thus, optimization of delivery method represents another critical axis for treatment optimization. Below we discuss the results of several studies that have specifically evaluated the effects of delivery route (Fig. 18.3).

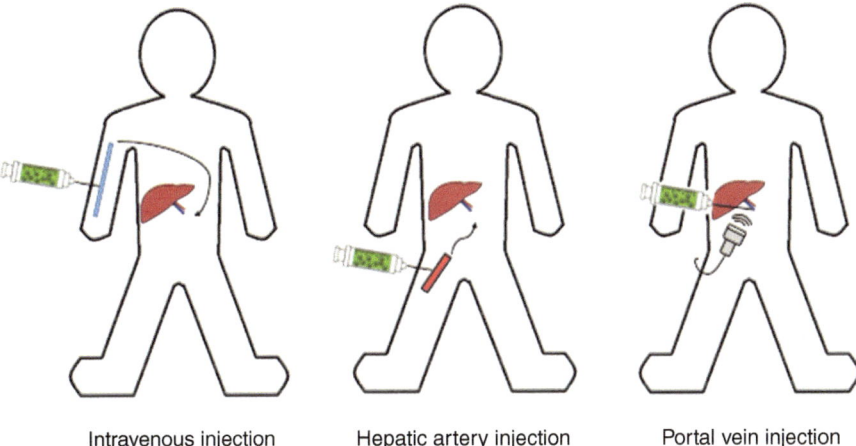

Intravenous injection   Hepatic artery injection   Portal vein injection

Fig. 18.3 Different injection routes used for delivery of stem cells. Intravenous injection is done through a peripheral vein. Hepatic artery injection is done by cannulation of the femoral artery. Portal vein injection is done percutaneously with ultrasound guidance

18.4.3 Peripheral Injection

Peripheral venous injection is the simplest delivery method, and no special equipment or personal is required. However, the drawback of peripheral injection is that stem cells are then subject to the first pass effect. That is, stem cells may implant into tissues other than the liver due to the fact that they have to traverse the entire circulatory system prior to reaching the liver [76, 90]. Stem cells have been delivered in this fashion in both the preclinical models and clinical trials.

Preclinical studies have consistently shown beneficial effects via peripheral injections, but mixed results have been observed in the clinical realm. In preclinical animal models, peripheral injections are typically done via retro orbital or tail vein injection. Both methods have shown improvement in liver function and fibrosis [31, 32, 71, 91, 92]. Clinically, several studies using peripheral injection of stem cells have demonstrated improvements in Child-Pugh scores after administration of a number of different stem cell types [43, 45, 73, 75, 93, 94]. However, two additional studies that used peripheral injections found no benefit in liver function compared to placebo or standard of care [39, 95]. Notably, one of the studies that found no improvement in liver function also observed increased adverse effects [39].

18.4.4 Portal Vein Injection

Portal vein injection is performed using ultrasound guidance to percutaneously cannulate the portal vein in the same way a portal vein embolization is performed. This is done by sterile preparation of the abdomen followed by needle puncture through the skin and liver parenchyma until the portal vein is reached. Using the Seldinger technique, a catheter is inserted and stem cells are subsequently infused. Though relatively routine, this procedure has been associated with incidence of severe bleeding complications such as hemoperitoneum [96].

Similar to peripheral injections, animal models using the portal vein for injection of stem cells have consistently demonstrated positive effects on fibrosis and liver function [61, 91, 97, 98]. Clinically, improvements in liver function and liver growth have also been demonstrated. One case report and several small studies of 5–8 patients demonstrated improvements in liver function at 1 to 6 months after injection of stem cells [47, 72, 99, 100]. Two larger studies of 48 and 90 patients also demonstrated significant improvement in liver function at 4 and 6 months, respectively [86, 96]. Am Esch et al. evaluated liver growth in response to CD133+ cells during portal vein embolism for HCC. They found significantly more growth in liver segments II/III in patients that received CD133+ cells [44]. Though portal vein injection is an invasive procedure, it appears to have promising effects in both the preclinical and clinical settings and may be more effective than peripheral administration.

18.4.5   Hepatic Artery Injection

Hepatic artery infusion is performed the same as a transarterial chemoembolization (TACE) procedure. It involves cannulating the femoral artery using the Seldinger technique [84]. The catheter is then advanced to the hepatic artery and confirmed by fluoroscopy. One of the earliest studies from this technique was done in 2007 specifically to evaluate the safety of this approach in patients with cirrhosis. They found no adverse events in the 4 months following the procedure [84]. Adverse events via this method are extremely rare as similar to the TACE procedure. Only one study reported a case of hepatic artery dissection [82].

There are mixed results from patients that received stem cells through the hepatic artery, but a majority of studies demonstrated early benefit after injection. Lyra et al. performed an injection of CD34+ enriched bone marrow cells in patients with chronic liver disease and demonstrated a significantly improved Child-Pugh score and increased albumin score at 90 days. They did not see any major adverse events at 1 year out [83]. Peng et al. delivered autologous mesenchymal stem cells via the hepatic artery and found a significant improvement in ALB, total bilirubin, and MELD score in the first several weeks. These patients were followed out to 192 weeks and no adverse outcomes were observed [46]. Histologically, improvement in fibrosis after hepatic artery infusion of MSC has been observed at 3 and 6 months after transfusion [41, 74].

Most studies report early benefits from hepatic artery injection, but several studies demonstrated no superiority or adverse long-term outcomes. Spahr et al. demonstrated no significant improvement at 3 months with patients that received stem cell therapy via hepatic artery infusion when compared to patients that received normal medical treatment [42]. The only negative long-term outcomes that were observed from hepatic artery injection was at 10 years in which there was a higher risk of

HCC [38]. Similar to the other injection methods, hepatic artery injections appear to demonstrate an improvement in liver function and fibrosis early on, but this does not appear to be sustained long term.

18.4.6 Direct Comparison of Injection Routes

While a majority of studies only deliver stem cells through one route, there are several studies, in both animals and humans, in which multiple injection routes are used. Animal studies have compared portal vein and peripheral vein injection methods [90, 97, 98]. Liang et al. found that MSC infused via the portal vein had higher rates of engraftment in both injured and non-injured liver compared to peripheral vein injections [90]. Two studies evaluated liver function after injection of MSC. Injection via the portal vein and peripheral veins both had improved liver function, and there was no significant difference between the two injection routes. This may suggest the injection site is not important when injecting MSC, but it remains unclear how this may extrapolate to other stem cell populations [97, 98].

Clinically, several studies have used multiple injection routes as a result of clinical circumstances, but not for direct comparison. Kharaziha et al. performed a study of eight patients in which six received portal vein injection and the remaining two received peripheral injections due to portal vein thrombosis. Overall these patients had improvement in LFTs, but a direct comparison between the two injection methods was not possible with the low patient numbers [72]. Levicar et al. injected five patients with CD34+ cells; three of these patients were injected through the portal vein and the other two through the hepatic artery [101]. There is no clear reason discussed for why they chose separate delivery routes, but four of these patients had an initial improvement in bilirubin at 1 month. Gordon et al. also looked at five patients with three receiving injection via the portal vein and two receiving injection via the hepatic artery [100]. Again these groups were not differentiated, but overall three patients had improvement in bilirubin, while four had improvement in albumin. Positive results from these multiple injection routes demonstrate the promise of all of these different delivery methods. However, it remains to be seen if there is an optimal delivery route.

18.5 Future Directions

18.5.1 Ex Vivo Perfusion

Ensuring adequate delivery of stem cells to the liver is one of the underlying reasons why studies are looking at multiple delivery routes. One way in which we can ensure stem cells are reaching the liver and not being pulled out of circulation at other sites is through ex vivo perfusion. Ex vivo perfusion is an exciting new technology that is now making its way from the bench to the bedside. Using this technology, decellularized collagen scaffoldings can be created for cell engraftment in tissue engineering applications [102]. This scaffolding contains normal architecture, vascular integrity, and GAG proteins which may signal to stem cells for proper location and differentiation [103]. Clinically, ex vivo perfusion devices are already being used for organ rehabilitation prior to transplant. This is occurring in hearts, lungs, kidneys, and livers. The approach allows organs which would have not been transplantable to be assessed and potentially revitalized, thereby allowing them to be used safely for transplant [104]. Using this same technology, it may be possible to remove a patient's own liver and perfuse cells at high concentration and then reimplant it back into the same patient. Surgical techniques such as this are currently being applied for previously unrespectable tumors [105]. When tumors are deemed unresectable due to location or vascular involvement, some cases can be completed ex vivo during cold perfusion prior to auto-reimplantation. Ex vivo perfusion is quickly becoming available clinically, and this technology could be used to effectively deliver stem cells to the liver in future.

18.5.2 Tumorigenic Potential of Stem Cells

Stems cells have shown promise as a potential therapeutic option in liver disease, but their potential to give rise to tumors cannot be ignored [56, 106]. Some studies have attempted to address this concern, but due to the small number of studies and patients, it is difficult to draw a definitive conclusion. One study looked at 58 patients 3 months after receiving BMMC transplant and found no cases of hepatocellular carcinoma [42]. However, long-term outcomes have conflicting results among several studies. Peng et al. found patients that received MSC transplant had lower rates of HCC (1.9%) at 3 years compared to patients that only received standard medical care (8.6%) [46]. Contrary to this study, Wang et al. found a higher incidence of HCC at 10 years in patients that received MSC or HSC (47.8%) compared to standard treatment (21.7%) [38]. Based on the current data, it will be important to continue evaluating patients for increased incidences of tumor formation after stem cell therapy.

18.6 Summary

The current body of literature for stem cell therapy in liver disease has demonstrated promising results throughout a large diversity of studies. To optimize this treatment modality, the mechanism in which different stem cells are repairing or reversing liver damage will be imperative. This information will then best inform which etiology of liver disease each stem cell is best suited for. Once that is determined, the optimal delivery method to ensure stem cells are reaching the appropriate portion of the liver at the appropriate time can be determined. The prior work presented in the chapter has laid the groundwork to inspire these more nuanced studies which will hopefully allow stem cell therapy to be a new therapeutic option in liver disease.

Bibliography

1. Hansel MC, et al. The history and use of human hepatocytes for the treatment of liver diseases: the first 100 patients. Curr Protoc Toxicol. 2014;62:14 12 1–23.
2. Maroni L, et al. Functional and structural features of cholangiocytes in health and disease. Cell Mol Gastroenterol Hepatol. 2015;1(4):368–80.
3. Poisson J, et al. Liver sinusoidal endothelial cells: physiology and role in liver diseases. J Hepatol. 2017;66(1):212–27.
4. Tsuchida T, Friedman SL. Mechanisms of hepatic stellate cell activation. Nat Rev Gastroenterol Hepatol. 2017;14(7):397–411.
5. Wilson CL, et al. Quiescent hepatic stellate cells functionally contribute to the hepatic innate immune response via TLR3. PLoS One. 2014;9(1):e83391.
6. Roth K, Copple B, Albee R. Cross-talk among Kupffer cells and hepatic stellate cells is critical for Kupffer cell activation during liver injury. FASEB J. 2016;30(1_supplement):56.2.
7. Ishibashi H, et al. Liver architecture, cell function, and disease. Semin Immunopathol. 2009;31(3):399.
8. Michalopoulos GK, DeFrances MC. Liver regeneration. Science. 1997;276(5309):60–6.
9. Nadalin S, et al. Volumetric and functional recovery of the liver after right hepatectomy for living donation. Liver Transpl. 2004;10(8):1024–9.
10. Guglielmi A, et al. How much remnant is enough in liver resection? Dig Surg. 2012;29(1):6–17.
11. Narasipura SD, et al. P-selectin coated microtube for enrichment of CD34+ hematopoietic stem and progenitor cells from human bone marrow. Clin Chem. 2008;54(1):77–85.
12. Mahla RS. Stem cells applications in regenerative medicine and disease therapeutics. Int J Cell Biol. 2016;2016:6940283.
13. Chen JZ, et al. A selective tropism of transfused oval cells for liver. World J Gastroenterol. 2003;9(3):544–6.
14. Golding M, et al. Oval cell differentiation into hepatocytes in the acetylaminofluorene-treated regenerating rat liver. Hepatology. 1995;22(4 Pt 1):1243–53.
15. Rogler CE, et al. Triple staining including FOXA2 identifies stem cell lineages undergoing hepatic and biliary differentiation in cirrhotic human liver. J Histochem Cytochem. 2017;65(1):33–46.
16. Roskams T, et al. Hepatic OV-6 expression in human liver disease and rat experiments: evidence for hepatic progenitor cells in man. J Hepatol. 1998;29(3):455–63.
17. Theise ND, et al. The canals of Hering and hepatic stem cells in humans. Hepatology. 1999;30(6):1425–33.
18. Turner R, et al. Human hepatic stem cell and maturational liver lineage biology. Hepatology. 2011;53(3):1035–45.
19. Lu WY, et al. Hepatic progenitor cells of biliary origin with liver repopulation capacity. Nat Cell Biol. 2015;17(8):971–83.
20. Bird TG, Forbes SJ. Two fresh streams to fill the Liver's hepatocyte pool. Cell Stem Cell. 2015;17(4):377–8.
21. Cardinale V, et al. The biliary tree--a reservoir of multipotent stem cells. Nat Rev Gastroenterol Hepatol. 2012;9(4):231–40.
22. Carpino G, et al. Stem/progenitor cell niches involved in hepatic and biliary regeneration. Stem Cells Int. 2016;2016:3658013.
23. Theise ND, et al. Liver from bone marrow in humans. Hepatology. 2000;32(1):11–6.
24. Alison MR, et al. Hepatocytes from non-hepatic adult stem cells. Nature. 2000;406(6793):257.
25. Perz JF, et al. The contributions of hepatitis B virus and hepatitis C virus infections to cirrhosis and primary liver cancer worldwide. J Hepatol. 2006;45(4):529–38.
26. Asrani SK, et al. Burden of liver diseases in the world. J Hepatol. 2019;70(1):151–71.
27. Yadav A, Vargas HE. Care of the patient with cirrhosis. Clin Liver Dis (Hoboken). 2015;5(4):100–4.

28. Rossle M, et al. New non-operative treatment for variceal haemorrhage. Lancet. 1989;2(8655):153.
29. Farkas S, Hackl C, Schlitt HJ. Overview of the indications and contraindications for liver transplantation. Cold Spring Harb Perspect Med. 2014;4(5):a015602.
30. Tsolaki E, et al. Hematopoietic stem cells and liver regeneration: differentially acting hematopoietic stem cell mobilization agents reverse induced chronic liver injury. Blood Cells Mol Dis. 2014;53(3):124–32.
31. Nakamura T, et al. Significance and therapeutic potential of endothelial progenitor cell transplantation in a cirrhotic liver rat model. Gastroenterology. 2007;133(1):91–107 e1.
32. Sakaida I, et al. Transplantation of bone marrow cells reduces CCl4-induced liver fibrosis in mice. Hepatology. 2004;40(6):1304–11.
33. Talens-Visconti R, et al. Hepatogenic differentiation of human mesenchymal stem cells from adipose tissue in comparison with bone marrow mesenchymal stem cells. World J Gastroenterol. 2006;12(36):5834–45.
34. Reid LM, et al. Long-term cultures of normal rat hepatocytes on liver biomatrix. Ann N Y Acad Sci. 1980;349:70–6.
35. Dhawan A. Clinical human hepatocyte transplantation: current status and challenges. Liver Transpl. 2015;21(Suppl 1):S39–44.
36. Ogoke O, Oluwole J, Parashurama N. Bioengineering considerations in liver regenerative medicine. J Biol Eng. 2017;11:46.
37. Fox IJ, et al. Treatment of the Crigler-Najjar syndrome type I with hepatocyte transplantation. N Engl J Med. 1998;338(20):1422–6.
38. Wang MF, et al. Efficacy and safety of autologous stem cell transplantation for decompensated liver cirrhosis: a retrospective cohort study. World J Stem Cells. 2018;10(10):138–45.
39. Newsome PN, et al. Granulocyte colony-stimulating factor and autologous CD133-positive stem-cell therapy in liver cirrhosis (REALISTIC): an open-label, randomised, controlled phase 2 trial. Lancet Gastroenterol Hepatol. 2018;3(1):25–36.
40. Ma XR, et al. Transplantation of autologous mesenchymal stem cells for end-stage liver cirrhosis: a meta-analysis based on seven controlled trials. Gastroenterol Res Pract. 2015;2015:908275.
41. Jang YO, et al. Histological improvement following administration of autologous bone marrow-derived mesenchymal stem cells for alcoholic cirrhosis: a pilot study. Liver Int. 2014;34(1):33–41.
42. Spahr L, et al. Autologous bone marrow mononuclear cell transplantation in patients with decompensated alcoholic liver disease: a randomized controlled trial. PLoS One. 2013;8(1):e53719.
43. El-Ansary M, et al. Phase II trial: undifferentiated versus differentiated autologous mesenchymal stem cells transplantation in Egyptian patients with HCV induced liver cirrhosis. Stem Cell Rev Rep. 2012;8(3):972–81.
44. am Esch JS, et al. Infusion of CD133+ bone marrow-derived stem cells after selective portal vein embolization enhances functional hepatic reserves after extended right hepatectomy: a retrospective single-center study. Ann Surg. 2012;255(1):79–85.
45. Saito T, et al. Potential therapeutic application of intravenous autologous bone marrow infusion in patients with alcoholic liver cirrhosis. Stem Cells Dev. 2011;20(9):1503–10.
46. Peng L, et al. Autologous bone marrow mesenchymal stem cell transplantation in liver failure patients caused by hepatitis B: short-term and long-term outcomes. Hepatology. 2011;54(3):820–8.
47. Nikeghbalian S, et al. Autologous transplantation of bone marrow-derived mononuclear and CD133(+) cells in patients with decompensated cirrhosis. Arch Iran Med. 2011;14(1):12–7.
48. Thomson JA, et al. Embryonic stem cell lines derived from human blastocysts. Science. 1998;282(5391):1145–7.
49. O'Donoghue K, Fisk NM. Fetal stem cells. Best Pract Res Clin Obstet Gynaecol. 2004;18(6):853–75.

50. Tsolaki E, Yannaki E. Stem cell-based regenerative opportunities for the liver: State of the art and beyond. World J Gastroenterol. 2015;21(43):12334–50.
51. Zhang Z, Wang FS. Stem cell therapies for liver failure and cirrhosis. J Hepatol. 2013;59(1):183–5.
52. Kwak KA, et al. Current perspectives regarding stem cell-based therapy for liver cirrhosis. Can J Gastroenterol Hepatol. 2018;2018:4197857.
53. Basma H, et al. Differentiation and transplantation of human embryonic stem cell-derived hepatocytes. Gastroenterology. 2009;136(3):990–9.
54. Moriya K, et al. Embryonic stem cells develop into hepatocytes after intrasplenic transplantation in CCl4-treated mice. World J Gastroenterol. 2007;13(6):866–73.
55. Yamamoto H, et al. Differentiation of embryonic stem cells into hepatocytes: biological functions and therapeutic application. Hepatology. 2003;37(5):983–93.
56. Chinzei R, et al. Embryoid-body cells derived from a mouse embryonic stem cell line show differentiation into functional hepatocytes. Hepatology. 2002;36(1):22–9.
57. Oertel M, et al. Purification of fetal liver stem/progenitor cells containing all the repopulation potential for normal adult rat liver. Gastroenterology. 2008;134(3):823–32.
58. Dabeva MD, et al. Proliferation and differentiation of fetal liver epithelial progenitor cells after transplantation into adult rat liver. Am J Pathol. 2000;156(6):2017–31.
59. Khan AA, et al. Human fetal liver-derived stem cell transplantation as supportive modality in the management of end-stage decompensated liver cirrhosis. Cell Transplant. 2010;19(4):409–18.
60. Oertel M, et al. Cell competition leads to a high level of normal liver reconstitution by transplanted fetal liver stem/progenitor cells. Gastroenterology. 2006;130(2):507–20; quiz 590.
61. Yovchev MI, et al. Repopulation of the fibrotic/cirrhotic rat liver by transplanted hepatic stem/progenitor cells and mature hepatocytes. Hepatology. 2014;59(1):284–95.
62. Lagasse E, et al. Purified hematopoietic stem cells can differentiate into hepatocytes in vivo. Nat Med. 2000;6(11):1229–34.
63. Lorenzini S, et al. Stem cell mobilization and collection in patients with liver cirrhosis. Aliment Pharmacol Ther. 2008;27(10):932–9.
64. King A, et al. Sphingosine-1-phosphate prevents egress of hematopoietic stem cells from liver to reduce fibrosis. Gastroenterology. 2017;153(1):233–248 e16.
65. Shu SN, et al. Hepatic differentiation capability of rat bone marrow-derived mesenchymal stem cells and hematopoietic stem cells. World J Gastroenterol. 2004;10(19):2818–22.
66. Maleki M, et al. Comparison of mesenchymal stem cell markers in multiple human adult stem cells. Int J Stem Cells. 2014;7(2):118–26.
67. Nauta AJ, Fibbe WE. Immunomodulatory properties of mesenchymal stromal cells. Blood. 2007;110(10):3499–506.
68. Le Blanc K, Mougiakakos D. Multipotent mesenchymal stromal cells and the innate immune system. Nat Rev Immunol. 2012;12(5):383–96.
69. Poggi A, Zocchi MR. Immunomodulatory properties of mesenchymal stromal cells: still unresolved "Yin and Yang". Curr Stem Cell Res Ther. 2019;14(4):344–50.
70. Abdel Aziz MT, et al. Therapeutic potential of bone marrow-derived mesenchymal stem cells on experimental liver fibrosis. Clin Biochem. 2007;40(12):893–9.
71. Tang WP, et al. Splenectomy enhances the therapeutic effect of adipose tissue-derived mesenchymal stem cell infusion on cirrhosis rats. Liver Int. 2016;36(8):1151–9.
72. Kharaziha P, et al. Improvement of liver function in liver cirrhosis patients after autologous mesenchymal stem cell injection: a phase I-II clinical trial. Eur J Gastroenterol Hepatol. 2009;21(10):1199–205.
73. Liang J, et al. Effects of allogeneic mesenchymal stem cell transplantation in the treatment of liver cirrhosis caused by autoimmune diseases. Int J Rheum Dis. 2017;20(9):1219–26.
74. Suk KT, et al. Transplantation with autologous bone marrow-derived mesenchymal stem cells for alcoholic cirrhosis: phase 2 trial. Hepatology. 2016;64(6):2185–97.

75. Zhang Z, et al. Human umbilical cord mesenchymal stem cells improve liver function and ascites in decompensated liver cirrhosis patients. J Gastroenterol Hepatol. 2012;27(Suppl 2):112–20.

76. Amer ME, et al. Clinical and laboratory evaluation of patients with end-stage liver cell failure injected with bone marrow-derived hepatocyte-like cells. Eur J Gastroenterol Hepatol. 2011;23(10):936–41.

77. Asahara T, et al. Isolation of putative progenitor endothelial cells for angiogenesis. Science. 1997;275(5302):964–7.

78. Taniguchi E, et al. Endothelial progenitor cell transplantation improves the survival following liver injury in mice. Gastroenterology. 2006;130(2):521–31.

79. Scholten D, et al. The carbon tetrachloride model in mice. Lab Anim. 2015;49(1 Suppl):4–11.

80. Piscaglia AC, et al. Granulocyte-colony stimulating factor promotes liver repair and induces oval cell migration and proliferation in rats. Gastroenterology. 2007;133(2):619–31.

81. Akahoshi T, et al. Laparoscopic splenectomy with peginterferon and ribavirin therapy for patients with hepatitis C virus cirrhosis and hypersplenism. Surg Endosc. 2010;24(3):680–5.

82. Couto BG, et al. Bone marrow mononuclear cell therapy for patients with cirrhosis: a phase 1 study. Liver Int. 2011;31(3):391–400.

83. Lyra AC, et al. Infusion of autologous bone marrow mononuclear cells through hepatic artery results in a short-term improvement of liver function in patients with chronic liver disease: a pilot randomized controlled study. Eur J Gastroenterol Hepatol. 2010;22(1):33–42.

84. Lyra AC, et al. Feasibility and safety of autologous bone marrow mononuclear cell transplantation in patients with advanced chronic liver disease. World J Gastroenterol. 2007;13(7):1067–73.

85. Takami T, Terai S, Sakaida I. Novel findings for the development of drug therapy for various liver diseases: current state and future prospects for our liver regeneration therapy using autologous bone marrow cells for decompensated liver cirrhosis patients. J Pharmacol Sci. 2011;115(3):274–8.

86. Salama H, et al. Autologous CD34+ and CD133+ stem cells transplantation in patients with end stage liver disease. World J Gastroenterol. 2010;16(42):5297–305.

87. Higgs MR, Chouteau P, Lerat H. 'Liver let die': oxidative DNA damage and hepatotropic viruses. J Gen Virol. 2014;95(Pt 5):991–1004.

88. Mengshol JA, Golden-Mason L, Rosen HR. Mechanisms of disease: HCV-induced liver injury. Nat Clin Pract Gastroenterol Hepatol. 2007;4(11):622–34.

89. Eipel C, Abshagen K, Vollmar B. Regulation of hepatic blood flow: the hepatic arterial buffer response revisited. World J Gastroenterol. 2010;16(48):6046–57.

90. Liang L, et al. Therapeutic potential and related signal pathway of adipose-derived stem cell transplantation for rat liver injury. Hepatol Res. 2009;39(8):822–32.

91. Zhan Y, et al. Differentiation of hematopoietic stem cells into hepatocytes in liver fibrosis in rats. Transplant Proc. 2006;38(9):3082–5.

92. Jang YY, et al. Hematopoietic stem cells convert into liver cells within days without fusion. Nat Cell Biol. 2004;6(6):532–9.

93. Aab A, et al. Search for patterns by combining cosmic-ray energy and arrival directions at the Pierre Auger Observatory. Eur Phys J C Part Fields. 2015;75(6):269.

94. Terai S, et al. Improved liver function in patients with liver cirrhosis after autologous bone marrow cell infusion therapy. Stem Cells. 2006;24(10):2292–8.

95. Mohamadnejad M, et al. Randomized placebo-controlled trial of mesenchymal stem cell transplantation in decompensated cirrhosis. Liver Int. 2013;33(10):1490–6.

96. Salama H, et al. Autologous hematopoietic stem cell transplantation in 48 patients with end-stage chronic liver diseases. Cell Transplant. 2010;19(11):1475–86.

97. Song YM, et al. Effects of bone marrow-derived mesenchymal stem cells transplanted via the portal vein or tail vein on liver injury in rats with liver cirrhosis. Exp Ther Med. 2015;9(4):1292–8.

98. Truong NH, et al. Comparison of the treatment efficiency of bone marrow-derived mesenchymal stem cell transplantation via tail and portal veins in CCl4-induced mouse liver fibrosis. Stem Cells Int. 2016;2016:5720413.
99. Gasbarrini A, et al. Rescue therapy by portal infusion of autologous stem cells in a case of drug-induced hepatitis. Dig Liver Dis. 2007;39(9):878–82.
100. Gordon MY, et al. Characterization and clinical application of human CD34+ stem/progenitor cell populations mobilized into the blood by granulocyte colony-stimulating factor. Stem Cells. 2006;24(7):1822–30.
101. Levicar N, et al. Long-term clinical results of autologous infusion of mobilized adult bone marrow derived CD34+ cells in patients with chronic liver disease. Cell Prolif. 2008;41(Suppl 1):115–25.
102. Gilbert TW, Sellaro TL, Badylak SF. Decellularization of tissues and organs. Biomaterials. 2006;27(19):3675–83.
103. Hassanein W, et al. Recellularization via the bile duct supports functional allogenic and xenogenic cell growth on a decellularized rat liver scaffold. Organogenesis. 2017;13(1):16–27.
104. Akateh C, et al. Normothermic ex-vivo liver perfusion and the clinical implications for liver transplantation. J Clin Transl Hepatol. 2018;6(3):276–82.
105. Hwang R, Liou P, Kato T. Ex vivo liver resection and autotransplantation: an emerging option in selected indications. J Hepatol. 2018;69(5):1002–3.
106. Blum B, Benvenisty N. The tumorigenicity of human embryonic stem cells. Adv Cancer Res. 2008;100:133–58.

Chapter 19
Stem Cell Therapy for Lymphedema

Dylan McLaughlin, Angela Cheng, and Luke Brewster

19.1 Introduction

The lymphatic system is critical to volume hemostasis and is primarily responsible for the return of interstitial fluid and lymph products such as proteins and immune cells from tissues back into circulation via drainage into the central venous system. Originating distally, lymphatic drainage is segmental moving distal to proximal, and superficial to deep, through well-defined paths parallel to the venous system and typically terminates into venous system in the left neck via the thoracic duct. Like veins, lymphatics are typically low pressure systems that must overcome gravity and do not have the pumping assistance that arteries do from the left ventricle. Unlike veins, which are composed of three layers (intima, media, and adventitia), lymphatic vessels are relatively porous (enabling proteins to passively return with interstitial fluid) and lined with lymphatic endothelial (and sometimes smooth muscle) cells (LEC) that can contract in coordination with lymphatic valves to help move lymph forward. Such contractions are informed by both pressure and wall shear stress [1, 2].

D. McLaughlin
Emory University, Department of Surgery, Vascular Surgery and Endovascular Therapy, Atlanta, GA, USA

A. Cheng
Emory University, Department of Surgery, Division of Plastic and Reconstructive Surgery, Atlanta, GA, USA

L. Brewster (✉)
Emory University, Department of Surgery, Vascular Surgery and Endovascular Therapy, Atlanta, GA, USA

Atlanta VA Medical Center, Surgical and Research Services, Decatur, GA, USA

Georgia Institute of Technology, Institute for Bioengineering and Bioscience, Atlanta, GA, USA
e-mail: lbrewst@emory.edu; luke.brewster@va.gov

© Springer Nature Switzerland AG 2021
T. P. Navarro et al. (eds.), *Stem Cell Therapy for Vascular Diseases*,
https://doi.org/10.1007/978-3-030-56954-9_19

Lymphedema is classified as primary or secondary. Primary lymphedema is predominantly found in females and typically classified by timing of onset: congenital (less than 2 years of age), praecox (between 2 years and 35 years of age) (Fig. 19.1), or tarda (after 35 years of age) (Fig. 19.2). In primary lymphedema, there have been a number of genetic targets identified. Mutations in GATA2, a transcription factor, and BRG1 (SMARCA4), a transcription activator, and defects in both VEGF and FAT4 genes lead to lymphedema in mouse models [3]. In Hennekam syndrome, FAT4 mutations contribute to the intestinal lymphectasia and the peripheral lymphedema secondary to defects in lymphatic valve formation [4]. The genes FAT4 and Dachsous1 both contribute to lymphatic valve formation, and mutations in these genes promote lymphedema [5].

The identification of these pathways may be important to reparative strategies for patients, but also to inform the complex mechanisms disrupted during the onset and progression of lymphedema. Such discoveries not only aid in identifying other causes of primary lymphedema, but also inform the mechanism of lymphedema development. By immortalizing cells from affected patients, one can test novel therapeutics in vitro but in a translational manner. For example, patient-derived inducible pluripotent stem cells (iPSC) have been explored as they relate to

Fig. 19.1 Preoperative picture of a patient with primary lymphedema who had become wheelchair bound by the condition

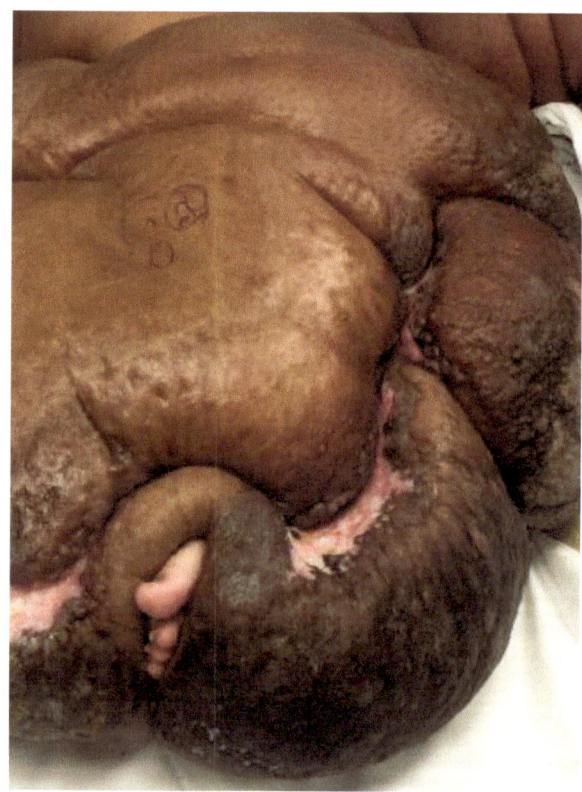

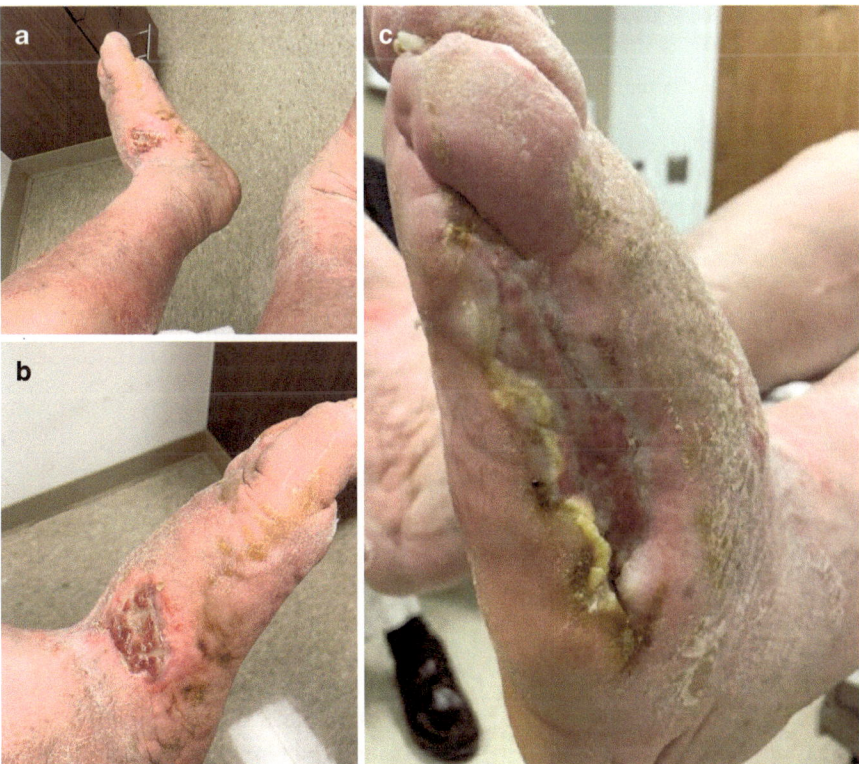

Fig. 19.2 Representative picture of a patient with primary lymphedema and wounds that were precipitated by weeping of fluid during a cellulitis episode. (**a**) Picture of leg. (**b**) Picture of foot and wound on dorsal surface. C) Lateral foot wound and pathognomonic swelling of toes

GATA2-deficient lymphedema. Such modeling systems hold promise for translational testing of rare genetic diseases [6].

Secondary lymphedema is the most common type of lymphedema, and it occurs after traumatic injury (surgical operations, radiation, etc.) or infection (filiariasis). In secondary lymphedema, lymphatic vessel obstruction occurs from injury to the lymph vessel architecture. Worldwide infection is the most common cause of secondary lymphedema, but in more developed countries, secondary lymphedema is commonly seen after surgery (e.g., lymphadenectomy for breast cancer) or other tissue trauma (radiation). Secondary lymphedema occurs in 20% of women who survive breast cancer [7].

Clinical staging of lymphedema has been established by the International Congress of Lymphology [8] to assist in the classification of patients and to inform a better understanding of the published literature (Table 19.1).

Lymphedema has a significant impact on quality of life [9], and quality of life in lower extremity lymphedema has been reported to be lower than for upper extremity disease [10]. For the purposes of this chapter, we will attempt to incorporate the data

Table 19.1 Clinical grading system for lymphedema

Stage	Criteria
Latent phase	Fluid accumulation and lymphatic fibrosis; no edema seen clinically
Grade I	Pitting edema (protein-rich fluid accumulation) that improves with elevation; no clinical evidence of fibrosis
Grade II	Non-pitting edema that does not improve with elevation; moderate to severe fibrosis on clinical exam
Grade III	Persistent edema with lymphostatic elephantiasis

that exists and segregate our analysis according to primary and secondary as well as upper or lower extremity lymphedema.

19.2   Diagnosis and Current Treatments

Lower extremity swelling is a common presenting symptom for patients in a vascular clinic. Diagnosis of lymphedema relies heavily on history and physical examination to distinguish it from other causes of limb swelling such as venous insufficiency, right heart failure, myxedema, and obesity [11]. Pathognomonic swelling of the affected extremity (10% swelling difference) into the digits is the key findings of lymphedema [12]. However, early diagnosis of lymphedema is more difficult, and in order to prevent future morbidity, some recommend lowering the swelling threshold in patients preparing for breast cancer treatment [13].

In addition to physical exam and clinical acumen, multiple imaging modalities exist to assist in diagnosing lymphedema. MRI localizes the level of edema allowing differentiation of limb swelling. Cutaneous edema is typical of lymphedema. More invasive diagnostic testing includes lymphoscintigraphy and lymphangiography; here a positive test is identified by pooling of lymph or increased transit time. Both modalities allow evaluation of lymph vessels for patency but come with certain risks.

19.2.1   Medical Management

The mainstays of patient management include: skin hygiene (keeping clean and moisturized (low pH lotions), basic exercise/rehabilitation (walking, yoga, bicycling), and complete decongestive therapy (CDT) [8].

Secondary recommendations include pneumatic compression devices, but these are not recommended in the absence of compression therapy [8, 14]. In addition to these standard therapies, it is important to manage associated medical comorbidities (e.g., obesity) as they may affect the clinical course of the patient's lymphedema and also may affect the type and consistency of treatment received by providers [15]. Additional medical therapies including medications are well summarized by the Lymphology Society in 2016 guidelines [8].

19.2.2 Surgical Management

Surgical options for managing lymphedema are divided broadly into ablative or physiologic procedures. Ablative operations include tissue reduction procedures as described originally by Dr. Charles and Dr. Homans. Here, subcutaneous tissue is removed and the skin is laid upon the fascia [16, 17]. This operation is typically reserved for patients with refractory and severe disease (Fig. 19.3). Given the amount of tissue removed and requirement for skin grafting, a number of complications are related to this operation [18, 19].

Today, lymphatic reconstruction with either lympho-lymphatic, lympho-venous, or lymphaticovenular bypasses is more common [20–22]. These operations can be expected to yield modest volume reductions (less than 50%) but are associated with symptomatic improvement [21, 23, 24]. Lymph node transfer, whereby a healthy

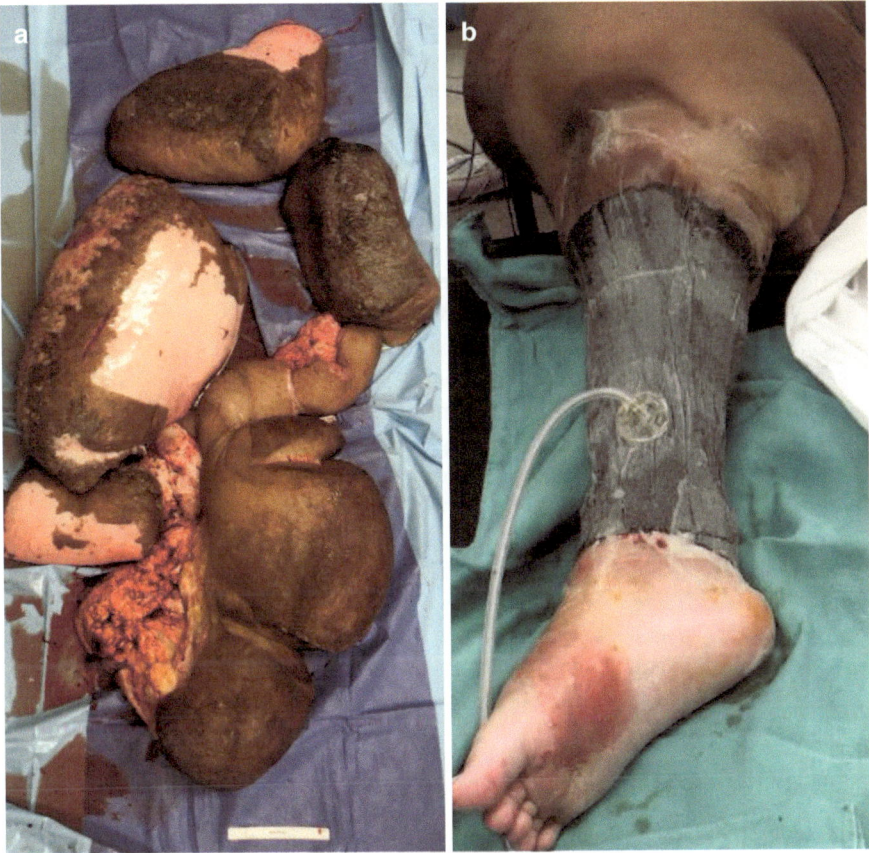

Fig. 19.3 Postoperative picture of patient with primary lymphedema who underwent a Charles procedure and skin grafting from excised tissue. (**a**) Excised tissue from which donor skin was taken. (**b**) Wound vac dressing over the skin graft on the affected leg

donor lymphatic segment is used as a bypass of dysfunctional lymphatic drainage, is another operative technique that yields similar volume reduction in selected patients [25–27], but it is more morbid than lymph-venous bypass and may cause donor site lymphedema [28, 29–31]. Donor site lymphedema may be predicted (and avoided) by preoperative lymphatic mapping [32]. Finally in patients with non-pitting lymph-edema, liposuction itself may also be of some benefit, but patients still require CDT [8].

Systematic reviews of the world literature suggest that lympho-venous anasto-mosis is the most appropriate operation for middle staged lymphedema [33]. Such techniques typically require advanced training in supermicrosurgical techniques [34].

19.3 Regenerative Technologies and Novel Pharmacotherapies

19.3.1 Pathologic Overview and Lineage Specific Techniques

In order to help design intelligent regenerative strategies, certain molecular path-ways that are important to lymphangiogenesis have been identified. VEGF-C is of particular importance in stimulating LEC migration, proliferation, and function [35]. In addition, granulocyte colony-stimulating factor (G-CSF) is a potent angio-gen expressed by many stem cells that may be useful in lymphedema therapies [36], and AKT signaling pathways may be manipulated to steer adipose-derived stem cell differentiation to LEC via IL-7 [37].

Lymphangiogenesis can also be promoted by hypoxia via MFN1 and MFN2 signaling [38], and cell-cell signaling via VE-cadherin and alpha-catenin interaction can specifically promote differentiation of hematopoietic progenitors to the lym-phatic lineage [39]. Here, lymphatic-specific genetic markers are critical to meth-odologic understanding of lymphangiogenesis. Such markers include Prox1, Podoplanin, LYVE1, and VEGFR3. Prox1 is found to be the primary driver earlier in the differentiation pathway into stable LEC and lymph vessel architecture [40]. Prox1 expression is upstream to these other lymphatic markers.

In the same manner that lymphedema is relatively less well studied than arteries and veins [41], there are relatively few cellular studies related to lymphedema. A recent review of cellular therapy for lymphedema found only 19 (11 animal; 7 human) published studies from 2008 to 2018 [42].

19.3.2 Current Status of Preclinical Research for Lymphedema

In 2017, Tian et al. identified that leukotriene B4 (LTB4) antagonism was a potential therapy for lymphedema. This work pulled together many of leading scientists in lymphology. After identifying higher LTB4 in their animal model and in patients with lymphedema, they identified bimodal behavior of LTB4 with pro-lymphangiogenic effects in vitro at lower concentrations (1–10 nM) and anti-lymphangiogenic effects at higher concentrations (200–400 nM). These effects were regulated by VEGFR3 and notch signaling. The use of bestatin to block this pathway is currently in clinical trial [43].

Adipose-derived MSCs promote lymphatic differentiation and maturation via VEGF-C induction of lymphatic gene expression [44]. VEGF-C preferentially drives lymphangiogenesis over angiogenesis in ex vivo mosue models, such as the dual aortic ring and thoracic duct assay [45]. These studies demonstrate that VEGF-C is the primary driver of lymphatic differentiation. VEGF-C stimulates adipose-derived stem cells to promote lymphangiogenesis in a paracrine manner. VEGF-C signaling also increases the overall number of adipose-derived MSCs [46]. Similarly, MSCs also promote lymphatic drainage and can be directed to sites of damage by VEGF-C [47].

However, the ability of MSCs to promote lymphangiogenesis and stimulate LECs is more complex than VEGF-C pathways [48, 49]. Physiologically, MSC administration in mice decreases edema in tail and hindlimb lymphedema models [47, 50–54]. Another group found that the combined injection of MSCs and VEGF-C reduced edema in a rabbit hindlimb lymphedema model by 60 days after treatment [55]. Importantly the potential reversibility of lymphedema and complex inflammatory mechanisms was demonstrated in an adoptive transfer experiment of T regulatory cells [56].

Platelet-rich plasma combined with stem cell injection improved lymphedema by restoring disrupted lymphatic channels and promoting lymphatic vessel regeneration in a mouse model [50]. This early study suggests treatment of lymphedema with stem cell therapy in conjunction with growth factors is feasible. We have found similar results in preclinical work using human platelet lysate to promote MSC regenerative activity in vitro and in vivo using preclinical murine models of hindlimb ischemia (Fig. 19.4) [57].

19.3.3 Current Status of Translational Research

Transplantation of stem cells stimulates angiogenesis and lymphangiogenesis in both in vitro and in vivo lymphedema models. These cells promoted survival and function of transplanted lymph nodes and improved lymphatic flow through regeneration of capillary and pre-collector vessel growth, restoring collector vessels and increasing vascular supply to lymphatic structures. This provides a functional mechanism for stem cell transplantation in conjunction with standard lymphedema therapies [58]. Still translation to clinical benefit will need to consider some key differences in lymphedema patients that are not easily replicated in preclinical models.

Chronic lymphedema causes skin changes by inducing chronic inflammatory response secondary to volume overload. This response promotes fibrosis and impairs regenerative and immunogenic capacity of surrounding tissue [59]. Management of

MSC assay (day 2)

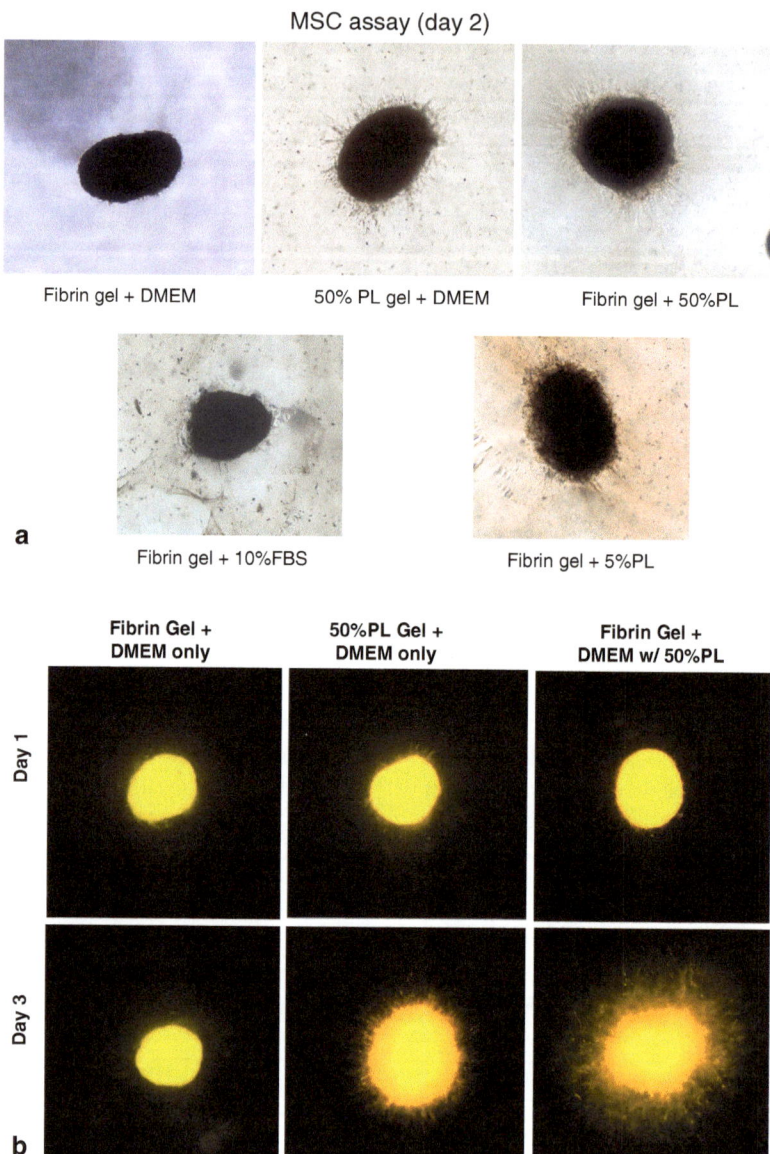

Fig. 19.4 Combinatorial benefits of biomaterials and platelet lysate on MSC behavior. (**a**) Representative images of MSC pellets under different conditions. Here a hydrogel made of human PL was superior to fibrin as a standalone hydrogel during culture in a basal culture medium (DMEM). The addition of exogenous PL to fibrin led to the most robust MSC invasion of the gels. (**b**) Fluorescent imaging of MSC pellets under select conditions demonstrates the same gains in MSC invasion. (**c**) Quantification of this effect at different time points demonstrating significantly greater MSC invasion over time in hydrogel + PL media supplement. DMEM Dulbecco's Modified Eagle Medium, FBS fetal bovine serum, PL human platelet lysate. PL is a liquid that can be used as a replacement for xenogenic serum like FBS. We have demonstrated that it can also be manipulated into gel form. *P < .05. **P < .01

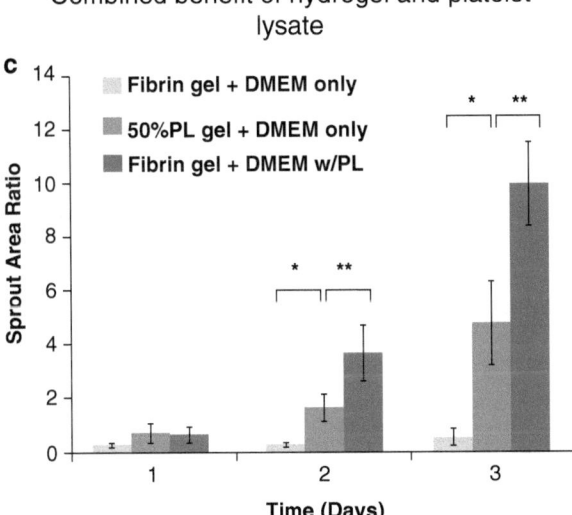

Fig. 19.4 (continued)

lymphedema before it progresses to chronic stages may prevent these inflammatory changes and subsequent skin changes and decreased wound healing. However, regenerative strategies may be hampered by these same chronic insults.

Additionally, adipocytes inhibit angiogenesis [60]. This is important for two reasons. First, adipose-derived MSCs in patients with lymphedema have altered differentiation capacity with a shift in adipogenic lineage at the cost of vasculogenic lineage [61]. Second, the increasing adiposity with age may limit the lymphatic repair in adipose tissue. Further, MSCs from patients with systemic disease (e.g., diabetes) have been reported to have diminished proliferative capacity, even when harvested from well perfused tissue [62]. However, our group has identified ways of improving proliferative capacity of these MSCs, and we have identified pathway-specific defects in these cells that can be therapeutically corrected with human platelet lysate administration [63, 64]. In addition, we have found that the secretomes from MSCs cultured from bone marrow and adipose tissue from the same patients were very similar [63].

In research specific to lymphedema, adipose-derived MSCs promote lymphangiogenesis in conjunction with lymph node transfer by restoring lymphatic flow and drainage [51]. These stem cells increase the number of lymphatic vessels, thus improving flow with the potential to decrease limb size and edema volume. They also have been reported to preferentially increase the collecting vessels [52].

19.3.4   Current Status of Clinical Research

Ketoprofen has been proposed as a pharmacologic treatment with benefit in decreasing by half skin thickness. However, there was no benefit identified to limb volume or other study endpoints [65]. One particularly promising drug therapy has been testing leukotriene inhibition, which decreased skin thickness and histopathologic staging in a select group of lymphedema patients [65]. Surprisingly, the role of cell therapies in abrogating prolonged inflammation in lymphedema has not yet been studied, but it is thought to be important in other vascular diseases [66].

Meta-analysis of publications that add regenerative therapies to surgical treatment of lymphedema could only identify studies where lymph node transplantation operations were used (in conjunction with adipose-derived stem cells or growth factor delivery) [42, 67]. Such publications identified a paucity of data regarding outcomes. In fact, there was only one randomized controlled study using bone marrow-derived mononuclear cells for lower limb lymphedema. This trial non-selectively included only primary lymphedema patients (inclusion of clinical stages up to stage III), and none of the recruited patients had venous reflux. If the initial biopsy showed lymphatic hyperplasia, patients were also excluded. The treatment group was not blinded and received GCSF injection prior to the BM harvest. The cells were isolated and delivered subcutaneously fresh along the superficial veins of the leg and the ankle/foot interspaces. All treatment patients also received compression therapy. The comparison group only received compression therapy. The treatment group had complications of biopsy site hematoma (10%) and superficial infection (15%), but they also had decreased ankle circumference measurements, an increase in lymphatic capillaries, and a subjective improvement in pain and walking [68].

For secondary lymphedema, women with history of lymphadenectomy and radiation therapy for breast cancer were recruited for liposuction and cell-assisted lipotransfer into the axilla with fat grafting. At 4 months, patients were found to no longer require compression therapy daily and had decreases in wrist, lower arm, and upper arm circumference [69]. At 1 year follow-up, patients reported improved outcomes with half of patients requiring less symptomatic treatment. However, there was no objective clinical change in lymphedema [70]. Similarly, a prospective study demonstrated that a one-time injection of stem cells decreased limb volume in lymphedema versus compression therapy for women with lymphedema secondary to mastectomy [71]. This study is limited by its small sample size of 10 women in each study arm. However, it too demonstrated favorable results.

19.4 Conclusions

Stem cells are unique in their ability to promote tissue repair and regeneration. The data to date suggests that adult MSCs have a potential role in the treatment of lymphedema. MSCs provide stromal and paracrine signaling of existing and recruited cells in/to the site of injury. Such testing requires better preclinical models and more refined clinical trialing that segregate type of lymphedema and clinical staging. Perhaps more importantly, there needs to be a call to action for this disease in a broad manner because there is both a lack of knowledge into the treatment of this disease and a lack of interest and funding to pay for the proven therapies for persons with lymphedema. In fact, for a common disease, medical students get on average <30 min on this topic, and funding for compression therapy is literally requiring an act of Congress (Lymphedema Treatment Act) [41].

Regardless of opinion, the spread of regenerative therapies will be dependent on the boldness of investigators and willingness of patients to participate in next-generation studies. Given the morbidity patients experience with lymphedema, combined with the relatively superficial location of disease, it is reasonable to suspect a much needed growth in the investigation of stem cell therapies for the treatment of lymphedema in the near future.

Acknowledgments Dr. Brewster's data and time on this chapter was supported in part by his research funding from the NIH and VA; NHLBI R01HL143348; VABLRD IO1BX004707; and VARRD I21RX003188. The authors are grateful to the academic support of Emory University's Department of Surgery, including our leadership, Drs. John F. Sweeney, Grant Carlson, and Will Jordan.

References

1. Kornuta JA, Nepiyushchikh Z, Gasheva OY, Mukherjee A, Zawieja DC, Dixon JB. Effects of dynamic shear and transmural pressure on wall shear stress sensitivity in collecting lymphatic vessels. Am J Physiol Regul Integr Comp Physiol. 2015;309(9):R1122–34.
2. Mukherjee A, Hooks J, Nepiyushchikh Z, Dixon JB. Entrainment of lymphatic contraction to oscillatory flow. Sci Rep. 2019;9(1):5840.
3. Singh AP, Foley J, Tandon A, Phadke D, Karimi Kinyamu H, Archer TK. A role for BRG1 in the regulation of genes required for development of the lymphatic system. Oncotarget. 2017;8(33):54925–38.
4. Alders M, Al-Gazali L, Cordeiro I, et al. Hennekam syndrome can be caused by FAT4 mutations and be allelic to Van Maldergem syndrome. Hum Genet. 2014;133(9):1161–7.
5. Pujol F, Hodgson T, Martinez-Corral I, et al. Dachsous1-Fat4 signaling controls endothelial cell polarization during lymphatic valve morphogenesis-brief report. Arterioscler Thromb Vasc Biol. 2017;37(9):1732–5.
6. Jung M, Cordes S, Zou J, et al. GATA2 deficiency and human hematopoietic development modeled using induced pluripotent stem cells. Blood Adv. 2018;2(23):3553–65.
7. DiSipio T, Rye S, Newman B, Hayes S. Incidence of unilateral arm lymphoedema after breast cancer: a systematic review and meta-analysis. Lancet Oncol. 2013;14(6):500–15.
8. Executive C. The diagnosis and treatment of peripheral lymphedema: 2016 consensus document of the International Society of Lymphology. Lymphology. 2016;49(4):170–84.
9. Kim SI, Lim MC, Lee JS, et al. Impact of lower limb lymphedema on quality of life in gynecologic cancer survivors after pelvic lymph node dissection. Eur J Obstet Gynecol Reprod Biol. 2015;192:31–6.
10. Cromwell KD, Chiang YJ, Armer J, et al. Is surviving enough? Coping and impact on activities of daily living among melanoma patients with lymphoedema. Eur J Cancer Care (Engl). 2015;24(5):724–33.
11. Rockson SG. Lymphedema. Vasc Med. 2016;21(1):77–81.
12. Armer JM, Stewart BR. A comparison of four diagnostic criteria for lymphedema in a post-breast cancer population. Lymphat Res Biol. 2005;3(4):208–17.
13. Stout Gergich NL, Pfalzer LA, McGarvey C, Springer B, Gerber LH, Soballe P. Preoperative assessment enables the early diagnosis and successful treatment of lymphedema. Cancer. 2008;112(12):2809–19.

14. Desai SS, Shao M. Vascular outcomes C. Superior clinical, quality of life, functional, and health economic outcomes with pneumatic compression therapy for lymphedema. Ann Vasc Surg. 2019;63:298.

15. Son A, O'Donnell TF Jr, Izhakoff J, Gaebler JA, Niecko T, Iafrati MA. Lymphedema-associated comorbidities and treatment gap. J Vasc Surg Venous Lymphat Disord. 2019;7(5):724–30.

16. Miller TA. A surgical approach to lymphedema. Am J Surg. 1977;134(2):191–5.

17. Charles RH. The surgical treatment of elephantiasis. Ind Med Gaz. 1901;36(3):84–99.

18. Kobayashi MR, Miller TA. Lymphedema. Clin Plast Surg. 1987;14(2):303–13.

19. Mavili ME, Naldoken S, Safak T. Modified Charles operation for primary fibrosclerotic lymphedema. Lymphology. 1994;27(1):14–20.

20. Campisi C. Use of autologous interposition vein graft in management of lymphedema: preliminary experimental and clinical observations. Lymphology. 1991;24(2):71–6.

21. Chang DW. Lymphaticovenular bypass for lymphedema management in breast cancer patients: a prospective study. Plast Reconstr Surg. 2010;126(3):752–8.

22. Ho LC, Lai MF, Kennedy PJ. Micro-lymphatic bypass in the treatment of obstructive lymphoedema of the arm: case report of a new technique. Br J Plast Surg. 1983;36(3):350–7.

23. Koshima I, Inagawa K, Urushibara K, Moriguchi T. Supermicrosurgical lymphaticovenular anastomosis for the treatment of lymphedema in the upper extremities. J Reconstr Microsurg. 2000;16(6):437–42.

24. Chang DW, Suami H, Skoracki R. A prospective analysis of 100 consecutive lymphovenous bypass cases for treatment of extremity lymphedema. Plast Reconstr Surg. 2013;132(5):1305–14.

25. Raju A, Chang DW. Vascularized lymph node transfer for treatment of lymphedema: a comprehensive literature review. Ann Surg. 2015;261(5):1013–23.

26. Cheng MH, Chen SC, Henry SL, Tan BK, Lin MC, Huang JJ. Vascularized groin lymph node flap transfer for postmastectomy upper limb lymphedema: flap anatomy, recipient sites, and outcomes. Plast Reconstr Surg. 2013;131(6):1286–98.

27. Lin CH, Ali R, Chen SC, et al. Vascularized groin lymph node transfer using the wrist as a recipient site for management of postmastectomy upper extremity lymphedema. Plast Reconstr Surg. 2009;123(4):1265–75.

28. Gianesini S, Obi A, Onida S, et al. Global guidelines trends and controversies in lower limb venous and lymphatic disease: narrative literature revision and experts' opinions following the vWINter international meeting in phlebology, lymphology & aesthetics, 23-25 January 2019. Phlebology. 2019;34(1 Suppl):4–66.

29. Patel KM, Lin CY, Cheng MH. A prospective evaluation of lymphedema-specific quality-of-life outcomes following vascularized lymph node transfer. Ann Surg Oncol. 2015;22(7):2424–30.

30. Pons G, Masia J, Loschi P, Nardulli ML, Duch J. A case of donor-site lymphoedema after lymph node-superficial circumflex iliac artery perforator flap transfer. J Plast Reconstr Aesthet Surg. 2014;67(1):119–23.

31. Viitanen TP, Maki MT, Seppanen MP, Suominen EA, Saaristo AM. Donor-site lymphatic function after microvascular lymph node transfer. Plast Reconstr Surg. 2012;130(6):1246–53.

32. Dayan JH, Dayan E, Kagen A, et al. The use of magnetic resonance angiography in vascularized groin lymph node transfer: an anatomic study. J Reconstr Microsurg. 2014;30(1):41–5.

33. Carl HM, Walia G, Bello R, et al. Systematic review of the surgical treatment of extremity lymphedema. J Reconstr Microsurg. 2017;33(6):412–25.

34. Pappalardo M, Chang DW, Masia J, Koshima I, Cheng MH. Summary of hands-on supermicrosurgery course and live surgeries at 8th world symposium for lymphedema surgery. J Surg Oncol. 2019;121:8.

35. Rauniyar K, Jha SK, Jeltsch M. Biology of vascular endothelial growth factor C in the morphogenesis of lymphatic vessels. Front Bioeng Biotechnol. 2018;6:7.

36. Iwata Y, Fujimoto Y, Morino T, et al. Effects of stem cell mobilization by granulocyte colony-stimulating factor on endothelial function after sirolimus-eluting stent implantation: a double-blind, randomized, placebo-controlled clinical trial. Am Heart J. 2013;165(3):408–14.

37. Sun Y, Lu B, Deng J, et al. IL-7 enhances the differentiation of adipose-derived stem cells toward lymphatic endothelial cells through AKT signaling. Cell Biol Int. 2019;43(4):394–401.

38. Lee CY, Kang JY, Lim S, Ham O, Chang W, Jang DH. Hypoxic conditioned medium from mesenchymal stem cells promotes lymphangiogenesis by regulation of mitochondrial-related proteins. Stem Cell Res Ther. 2016;7:38.

39. Dartsch N, Schulte D, Hagerling R, Kiefer F, Vestweber D. Fusing VE-cadherin to alpha-catenin impairs fetal liver hematopoiesis and lymph but not blood vessel formation. Mol Cell Biol. 2014;34(9):1634–48.

40. Deng J, Dai T, Sun Y, et al. Overexpression of Prox1 induces the differentiation of human adipose-derived stem cells into lymphatic endothelial-like cells in vitro. Cell Reprogram. 2017;19(1):54–63.

41. Rockson SG. Lymphatic medicine: paradoxically and unnecessarily ignored. Lymphat Res Biol. 2017;15(4):315–6.

42. Chen CE, Chiang NJ, Perng CK, Ma H, Lin CH. Review of preclinical and clinical studies of using cell-based therapy for secondary lymphedema. J Surg Oncol. 2019;121:109.

43. Tian W, Rockson SG, Jiang X, et al. Leukotriene B4 antagonism ameliorates experimental lymphedema. Sci Transl Med. 2017;9(389):eaal3920.

44. Strassburg S, Torio-Padron N, Finkenzeller G, Frankenschmidt A, Stark GB. Adipose-derived stem cells support lymphangiogenic parameters in vitro. J Cell Biochem. 2016;117(11):2620–9.

45. Wang S, Yamakawa M, Santosa SM, et al. Quantification of angiogenesis and lymphangiogenesis in the dual ex vivo aortic and thoracic duct assay. Protein Pept Lett. 2019;27:30.

46. Yan A, Avraham T, Zampell JC, Haviv YS, Weitman E, Mehrara BJ. Adipose-derived stem cells promote lymphangiogenesis in response to VEGF-C stimulation or TGF-beta1 inhibition. Future Oncol. 2011;7(12):1457–73.

47. Conrad C, Niess H, Huss R, et al. Multipotent mesenchymal stem cells acquire a lymphendothelial phenotype and enhance lymphatic regeneration in vivo. Circulation. 2009;119(2):281–9.

48. Takeda K, Sowa Y, Nishino K, Itoh K, Fushiki S. Adipose-derived stem cells promote proliferation, migration, and tube formation of lymphatic endothelial cells in vitro by secreting lymphangiogenic factors. Ann Plast Surg. 2015;74(6):728–36.

49. Saijo H, Suzuki K, Yoshimoto H, Imamura Y, Yamashita S, Tanaka K. Paracrine effects of adipose-derived stem cells promote lymphangiogenesis in irradiated lymphatic endothelial cells. Plast Reconstr Surg. 2019;143(6):1189e–200e.

50. Ackermann M, Wettstein R, Senaldi C, et al. Impact of platelet rich plasma and adipose stem cells on lymphangiogenesis in a murine tail lymphedema model. Microvasc Res. 2015;102:78–85.

51. Hayashida K, Yoshida S, Yoshimoto H, et al. Adipose-derived stem cells and vascularized lymph node transfers successfully treat Mouse Hindlimb secondary lymphedema by early reconnection of the lymphatic system and lymphangiogenesis. Plast Reconstr Surg. 2017;139(3):639–51.

52. Yoshida S, Hamuy R, Hamada Y, Yoshimoto H, Hirano A, Akita S. Adipose-derived stem cell transplantation for therapeutic lymphangiogenesis in a mouse secondary lymphedema model. Regen Med. 2015;10(5):549–62.

53. Hwang JH, Kim IG, Lee JY, et al. Therapeutic lymphangiogenesis using stem cell and VEGF-C hydrogel. Biomaterials. 2011;32(19):4415–23.

54. Shimizu Y, Shibata R, Shintani S, Ishii M, Murohara T. Therapeutic lymphangiogenesis with implantation of adipose-derived regenerative cells. J Am Heart Assoc. 2012;1(4):e000877.

55. Zhou H, Wang M, Hou C, Jin X, Wu X. Exogenous VEGF-C augments the efficacy of therapeutic lymphangiogenesis induced by allogenic bone marrow stromal cells in a rabbit model of limb secondary lymphedema. Jpn J Clin Oncol. 2011;41(7):841–6.

56. Gousopoulos E, Proulx ST, Bachmann SB, et al. Regulatory T cell transfer ameliorates lymphedema and promotes lymphatic vessel function. JCI Insight. 2016;1(16):e89081.

57. Robinson ST, Douglas AM, Chadid T, et al. A novel platelet lysate hydrogel for endothelial cell and mesenchymal stem cell-directed neovascularization. Acta Biomater. 2016;36:86–98.

58. Beerens M, Aranguren XL, Hendrickx B, et al. Multipotent adult progenitor cells support lymphatic regeneration at multiple anatomical levels during wound healing and lymphedema. Sci Rep. 2018;8(1):3852.
59. Tashiro K, Feng J, Wu SH, et al. Pathological changes of adipose tissue in secondary lymph-oedema. Br J Dermatol. 2017;177(1):158–67.
60. Kondo K, Shintani S, Shibata R, et al. Implantation of adipose-derived regenerative cells enhances ischemia-induced angiogenesis. Arterioscler Thromb Vasc Biol. 2009;29(1):61–6.
61. Levi B, Glotzbach JP, Sorkin M, et al. Molecular analysis and differentiation capacity of adipose-derived stem cells from lymphedema tissue. Plast Reconstr Surg. 2013;132(3):580–9.
62. Lee HC, An SG, Lee HW, et al. Safety and effect of adipose tissue-derived stem cell implantation in patients with critical limb ischemia. Circ J. 2012;76(7):1750–60.
63. Chadid T, Morris A, Surowiec A, et al. Reversible secretome and signaling defects in diabetic mesenchymal stem cells from peripheral arterial disease patients. J Vasc Surg. 2018;68(6S):137S–151S e132.
64. Morris AD, Dalal S, Li H, Brewster LP. Human diabetic mesenchymal stem cells from peripheral arterial disease patients promote angiogenesis through unique secretome signatures. Surgery. 2018;163(4):870–6.
65. Rockson SG, Tian W, Jiang X, et al. Pilot studies demonstrate the potential benefits of antiinflammatory therapy in human lymphedema. JCI Insight. 2018;3(20):e123775.
66. Powell RJ, Marston WA, Berceli SA, et al. Cellular therapy with Ixmyelocel-T to treat critical limb ischemia: the randomized, double-blind, placebo-controlled RESTORE-CLI trial. Mol Ther. 2012;20(6):1280–6.
67. Forte AJ, Boczar D, Huayllani MT, Cinotto GJ, McLaughlin S. Targeted therapies in surgical treatment of lymphedema: a systematic review. Cureus. 2019;11(8):e5397.
68. Ismail AM, Abdou SM, Abdelnaby AY, Hamdy MA, El Saka AA, Gawaly A. Stem cell therapy using bone marrow-derived mononuclear cells in treatment of lower limb lymphedema: a randomized controlled clinical trial. Lymphat Res Biol. 2018;16(3):270–7.
69. Toyserkani NM, Jensen CH, Sheikh SP, Sorensen JA. Cell-assisted Lipotransfer using autologous adipose-derived stromal cells for alleviation of breast cancer-related lymphedema. Stem Cells Transl Med. 2016;5(7):857–9.
70. Toyserkani NM, Jensen CH, Tabatabaeifar S, et al. Adipose-derived regenerative cells and fat grafting for treating breast cancer-related lymphedema: Lymphoscintigraphic evaluation with 1 year of follow-up. J Plast Reconstr Aesthet Surg. 2019;72(1):71–7.
71. Maldonado GE, Perez CA, Covarrubias EE, et al. Autologous stem cells for the treatment of post-mastectomy lymphedema: a pilot study. Cytotherapy. 2011;13(10):1249–55.

Index

© Springer Nature Switzerland AG 2021
T. P. Navarro et al. (eds.), *Stem Cell Therapy for Vascular Diseases*,
https://doi.org/10.1007/978-3-030-56954-9